Elderly Medicine
A Training Guide

Commissioning Editor: Timothy Horne
Development Editors: Linda Bennett, Lulu Stader
Project Manager: Joannah Duncan
Design Direction: Erik Bigland
Illustrators: Richard Morris, Alexa Rutherford
Illustration Manager: Merlyn Harvey

Elderly Medicine
A Training Guide

SECOND EDITION

Edited by

Gurcharan S. Rai
*Whittington Hospital,
London, UK*

Graham P. Mulley
*St James's University Hospital,
Leeds, UK*

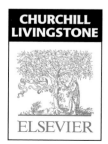

CHURCHILL
LIVINGSTONE

ELSEVIER

EDINBURGH LONDON NEW YORK OXFORD PHILADELPHIA ST LOUIS SYDNEY TORONTO 2007

MT

CHURCHILL
LIVINGSTONE
ELSEVIER

An imprint of Elsevier Limited

First edition 2002
Second edition 2007

ISBN-13: 978-0-443-10302-5

British Library Cataloguing in Publication Data
A catalogue record for this book is available from the British Library

Library of Congress Cataloging in Publication Data
A catalog record for this book is available from the Library of Congress

Notice
Knowledge and best practice in this field are constantly changing. As new research and experience broaden our knowledge, changes in practice, treatment and drug therapy may become necessary or appropriate. Readers are advised to check the most current information provided (i) on procedures featured or (ii) by the manufacturer of each product to be administered, to verify the recommended dose or formula, the method and duration of administration, and contraindications. It is the responsibility of the practitioner, relying on their own experience and knowledge of the patient, to make diagnoses, to determine dosages and the best treatment for each individual patient, and to take all appropriate safety precautions. To the fullest extent of the law, neither the Publisher nor the Authors assume any liability for any injury and/or damage to persons or property arising out of or related to any use of the material contained in this book.

The Publisher

Printed in China

Contents

Preface

Almost two-thirds of hospital beds are occupied by people aged 65 years and older, and this is the most important group in the rising number of hospital admissions. Geriatric medicine has been a well-recognized and popular medical specialty for some time now. Most textbooks on geriatric medicine and gerontology are written either as reference works or are aimed at recently qualified doctors. The first edition of this book concentrated not only on mainstream themes, but also on topics that may not always get the attention that they deserve, and those which may perplex the novice and the experienced clinician alike. The book was designed to serve as a guide primarily for trainees in geriatric medicine, but also proved useful for trainees in general medicine and other specialties as well as consultants in both general and geriatric medicine in the UK and Europe, America, Australasia and elsewhere.

Since the publication of the first edition of this book in 2002 we have had the publication of the National Service Framework for Older People with a commitment to abolish ageism, new guidelines on cardiopulmonary resuscitation and the Mental Capacity Act, which received the Royal Assent this year. In addition, the curriculum for trainees in geriatric medicine has been updated by the Specialty Advisory Committee for Geriatric Medicine on behalf of the Joint Committee for Higher Medical Training of the Royal Colleges of Physicians. The updated chapters take into account these changes as well as any new evidence that has been published.

Based on comments made by colleagues, we have included new chapters on frailty, prevention and health promotion, contractures, driving and the older person, therapeutics, carers and how to investigate an older patient.

The aims of the book remain the same:

1. To provide a learning guide based on the curriculum in geriatric medicine prepared by the Royal Colleges of Physicians
2. To provide a practical approach to the management of common problems encountered in elderly people

Although it is written primarily for medical trainees in geriatric medicine, this book should prove useful to many others involved in caring for older people, whether in the UK or elsewhere.

We are delighted that so many of the authors of chapters for the first edition have contributed updated pieces for the second edition. We also welcome new contributors, who have written with authority, clarity and panache.

Gurcharan Rai
Graham Mulley

Contributors

Katja Adie
Specialist Registrar in Health Care for the Elderly and General Internal Medicine, Derriford Hospital, Truro, UK
5. Developing and planning services

Nick Balcombe
Consultant Physician/Geriatrician, Hospital of St Cross, Rugby, UK
57. Research and audit

Sube Banerjee
Professor of Mental Health and Ageing, Institute of Psychiatry, King's College, London, UK
17. Old age psychiatry

James A. Barrett
Consultant Physician, Wirral Hospital and Honorary Professor of Health Care of Older People, Liverpool John Moores University, Wirral, UK
32. Faecal incontinence and constipation

Nigel S. Beckett
Consultant Physician/Geriatrician, Imperial College School of Medicine, London, UK
25. When to treat hypertension

Peter Belfield
Consultant Physician, Leeds General Infirmary, Leeds, UK
49. All you need to know about management in one chapter

Gerry C. J. Bennett (Deceased)
Professor/Consultant Physician, Barts and the London NHS Trust, London, UK
48. Education

David Berridge
Consultant Vascular Surgeon, Leeds General Infirmary, Leeds, UK
26. Abdominal aortic aneurysm and peripheral vascular disease

Fiona Boyd
Consultant Physician, Treliske Hospital, Truro, UK
46. Nutrition

Alex Brown
Consultant for the Elderly, St Luke's Hospital, Bradford, UK
50. Preparing for a consultant post
47. Percutaneous endoscopic gastrostomy (PEG) feeding

Lydia Chambers
Specialist Registrar in Old Age Psychiatry, South London and Maudsley NHS Trust , London, UK
17. Old age psychiatry

Michael J. Cheesbrough
Retired Consultant Dermatologist, Huddersfield Royal Infirmary, Huddersfield, UK
43. Pruritis
44. Leg ulcers

Marcus Chesterfield
Specialist Registrar in Geriatric Medicine, The Royal Hampshire County Hospital, Winchester, UK
7. Medical ethics and the law

Jacqueline C. T. Close
Consultant Physician, Prince of Wales Hospital and Prince of Wales Medical Research Institute, University of New South Wales, Australia
14. Falls and instability

Rónán Collins
Consultant Physician in Geriatric Medicine, Adelaide and Meath Hospital, Dublin, Republic of Ireland
11. Carers

Nick Coni
Consultant Physician (retired), Addenbrooke's Hospital, Cambridge, UK
56. Professional issues

Martin J. Connolly
Professor in Geriatric Medicine, North Shore Hospital, Takapuna, New Zealand
30. Respiratory rehabilitation

Oliver J. Corrado
Consultant in Geriatric Medicine, Leeds General Infirmary, Leeds, UK
45. Preventing infections

Colin Currie
Consultant Physician/Lead Clinician, Astley Ainslie Hospital, Edinburgh, UK
15. Orthogeriatric care

Keren Davies
Consultant Physician, Barts and the London NHS Trust, London, UK
48. Education

Paul Diggory
Consultant Physician in Elderly Care Medicine, Mayday University Hospital, Surrey, UK
41. Ophthalmology

Teresa Donnelly
Specialist Registrar in Geriatric Medicine, King's College Hospital, London, UK
21. Therapeutics

Ian Eardley
Consultant Urologist, St James's University Hospital, Leeds, UK
33. Prostate diseases

Jim Eccles
Consultant Physician, St James's University Hospital, Leeds, UK
7. Medical ethics and the law

John W. Feightner
Professor of Family Medicine, University of Western Ontario, London, Ontario, Canada
8. Prevention and health promotion

Emily Feilding
Specialist Registrar in Geriatric Medicine, Wythenshawe Hospital, Manchester, UK
2. Social gerontology

Roger M. Francis
Professor of Geriatric Medicine, Freeman Hospital, Newcastle upon Tyne, UK
36. Management of osteoporosis

Wendy Franks
Consultant Ophthalmologist, Moorfields Eye Hospital, London, UK
41. Ophthalmology

Mary Garthwaite
Urology Research Fellow, St James's University Hospital, Leeds, UK
33. Prostate diseases

Jim George
Consultant Physician/Clinical Director, Cumberland Infirmary, Carlisle, UK
24. Gait disorders

Mahendra Gonsalkorale
Consultant Physician (Retired), Westward, Sale, UK
20. Clinical aspects of pressure sores

Karen M. Goodman
Consultant Physician, Care of the Elderly, Calderdale Royal Hospital, Halifax, UK
35. Sexuality and ageing

Margot Gosney
Professor of Elderly Care Medicine, University of Reading, Reading, UK
40. Cancer in old age

Rosaire Gray
Consultant Physician in Geriatric and General Medicine and Cardiology, Whittington Hospital, London, UK
34. Urinary tract infections

Keith Harkins
Consultant Physician in Elderly Medicine, Wythenshawe Hospital, Manchester, UK
2. Social gerontology

Rowan H. Harwood
Professor of Geriatric Medicine, Nottingham City Hospital, Nottingham, UK
51. Time management and organizing paperwork
52. Dealing with complaints
53. Maintaining morale
54. Keeping up to date
55. Making the most of information technology (IT)

Stephen Jackson
Professor of Clinical Gerontology, Dulwich Hospital, London, UK
21. Therapeutics

Rhian Jones
Specialist Registrar in Geriatric and General Medicine, Leeds General Infirmary, Leeds, UK
45. Preventing infections

Suzanne Kite
Consultant Physician in Palliative Care, Leeds General Infirmary, Leeds, UK
16. Palliative care

Peter Langhorne
Professor of Stroke Medicine, Glasgow Royal Infirmary, Glasgow, UK
19. Management of stroke

Joanna Lawson
Associate Specialist, Newcastle upon Tyne Hospitals NHS Trust, Newcastle upon Tyne, UK
23. Syncope and dizziness

Stephen R. Lord
Associate Professor and Principal Research Fellow, Prince of Wales Medical Research Institute, Sydney, Australia
14. Falls and instability

Shona McIntosh
Consultant Physician in Elderly and Vascular Medicine, St James's University Hospital, Leeds, UK
23. Syncope and dizziness

Douglas G. MacMahon
Consultant Physician, Camborne-Redruth Hospital, Redruth, UK
5. Developing and planning services

Anis Mamun
Consultant Physician, Medway Maritime Hospital, Gillingham, UK
27. The management of atrial fibrillation in the older patient

Alan Martin
Specialist Registrar in Geriatric Medicine, Beaumont Hospital, Dublin, Republic of Ireland
10. Driving assessment

Finbarr C. Martin
Consultant Physician/Geriatrician, Guys and St Thomas' Hospital, London, UK
1. Biological ageing – its relevance to geriatricians

Jolyon Meara
Senior Lecturer in Geriatric Medicine, Cardiff University, Glan Clwyd Hospital, Rhyl, North Wales
22. The management of Parkinson's disease

Rob Morris
Consultant Physician in Care of the Elderly, Nottingham City Hospital, Nottingham, UK
55. Making the most of information technology

Graham P. Mulley
Professor, Department of Elderly Medicine, St James's University Hospital, Leeds, UK
3. Clinical ageing
4. Investigating older patients

Catherine O'Doherty
Consultant Physician in Palliative Care, Basildon Hospital, Basildon, UK
16. Palliative care

Desmond O'Neil
Professor, Department of Medical Gerontology, Adelaide and Meath Hospital, Dublin, Republic of Ireland
10. Driving assessment

Chris Patterson
Consultant Physician, St Luke's Hospital, Bradford, UK
50. Preparing for a consultant post

Christopher Patterson
Professor of Geriatric Medicine, McMaster University, Hamilton, Ontario, Canada
8. Prevention and health promotion

Jane E. Preston
Senior Lecturer in Biogerontology, King's College London, London, UK
1. Biological ageing – its relevance to geriatricians

Christopher I. M. Price
Clinical Senior Lecturer of Medicine, Wansbeck General Hospital, Northumberland, UK
37. Painful shoulder

Gurcharan S. Rai
Consultant Physician, Care of Older People, Whittington Hospital, London, UK
3. Clinical ageing
4. Investigating older patients
7. Medical ethics and the law
28. Asthma and chronic obstructive pulmonary disease

Shilpa Raje
Specialist Registrar in Geriatric Medicine, The University College London Hospitals, London, UK
13. Urinary incontinence

Scott Ramsay
Consultant Physician, Medicine for the Elderly, St John's Hospital, Liverpool, UK
19. Management of stroke

Kenneth Rockwood
Kathryn Allen Weldon Professor of Alzheimer Research, Camp Hill Hospital, Halifax, Canada
9. Overview of complexity/co-morbidity

T. A. Roper
Consultant Physician, Seacroft Hospital Community Unit, Leeds, UK
42. Hearing disorders

Gudrun Seebass
Consultant Physician, Huddersfield Royal Infirmary, Huddersfield, UK
39. Contractures

Alan J. Sinclair
Associate Dean and Professor of Medicine, University of Bedfordshire, Luton, UK
57. Research and audit

Alison South
Specialist Registrar, St James's University Hospital, Leeds, UK
18. Rehabilitation

Branwell Spencer
Consultant Physician in Elderly Medicine, Arrowe Park Hospital, Wirral, UK
6. Community geriatric care

Kevin Stewart
Consultant Physician in Geriatric Medicine, The Royal Hampshire County Hospital, Winchester, UK
7. Medical ethics and the law

Sheldon Stone
Senior Lecturer/Consultant Physician in Geriatric Medicine, Royal Free Hospital, London, UK
45. Preventing infections

Charlie Teale
Consultant Physician, St James's University Hospital, Leeds, UK
29. Tuberculosis

Helen Terry
Consultant Physician, Care of the Elderly, St Luke's Hospital, Bradford, UK
47. Percutaneous endoscopic gastrostomy (PEG) feeding

Anita J. Thomas
Consultant Physician in Acute Medicine and Care of the Elderly, Plymouth Hospital NHS Trust, Plymouth, UK
46. Nutrition

Susan Thomas
Health Policy Adviser, Royal College of Nursing, London, UK
5. Developing and planning services

Adrian Wagg
Senior Lecturer/Consultant Physician in Geriatric Medicine, The University College London Hospitals, London, UK
13. Urinary incontinence

Barbara Wall
Formerly Senior Lecturer, The London Foot Hospital & School of Podiatric Medicine, London, UK
38. Foot disorders

Angus Walls
Professor of Restorative Dentistry, University of Newcastle upon Tyne, Newcastle upon Tyne, UK
31. Oral health

Eric White
Consultant Physician, Care of the Elderly, St Luke's Hospital, Bradford, UK
12. Ethnic elders

Mark Wilcox
Consultant/Clinical Director of Microbiology, Director of Infection Prevention and Control, Professor of Medical Microbiology, Leeds General Infirmary, Leeds, UK
45. Preventing infections

C. P. Wilkinson
Specialist Registrar, St James's University Hospital, Leeds, UK
12. Ethnic elders

John Young
Professor and Consultant Physician, St Luke's Hospital, Bradford, UK
18. Rehabilitation

Rosemary Young
Senior Social Worker (elderly), Leeds General Infirmary, Leeds, UK
11. Carers

PART 1

General themes

Chapter 1

Biological ageing – its relevance to geriatricians

Finbarr C. Martin and Jane E. Preston

INTRODUCTION

The early pioneers of geriatric medicine were not much concerned about the biology of ageing. On the contrary, progress was made by identifying treatable disease and disability in the face of the widespread nihilism and general neglect by doctors and society of illness in old age. The inevitability of decline in later years was challenged. Geriatric medicine went on to recognize that illness might present in an atypical way and that diseases might behave and respond differently in later life. However, it was not necessary to know the meaning or mechanisms of biological ageing in order to be a competent geriatrician.

Have things changed? Most of our work is still concerned with diseases, which may cause premature death. They result from environmental factors such as accidents, infection, carcinogens and so on, with genetic and life-course differences contributing to the considerable variability observed between individuals. We recognize age-related increased incidences of cardiovascular disease, dementia, some cancers and infections but neither the preventative health approaches nor treatments have been acclaimed as anti-ageing measures. We have also learnt about the important loss of functional reserve in older patients. Remedial therapies and other rehabilitative approaches strive to restore reserve lost through illness or injury.

Rowe and Kahn (1987) described the distinction between 'usual' and 'successful' ageing in 1987.

They drew attention to the spectrum observed among older people. At one end are those who remain generally well and independent until a sudden natural death. At the other are those who accumulate greater degrees of impairments, frailty, and often a period of disability followed by premature death. Increasingly it has been recognized that age-related impairments, universal but highly variable in degree, are the product of numerous interacting factors: maternal health, genes, lifestyle, socioeconomics as well as ageing-associated molecular damage. While this 'usual' ageing state is often accompanied by well-defined and potentially avoidable diseases, it also contributes directly to the frailty, which is predictive of loss of functional capacity. The traditional view that sought to separate ageing from pathology absolutely, is no longer tenable. While the claims of the anti-ageing movement remain largely money-making fiction, biological gerontology is now shedding light on the relationships between ageing, frailty and death, and suggesting new treatment possibilities.

In this chapter we will briefly address several questions:

- What is ageing and how did it evolve?
- Is there an ageing clock?
- What are the cellular mechanisms of ageing?
- How do these changes relate to the diseases of old age and their treatments?
- How does frailty relate to ageing?

DEVELOPMENT, AGEING AND DEATH

The survival curves of populations in developed and most developing countries now approach the rectangular shape, which happens when chronological age becomes the predominant predictor of incident death. Although increasing chance of death is the defining characteristic of ageing, the biological details of the relationship are not clear. In human societies with long life expectancies, the onset of maturity coincides with the nadir of the age-specific mortality curve, but there is no evidence of an overall controlling 'clock' governing the pace of changes observed over time. Rather, the molecular physicochemical changes in cells, tissues and physiological systems which are commonly regarded as ageing, do not begin after a set time period of life but accumulate gradually during the process of living. Indeed some, such as glycated cross-linkages in collagen, can develop in the test-tube as well as in the living cell.

These ageing changes (described more fully later) lead to a reduced capacity to repair damage and reduced functional homeostasis, but their relationship to death is not established. The processes going on in cases of 'quiet death', without evident overwhelming disease, are often uncertain, but limiting the term 'ageing' to the physical changes which link clearly to death would be to restrict its meaning severely. So we are left without a clear-cut definition. The consensus in biological gerontology is to view ageing *as those changes that deviate from the state presumed to be advantageous in terms of optimal reproductive capacity*. This makes sense from an evolutionary viewpoint.

THE EVOLUTION OF AGEING

Not all organisms age. For example, single cell organisms reproduce by division without having undergone the range of ageing changes seen in multicellular organisms. As life forms have become more complex, ageing has emerged. Most animals in the wild, like humans until several hundred years ago, live no more than 50% of their potential lifespan. For most animal populations, ageing has played little or no part in shaping their survival curve. Their maximum lifespan potential has evolved through generations of predominantly young animals living short lives,

not as a result of selective survival and reproduction of long-lived animals. The actual achievement by individual animals of their potential maximum lifespan was so rare as to exert little or no direct evolutionary pressure. Instead, natural selection has favoured genotypes that produce fitness to reproduce successfully during young adulthood, but has simultaneously incorporated phenotype changes which add up to ageing, with a maximum lifespan built in. Ageing has not evolved 'in' so much as *not* been evolved 'out'. It has not evolved 'for itself' but as a consequence of other characteristics which did evolve through preferential selection under evolutionary pressure. It is the preservation of animals in captivity or humans through relatively recent cultural developments that has resulted in ageing becoming more common and therefore highly relevant.

Central to this argument is that the tissues in multicellular animals show specialization. The tissues concerned with maintenance of present life, the soma, are separate from the tissues concerned with propagation through inheritance, the germ line. Evolutionary pressure applies to prevent or reverse deleterious changes only in so far as they impede the fitness of the animal in evolutionary terms, i.e. the ability to produce robust offspring who survive to reproduce.

In conditions of finite environmental resources (food, etc.) and high risk of 'premature' death (e.g. through predation, cold and infection), the evolution of form and function capable of reaching this fitness involves a number of compromises in the best use of biological energy. In Kirkwood and Cremer's 'Disposable Soma' theory (Kirkwood 2005), the separation of the germ line from other cells in the body has allowed the selection of mechanisms for specific accurate preservation of the germ line, but at the expense of biological work to preserve the soma. Embryonic stem cells are more able to resist ageing changes (such as oxidative damage described below) than differentiated somatic cells. Since the soma and the genetic material in the cells of the soma are not available for inheritance, preserving them for immortality in the face of inevitable death through predation, accident or deprivation is energy wasted.

Rather, evolution has favoured strategies which have devoted energy and resources to enabling the soma to attain reproductive fitness with the germ line safe from damage. It is apparent, however, that this protection of the germ line is not absolute as, for example, increased parental age is associated with an increased risk of a Down's syndrome child. There are several features evident in the germ-cell line, e.g. the ovary, which may result in enhanced protection for the genetic material compared to those present in the cells of other tissues. It would be expected from this theory that the cellular mechanisms to protect the soma from damage would be better developed in species likely to live longer. Thus animals which have adapted to their environment sufficiently to enable more of them to survive longer, e.g. primates, would be expected to have evolved more successful anti-ageing mechanisms to protect the soma. Available evidence confirms this prediction.

IS THERE A GENETIC BIOLOGICAL CLOCK?

The genetic contribution to ageing has prompted *programmed ageing theories*, attractive because they suggest the presence of an ageing gene, which if we look hard enough may be isolated and modified in favour of longevity. The reality is proving far more complex. Some facts point towards the genetic influences on maximum lifespan being restricted to relatively few genes. For example, longevity is species-specific and even closely related and therefore genetically similar species can have substantially different longevity associated with their adaptation to distinct environmental features, even when protected from predators or deprivation. Second, conditions such as Werner's syndrome, which is due to genetic mutation sufficiently specific to produce a dramatic fast-ageing syndrome, with a life expectancy of about 40 years, do not prevent normal intrauterine and early life development. On the other hand, only about a quarter of the variation of lifespan in humans is inherited (McGue et al 1993) and there is up to a three-fold variation in the lifespan of genetically identical nematodes which are bred together. Of course, as a result of continuous random damage, they do not remain identical.

Taking a broader interpretation of ageing, including changes not necessarily associated with death, an estimated two-thirds of the genome is implicated. A major factor lies in the build-up of random damage, which is left unrepaired by (genetically directed) inefficient cellular 'somatic housekeeping' mechanisms (as predicted by the disposable soma theory). In 1964, Strehler (1964) proposed that the term 'ageing' should be reserved for those changes that occur gradually and universally, not only in particular living circumstances, although universality must allow for some within-species variability. Gradualness may not be evident at the functional level, as thresholds of functionality may be reached through less obvious incremental change at a more fundamental level. As already discussed above, Strehler's proposition of 'intrinsic ageing' is inherently unsatisfactory because ageing is a product of living, a dynamic relationship between a biological organism and the environment.

THE CELLULAR MECHANISMS OF AGEING

The following overview will be confined to three areas where research is making a major contribution to our understanding of ageing and disease at the cellular and molecular levels:

- Oxidative stress
- Protein glycation
- Cell senescence

It should, however, be kept in mind that there are over 300 theories for contributors to these processes.

Oxidative stress

The *free radical theory of ageing* has evolved since first proposed and developed by Harman in the 1950s as a cause of ageing and disease. Free radicals are now considered key in the development of age-related pathophysiology (Harman 1998).

Oxidative stress occurs when the production of reactive oxygen species (ROS) – including free radicals – exceeds the available antioxidant 'defence' systems. The most common ROS in mammals are the superoxide anion, hydrogen peroxide, the hydroxyl radical and nitric oxide radical. ROS come from a variety of sources, primarily the mitochondria, which form superoxide free radical anions alongside adenosine triphosphate (ATP), both being products of oxidative phosphorylation. Other sources include the macrophages, particularly during chronic infections, the peroxisomes involved in lipid degradation and cytochrome P450 involved in drug detoxification. Some support for the importance of oxidative stress in the development of ageing comes from Rubner's rule. This derives from the observation that mammalian species metabolize a similar number of calories per gram per lifespan, suggesting that the results of oxidative metabolism on cells confer a maximum lifespan via the consequences of oxidative damage. To date, post-weaning calorie restriction is the only consistent technique of prolonging lifespan in laboratory animals, though at the expense of fertility.

Interaction of ROS with deoxyribonucleic acid (DNA), both mitochondrial and nuclear, can result in breaks in the sugar–phosphate backbone resulting in mutations or deletions – especially in the mitochondria, where DNA repair mechanisms are less efficient than in the nucleus. Damage accumulates over time and may be passed on to daughter cells, the process continuing until oxidative phosphorylation is compromised, ATP production declines and cells begin to die. The outcome in vascular system endothelial cells is production of adhesion molecules by dying cells. These attract neutrophils and macrophages in a local inflammatory reaction, in which hydrogen peroxide is released. This additional ROS load further damages the compromised cell as well as the extracellular matrix and surrounding cells, resulting in a cascade of oxidative stress.

In the skin, photon-induced free radicals causing local inflammation may result in a similar oxidative stress cascade. In many tissues, these mechanisms may also be initiated by infection, smoking, and advanced glycosylation end products (AGEs) following sugar–protein interaction, seen particularly in long-lived cell types such as neurones. Indeed, brain tissue is particularly vulnerable to the effects of sustained mitochondrial damage and reduced ATP availability, with affected cells dying by apoptosis, or the fatal 'excitotoxicity' cascade in those cells with N-methyl-D-aspartate (NMDA) receptors such as in the hippocampus dentate gyrus (Kowaltowski 2000).

An alternative fate for cells with specific nuclear DNA mutation following oxidative stress may be transformation into an immortal cell line and the beginning of a tumour.

Experimental attempts or chance mutations, which shift the balance away from oxidative stress by increasing antioxidant levels, have had some limited influence on maximum lifespan. There are few effects in mammals, but the fruit fly *Drosophila melanogaster* shows increased maximum lifespan following mutations enhancing the antioxidant enzyme activity of superoxide dismutase (SOD) and catalase. Increase in SOD in humans is seen with Down's syndrome. Rather than affording protection, the brain tissue shows greater than expected free radical damage because SOD converts superoxide radicals into hydrogen peroxide. Without elevation of catalase or glutathione peroxidase, the final neutralization step to water is not completed.

Potential implications for clinical practice

Diets rich in vegetables and fruits are associated with lower rates of a number of chronic diseases, including cancer, cardiovascular disease, diabetes mellitus and age-related macular degeneration. The potentially beneficial antioxidant effects of the minerals zinc and selenium or vitamins A, C and E have been proposed as an explanation. Antioxidants can reduce progression of atherosclerosis in in-vitro experiments and animal models, but overall the clinical trials (including the HOPE study of vitamin E reported in 2000) have not shown benefit.

Similarly, clinical trials of antioxidants did not prevent development of age-related macular degeneration (Evans & Henshaw 2000) or show consistent benefit in preventing cataract. Although free radical formation may contribute to brain cell damage in Alzheimer's disease, the only randomized controlled trial with vitamin E produced mixed results, insufficient to confirm effectiveness (Tabet et al 2000). A recent Cochrane review of clinical trials assessing beta-carotene, vitamins A, C and E and selenium came to the conclusion that there are no significant effects of antioxidant supplementation on the incidence of gastrointestinal cancers.

Protein modification by glycation

Many forms of protein modification occur increasingly with age. These include oxidative damage and addition of excess phosphate groups, which may be factors in both the slowing of new protein synthesis in later life, and causation of specific diseases such as Alzheimer's disease (AD). A major, well-characterized contributor to post-translational change is modification by glycation and the formation of AGEs as the end result of a series of spontaneous reactions between any protein and local sugar molecules, particularly ribose in ribonucleic acid (RNA) and fructose. The final steps of the reaction sequence are further encouraged by oxidative stress and result in a toxic aggregation of protein, which resists being broken down by the cells. This is the explanation for the harmless yellowing hue of ageing nails and cornea, but also can cause functional damage to many affected proteins. Protein glycation is most marked in the persistent hyperglycaemia of diabetes mellitus, where it plays a part in end organ damage.

In Alzheimer's disease, glycated tau protein may stabilize paired helical fragments contributing to the neurofibrillary tangles. AGEs also play a role in amyloid plaque formation and activation of microglia (Munch et al 1998). AGEs also contribute to development of atherosclerosis, macular degeneration, cataract formation and nephropathy.

Given the well-reported detrimental effects of both oxidative stress and protein glycation, it is perhaps not surprising that recent research on animal longevity provides tantalizing links between the two sets of theories. The microscopic worm (C. elegans) is used as a model of ageing. Mutation of genes for insulin receptor subunits and the associated downstream intracellular messengers have resulted in the worm's maximum lifespan doubling. It has also illustrated a link between glucose metabolism and ageing. Furthermore, mammals reared under conditions of caloric restriction produce fewer mitochondrial reactive oxygen species, supporting the correlation between ageing, health and ROS generation. However, addition of insulin reverses the positive effects of caloric restriction on ROS generation,

increasing mitochondrial ROS to levels above control (Lambert et al 2004). This effect may prove to be relevant to human diabetes mellitus, metabolic syndrome and ageing.

Potential implications for clinical practice

Research to counter the effects of AGEs has concentrated with some success on preventing their formation (Rahbar et al 1999), cleaving formed cross-links with AGE 'breakers' or reducing oxidative stress, for example with oestrogen or nonsteroidal antiinflammatory drugs. Although these studies are only in the very early stages of research as possible therapies, there are potential benefits across a range of age-related diseases.

Cell senescence and loss of telomeres

In the early 1960s, Hayflick and Moorhead made the observation that cells in culture could undergo only a limited number of cell divisions (the 'Hayflick limit'). Further research showed that cultured fibroblasts from old donors could undergo fewer cell divisions than those from young donors, that cells frozen for extended periods could 'remember' how many divisions they had left and that senescent cells which had stopped dividing could be identified in vivo. These studies, and others, were interpreted as evidence of a 'biological clock'. This clock is capable of counting and limiting the number of cell divisions, sufficient for the animal to reach healthy reproductive maturity but lowering the risk of immortal cell lines becoming cancerous.

The 'clock' turns out be the telomere end regions of DNA, which shorten with each cell division. Telomeres consist of repeat sequences of DNA, which shorten during DNA replication because polymerase is not able to copy fully to the end of the 3' strand of linear DNA. Because of the limitation, repeated cell replication results in progressive damage. When the telomeres are sufficiently eroded, cells stop dividing. An additional factor is that free radical damage acts to accelerate telomere loss, resulting in early cell senescence in conditions of oxidative stress. Telomeric DNA may therefore be regarded as a 'stress sensor'. As yet, the exact mechanism linking telomere loss to cessation of cell division is unclear, but the cells do not then die. Rather, they are senescent and at the end of their replicative lifespan.

Detection of senescent cells in vivo poses technical difficulties but studies have implicated them in the cornea, blood vessels and skin. Tissue ageing may result from the limited regenerative potential of tissues that contain large numbers of senescent cells. These may particularly occur if the affected tissue has a naturally high turnover, such as in the immune system or in the vascular endothelium, skin or cornea where cell replication is a necessary response to damage (Faragher & Kipling 1998). People with the fast-ageing Werner's syndrome display damaged DNA due to lack of helicase (required for DNA repair and mRNA formation), and in particular demonstrate shortened telomeres. Recent studies of this condition provide evidence that senescence may contribute to normal ageing of somatic cells (Kipling et al 2004). Telomeres from Dolly, the cloned sheep, were also shortened. This suggests that her biological age was greater than expected, and closer to that of her donor 'mother'. Indeed, her lifespan turned out to be short (for a sheep).

Potential implications for clinical practice

Immortal cells overcome the problem of telomere shortening with the enzyme telomerase, a ribonucleoprotein with an RNA template for elongating telomeres before replication. Most human cancers, all human germ-line cells and some stem cells contain the enzyme, and targeting of telomerase is being developed as a potential cancer therapy. Telomerase has also been artificially introduced into normal fibroblasts by viruses carrying the gene (transfection), resulting in extended lifespan in vitro but still with normal phenotype and karyotype, raising the future possibility of extension of replicative lifespan in vivo.

AGEING AND FRAILTY

The route to frailty is not only through identifiable disease. The concept of frailty has developed significantly in recent years, incorporating a biological model that includes sarcopenia, neuroendocrine decline, and immune dysfunction (Bortz

2002). A quantifiable frailty phenotype has been described by Fried et al (2001), with clinical predictability for disability and death. The relationship between frailty and ageing is attracting increasing research interest and debate. This phenotype is more prevalent in older women than men, is multifactorial in origin, but is also associated with age-associated increases in interleukin-6 (IL-6), a proinflammatory cytokine, linked to poor health outcomes in older adults.

Oxidative stress triggers IL-6 production and antioxidant micronutrients play a critical role in decreasing this inflammatory response. It is therefore intriguing that in the longitudinal Baltimore Women's Health and Aging Study, low baseline antioxidant levels were associated with both higher IL-6 levels and 5-year mortality rates (Walston et al 2006).

CONCLUSION

- From evolutionary and historical perspectives, ageing is new.
- The reality of old age for each individual is a mixture of the universal but variable age-associated changes and specific diseases. Together these contribute to frailty or disability.
- Some age-associated disease processes are multifactorial, with age-associated processes such as oxidative stress damage and glycation playing a part.
- The metabolic characteristics associated with the frailty phenotype may also prove to be closely linked to ageing changes but are also partly avoidable, through activity or lifestyle modification.

Elucidation of these fascinating inter-relationships seems set to enrich the future clinical practice of geriatric medicine.

REFERENCES

*** Essential reading; ** recommended reading; * interesting but not vital

Bortz W M 2002 A conceptual framework of frailty: a review. Journals of Gerontology Series A, Biological Sciences and Medical Sciences 57:M283–288

Evans J R, Henshaw K 2000 Antioxidant vitamin and mineral supplementation for preventing age-related macular degeneration. The Cochrane Database of Systematic Reviews 2. Art. No.: CD000253. DOI: 10.1002/14651858.CD000253 *

Faragher R G A, Kipling D 1998 How might replicative senescence contribute to human ageing? Bioessays 20:985–991 **

Fried L P, Tangen C M, Walston J et al 2001 Frailty in older adults: evidence for a phenotype. Journals of Gerontology Series A, Biological Sciences and Medical Sciences 56:M146–156 **

Harman D 1998 Extending functional lifespan. Experimental Gerontology 33:95–112 ***

Kipling D, Davis T, Ostler E L et al 2004 What can progeroid syndromes tell us about human aging? Science 305:1426–1431 *

Kirkwood T B 2005 Understanding the odd science of aging. Cell 120:437–447 ***

Kowaltowski A J 2000 Alternative mitochondrial functions in cell physiopathology: beyond ATP production. Brazilian Journal of Medical and Biological Research 33:241–250 *

Lambert A J, Wang B, Merry B J 2004 Exogenous insulin can reverse the effects of caloric restriction on mitochondria. Biochemical and Biophysical Research Communications 316:1196–1201 **

McGue M, Vaupel J W, Holm N et al 1993 Longevity is moderately heritable in a sample of Danish twins born 1870–1880. Journal of Gerontology 48:B237–244 *

Munch G, Schinzel R, Loske C et al 1998 Alzheimer's disease: synergistic effects of glucose deficit, oxidative stress and advanced glycation endproducts. Journal of Neural Transmission 105:439–461 *

Rahbar S, Yernini K K, Scott S et al 1999 Novel inhibitors of advanced glycation endproducts. Biochemical and Biophysical Research Communications 262:651–656 *

Rowe J W, Kahn R L 1987 Human aging: usual and successful. Science 237:143–149 ***

Strehler B L 1964 Time, cells and life. Academic Press, New York and London **

Tabet N, Birks J, Grimley Evans J et al 2000 Vitamin E for Alzheimer's disease. The Cochrane Database of Systematic Reviews 4:CD002854 *

Walston J, Xue Q, Semba R D et al 2006 Serum antioxidants, inflammation, and total mortality in older women. American Journal of Epidemiology 163:18–26 ***

RECOMMENDED READING

Rose M R 2004 Will human ageing be postponed? In: The science of staying young. Scientific American special edition, p 24–29 (http://www.sciam.com)

SELF-ASSESSMENT QUESTIONS

Are the following statements true or false?

1. The following describes the genetic basis of longevity on humans:
    a. Individual lifespan depends largely on maternal genetic inheritance
    b. About a quarter of the variation of lifespan in humans is inherited
    c. Relatively few genes determine the individual lifespan
    d. Differential ability to counteract the effect of telomere shortening explains most of the individual variation observed

2. Cellular senescence occurs because:
    a. People do not have sufficient antioxidants in their diets
    b. Insufficient proteins are available for cell proliferation
    c. Cells undergo apoptosis as a result of mitochondrial damage
    d. DNA replication and free radical damage erode the telomeres

Chapter 2

Social gerontology

Keith Harkins and Emily Feilding

Social gerontology is the study of the social aspects of ageing. The purpose of this brief chapter is to give an insight into some of the issues surrounding the subject, and to stimulate thought about them.

There are 11 014 000 pensioners in the UK, accounting for about 16% of the total population. The data quoted in this section are taken from several sources, mainly governmental surveys, and these generally equate 'elderly' with being retired. This rather inadequate definition of old age demonstrates the difficulty in determining what it is to be an elder in our society, and reflects the fact that this group of people are heterogeneous, and at least as diverse a population as any other age group.

DEMOGRAPHICS

There have been large increases in the numbers of elderly people in recent years, which mirrors their increasing life expectancy (see Table 2.1). There are currently more people aged 70 and 80 years than ever before.

It is the over-75s who are increasing in number most, both as a proportion of the total population and in absolute terms. It is expected that the total number of elderly people will plateau, but the proportion of very old will increase. At the time of writing there are around 10 000 people aged 100 years and over; this is expected to rise to 136 000 by 2051.

Table 2.1 Life expectancy at year of birth (UK)		
	Men	Women
12th century	35	35
1841	40	42
1931	58	62
1961	67	73
2002	76	81
2051	84	88

These demographic changes may have important implications for both health and social services. There is an assumption that an older population will create heavier demands on such services, but as longevity has improved, so has the overall health of the population at any given age. While this healthy life expectancy is increasing, it is at a slower rate than total life expectancy.

ATTITUDES

'All would live long, none would grow old'
(Benjamin Franklin)

The care that a society takes of its elders has been held up as a measure of its civilization.

'... The way in which a society behaves toward its old people uncovers the naked, and often carefully hidden, truth about its real principles and aims.'

(Simone de Beauvoir in *The Coming of Age*)

‌‌

Treating older people with a lack of respect is thought of as being a modern western phenomenon, but this is not so. Many primitive societies, especially those who lived where resources were scarce, abandoned their elderly, such as the Eskimos who sent their elderly paddling off alone in a canoe. Agrarian societies, however, were more likely to value the wisdom and experience of older people. In western society, respect for elderly people is thought to have deteriorated around the time of the industrial revolution, when times were hard, and the young people were doing new jobs of which their elders had no experience or knowledge.

Young people generally have a negative opinion about what it means to be old. Surveys in the UK and the USA found that older people tended to be viewed as 'doddery but dear'. While older people were considered to be more moral and amiable than younger people, they were seen as frail, pitiable and rarely enviable. Old age is viewed as a time of loss, poor health, and social isolation.

The expectations of younger generations are that they will feel unwanted and lonely in their old age. The truth, however, is that in general, old people have quite a good time.

Although the old take part in less social activities than the young, only about a half feel that they are missing out on anything. The biggest fear that the over 71-year-olds cite is losing their independence (IndependentAge & MORI 2005) – a greater fear than loneliness or financial worries.

Most elderly people function well in society, and the negative aspects of ageing are much less of a problem in the eyes of old people than we expect them to be. It is unusual for elderly people to complain about either their standard of living or financial situation, despite their relative poverty in modern-day society. Perhaps they are now better off than they used to be, even if they are not wealthy in relation to others in our community.

It is a rarity for elderly people to feel rejected by their family. Although the overall contact with families reduces with advancing age (with contemporaries dying off) and half of elderly subjects have no close family nearby, most elderly people who have taken part in surveys are happy with the level of contact from their families. The quality of social relationships tends to improve with age.

A third of younger people claim to want their elderly parents to live with them. However, only one in eight of those over 65 years actually want to live with their children.

RETIREMENT AND PENSIONS

'Retirement kills more people than hard work ever did'
(Malcolm Forbes)

The concept of retirement is relatively new. Until the late 19th century, people used to work until they were physically incapable of continuing their job. In 1859, civil servants became the first occupational group in the UK to receive a pension. Pensions were introduced to increase economic efficiency and increase employment for younger workers, rather than for the welfare of older workers. It was not until 1908 that Lloyd George introduced the non-contributory means-tested state benefit for those over 70 years.

The timetable for the introduction of pensions in the UK was:

- 1859 – First pension scheme for civil servants
- 1908 – First non-contributory means-tested pension introduced in the UK for over-70s
- 1925 – Age for qualifying for a pension reduced to 65 years
- 1940 – Age for women qualifying for a pension reduced to 60 years
- 2010 – Age for women qualifying for a pension to be increased to 65 years

Since the 1970s there has been an increasing trend to retire early. Many workers have planned this and voluntarily opt to leave work early. Others are forced into early retirement by changes in the job market.

The predicted financial cost of providing pensions to a growing elderly population is causing a great deal of concern as a 'pensions crisis' looms. Many final salary pension schemes have been closed to new employees, and there are proposals to increase the retirement age. It remains to be seen how plans to deal with this will develop.

FINANCES

'In a country well governed poverty is something to be ashamed of.'

(Confucius)

There are enormous variations of income between the poorest and richest pensioners. At one end of the spectrum there are younger pensioners who are more likely to be half of a couple, have an occupational pension and have more disposable income. At the other, more elderly pensioners (usually single women) are more likely to be solely dependent on state benefits, and subsequently struggle to get by (see Table 2.2).

Despite the average wealth (income and non-housing assets) of the over-50 population being £40000, half have less that £12000 and a quarter have less than £1500.

Here are some basic facts and figures:

■ 47% of pensioners are liable to pay income tax
■ 1.5% pay higher rate income tax
■ 50% of pensioners receive at least three-quarters of their income from state benefits
■ 17% of pensioners receive all their income from state benefits
■ The average pensioner household receives 51% of its income from state benefits

About 50% of pensioners also rely on means-tested benefits, such as income support, housing benefit and council tax benefit, to supplement their pension. In addition to these, there are between 400000 and 700000 pensioners who are entitled to these benefits but do not claim them. The reasons for this are not clear.

About 20% of pensioners receive disability benefits such as attendance allowance or disability living allowance. Again, the take-up of these benefits is low, with about 50% of those who are entitled to them not claiming the benefits.

Occupational pensions, which are becoming more common and more important, account for 27% of pensioners' incomes. The median value of these is £53 a week.

In summary, there are a few wealthy pensioners, who tend to be younger. Nearly half have moderate incomes, sufficient for them to need to pay income tax. The remaining half are reliant on state benefits and have income below the income tax threshold. There is a strong correlation between wealth and health.

HOUSING

'Be nice to your kids – they'll be choosing your nursing home'

Elderly people do have an advantage over the young in that they are more likely to have paid off their mortgage and have a solid asset in their house. The very old, though, are more likely to rent. There is often a problem with the condition of the houses in which elderly people live. The comfort of their home can be particularly important for the elderly because they spend more time there. In 2001 more than a million households containing a person over 75 years failed the 'Decent Homes Standard' in the English Housing Survey.

Elderly people are more likely to live in houses that are energy inefficient, and are less likely to have central heating. To keep warm, the average pensioner needs to spend 18% of income on heating. The average amount actually spent by pensioners on heating is about 10%. This may be one explanation of why the excess number of winter deaths in the UK is high compared with other European countries.

Some facts about the housing of pensioners in Britain:

■ 2% live in nursing homes
■ 3% live in residential homes
■ 5% live in sheltered housing
■ 18% of over-85s lived in institutional care in 2001 (23% in 1991)

Table 2.2 Average gross income per week		
	Non retired	Retired
Single man	£405	£248
Single woman	£349	£178
Couple	£382	£376

- 71% of women over 85 years live alone, as do 42% of single men over 85 years.
- 58% of homeowners who have paid off their mortgage are over 65 years

More older people live in rural areas than urban, and this is expected to rise in the next few decades. This can present its own problems in terms of local services. For example, 12% of all rural households are more than 12 km from a doctor's surgery. People over 75 years are most likely to report difficulties in accessing local amenities.

Circumstances often arise where houses, in which people have lived for many years, become unsuitable for their needs because, for example, of increasing disability. For those who decide to move from their home, finding suitable alternatives can be difficult. There is a lack of suitable housing and, especially for owner-occupiers, access to local authority or housing association accommodation may be restricted.

There is a relatively small proportion of the elderly population in residential or nursing homes, although living in a care home becomes more likely the older a person becomes. Women are more likely to live in a communal establishment than men. Elderly people are reluctant to even consider a move to residential care, as they believe it will lead to a decline in their quality of life and that these homes are simply places for them to die. Carers may also resist a move, seeing it as failure on their part. Two-thirds of admissions to residential care follow a hospital admission or occur after living with someone else. Often considerable pressure is placed upon older people in order to persuade them to move into care.

ELDER ABUSE

The abuse of elderly people is not a new phenomenon – it was first described in the medical literature in the mid-1970s, when the term 'granny battering' was used. Despite over 20 years of awareness, the issue of elder abuse has been relatively ignored in comparison with other forms of abuse, such as violence against women or child abuse.

Elder abuse encompasses physical, psychological, and financial mistreatment of elderly people, in addition to passive and active neglect.

Although the prevalence is impossible to quantify accurately because of problems of definition and reliability of information, community studies from both sides of the Atlantic suggest a prevalence of all types of abuse of around 3–5% of elderly people, which is probably an underestimate. Physical abuse accounts for about half of this.

Most elder abuse occurs at home, but when abuse does occur in care homes, the results can be disastrous as the abuse can become institutionalized and endemic. Such abuse has been the cause of many inquiries, but in spite of these, lessons do not seem to have been learnt and institutional scandals continue to occur with shocking regularity.

ETHNIC ELDERS

In the UK, one of the major social changes in the late 20th century was large-scale immigration, mainly from Commonwealth countries. There are proportionately fewer elderly people from these groups compared to the indigenous population, but this is likely to rise as the cohort of young immigrants graduate into retirement age.

The elderly people from these ethnic groups are disadvantaged in several ways:

- They are less likely to have built up an occupational pension and are more likely to be living in poverty than white elders
- They tend to have more chronic ill health than their white contemporaries
- They are less likely to have access to appropriate health and social services

Hospitalization can be unpleasant for anyone, but it can be especially difficult if the hospital routine is not understood, the food is unsuitable, and language barriers prevent proper communication. The concept of rehabilitation is also difficult for some ethnic elders to grasp, particularly where the traditional illness behaviour is to take to one's bed, and wait to either recover or die. Careful explanations to both the patient and their families about the principles of modern-day geriatric rehabilitation are needed to ensure the patients' understanding and cooperation.

REFERENCES

*** Essential reading; ** recommended reading; * interesting but not vital

IndependentAge and MORI 2005 Attitudes to ageing: a survey by IndependentAge and MORI. Online. Available: http://www.independentage.org.uk *

RECOMMENDED READING

Age Concern. *Age Concern England regularly produces policy documents about current issues concerning older people. These are easy to read, up to date and very relevant.* **
Aiken L R 1995 Aging: an introduction to gerontology. Sage Publications, London ***
Bond J, Coleman P, Peace S (eds) 1993 Aging in society. Sage Publications, London ***
de Beauvoir S 1970 Old age. Andre Deutsch and Weindenfeld and Nilcolson, London *
English House Condition Survey 2003. Online. Available: http://www.odpm.gov.uk *

National Office of Statistics: Focus on older people. Online. Available: http://www.statistics.gov.uk/focuson/olderpeople ***
Victor C R 1994 Old age in modern society. Chapman & Hall, London **

SELF-ASSESSMENT QUESTIONS

Are the following statements true or false?

1. With regards to retired people in the UK:
   a. They are more religious than younger people
   b. They spend more time on computers than younger age groups
   c. They hardly ever do voluntary work
   d. They are invariably good at dominoes

2. In the UK, elderly women:
   a. Have always had a longer life expectancy than men
   b. Are more likely to live alone than elderly men
   c. Account for three-quarters of the over-75s
   d. Drink over half of the total volume of sherry consumed in the UK each year

Chapter 3

Clinical ageing

Gurcharan S. Rai and Graham P. Mulley

It ought to be lovely to be old
To be full of peace that comes of experience
And wrinkled ripe fulfilment
The wrinkled smile of completeness that follows
*   a life*
Lived undaunted and unsoured with accepted
*   lies.*
If people lived without accepting lies
They would ripen like apples, and be scented like
*   pippins*
In their old age

                (D H Lawrence in *Beautiful Old Age*)

CLINICAL PRESENTATION OF ILLNESS IN OLD AGE

An assessment of an ill young person should lead to a unifying single diagnosis. While such an approach can also be true for older people some sick old people differ in their presenting features from younger persons. What are these differences? A helpful mnemonic is 'NAMES'.

- Non-specific presentation
- Atypical or uncommon presentation
- Multiple pathologies or diagnoses
- Erroneous attribution of symptoms to old age
- Single pathology/illness can lead to catastrophic consequences

NON-SPECIFIC PRESENTATION

The first President of the British Geriatrics Society, Trevor Howell, described five great problems often encountered in aged patients. These 'dragons' usually carried a poor prognosis and made caring for older people ardous. They were:

- Confusion
- Incontinence
- Contractures of joints
- Bedsores and other ulcers
- Falls

Bernard Isaacs continued the mythological theme by describing the 'Giants of Geriatric Medicine' (instability (falls), immobility, intellectual impairment and incontinence) and recently geriatricians have added 'iatrogenic illness' to make the five 'I's of geriatrics (Box 3.1). These may be the only presenting features of illness. With such non-specific

Box 3.1   Five 'I's
Incontinence
Instability
Immobility
Intellectual failure
Iatrogenic disease (which can cause any of the above non-specific symptoms)

presentation, differential diagnosis is broad and the doctor has to use all available information from the history (which may have to be sought from a third party), carry out a full examination and appropriate investigations to find the cause of vague symptoms. A physician looking after an elderly patient not only requires medical knowledge but also observational, listening and deductive skills.

ATYPICAL OR UNCOMMON PRESENTATION

Atypical or uncommon symptoms may replace the commonly stated features of illness listed in textbooks. Myocardial infarction may present with shortness of breath or a fall resulting from a cardiac arrhythmia or hypotension. Pneumonia or other serious infections may not give rise to a temperature or a rise in white cell count in an older person. Peptic ulcer perforation in an older person can be asymptomatic and the diagnosis may be made by examination of the chest X-ray.

MULTIPLE PATHOLOGIES

With ageing there is an increasing tendency for many pathologies. The main factors that contribute to the development of multiple diseases include:

1. An age-related increase in incidence of common disorders, e.g. hypertension, osteoarthritis, diabetes mellitus, vascular disease, dementia
2. Disturbance of the immune system leading to increased chances of cancer and hypothyroidism
3. The increased likelihood of an illness affecting one system leading to disorder in another, e.g. a respiratory infection leading to the development of atrial fibrillation and heart failure
4. Vascular diseases – these may develop gradually and during the latent period an acute illness may develop
5. Immobility which is associated with many neurological or musculoskeletal disorders and may lead to an increased risk of developing

complications such as falls, urinary incontinence, infections, pressure sores, deep vein thrombosis and pulmonary embolism.

ERRONEOUS ATTRIBUTION OF SYMPTOMS IN OLD AGE

Not only doctors but elderly people themselves may mistakenly attribute non-specific signs and symptoms to old age. An elderly person may say 'it is my age, Doctor' or 'I am only here because my daughter is worried'. The doctor may find one or more physical underlying causes for the symptoms.

SINGLE ILLNESS/PATHOLOGY LEADING TO CATASTROPHIC CONSEQUENCES

While a simple illness (such as an influenza) may produce symptoms that last for a few days in a young person, in some older people it can lead to a cascade of events that can have dire consequences (Fig. 3.1).

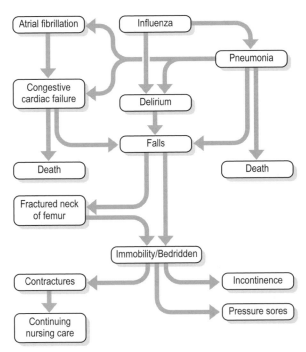

Figure 3.1 Cascade of events as a result of influenza.

A pathological process does not just lead to abnormality of one or more organs of the body but has consequences for the individual as a whole, leading to physical, psychological, functional and social problems. The functional decline of acute illness can be made worse by hospitalization and the organization of acute units for older patients should be designed to prevent or reverse this dysfunction.

In 1980 the WHO published the International Classification of Impairments, Disabilities and Handicaps (ICIDH) and defined:

- *Impairment* as any loss or abnormality of psychological, physiological, or anatomical structure or function (for example, shortness of breath or weakness in a limb)
- *Disability* as any restriction or lack of ability to perform a task or activity within the range considered as normal activity (e.g. walking, dressing)
- *Handicap* as the social disadvantage suffered by an individual as a result of ill health compared with what is normal for someone of the same age, sex and background

Therefore disability is about activity; handicap involves participation.

While definitions can differentiate between symptoms, impairments, disabilities and handicaps, in reality they are intrinsically linked. The effect of an intervention to influence one will affect the others (an exception being some handicaps, which may be altered by an intervention without disability or impairment being affected – an example of this is provision of a stairlift for someone who has difficulty climbing stairs

---

In 2001 WHO moved away from the impact of diseases or other health problems to 'components of health' defining what constitutes health and the concepts include:

- Body functions, body structures and impairments
- Activities and participation covering a full range of life areas
- Environmental factors that make up the physical, social and attitudinal environment

---

because of osteoarthritis of the hip). Such an action will not improve the symptom of pain, nor will it improve mobility on a level surface.

MULTI–DISCIPLINARY ASSESSMENT

Complex disability in relation to impairment and handicap requires the full and thorough assessment of an individual by not only a physician but also other professionals. The roles of these professionals are to implement rehabilitation in order to achieve maximum recovery, function and well-being with decline in handicap, disability and impairment. If handicap or disability cannot be abolished then the team's role should be to ensure that individuals are able to live as independent a life as possible with the support of individuals or aids and adaptations and services that meet their needs (see Ch. 18 on rehabilitation). In attempting to meet the physical and psychological needs of an individual, it is important to remember that professionals' actions should:

1. Reduce the individual's distress
2. Improve the individual's well-being
3. Improve the individual's quality of life (people themselves are the best judges of an outcome of a 'life worth living')

RECOMMENDED READING

Hodkinson H M 1973 Non-specific presentation of illness. British Medical Journal 4:94

Horan M A 2000 Presentation of disease in old age. In: Tallis R, Fillit H M, Brocklehurst J C (eds) Textbook of geriatric medicine and gerontology. Churchill Livingstone, Edinburgh, p 201–206

Howell T H 1975 Old age – some practical points in geriatrics. H K Lewis, London

Issacs B 1975 The Giants of geriatric medicine. Inaugural lecture, University of Birmingham

Issacs B 1981 Is geriatrics a specialty? In: Arie T (ed) Health care of the elderly. Croom Helm, Beckenham, p 224–235

Issacs B, Livingstone M, Neville Y 1972 Survival of the unfittest. Routledge and Kegan Paul, London

World Health Organization 1980 International classification of impairments, disabilities and handicaps. WHO, Geneva

World Health Organization 2001 International classification of functioning, disability and health (ICF). WHO, Geneva

SELF-ASSESSMENT QUESTIONS

Are the following statements true or false?

1. 'Giants of Geriatric Medicine' include:
   a. 'Social' problems
   b. Instability
   c. Multiple pathologies
   d. Lack of pyrexia in pneumonia

2. An elderly person with thrombosis of the left middle cerebral artery may have the following handicap:
   a. Weakness of right arm
   b. Weakness of right leg
   c. Dysphasia
   d. Inability to write letters

Chapter 4

Investigating older patients

Gurcharan S. Rai and Graham P. Mulley

'Geriatric medicine started with the concept that old age is not a disease; this led to the conclusion that accurate diagnosis of illness in older people is essential.'

(Sir William Ferguson Anderson [Anderson 1981])

INTRODUCTION

The first geriatricians sometimes had difficulty persuading colleagues to do even basic investigations on elderly patients. Discriminating against old people by restricting access to diagnostics is now unacceptable. Indeed, an important role of geriatricians nowadays is to protect their patients from being subjected to tests that might be burdensome, unpleasant or unlikely to alter management.

PRINCIPLES OF INVESTIGATION

WHY INVESTIGATE?

A detailed history and physical examination will often suggest a diagnosis, but objective confirmation is important, especially if the history is imprecise, the symptoms atypical or the signs difficult to elicit or interpret.

The confirmation of a diagnosis by investigations can:

- Explain the cause of a patient's symptoms
- Reassure them about conditions they do not have
- Prevent the patient being subjected to further tests
- Enable the doctor to give treatment, which may cure or modify the disease, or increase the duration or improve the quality of the patient's life
- Perhaps allow prognostication
- Trigger the delivery of help (palliative, domestic, financial) to those with serious illnesses

WHY *NOT* INVESTIGATE?

Tests may be requested that are not only futile but may result in anxiety or unnecessary or potentially harmful treatments. Examples are routine swabbing of wounds for microbiology (see pressure sores in Ch. 20), sending 'routine' catheter specimens of urine (see Ch. 34 on urinary tract infections), repeating cardiac echos, and requesting thyroid function tests in acutely ill old patients. Other tests may not alter management, for example, a neurosurgeon is unlikely to operate on a patient with advanced dementia who has a subdural haematoma.

Investigations that are unnecessary include echocardiography in patients with normal chest

X-rays and electrocardiograms (ECGs), and most electroencephalograms (EEGs) (unless done at the time of a seizure).

Investigations should be carefully considered in patients with complex co-morbidity, serious disabilities and advanced cognitive impairment. Of course, those with such problems should not be denied potentially useful investigations but the wise clinician will weigh up technical, philosophical and individual considerations before requesting a particular test. We should balance our wish for diagnostic certainty with the practical utility of seeking a diagnosis (Caird & Judge 1979). Patients' individual wishes must be taken into account: they may be frightened of needles, find computed tomography (CT) scans claustrophobic or be troubled by the noise of a magnetic resonance imaging (MRI) scanner.

A PRACTICAL APPROACH

The co-existence of acute and chronic diseases makes it appropriate to create a summary list of symptoms and their causes. Investigations should be targeted at those that are likely to prove useful and likely to improve well-being. The patient's preferences, fears and priorities must be considered.

The presence of cognitive impairment raises the important issue of consent to investigation. As physicians, it is our duty to follow ethical principles of *beneficence (do good)* and *non-maleficence (do no harm)*: we should do only those investigations that are likely to be beneficial to patients (see Ch. 7 on medical ethics and the law). They should yield useful information that will help to plan treatment (or indicate that no therapy is indicated) and cause little or no discomfort (Caird & Judge 1979). In patients who lack capacity, we should invoke the principle of *best interests*.

Not all problems are reversible or modifiable and, near the end of life, one has to question the value of subjecting an older person to invasive investigations. Decision making at such a crucial time should involve open and frank discussion with the patient (if competent), the family and other health professionals.

INVESTIGATING AN OLDER PATIENT

Taking into account the principles outlined above and knowledge of the medicine of old age, it is possible to divide investigations into three groups: essential, useful and targeted.

ESSENTIAL INVESTIGATIONS

These should be done in virtually all ill elderly patients referred to a geriatrician. They are likely to yield useful results or lead to explanations for non-specific, silent or atypical presentations of disease. These investigations should include:

■ Full blood count
■ Erythrocyte sedimentation rate (ESR) or plasma viscosity
■ Urea and creatinine
■ Urinalysis, particularly for the presence of blood, which may be the first manifestation of bladder or renal cancer)
■ Chest X-ray, which may reveal a symptomless neoplasm, reactivated TB, unsuspected consolidation, or pulmonary oedema in someone with left ventricular failure who is 'failing to thrive'
■ ECG, which may show an unsuspected recent or old myocardial infarction; an acute coronary event may present with falls or delirium but with no chest pain

USEFUL INVESTIGATIONS

Investigations that are useful or helpful because abnormalities can indicate presence of a systemic illness or a disease of a particular organ without the classical clinical features include:

■ Thyroid function tests – elderly patients with thyroid disease may not exhibit symptoms and signs of thyroid disease (Lloyd & Goldberg 1961)
■ Liver function tests – these can be abnormal with painless gallstones or in association with a pyrexial illness or an occult infection (James 1998)
■ Calcium and phosphate – hypercalcaemia may be a first sign of malignancy and in elderly patients is more often associated with neuro-

psychiatric symptoms, such as delirium or cognitive impairment

■ Random glucose – high renal threshold for glucose in some old people means that those with diabetes mellitus may not have osmotic symptoms (thirst, polydipsia, polyuria), and insidious presentation in these patients can delay diagnosis (Sinclair 2001)

TARGETED INVESTIGATIONS

Some investigations should be targeted at the clinical problem or disease suspected, balancing this with benefits and risks of the test. Examples of these include:

■ CT pneumocolon for suspected colonic carcinoma – this investigation is replacing barium enema, which was sometimes not well tolerated and was distressing for frail old people
■ 24 Holter monitoring for suspected arrythmias in a patient with unexplained syncope
■ ESR or plasma viscosity for suspected polymyalgia rheumatica or myeloma

HOW FAR SHOULD AN OLDER PERSON BE INVESTIGATED?

The decision to investigate an individual should take into consideration the:

■ Individual's wishes – taking into account the individual rights of the patient under the Human Rights Act
■ Individual's health at the time of presentation, i.e. presence of co-morbid disease/s and presence of disabilities or handicaps
■ Presence of cognitive impairment
■ Benefits and risks of investigations
■ Availability of curative treatment
■ Life expectancy

Balancing the influence of these factors with the duty of doctors to do their best for patients can prove to be very difficult; open discussion with patients (if they are competent) or with relatives (if they lack capacity) and with other professionals can be valuable. On occasion, the doctor may have to ask for a second opinion from a colleague, particularly where it is proving difficult to reach a decision that is acceptable to other professionals or informal caregivers.

Key points

■ The decision to investigate an elderly patient should take into account basic principles of medical ethics, i.e. autonomy, beneficence and non-maleficence as well as futility.
■ In practice it is possible to divide investigations into *essential* (those that should be performed in virtually all ill elderly patients), *useful* (because they may indicate the presence of a systemic illness or a disease without classical clinical signs) and *targeted* (at the clinical problem or disease suspected).

REFERENCES

Anderson W F 1981 The evolution of services in the United Kingdom. In: Kinnard J, Brotherston Sir J, Williamson J (eds) The provision of care for the elderly. Churchill Livingstone, Edinburgh, p 117–123

Caird F I, Judge T G 1979 Assessment of the elderly patient, 2nd edn. Pitman Medical, Tunbridge Wells

James O F W 1998 The liver. In: Tallis R, Fillit H, Brocklehurst J C (eds) Brocklehurst's textbook of geriatric medicine and gerontology, 5th edn. Churchill Livingstone, Edinburgh, p 841–859

Lloyd W A, Goldberg I J L 1961 Incidence of hypothyroidism in the elderly. British Medical Journal 2:1256–1259

Sinclair A J 2001 Issues in the initial management of type 2 diabetes. In: Sinclair A J, Finucane P (eds) Diabetes in old age, 2nd edn. John Wiley & Sons, Chichester, p 155–164

RECOMMENDED READING

*** *Essential reading;* ** *recommended reading;* * *interesting but not vital*

Adler B J, Stott D J 2003 How far to investigate older people? Clinical Medicine 3:418–422 ***

Hodkinson H M 1977 Biochemical diagnosis of the elderly. Chapman & Hall, London *

Wright W B 1978 How to investigate an old person. Lancet ii:419–420 **

SELF-ASSESSMENT QUESTIONS

1. An 89-year-old patient, who is very dependent on nursing staff for all his basic needs because of advanced dementia, is admitted from a nursing home with clinical features of a left middle cerebral artery territory infarction. Essential investigations reveal that he has haemoglobin of 9.1 g/dL with a blood film showing hypochromia and microcytosis.
   a. Should he have a CT head scan within 24 hours (as recommended by the National Stroke Guidelines)?
   b. Should his iron deficiency anaemia be investigated with endoscopy and colonoscopy?

Are the following true or false?

2. An older patient referred to a geriatrician should have the following investigations:
   a. Chest X-ray
   b. Abdominal X-ray
   c. Troponin level to detect a silent myocardial infarction
   d. Full blood count
   e. Ferritin level

Chapter 5

Developing and planning services

Douglas G. MacMahon, Katja Adie and Susan Thomas

INTRODUCTION

High quality services for older people do not just happen – they must be planned. Developing such services requires awareness of many aspects of health and social care, and an appreciation of both national and local political, economic and sociological factors, as well as a prediction of how they may change. This should be translated into local action, taking account of such factors as geography, transport, culture and resources.

This is a particularly difficult time to be advising on service planning in the UK. Primary care and community services have undergone further reorganization (DoH 2006), and commissioning of secondary care is now being undertaken by organizations that have themselves seen enormous changes in the last 5 years, with even more changes expected. These changes will produce challenges and opportunities for service planning, and so sensible clinicians will discern the opportunities while watching out for the threats. Whatever may change, one basic factor will continue to be present: there will always be elderly people in need of good care, no matter how organizations and technologies change.

Evidence-based medicine and clinical governance place an increasing emphasis on the use of interventions proven to improve patient outcome in the most cost-effective way. Primarily, this is driven by limited resources; finite budgets have

to deal with competing claims. Decision makers must maximize what society gains from healthcare investments. However, many of our patients do not present with a single diagnosis. They therefore differ from patients included in most clinical trials on which evidence rests. First, many will have multi-system disease(s). Second, their social environments may be precarious, and may have as important an impact on their discharge plans as their medical condition. Third, a functional approach is usually required rather than a strictly medical one. Fourth, it may be difficult to show clear benefits from some components of many of the commonly deployed interdisciplinary interventions. This will have implications for older patients when commissioners of services are allocating scarce funds and demanding evidence of effectiveness.

In this chapter we will investigate these themes. The reader is invited to consider not only how these topics impinge on their current activities, but also to reflect on their own practice.

THE CHANGING ENVIRONMENT AND THE NEED FOR SERVICES

LIFE EXPECTANCY

Global life expectancy at birth is projected to increase by 19 years for men and 17 years for women between 2000 and 2100, reaching levels of

81 and 84 years, respectively. As life expectancy levels continue to rise, the rate of increase slows, so that women may gain 8 years of life between 2100 and 2200, and men 9 years. Gains during 2200 to 2300 will be 5 years for each sex, resulting in projected 'final' life expectancies at birth of 97 for women and 95 for men at the end of the 23rd century (United Nations Department of Economic and Social Affairs 2003).

In the UK by 2030, the number of people over 65 years will have more than doubled. Within the overall rise, it is the number of very elderly people (i.e. over 85 years) that shows the greatest increase (almost tripling), whereas the increase in younger cohorts is more modest. The population under 65 years is predicted to remain constant, causing a massive shift in the balance between young and old. The nature of the economically-dependent population is changing dramatically. By 2150 it will entail mostly elderly people whose support may have to depend either directly or indirectly on younger generations – unless the period of economically productive life is extended or sound mechanisms for funding of pensions are in place.

Increasing life expectancy is often portrayed as a problem. However, in many ways it is a marker of the success of a number of strategies affecting the whole population. It is a fallacy to claim a strong relationship between survival and better medical care. Rather, increased life expectancy is largely the result of better sanitation, better housing, preventative health measures (particularly immunization against common childhood killers, but also treatment of hypertension and reduction of smoking), and improved financial status. Technical advances in medical management have until recently made only relatively minor contributions.

LONG-TERM CONDITIONS

Long-term conditions affect the lives of six in ten adults in England, but chronic illnesses are commonest in older people, affecting two-thirds of those aged over 75 years (2.64 million people), 45% of whom have more than one long-term condition. Long-term conditions also have an impact on NHS activity, accounting for 80% of consultations with GPs, 40% of out-patient activity and 80% of hospital in-patient bed days (ONS survey 2002–2003). Long-term conditions represent a challenge for the NHS, but the problem is growing because of increasing obesity, more sedentary lifestyles and an ageing population. As the World Health Organization noted (WHO 2004):

'[This trend] places new long-term demands on health care systems. Not only will chronic conditions be the leading cause of disability throughout the world by 2020; if not successfully managed they will become the most expensive problems faced by our health care system.'

The concept of *disability-free life expectancy* is important: any measure that extends the time spent living with disability will lead to increased demand on services. Thus, reduced mortality from stroke, for example, may paradoxically increase service demands for rehabilitation and longer-term care.

DEMAND ON SERVICES

The decline of the extended family could lead to a relative lack of informal carers (see Ch. 11 on carers), so that more formal services will be required to replace those that previous generations would have provided from within the family. When taken in conjunction with an increased dependency ratio, the implications for rationing of resources (or increasing revenue, e.g. by insurance or taxes) are considerable. In some cases, voluntary organizations have stepped in to provide help to older people; in others, there is a balance between voluntary, statutory and independent sector providers. Changes in professional activities lead to altered staffing and service delivery, e.g. the need for CT scanning and swallowing assessments after stroke increases the requirement for access to a scanner and increases demands for speech and language therapists. Clinical governance demands that services must meet agreed criteria, which will be rigorously audited.

Key points

- The number of elderly people is increasing, with an increased dependency ratio.
- Many of these people have long-term conditions.
- Increasing life expectancy and decline of the extended family will increase demand on services.
- Service redesign and innovation will inevitably be required.

THE POLITICAL ARENA

In contrast to the USA, the 'grey' movement in the UK has had limited success in persuading politicians to adopt a policy framework that is friendly to older people.

The Survey of Health, Ageing and Retirement in Europe (SHARE; Börsch-Supan et al 2005) showed that northern Europeans are healthier and wealthier but southern Europeans live longer. Those with better education are usually fitter and rich people are generally healthier. Improved geriatric care should help to ensure the financial viability of healthcare systems. To fulfil the aims of a healthier old age, greater emphasis is needed on public health and maintaining well-being.

Within the UK, differences are developing between the nation countries. For example, the devolved Scottish assembly has agreed to fund nursing care in full, whereas the British Parliament (covering England and Wales in this context) will only fund the nursing element of care. Whether any of the political parties will address this disparity in future remains unclear, especially as the major problem caused by the 'pensions gap' continues to grow (caused by the same demographic tensions – fewer working people paying for a growing elderly population).

With the current political agenda, the Department of Health has prioritized the management of long-term conditions. In reality, there are special problems in delivering personal health services for people with long-term conditions: 50% of people have not been informed about their treat-ment options, 25% do not have a care plan, 50% do not have a self-care plan and 50% of medicines are not taken as intended (DoH 2005a). Many factors contribute to these deficiencies, but lack of coordination between health and social care professionals and within primary, secondary and tertiary healthcare, is a major factor. The aim is to improve health outcomes for people with long-term conditions by offering a personalized care plan for vulnerable people most at risk; to reduce emergency bed days by 5% by 2008 through improved care in primary care and community settings for people with long-term conditions (DoH 2005a); and to improve access to services, ensuring that by 2008 no one waits more than 18 weeks from GP referral to hospital treatment, including all diagnostic procedures and tests.

This aim is to be achieved through a new model of care that helps to empower and inform patients, and creates prepared and proactive health and social care teams. The process of change is beginning in the infrastructure of health and social care, where decision support tools and clinical information systems are being designed to support care delivery. Case management and disease management are central, but supported self-care and the promotion of better public health are also key contributors to the delivery of care. Crucially, the intention is to match care to need. Case management will be directed towards the 5% of people with multiple co-morbidities, who currently account for 42% of hospital bed days. Case management may be helpful because it will enable the identification of patients with the most complex problems in order to provide proactive care to those with the highest burden of disease. The aim is a smooth patient journey through all parts of the health and social care system. The care plan for each patient will be coordinated by a community matron, who will use case management techniques to reduce unplanned hospital admissions caused by poor disease control and lack of effective prevention and support. People who are less vulnerable but who are still at risk will be cared for through a disease-management approach, while stable patients will be encouraged to manage their own care through approaches such as the Expert Patient Programme (DoH

2005a). Public health promotion will be used to help to maintain the health of the general population. This changing approach is a key part of Government policy on health and social care, which emphasizes choice and a move towards a patient-led NHS (DoH 2005a,b). Similarly, the need to tackle health inequalities is central to policy (DoH 2005c) and in this context personal health services have a major role in promoting equality. This is because these services have a relatively greater impact on severity than on incidence, and inequities in the severity of health problems are even greater than inequities in the incidence of health problems.

Key points

- The ageing population and shrinking workforce are major challenges for European societies.
- Health inequalities and the 'pension gap' are increasing in the UK and Europe.
- Solutions are needed to secure access to high quality healthcare for all and to manage the economical implications of ageing.
- Long-term conditions are now a political priority in England.
- Case management is seen as the model to improve care for those with complex conditions.

THE NEEDS OF OLDER PATIENTS

When older people become ill, the service and treatment that they receive should take account of their special problems and should meet their expectations and wishes. Access to the most effective interventions for their condition should be based on need rather than age (DoH 2001, 2004).

Older patients do have some differing needs from younger ones, but not just as a result of their age. Some diseases are more prevalent in the ageing population. While many will present in a textbook fashion, unusual presentations and also multiple disabilities are common with advancing age. In addition, side-effects of medication become increasingly common. Older people take longer to recover from acute illnesses and often develop non-specific functional difficulties (such as mobility problems, confusional states and incontinence) when ill. Nevertheless, a central tenet of geriatric medicine is that much illness and disability in old age is treatable and sometimes reversible.

Elderly patients in particular may benefit from specialist services such as coronary care units, endoscopy and haemodialysis, and the removal of age barriers to those services is progressing (Royal College of Physicians 2000). The risks and benefits of therapeutic interventions may differ at different ages. For instance, older age groups are the greatest beneficiaries in the prevention of stroke through treatment of hypertension (Kuo et al 2004).

Chronological age per se is a poor proxy for biological age. Ageism cannot be condoned in any area of medical care. The key test is to suggest whether all ages are included and/or excluded and, if designed specifically for the elderly, whether specialist medical, nursing and therapy staff with experience in geriatric practice are involved.

The involvement of patients, carers and the public in health decision-making is at the heart of modernizing the NHS (DoH 2001). Although this may lead to an increased demand on resources in the educational phase, it may help patients to manipulate their own therapy and so attend specialists less often; this has implications for service provision. Professionals are becoming facilitators and partners rather than authorities, and contribute to the development of self-help networks and individual self-care. Innovations such as 'Expert Patients' (DoH 2005a) and the greater use of information technology, when coupled with greater expectations from patients and carers, will alter the pattern of services.

Key points

- Many older patients have complex health needs and benefit from specialist services.
- Chronological age per se is a poor proxy for biological age.
- Increased patient expectations and patient involvement may have an impact on healthcare provision.

MODELS OF SERVICES AND HOW THEY MAY CHANGE

In the UK, health services are divided into primary, secondary and tertiary care. A comprehensive service will consider the provision of facilities to cater for a variety of scenarios. At their most intense and technological, this will be tertiary care. Since this differs little from the same services for younger patients, we shall give no further consideration to tertiary care. Traditionally, medical emergencies have been handled in secondary care, and various models and configurations have emerged both around the acute intake and between acute and rehabilitation wards. Arguably, chronic disease management and prevention are at least as important – if not more so – than the tip of the iceberg that acute admissions represent and there is now increasing focus on managing patients outside hospital.

All models should be capable of organizing a comprehensive geriatric assessment (CGA), with components drawn from physical, social, psychological, economic, functional and environmental aspects. The evidence base for the efficacy of the CGA in geriatric medicine is growing, indicating benefits relating to functional status, quality of life, length of hospital stay, rates of readmission and institutionalization in different healthcare environments, although no influence on survival has yet been demonstrated (British Geriatrics Society 2003).

ACUTE TREATMENT

There are three main service patterns that describe the division of the acute medical intake between geriatric medicine and general medicine (Beresford 1993):

- Needs-related model
- Age-defined model
- Integrated model

Needs-related model

Non-geriatricians select patients for admission to the geriatric unit. Selection may be undertaken by medical staff in the Accident and Emergency Department following preliminary assessment and may result in referral either to geriatric or general medical services. Particular problems (e.g. delirium or recurrent falls) may be identified as automatically appropriate for geriatric care.

Age-defined model

All medical patients above a certain age threshold referred to hospital are admitted to the geriatric service, the commonest defining age being around 75 years (but this varies from 65 to 85 years).

Integrated model

Physicians with special responsibility for elderly people serve as members of multi-consultant medical teams, take equal part in acute medical emergency work and are also responsible for providing specialist geriatric services (including rehabilitation, long-stay, day hospital, out-patient and community liaison work, e.g. with community matrons or rapid assessment community teams). A consultant physician in the specialty of geriatric medicine shares a team of junior doctors with other general medical colleagues.

No single model of care has been shown to be the superior (Royal College of Physicians 2000). There are arguments strongly in favour of separating the extremes of presentation, e.g. coronary care units for patients with acute myocardial infarction and overnight stay wards for deliberate self-harm. There are less persuasive arguments concerning the more common presentations of many elderly patients, some of whom may require intensive investigation and treatment, others needing less intense, but more protracted rehabilitation. Length of stay tends to increase with age, partly because of the difficulties in managing complex concurrent conditions, which tend to predominate in older people, but also because of the time required to rehabilitate and to organize effective discharge.

Whether all older patients should share facilities with their younger counterparts is more contentious. Most hospitals will provide some specialized elderly beds, in which the specialist geriatric team cares for those patients. People aged 65 years and above occupy almost two-thirds of beds. Over 40% of patients aged 65 years or more with disability, who number 1.3 million in England and Wales, will require admission to an acute hospital over a 2-year period (Royal College of Physicians 2000). They are one of the major reasons for the rise in the number of emergency admissions. Unless a hospital dedicates a similar proportion of its wards to acute geriatric medicine, many elderly patients will be cared for in general medical or other medical subspecialty wards. This can be advantageous if this is an appropriate specialty, but can lead to misplacement, delayed assessment and discharge planning.

Some departments separate their acute and rehabilitation facilities, others have them combined. There is controversy on the value of combining acute with rehabilitation, or keeping them separate and distinct. The argument is not quite as polarized as it may appear, and in practice most wards will fulfil a mixture of roles. However, the argument in favour of combining is largely predicated on efficiency, and the injection of a rehabilitation culture early in the admission. The argument against can be summed up in two main phrases – the incapacity of a rehabilitation unit to cope with the increasingly more technical acute end of the spectrum of disease, and with the squeezing out of rehabilitation from the acute environment. All facilities should have adequate provision of staff, equipment and finance so that patients can receive high quality care when they most need it and wherever they are cared for.

Key points

■ There is a wide variety of models of service provision.
■ Length of hospital stay increases with age due to complex conditions and time taken to rehabilitate.
■ Adequate resourcing (people, facilities and money) is a cornerstone of effective patient care and rehabilitation.

SECONDARY PREVENTION AND DISEASE MANAGEMENT

With the launch of the National Service Framework (NSF) for Older People in 2001, the health and social care system has focused on the needs of older people (DoH 2001). The NSF aims to promote independence and well-being and provide support at home or in other community settings. Services should be designed around the needs and choices of patients and service users (DoH 2004). The four underpinning principles are: person-centred care, joined-up services, a timely response to needs and promotion of health and active life.

Person–centred care

There are many possible ways in which older people may gain access to diagnostic, therapeutic and rehabilitation facilities. Each has its own virtues, and none has a universally agreed service, being at least partly dependent on local staffing, preferences, personalities and the use of resources. *Most important is promoting a person-centred approach, treating the older person with dignity and rooting out age discrimination.* Future developments will include more control being passed to the service users through direct payment for social care, greater choice and responsibility for self-care. This will require fair and consistent assessment of needs with budgets devolved either as direct payment to social service users or to practitioners, who will work with service users to align service response to user priorities. User involvement may take many forms, including consultation, providing information, establishing user satisfaction and participation in decision-making.

Provision of information is pivotal to user choice. Older people may find it difficult to explore a range of needs if they have deficient knowledge of what is available. Information systems should meet users' needs by providing information on diagnosis, research evidence on treatments and details of local services. Beresford (1993) identified support for service users as including:

1. Support for personal development to increase users' confidence and assertiveness
2. Support to develop participative skills

3. Practical support, including information, advocacy and transport
4. Support for equal opportunities for access to care, regardless of age, race, gender, sexuality or disability (Queen's Printer of Acts of Parliament 2000)

Joined-up service

Bridging the gap between hospital and home is paramount for improving patient care. Initiatives include the single assessment process and integrated services for falls, stroke, mental illness and continence (DoH 2001). Traditionally, NHS and local authority services have worked alongside each other with varying degrees of collaboration. Differences in funding streams, political accountability, organizational structure and professional cultures have contributed to the creation of barriers between services. The Health Act 1999 (Hultberg et al 2005) relaxed some of the statutory boundaries and responsibilities between the two sectors with the aim of promoting collaboration. This legislation was permissive and not compulsory and partnerships between NHS and local authorities had to be underpinned by legal agreements to safeguard the probity of the partnership. By 2000, only 32 localities had plans to use the flexibilities and pooled budgets; by 2002 this had increased to 130 (DoH 2000). As well as establishing formal arrangements for the relationships between local NHS and local authority organizations, agreement also had to be reached about the new relationships and responsibilities of the commissioners and the providers in the partnership. Matters such as budget monitoring, information sharing and charges paid by users of the social care elements of services also had to be incorporated into contracts. Possible benefits include:

1. Highlighting areas of service duplication
2. Improved information flow
3. Bringing together fragmented services
4. Avoiding delayed discharges
5. Delivery of complex care packages for patients with particularly specialized needs

Among senior managers and politicians, budget pooling broadened their awareness of interdependencies with other agencies and professionals in promoting patients' welfare. However, these broadened perspectives were not shared immediately by professionals working at the frontline and evidence for improved cost-effectiveness of pooled budgets is not yet available (DoH 2000).

Timely response to needs

This has concentrated on rapid access to treatment and care following identification of need or at crisis. Service developments will focus on population screening, opportunistic case finding and anticipatory care, aiming at identification of problems at an earlier stage and intervention ahead of crisis (DoH 2004). People with complex needs will have these addressed by teams led by community matrons working across hospital, community and care service boundaries. As professional case managers, community matrons work in collaboration with social services and secondary healthcare. They will be nurses undertaking a challenging role that requires a combination of clinical and case management skills in order to plan, manage and coordinate the care of people with complex long-term conditions and high-intensity needs.

Primary and secondary care networks should be strengthened by a universal electronic record system, which enables sharing of information about needs and identification of responses. The continued investment in community services is vital – particularly in intermediate care – to provide an alternative for hospital admissions for appropriate patients and to support early discharge.

Intermediate care

The notion of intermediate care was first signalled in the National Beds Enquiry (Forster et al 1999). It became policy in the NHS Plan and is now being implemented in England through the NSF for Older People (DoH 2001). Intermediate care is conceived as a range of service models aimed at 'care closer to home' to be achieved by expansion and development of community health and social services. The two key principles are, first, to provide a genuine alternative to hospital admission for carefully selected patients and, second, to provide supported discharge for others. This includes the provision of opportunities for further assessment and rehabilitation of older people so that no older person is placed in a care home directly from an acute ward. Intermediate care schemes include community assessment and rehabilitation teams, residential re-ablement units, nurse-led units, hospital-at-home schemes and a revitalized role for community hospitals. Many services have been developed according to local need and tend to vary in capacity and content between districts.

The evidence base for intermediate care remains insufficient to allow firm conclusions. Most current models of intermediate care do not have adverse outcomes in terms of mortality, morbidity or readmission to hospital and early discharge models appear to improve the prospects of older people staying at home after discharge. A Cochrane review comparing the effectiveness of medical day hospital care for elderly patients with other forms of care concluded that day hospitals are more effective than no intervention, but have no advantage over the alternative forms of care (Shepperd & Iliffe 2005). A systematic review of the effectiveness of hospital-at-home schemes found that they are effective at reducing the length of hospital stay. However, this was offset by the increased duration of the hospital-at-home service (Griffiths et al 2004). The evidence for nurse-led units shows increased length of stay, and the possibility of increased mortality cannot be discounted (British Geriatrics Society 2004a). To date there are no published randomized controlled trials of community hospitals.

In conventional hospital care, the medical responsibility lies with the consultant, who may delegate to junior medical staff or other doctors. In the community, general practitioners perform most of these functions under their General Medical Services contract. Commissioning and provision of intermediate care services need high-level leadership with the support of both the NHS and social services and the independent sector in delivery (Royal College of Physicians 2000). It is therefore helpful for representatives of other departments and organizations to attend some clinical governance service review meetings. This ensures a wider ownership and promotes integration into other mainstream services. The

involvement of service users at both practice and policy levels is important to develop services that are user-friendly and responsive (British Geriatrics Society 2004b). Topics to be considered when reviewing intermediate care schemes, particularly when considering them alongside conventional geriatric services, include:

■ The need for the service in the context of other local service components
■ Medical and professional responsibility – who, how, and for what?
■ Liability – who offers vicarious liability and undertakes to cover this?
■ Training – what will be given, to whom, at commencement and thereafter?
■ Risk assessment – and responsibility for maintenance of clinical standards
■ Relationship between geriatric medicine and other hospital services (e.g. psychiatry of old age) and primary care
■ Re-admission arrangements
■ Medical assessment, reassessment, and arrangements for on-going care
■ Which staff are involved, staffing levels, and the skill mix
■ Opportunity costs, and cost shifting between NHS, social services and the service user
■ Sources of longer-term funding
■ Contractual incentives and disincentives

Promotion of health and active life

There has been a shift of emphasis towards health promotion in old age (DoH 2001, 2004) There is recognition of the value of maintaining good health, e.g. through diet, activity and exercise. The health services must focus on the contribution that this can make, and particularly to concentrate efforts on those most at risk. While setting up schemes to keep all older people fitter, the service also needs to restore fitness after illness.

Sedentary behaviour accelerates the physiological loss of functional ability. Forty per cent of people aged over 50 years in the UK are sedentary. Disability can be delayed by as much as 10 years through moderate physical activity, good nutrition and stopping smoking. Regular physical activity contributes to improvements in physical and psychological function. It contributes to a healthier, independent lifestyle by improving functional capacity and quality of life for older people.

The aim of standard eight of the NSF for Older People is to extend healthy life expectancy (DoH 2001). The April 2003 milestone included programmes to promote healthy ageing and to prevent disease in older people. The target to demonstrate year-on-year improvements in measures of health and well-being through flu immunization, smoking cessation and blood pressure control should ensure that many older people will benefit from health promotion interventions and that barriers such as ageism are removed. In one example of the efficacy of this approach, uptake of flu vaccination in the over 65 age group (DoH 2004) rose from 65% in 2000 to 71% in 2004.

Lifestyle influences morbidity. Among individuals aged 70–90 years, adherence to a Mediterranean diet and healthy lifestyle is associated with a more than 59% lower rate of all-causes and cause-specific mortality. Health, housing, transport, voluntary organizations and social care should all collaborate to ensure that older people enjoy their longevity as healthy active years by preventing or deferring loneliness, social isolation and immobility. Healthy ageing should be promoted among all groups, including those with disability or dementia as well as older carers, older people living alone and older homeless people. There are opportunities in:

1. Mass media campaigns
2. Information or education sessions
3. Management or organizational change strategies
4. Policy changes, e.g. improving the sociocultural environment to encourage people of specific gender or ethnicity to participate
5. Changes to traditional or existing programmes and provision of activities beyond traditional or existing programmes, e.g. 'Come and Try' initiatives (teaser or taster programmes)
6. Skill improvement programmes
7. Volunteer encouragement programmes

Good cooperation with primary care is important, as general practitioners are at the frontline in identification of asymptomatic disease and health promotion. Incorporating health promotion for elderly people in the Quality and Outcome Framework could act as an incentive for general practitioners.

Cancers are increasingly remediable to surgery or chemotherapy and are best identified early. Early identification of older people with dementia may ensure appropriate treatment and ongoing care for patients and their families. Similarly, early diagnosis and treatment of depression can improve quality of life in older people (Knoops et al 2004). Older people with chronic diseases such as hypertension, atrial fibrillation, arthritis, diabetes mellitus and Parkinson's disease should be identified to ensure appropriate review and follow-up. The National Service Framework for Long-term Conditions reinforces the promotion of health and active life through its eleven quality requirements (DoH 2005a).

Key points

- Provision of support, including information and advocacy should increase user confidence.
- Further evidence is needed for the efficacy of intermediate care strategies.
- Lifestyle modification and health promotion can lead to improved quality of life and reduce morbidity and mortality in older people.

REFERENCES

*** *Randomized controlled trials (RCTs) or pooled data from RCTs; ** cohort/long-term observational study, non-randomized trial; * prospective (short duration) survey/ consensus statement*

Beresford P 1993 A programme for change: current issues in user involvement. In: Beresford P, Harding Y (eds) A challenge to change: practical experiences of building user-led services. The National Institute for Social Work, London *

Börsch-Supan A, Brugiavini A, Jürges H et al 2005 Health, ageing and retirement in Europe. First results from the survey of health, ageing and retirement in Europe. Mannheim Research Institute for the Economics of Aging (MEA), Mannheim. Online. Available: http://www.share-project.org **

British Geriatrics Society 2003 Standards of medical care for older people. Expectations and recommendations. Compendium document 1.3. Online. Available: http://www.bgs.org.uk/Publications/Compendium/compend_1-3.htm **

British Geriatrics Society 2004a Intermediate care. Guidance for commissioners and providers of health and social care. Compendium document 4.2, Online. Available: http://www.bgs.org.uk/Publications/Compendium/compend_4-2.htm **

British Geriatrics Society 2004b Health promotion and preventative care. Compendium document 4.1. Online. Available: http://www.bgs.org.uk/Publications/Compendium/compend_4-1.htm **

Department of Health 2000 Shaping the future NHS: long term planning for hospitals and related services (national beds inquiry). DoH, London. Online. Available: http://www.dh.gov.uk/assetRoot/04/02/04/70/04020470.pdf **

Department of Health 2001 National Service Framework for Older People. Modern standards and service models. DoH, London. Online. Available: http://www.dh.gov.uk/Publicationsandstatistics/Publications/PublicationsPolicyAndGuidance/PublicationsPolicyAndGuidanceArticle/fs/en?CONTENT_ID=4010161&chk=6GV5oj **

Department of Health 2004 Better health in old age. DoH, London. Online. Available: http://www.dh.gov.uk/assetRoot/04/09/32/15/04093215.pdf *

Department of Health 2005a The National Service Framework for long term conditions. DoH, London. Online. Available: http://www.dh.gov.uk/Publicationsandstatistics/Publications/PublicationsPolicyAndGuidance/PublicationsPolicyAndGuidanceArticle/fs/en?CONTENT_ID=4105361&chk=jl7dri *

Department of Health 2005b Creating a patient-led NHS: delivering the NHS improvement plan. DoH, London. Online. Available: http://www.dh.gov.uk/Publicationsandstatistics/Publications/PublicationsPolicyAndGuidance/PublicationsPolicyAndGuidanceArticle/fs/en?CONTENT_ID=4106506&chk=ftV6vA *

Department of Health 2005c Tackling health inequalities: status report on the program for action. DoH, London. Online. Available: http://www.dh.gov.uk/Policyandguidance/HealthAndSocialCareTopics/HealtInequalities/fs/en **

Department of Health 2006 Our health, our care, our say. A new direction for community services. DoH, London. Online. Available: http://www.dh.gov/assetRoot/04/12/76/04/04127604.pdf **

Forster A, Young J, Langhorne P, for the Day Hospital Group 1999 Medical day hospital care for the elderly versus alternative forms of care. The Cochrane Database of Systematic Reviews 3. Art. No.: CD001730. DOI: 10.1002/14651858.CD001730 ***

Griffiths P D, Edwards M H, Forbes A et al 2004 Effectiveness of intermediate care in nursing-led in-patient units. The Cochrane Database of Systematic Reviews 4. Art. No.: CD002214. DOI: 10.1002/14651858.CD002214.pub2 ***

Hultberg E L, Glendinning C, Allebeck P et al 2005 Using pooled budgets to integrate health and welfare services: a comparison of experiments in England and Sweden. Health and Social Care in the Community 13:531–543 *

Knoops K T, de Groot L C P, Kromhout D et al 2004 Mediterranean diet, lifestyle factors, and 10-year mortality in elderly European men and women. The HALE Project. Journal of the American Medical Association 292:1433–1439 **

Kuo H K, Scandrett K G, Dave J et al 2004 The influence of outpatient comprehensive geriatric assessment on survival: meta-analysis. Archives of Gerontology and Geriatrics 39:245–254 **

Office for National Statistics (ONS) 2002–2003 General Household Survey. ONS, London. Online. Available: http://www.statistics.gov.uk **

Queen's Printer of Acts of Parliament 2000 Health Act 1999. The National Health Service. Queen's Printer of Acts of Parliament. Online. Available: http://www.opsi.gov.uk/acts/acts1999/19990008.htm *

Royal College of Physicians 2000 Working party reports: Management of the older medical patient. Online Publications. RCP, London. Online. Available: http://www.rcplondon.ac.uk/pubs/books/momp/wp_momp_part2.htm **

Shepperd S, Iliffe S 2005 Hospital at home versus in-patient hospital care. The Cochrane Database of Systematic Reviews 3. Art. No.: CD000356. DOI: 10.1002/14651858.CD000356.pub2 ***

United Nations Department of Economic and Social Affairs 2003 World population in 2300, ESA/P/WP.187 (Draft). United Nations, New York. Online. Available: http://www.un.org/esa/population/publications/longrange2/Long_range_report.pdf **

World Health Organization 2004 A strategy to prevent chronic disease in Europe: a focus on public health action. The CINDI Vision. WHO, Denmark. Online. Available: http://www.euro.who.int/document/E83057.pdf **

SELF-ASSESSMENT QUESTIONS

1. Are the following statements true or false?
   a. The proportion of people over 85 years in England is declining
   b. Reduced mortality will increase service demands
   c. Northern Europeans live longer than southern Europeans
   d. 5% of people with multiple co-morbidities account for 42% of hospital bed days
   e. Health professionals have embraced pooled budgets which bridge the gap between agencies

2. Are the following statements true or false?
   a. Intermediate care interventions have been shown to reduce admissions to acute hospitals and reduce care home placements
   b. 20% of people aged over 50 years in the UK are sedentary
   c. A Mediterranean diet and healthy lifestyle are associated with a 60% lower rate of mortality
   d. Geriatricians will become redundant with increasing specialized medical input and falling numbers of elderly care beds
   e. Involvement of patients, carers and the public in health decision-making will increase the cost of the NHS

3. Are the following statements true or false? The health and social needs of an older person:
   a. Are complex and benefit from specialist services
   b. Are dependent upon the principle of person-centred care
   c. Benefit from joined-up services
   d. Are best met by timely response from professionals
   e. Can be reduced by identifying asymptomatic disease

4. Are the following statements true or false? Life expectancy:
   a. Is an average which relates to all persons still alive at a given age
   b. At birth there is no difference between life expectancy of men and women
   c. At the age of 75 years, the life expectancy of a female is about 2.7 years longer than the life expectancy of a man of the same age in England
   d. The increase in life expectancy for men between 2100 and 2200 is expected to be 8 years
   e. Disability-free life expectancy is longer than healthy life expectancy

Chapter 6

Community geriatric care

Branwell Spencer

INTRODUCTION

In this chapter I will concentrate on exploring the reasons behind, the need for and the development of a more integrated role of the geriatrician within the community. There are compelling theoretical reasons why increasing the community role of geriatricians is a necessary advance and there are several major government papers which can be used to forward the case for a community geriatrician. The evidence of benefit in specific areas of community practice is increasing but is often meagre.

COMMUNITY GERIATRICS: WHAT IS IT?

All geriatricians have a role to play in community care – even if it is limited to domiciliary visits, day hospital and out-patient care. A definition of the 'community' should include all the various residences of older people, ranging from their own home to residential and nursing homes, with all the associated support services.

Unfortunately, with recent emphasis on acute hospital workload and the simultaneous decrease in NHS long-stay beds, geriatricians may be in danger of becoming removed from those areas of care on which geriatrics was founded. It is

increasingly important for geriatricians to maintain and develop services for older people outside hospital.

What constitutes the community?

1. Older people
2. Family and friends
3. Other informal carers
4. Nursing homes
5. Residential homes
6. Sheltered accommodation
7. Social services
8. Voluntary community services (independent or private)
9. General practitioners and primary care trusts
10. Day centres
11. Day hospitals
12. Specialist nurses, e.g. district nurses, Macmillan nurses and psychiatric community nurses
13. Therapy services

SOCIAL SERVICES PROVISION

Social services primarily assess the need for personal care and provision of financial support for residential and nursing home places. In essence, social workers act as gatekeepers. Some of the areas that they are responsible for are outlined in the following box.

Social services provision: areas of responsibility

1. Assessment of need for residential (independent or social services local authority accommodation) or nursing home
2. Review of financial ability to pay for care in long-stay facilities
3. Housing adaptation team
4. Equipment for daily living
5. Home care
6. Respite care
7. Day centres

Areas of health authority provision, voluntary services and private organizations within the community are outlined in the next three boxes.

Health authority provision: areas of responsibility

1. Nursing
2. Palliative care
3. Macmillan nurses
4. Continence services
5. Physiotherapy
6. Occupational therapy
7. Speech and language therapy
8. Chiropody
9. Dental services
10. Dietetics
11. Community pharmacists

Voluntary services in the community

Two main organizations coordinate the voluntary sector; the Council for Voluntary Services and the National Council for Voluntary Organizations.

Voluntary organizations include:

1. National general organizations (e.g. Age Concern and Help the Aged)
2. Disease– or disability-specific organizations (e.g. Parkinson's Disease Society, Alzheimer's Society)
3. Carers' organizations (e.g. Crossroads, Carers National Association)

4. Locally orientated organizations (e.g. Citizen Advice Bureau, Women's Royal Voluntary Service)
5. Culturally-based organizations
6. Hospices
7. Housing associations

Private organizations within the community

1. Most nursing and residential homes
2. Some home-care services
3. Live-in companions
4. Some domiciliary nursing services

THE BRITISH GERIATRICS SOCIETY VIEW OF THE CONSULTANT GERIATRICIAN'S ROLE IN THE COMMUNITY

The British Geriatrics Society (BGS) envisages two main types of consultant geriatrician. The first is the consultant physician with an interest in geriatric medicine. Responsibilities would include the care of general medical and geriatric patients. The consultant would usually also have a specialist interest within geriatric medicine, e.g. stroke, but a minor clinical commitment to community care. The second model would be a consultant geriatrician with an interest in community care who would be expected to take a lead role in community care and to develop links between primary and secondary care, while still having direct access to hospital beds. The BGS anticipates that each department should have at least one consultant with a considerable amount of time devoted to community work.

MAKING THE CASE FOR GERIATRICIANS WITH A SPECIAL INTEREST IN THE COMMUNITY

Recent changes in the politics and philosophy of healthcare have spurred major changes in the healthcare provision for sick elderly patients. Key among a number of government publications was the National Service Framework for older people published in 2001. This was a driver for expanding community care and increased involvement by geriatricians.

A CHANGING POPULATION

Since 1931 the number of people over 65 years has doubled. The number of those aged over 75 years is now 4.6 million and this is expected to rise to 6.3 million by 2030.

In the UK, life expectancy is increasing for both men and women at a faster rate than healthy life expectancy (www.statistics.gov.uk). More of us will live longer but we may spend a longer amount of time in ill health. Figures comparing 1981 with 2001 illustrate increasing life expectancy between 1981–2001 with an average extra 4.8 years of life for men and 3.6 years for women, but an even greater increase in years in poor health (men in 2001 living on average 8.7 years in poor health and women 11.6 years) (www.statistics.gov.uk).

CHANGES IN FAMILY STRUCTURE AND WORKING PRACTICES

Traditionally, women have been the main providers of informal care at home for sick and elderly relatives. In recent years, many women have moved from an unpaid caring role into paid employment, usually outside the home. This shift in working patterns has potentially reduced the pool of people available to provide care at home or at least decreased the amount of time available to them to fulfill a caring role. Changes in employment patterns have led increasingly to people moving away from home to work. The extended family, which was often able to provide support at home for a relative in times of crisis, is becoming less common.

Considerable numbers of these old people are becoming more frail and often require increased support. Yet there is a decreasing proportion of younger family and friends. National statistical data show that, in 2001, 2.8 million people over 50 years in private households provided unpaid care for family, friends or neighbours. One in four

of these carers provided over 50 hours a week (rising to 1 in 2 for the over 85s) (www.statistics.gov.uk). A greater proportion of older men than older women provided free care.

> **The availability of carers is affected by many variables:**
>
> 1. The increasing number of women at work
> 2. Increased divorce rates
> 3. Increased workforce mobility
> 4. Break up of the nuclear family
> 5. Delays in forming stable relationships

MEDICAL AND SURGICAL ADVANCES

Changes in medical practice (such as management of myocardial infarction) and surgical developments (such as laparoscopic surgery) have allowed more people to be treated with shorter in-patient stays. Indeed, from 1990 to 1995 the average length of stay in geriatric wards decreased from 36 to 20 days, with similar reductions evident in other specialties.

Shorter length of stay after an acute admission can make optimum discharge planning difficult. Previous work from the Audit Commission on discharge planning for fractured neck of femur shows that this is often poorly planned, resulting in delaying discharge or failure to provide appropriate rehabilitation opportunities (Audit Commission 1995).

RISING ACUTE HOSPITAL ADMISSIONS

The year-on-year increase of acute medical admission has led to the annual winter bed crisis. This leads to a pressure to return patients home even more rapidly – sometimes without proper assessment and support. Conversely, those not discharged home quickly may find themselves assessed before they have been fully rehabilitated and are placed on a waiting list for a nursing home. In 1995, up to 82% of medically fit patients had their discharges delayed because they were waiting for community support schemes (packages of care) or long-term care home placement

(BMA 1995). Recently, the government introduced a reimbursement system: after an assessment has been done and a care need agreed by social services, and if there are delays in provision of that care, then social services would reimburse the hospitals on a daily basis.

THE CHANGING NUMBERS AND NEEDS OF RESIDENTS IN NURSING HOMES

The UK Government wished to change the organization and funding of long-term care. In 1983, changes were made to the benefits system by topping up social service payments for long-term care in the UK. This led to a massive increase in nursing and residential home beds in the independent sector. In England, the numbers of private nursing homes and voluntary sector nursing home beds increased from 18 200 in 1982 to 148 500 in 1994. The number of NHS beds fell from over 200 000 in 1981 to 130 000 in 2001. This increase in publicly-funded private nursing and residential home places was very costly.

Although the percentage of the older population in long-term care remains low (about 5% of those over 65 years), the total number of older people in nursing homes is rising and their increasing frailty requires more nursing staff and, increasingly, the need for more technical nursing skills (such as management of percutaneous endoscopic gastrostomy tubes and syringe drivers).

It is therefore imperative that nurses in nursing homes are fully trained and updated to enable them to provide quality care for their residents. This has major funding and recourse implications.

RISKS OF HOSPITAL ADMISSION TO THE MOST VULNERABLE PATIENT GROUPS

Advantages of hospital admission include rapid access to specialist medical advice, specialist nursing skills, specialist investigations and hospital records. Admission to hospital is not without its risks and dangers, ranging from injuries to hospital-acquired infections. In some cases, admission to hospital may be inappropriate and possibly the patient could be managed just as well (or even better) in a non-hospital setting. Some long-stay patients admitted to hospital may do less well than if they were managed in the nursing home; they often require relatively basic interventions to manage their acute illness (Spencer et al 1998, Turrell & Castleden 1999).

WHO CARES FOR RESIDENTS IN LONG-TERM CARE

The 1990 Community Care Act states that the health needs of an individual should be met by appropriate expertise, wherever they live. Some of these patients may be best managed by geriatricians whose core skills include the assessment and management of older people with multiple pathology and disability associated with chronic illness. The increased number of nursing home beds and the diminution of NHS long-term beds has reduced the input of consultants in continuing care. The major responsibility for planning and provision has been transferred to nurses and managers. General practitioners play a vital role in individual patient management, though many have had little or no training in elderly medicine.

Summary: implications of medical and social changes

An increasing proportion of older people who traditionally have been supported by the geriatrician in hospital are now in need of additional specialist support and services. Many are now based in the community.

PROJECTIONS FOR DEMAND OF LONG-TERM CARE

In Britain, less than 5% of the those aged over 65 years are in long-term care and even in the over-85s the figure is only 29%.

Presently there are about 480 000 older people in care homes, i.e. about 1 in 20 of all elderly people. Pressures on social services mean that care provision is being focused increasingly on a smaller number of increasingly dependent people. With more of the older and frailer people in the population, there is a real danger that they may not get the care they need.

AN OVERVIEW OF KEY GOVERNMENTAL PAPERS AND POLICIES

There have been several documents that focus on the need for changes in health service provision and provide political weight to the expansion of the community role of geriatricians.

COMMUNITY CARE ACT 1990

The widespread proliferation of independent nursing and residential homes in the early 1980s led to a spiraling increase in long-term care costs (DoH 1995, Laing 1995) and prompted the publication of the Community Care Act 1990.

The long-term care budget was therefore transferred to social services and managed locally, along with the responsibility for assessment for long-term care placement. The expansion of social services-funded long-term placements enabled easier discharge from hospital and allowed hospitals to close long-term care beds. Attempts to address these inequities were the force behind the publication of the Continuing Care Act 1996.

NHS RESPONSIBILITIES FOR MEETING CONTINUING CARE NEEDS

The Continuing Care Act 1996

One of the effects of the Community Care Act was the large scale closure of long-stay NHS beds but there was marked regional variation in the extent to which this happened. This led to a regional lottery as to whether long-term care was to be provided free on the NHS or whether an individual's assets were to be used to pay for independent nursing or residential home placement.

There was recognition that some individuals in nursing homes would have previously received free long-term care in long-stay hospital wards. A system of ongoing NHS funding was introduced for patients whose health problems were the main reason for their care needs.

All people who require any form of ongoing social care or long-term residential or nursing care should be assessed against a set of six eligibility criteria as to whether they have a continuing *healthcare* need. Those individuals who fulfill the criteria are entitled to ongoing NHS funding of their care needs.

Difficulties have arisen because there is no national standard and authorities have applied the criteria in different ways. This led to complaints to the Ombudsman with subsequent review of individual cases and process. Recently the Government has announced its intention to draw up national standards for continuing healthcare.

'With respect to old age' – a Royal Commission report into long-term care 1999

The Royal Commission into long-term care was established by the Labour party to examine the short- and long-term options for the funding of long-term care for elderly people.

One of the inequities within the previous nursing care provision in the community was that if you could be cared for at home or in hospital, then nursing care was free. If you lived in a nursing home, then you had to pay for your nursing care (after financial means-testing).

The Government decided that for England and Wales, the *nursing* component of care in nursing homes would be paid for by the state. However, defining what exactly is 'nursing care' for an individual has not been straightforward.

Living and personal care costs, however, were to remain means-tested in England and Wales, but not in Scotland, where the Scottish Parliament decided that the state would pay for this.

National Service Framework (NSF) for Older People 2001

Intermediate care was first mentioned in the NHS Plan in 2000 (DoH 2000). It merited a whole chapter in the NSF where its stated aim is that intermediate care should:

'Provide integrated services to promote faster recovery from illness, prevent unnecessary acute hospital admissions, support timely discharge and maximise independent living'

A stimulus for the development of intermediate care was the Audit Commission report of 1997 (Audit Commission 1997). Inadequate investment in preventative and rehabilitation services led to unplanned admission of older people to hospital and premature admissions to long-term care. Additionally, the National Beds Inquiry (www. doh.gov.uk) concluded that for older people, around 20% of bed days in hospital would not be needed if alternative facilities were in place.

Intermediate care services should (NSF 2001):

■ Involve multiagency working (social services, primary care, secondary care, private or voluntary services)
■ Follow a thorough assessment of needs
■ Have a treatment plan
■ Have agreed expected outcomes
■ Have input from a multidisciplinary team
■ Have equity of access to secondary care using clear protocols
■ Be performance managed and have ongoing evaluation of outcomes
■ Be acceptable to adult users of all ages

Additionally:

■ Intermediate care services are usually limited to 6 weeks, after which the patients may incur financial charges for services provided

---

The evidence for the benefits of intermediate care

The evidence for the benefits of intermediate care services is patchy. For defined groups with specific rehabilitation needs and disease-specific community support, there is evidence that there are benefits (examples of these are given later).

What is far less clear, because it has been studied less and is harder to evaluate, is the benefit for services that are generic, without a clearly-defined user group and involving a range of interventions.

A study from Leeds (Young et al 2005) was designed to evaluate newly introduced intermediate care service in that city. The researchers looked at frail elderly patients who had been admitted to hospital with falls, confusion, incontinence or poor mobility and then discharged with daily supportive care and rehabilitation at home. The clinical outcomes were similar to usual

care, but did not achieve strategic objectives of reducing long-term care and hospital use.

The Department of Health provides its own examples of what it considers to be good practice for intermediate care on its policy website.

Nurse–led discharge units
Evaluations of nurse-led discharge in-patient units after acute illness have shown that, though patients may be better prepared for discharge from hospital, outcomes are not improved over usual care and length of stay is prolonged. Cost analysis shows increased in-patient and total care costs (Griffiths et al 2001, 2004, Steiner et al 2001).

Rehabilitation in the community

Care home rehabilitation
There is some evidence to suggest that rehabilitation in care homes can divert patients from hospital without any adverse effect on well-being – but it does not appear to reduce the need for long-term care. There are too little research data for evidence-based decisions to be made in this area (Fleming et al 2004, Ward et al 2003).

Early discharge post stroke
There is now increasing evidence, including a Cochrane review, that early discharge and a well-coordinated rehabilitation programme at home after stroke is at least as good as any hospital-based rehabilitation programme. However, there are concerns about increased caregiver strain (Early Supported Discharge Trialists 2001).

Early discharge post fractured neck of femur
Early discharge schemes lead to shorter lengths of stay without worsening outcomes in selected patients. The overall length of rehabilitative care is increased (Handoll & Parker 2004).

Acute care–at–home schemes: specific conditions

Acute exacerbation of chronic obstructive pulmonary disease
Increasingly, acute exacerbations of chronic obstructive pulmonary disease (COPD) are being managed at home after assessment by intervention teams, who are able to provide nebulized

oxygen and antibiotic therapy. In selected cases, the outcome is similar to those hospitalized. Home care is preferred by most patients (Ram et al 2003, Yohannes & Connolly 2004).

Congestive cardiac failure

Evidence (mainly from abroad) shows that acute worsening of congestive cardiac failure can be managed at home and reduces hospital admission and improves functional New York Heart Association (NYHA) class. A Cochrane review found that the studies were poor and evidence that intensive community monitoring might reduce mortality and reduce admissions was inconclusive (Taylor et al 2005).

Deep venous thrombosis

With the development of low molecular weight heparins and simple subcutaneous dosing regimens, both distal and proximal deep vein thromboses (DVTs) can be managed at home with support from nursing teams and out-patient warfarinization protocols. Study evidence shows effectiveness and patient preference (Schraibman et al 2001).

Blood transfusion

Domiciliary blood transfusion is widely used both abroad and in the UK. It provides a safe and acceptable alternative to hospital admission.

Intravenous antibiotics

The development of once and twice daily intravenous antibiotics and the potential for long-stay intravenous lines mean that conditions requiring these interventions may now be managed at home, e.g. cellulitis not responding to oral agents (Asensio et al 2000, Grayson et al 1995).

Other areas

Parenteral nutrition and long-term ventilation are areas with potential for out-of-hospital care provision.

General hospital–at–home schemes

A systematic review of hospital-at-home schemes by Shepperd & Iliffe (2005) found lack of evidence

of benefit in clinical outcomes or cost benefits. The more recently published results of the Leicester hospital-at-home scheme showed significantly shorter hospital length of stay and no clinically important differences in health status. The case for hospital-at-home schemes remains unproved in terms of benefit over hospital treatment.

National research into intermediate care services

The Department of Health set up the National Intermediate Care Research Programme. Research was commissioned at three centres in England (Leeds, Leicester/Birmingham and Bradford/York Universities) to improve the understanding of costs and outcomes of intermediate care services.

The Leicester–Birmingham evaluation, 'A National Evaluation of the Costs and Outcomes of Intermediate Care for Older People' was published in January 2006 (Barton et al 2006). It concluded that there are wide variations on how intermediate care is being locally defined and that most areas are working towards integrating separate diverse individual services into a single system. Basic data collection and performance measures were often hard for areas to provide. Effective partnership working between primary care trusts and social services is the most important key in effective service development. Intermediate care services seem to provide additional care as well as substitutive care, and relationships between existing services and the limitations of some intermediate care services mean that intermediate care services are not being used effectively. At present, intermediate care services have had a limited impact on other services. Admission avoidance schemes are potentially the most cost effective and might produce better quality of life gains for users than supported discharge schemes, but there are concerns about delayed diagnosis. Residential schemes cost more than non-residential schemes but provide better quality of life and functional improvements in the short term.

Many of these conclusions will be familiar to geriatricians working within intermediate care and provide questions and directions for further research and service development.

Concerns about intermediate care

Intermediate care is not a new concept. Community services have long been developed, largely on an ad hoc basis, providing for a local need, with varying involvement of geriatricians. When developed and implemented properly and evaluated rigorously, intermediate care can potentially provide a valuable alternative tier of care, which is often appreciated by users and their families. What is not clear is whether it can deliver what policy-makers intended: a reduction in hospital admission rates, reduced length of stay and reduced use of long-term care placements. Intermediate care services must not be allowed to block appropriate access of old people to specialist secondary care skills and services. With an increasing number of hospital trusts struggling financially, there is a danger of developing in intermediate care at the expense of established services, on the unproven assumption that intermediate care is cheaper.

There should be appropriate and effective involvement of geriatricians both in service development and clinical input. It is important that we continue to remind commissioners that social functional decline often has an underlying medical cause, which needs to be diagnosed and managed. Effective communication must occur so that patient assessments include both clinical and social information.

Supporting people with long-term conditions: Department of Health 2005

The Government has recently published a document on the future management of long-term conditions. It comprises a three-tiered approach, with supported self-care at the base of the pyramid, disease-specific care management in the middle and case management at the top.

In case management, high-risk individuals form the caseload for a community matron, who is a case manager, involved in monitoring and managing their care – not just in the community, but during any hospital stay and during discharge planning.

This approach is moving away from traditionally reactive services to proactive illness prevention and integrated care planning between secondary and primary care.

The evidence for this approach comes largely from the USA and it is not clear to what extent the findings of reduced admission rate are applicable in the UK, which has a different style of social and healthcare provision. Indeed, a King's Fund review found that case management of a population – rather than high-risk individuals – may be effective in reducing institutional rates and mortality (but not hospital admission rates).

The role of assessment

An important component of intermediate care services and a key point of the Royal Commission into long-term care is the importance of the multidisciplinary team in comprehensive assessment.

The multidisciplinary assessment should:

1. Have a clear purpose
2. Be done at the right time
3. Provide accurate diagnosis and prognosis
4. Provide opportunity for rehabilitation
5. Reflect the wishes of the older person and informal carer
6. Provide clear communication with staff, patients and carers
7. Inform planning of future care

The timing of the assessment should be when the patient has recovered from their acute illness and is medically stable. There should be optimum rehabilitation. Placement in long-term care should not be seen as final, but open for review and reassessment. No individual should enter long-term care without detailed assessment, rehabilitation and treatment.

The effectiveness of geriatrician-led multidisciplinary assessment and management (compared with alternative hospital-based specialists and primary care teams) is now well established (Stuck et al 1993).

The increasing use of a single assessment process (such as Easycare) by health and social care staff might identify more easily those in need of a comprehensive assessment.

> **The dangers of not doing multidisciplinary assessment are:**
>
> 1. Inappropriate placement in nursing and residential care
> 2. Failure to maximize independence and quality of life
> 3. Poorly planned discharges
> 4. Increased readmission rates
> 5. Failure to recognize patients' wishes and concerns

Role of primary care groups and trusts

Previously, general practitioners in fund holding practices could commission whatever support services they felt necessary. In 1999, fund holding stopped and was replaced by the amalgamation of general practices into primary care groups, which later became primary care trusts (PCTs). PCTs were both service commissioners and service providers. Imminent government changes will see the amalgamation of PCTs into fewer, much larger groups which will just have a commissioning role.

General practitioners with a special interest in geriatrics

General practitioners often have individual areas of special interest, in a range of clinical specialties. Historically, they have provided the clinical care for residents in long-term care. With the expansion of community services and intermediate care, a role for the GP with a special interest in older people is evolving. Ideally, these posts should have clear working links with the local geriatricians. The new GP contract and the quality and outcome framework, which financially rewards practices achieving government targets in patient care and service, might stimulate further improvements in the care of older patients.

> **Roles of a geriatrician in the community:**
>
> 1. Working in a multiagency partnership to develop appropriate alternatives to hospital care
> 2. Effectively highlighting the importance of specialist medical input into intermediate care services
> 3. Assessment within the multidisciplinary team for appropriate home-care package or residential, nursing home care (long or short term)
> 4. Acute interventions for ill older people at home
> 5. Education in nursing and residential homes
> 6. Education and liaison with other concerned groups (e.g. social services, health authority and voluntary groups)
> 7. Liaison with GPs in primary care groups
> 8. Involvement in continuing healthcare decisions
> 9. Maintaining and developing effective links with secondary care services
> 10. Research into community care

DEVELOPING ALTERNATIVES TO HOSPITAL CARE

A key aim of community geriatrics must be to develop flexible and responsive health and social care schemes for older people.

> **Examples of possible alternatives to hospital care include:**
>
> 1. Intermediate care residential schemes
> 2. Intensive domiciliary support schemes
> 3. Community rehabilitation
> 4. Rapid response nursing teams
> 5. Hospital-at-home schemes
> 6. Community hospitals
> 7. Clinical service to individuals at home

PRACTICAL DIFFICULTIES IN COMMUNITY GERIATRICS

Geriatricians in training should ensure that they develop the skills needed for community care, gaining exposure to long-term care facilities, respite care and attachments to a geriatrician with an expertise in community care. This may be a problem in areas where community geriatric care may be less developed and the pressures on acute medical and geriatric service provision continue to be seen as a priority. The BGS has recognized this need for formal training in community geriatrics (www.jchmt.org.uk).

How you develop an integrated community geriatric job depends on the local services. It remains to be seen how the major reorganization across the primary and secondary care services in terms of commissioning and choice agenda will affect working practice. The imminent slowing of the funding stream from government to the health service will also have an impact on service development. Secondary care providers – as well as wanting to improve older people's services – may be keen to reduce in-patient hospital stays, giving the community geriatrician both opportunities and threats.

Ensure that in order to be effective, your job plan properly reflects the balance between hospital and community work. Service development can generate a lot of meetings. The development of closer working relationships and better understanding between the primary care trust, social services, nursing and residential homes and other care services are probably the most important things to allow the development of effective community services.

SUMMARY

Changing demographics and changes in healthcare and social policy mean that increasing numbers of older people will spend time in intermediate or other community care services. There is still a lack of evidence on which to base such a change in health and social service provision.

Some will embrace these changes; other will be sceptical of them. But, whatever your viewpoint, geriatricians need to be involved in order to pro-tect the healthcare of older people and develop services that are suitable for them – services in which we would all have confidence and be happy to use.

REFERENCES

Asensio O, Bosque M, Marco T et al 2000 Home intravenous antibiotics for cystic fibrosis. The Cochrane Database of Systematic Reviews 4. Art. No.: CD 001917. DOI: 10.1002/14651858.CD.001917

Audit Commission 1995 United they stand: coordinating care for elderly patients with hip fractures. HMSO, London

Audit Commission 1997 The coming of age: improving care services for older people. Audit Commission, London

Barton P, Bryan S, Glasby J et al 2006 A national evaluation of the costs and outcomes of intermediate care for older people. Online. Available: http://www.hs.le.ac.uk/nccsu/indexa.html

British Medical Association, Health Policy and Economic Research Unit 1995 Survey on the impact of the implementation of the community care reform: psychiatrists and geriatricians. British Medical Association, London

Department of Health 1995 House of Commons Health Committee: Long term care: NHS responsibilities for meeting continuing health care needs, vol.1, p VIII. HMSO, London

Department of Health 2000 Shaping the future NHS: Long term planning for hospitals and related services. Consultation document on the findings of the National Beds Inquiry. Online. Available: http://www.dh.gov.uk/en/Consultations/Closedconsultations/DH_4102910

Early Supported Discharge Trialists 2001 Services for reducing the duration of hospital care for acute stroke patients. (Cochrane review). The Cochrane Database of Systematic Reviews 2. Art. No.: CD 000443. DOI: 10.1002/14651858.CD000443

Fleming S, Blake H, Gladman J R et al 2004 A randomised controlled trial of a care home rehabilitation service to reduce long-term institutionalisation for elderly people. Age and Ageing 33:384–390

Grayson M L, Silvers J, Turnridge J 1995 Home intravenous antibiotic therapy. A safe and effective alternative to inpatient care. Medical Journal of Australia 162:249–253

Griffiths P, Harris R, Richardson G et al 2001 Substitution of a nursing-led inpatient unit for acute services: randomised controlled trial of outcomes and cost of nursing-led intermediate care. Age and Ageing 30:483–488

Griffiths P D, Edwards M H, Forbes A et al 2004 Effectiveness of intermediate care in nursing-led in-patient units. The Cochrane Database of Systematic Reviews 2. Art. No.: CD0002214. DOI: 10.1002/14651858.CD0002214

Handoll H, Parker M 2004 Early supported discharge followed by home based rehabilitation programmes. BMJ Clinical Evidence. Online. Available: http://www.clinicalevidence.com

Laing W 1995 Care of elderly people: market survey. 8th edn. Laing and Buisson, London

Ram F S F, Wedzicha J A, Wright J et al 2003 Hospital at home for acute exacerbations of chronic obstructive pulmonary disease. The Cochrane Database of Systematic Reviews 4. Art. No.: CD003573. DOI: 10.1002/14651858.CD003573

Schraibman I G, Milne A A, Royle E M 2001 Home versus in-patient treatment for deep vein thrombosis. The Cochrane Database of Systematic Reviews 2. Art. No.: CD003076. DOI: 10.1002/14651858.CD003076

Shepperd S, Iliffe S 2005 Hospital at home versus in-patient hospital care. The Cochrane Database of Systematic Reviews 3. Art. No.: CD000356. DOI: 10.1002/14651858.CD000356

Spencer B, Fook L, Turnbull C et al 1998 Acute admissions from nursing homes. British Geriatrics Society 27(supp1):46

Steiner A, Walsh B, Pickering R M et al 2001 Therapeutic nursing or unblocking beds? A randomised controlled trial of a post acute intermediate care unit. British Medical Journal 322:453–460

Stuck A E, Sui A L, Wiland G D et al 1993 Comprehensive geriatric assessment: a meta-analysis of controlled trials. Lancet 342:1032–1036

Taylor S, Bestall J, Cotter S et al 2005 Clinical service organisation for heart failure. The Cochrane Database of Systematic Reviews 2. Art. No.: CD002752. DOI: 10.1002/14651858.CD002752

Turrell A, Castleden M 1999 Improving the emergency medical treatment of older nursing-home residents. Age and Ageing 28:77–82

Ward D, Severs M, Dean T et al 2003 Care home versus hospital and own home environments for rehabilitation of older people. The Cochrane Database of Systematic Reviews 2. Art. No.: CD003164. DOI: 10.1002/14651858.CD003164

Yohannes A M, Connolly M R 2004 Current initiatives in the management of patients with chronic obstructive pulmonary disease: the NICE guidelines and the recent evidence base. Age and Ageing 33:419–421

Young J M, Robinson M, Chell S et al 2005 A whole system study of intermediate care services for older people. Age and Ageing 34:577–583

RECOMMENDED READING

Beales D 1998 Community care of older people. Radcliffe Medical Press, Oxford

Stevenson J, Spencer L 2002 Developing intermediate care: a guide for health and social service professionals. Kings Fund, London

Tallis R, Fillit H, Brocklehurst J (eds) 1998 Brocklehurst's textbook of geriatric medicine. Provision of care chapters. Churchill Livingstone, Edinburgh

Wade S 2003 Intermediate care of older people. Whurr, Chichester

Important publications

1990 National Health Service and Community Care Act 1990 (commencement No 7) order 1991, ISBM 0110133889

1995 Department of Health paper. NHS responsibilities for meeting continuing health care needs. http://www.dh.gov.uk/en/Publicationsandstatistics/Lettersandcirculars/Healthserviceguidelines/DH_4018189

1996 British Geriatrics Society. Standards of medical care for older people. Expectation and recommendation (revised 2003). Compendium document 1-3. http://www.bgs.org.uk/Publications/Compendium/compend_1-3.htm

1998 Clinical Standards Advisory Group. Community health care for older people. A committee report (Clark J, ed). Stationery Office, London

1999 With respect to old age. A report by the Royal Commission into Long Term Care. http://www.archive.official-documents.co.uk/document/cm41/4192/4192-00.htm

2000 The national plan: a plan for investment, a plan for reform. Department of Health, London. http://www.dh.gov.uk/en/Publicationsandstatistics/Publications/PublicationsPolicyAndGuidance/DH_4002960

2000 NSF: older people's services. http://www.dh.gov.uk/en/Publicationsandstatistics/Publications/PublicationsPolicyAndGuidance/DH_4003066

2002 Medical aspects of intermediate care. Royal College of Physicians. http://www.rcplondon.ac.uk/pubs/contents/cc4769b0-7ddl-46e2-85c6-87259cf8f48b.pdf

2002 Implementation of the NSF and intermediate care seen from geriatricians' and older people's perspective. Age Concern and the British Geriatrics Society. http://www.healthcarecommission.org.uk/_db/_documents/04001757.pdf

2003   Developing intermediate care to support reform
       of emergency care services Report of inter-
       mediate care working group. http://www.bgs.
       org.uk/Publications/Reference%20Material/
       ref4_intermediate_care_development.htm

2003   Interface between primary and secondary
       medical care in the new NHS in England: the
       care of frail older people by GPs and consultant
       geriatricians. http://www.bgs.org.uk/Publica
       tions/Compendium/compend_4-14.htm

2005   Supporting people with long-term conditions:
       An NHS and social care model to support local
       innovation and integration. Department of Health.
       http://www.dh/gov.uk/en/Publicationsand
       statistics/Publications/PublicationsPolicyAnd
       Guidance/DH_4100252

USEFUL WEBSITES

In addition to the usual medical websites, with which
you may be familiar, I would recommend the following:

http://www.kingsfund.org.uk
http://www.dh.gov.uk
http://www.statistics.gov.uk
http://www.performance.doh.gov.uk (includes lots of
social services statistics)

http://www.leeds.ac.uk/hsphr/hsc/research/eval_
intermediate.html (helpful website for national intermediate care project information)

SELF–ASSESSMENT QUESTIONS

Are the following statements true or false?

1. Consultants in elderly care with an interest in
   community geriatrics should:
   a. Have little recourse to hospital facilities
   b. May provide direct care for nursing home
      residents
   c. May provide clinical support to intermediate
      care services
   d. Have strong links with local general
      practitioners

2. Intermediate care:
   a. Has a robust evidence base of effectiveness
   b. Aims to provide a bridge between home and
      hospital
   c. Should be developed by geriatricians
   d. Is a new concept

Chapter **7**

Medical ethics and the law

Jim Eccles, Kevin Stewart, Marcus Chesterfield and Gurcharan S. Rai

LEGAL FRAMEWORKS FOR THE PROTECTION OF OLDER PEOPLE

'... the regimen I adopt shall be for the benefits of the patient according to my ability and judgement, and not for their hurt or for any wrong ...'

(Hippocrates 470–400 BC)

Both medical ethics and the law are concerned with the well-being of the individual – even though at times there may be conflict between what is regarded as the 'right thing to do' morally and what is regarded as 'right' in law. Despite the differences, both share one principle, i.e. respect for individuals' autonomous right to make decisions concerning themselves and to ensure there are safeguards for those who are not able to decide for themselves.

In clinical practice it is therefore important for doctors to understand principles of medical ethics and know how to apply them in clinical decision-making and have up-to-date knowledge of the law governing elderly subjects. There are five categories of legal procedures that offer protection to older people:

1. Procedures available for compulsory admission and treatment of patients with mental illness
2. Procedures available for use with patients who do not have a psychiatric illness but are considered to be at risk in their homes
3. Legislation governing provision of care and services for older people
4. Legal procedures for financial protection of older people
5. Anticipated developments in legal protection

LEGAL PROCEDURES AVAILABLE FOR COMPULSORY ADMISSION AND TREATMENT OF PATIENTS WITH A PSYCHIATRIC ILLNESS

Mental Health Act 1983

Introduction

The Mental Health Act can be used for patients with any formal mental illness, including delirium and dementia. It is unusual to use the Act for such patients, as treatment can be given under Common Law in the patient's best interests. Furthermore, treatment under the Act only applies to treatment of the mental illness itself and not to any coexisting physical illness. Having said this, it is possible to treat the physical illness which is the cause of a symptom of a mental illness. For example, under the Act it is possible to force-feed a patient with anorexia nervosa, but not to amputate a gangrenous leg because a person has schizophrenia.

Although doctors have the power to recommend compulsory admission under the Act, social workers or relatives have the main right to make a formal application.

Definitions included in the Act

- Mental disorder – mental illness, arrested or incomplete development of mind, psychopathic disorder and other disorder or disability of mind
- Mental impairment – impairment of intelligence and social functioning
- Severe mental impairment – a state of arrested or incomplete development of mind which includes severe impairment of intelligence and social functioning and is associated with abnormally aggressive or seriously irresponsible conduct on the part of the person concerned
- Psychopathic disorder – a persistent disorder or disability of mind which results in abnormally aggressive or seriously irresponsible conduct on the part of the person concerned
- Duties of approved social workers:
  - to gather information and coordinate the assessment process
  - to safeguard the civil liberties of the patient
  - to ensure that admission to hospital or guardianship is appropriate
  - to ensure that the necessary treatment recommended by the approved doctors is the least restrictive of all options

Provisions of the Act

Section 2   Under this section, a person can be formally admitted to hospital for assessment, observation and subsequent treatment.

- The application for this can be made by the patient's relative, a social worker or a person given power to act on the patient's behalf on recommendations of two registered medical practitioners
- The assessment period lasts for 28 days
- The grounds for application are: (i) the patient is suffering from a mental disorder of a nature and degree which warrants detention for assessment (or assessment followed by treatment) and, (ii) the detention is in the interests of the patient him or herself (health and safety) or for the protection of other people
- In case of urgent need, an application can be made on the recommendation of one practitioner

Section 3   This allows admission for compulsory treatment of mental disorder or illness for 6 months. The grounds for application include:

- The treatment is necessary for the health and safety of the patient and others
- The person has a mental illness, severe mental impairment, or psychopathic disorder, the nature of which makes it appropriate to receive treatment
- The treatment is likely to alleviate or prevent deterioration of the condition

The application procedure is similar to that for sectioning under section 2, except that under section 3 the nearest relative must be consulted when an applicant is a social worker.

Section 4   Under section 4 of the Mental Health Act 1983, a person can be admitted as an emergency by reason of 'urgent necessity' and, for this, only one medical recommendation is required.

- If they cannot cope with the patient's behaviour, social workers or relatives may ask for this
- There must be an immediate significant risk to the patient or others
- The doctor recommending emergency treatment should, if practicable, have known the patient before and have seen him or her in the previous 24 hours
- The period of detention is a maximum of 72 hours, but this can be converted to 28 days by seeking a second specialist opinion
- The patient has no right of appeal during the first 72 hours

Section 5   This section provides holding power for a doctor or a nurse for forcibly detaining informal patients for up to 6 hours. The consultant (or deputy) can enforce the detention for 72 hours. This applies to patients receiving in-patient treatment but not for patients being treated in the out-patient clinic or day hospital.

Under section 5(2), the medical practitioner responsible for treating a patient can make an application to detain the patient in hospital by writing a report to the hospital managers. If the medical practitioner in charge of clinical care of a patient is likely to be absent, they can nominate another in their absence.

Under section 5(4) (nurse's holding power), a nurse can detain patients who are receiving treatment for mental disorder as an in-patient in a hospital if the nurse feels that it is necessary to do so for their safety or for the safety of others and it is not practicable to get a doctor to attend to the patient for the purposes of preparing the report for application. The nurse can detain the patient in hospital for 6 hours.

Section 7 – Guardianship

This section allows the local authority (or a relative accepted by the local authority) to act as 'guardian' of a person with a mental disorder, mental illness or mental impairment and therefore provide community care. It may be used where there is conflict between the wishes of the relative and what is considered to be in the best interests of the patient. The guardian has the power to:

- Require an individual to live in a particular place
- Require access to be given to doctors, social workers and others at any place where the individual lives
- Attend a particular place for treatment

For this section to work effectively cooperation is required: the social worker does not have the authority to remove patients from their home if they refuse to do so and this can cause major difficulties for the appointed 'guardian'. To enforce this section, signatures of two registered practitioners (one of whom should be a specialist) are required.

The maximum duration is 6 months but it is renewable for a further 6 months, then year to year.

Section 117

This applies to people detained under section 3 and section 37 of the Mental Health Act 1983. Under this, the local authority as well as the health authority has a duty to carry out joint assessment and provide services.

The Mental Health Commission

The Mental Health Commission has responsibility for overseeing the treatment of compulsorily-detained patients and for dealing with complaints from detained people, as well as their carers.

Restraint of elderly patients

Freedom of movement is an important basic right enforceable through a writ of *habeas corpus* (Latin for 'you should have the body'). The clinical use of restraint raises moral and ethical dilemmas – particularly when individuals are confused and not competent to make a decision for themselves.

While it is usually morally unjustifiable to restrain an elderly patient, there may be a case for using restraint in the case of patients who, because of their mental condition, are at risk of harming themselves. Under these circumstances, the law may permit such an action as long as it is being performed in the best interests of the patient. (In mental health care, under section 5(4) of the Mental Health Act, a nurse may be allowed to use the minimum force necessary to prevent a patient from leaving the hospital.)

PROCEDURES FOR USE IN PATIENTS WHO DO NOT HAVE ACUTE PSYCHIATRIC ILLNESS BUT WHO ARE CONSIDERED TO BE AT RISK IN THEIR HOMES

National Assistance Act 1948 section 47

Under this section the local authority can seek an order from a magistrate to remove an individual who is considered to be at severe risk at home. For this section the person does not need to have a mental disorder or mental illness. Application can be made by a social worker, provided it is supported by a community physician. The grounds should include:

- A person who is suffering from a grave and chronic disease, or being aged, infirm or physically incapacitated, is living in unsanitary conditions
- Is unable to look after him or herself and is not receiving proper care and attention from others

An example is a person with a fracture who cannot look after himself. The living conditions are deteriorating, yet the patient refuses to go to hospital.

Relatives do not have any say in this and the patient has a limited right of appeal.

LEGISLATION GOVERNING PROVISION OF CARE AND SERVICES FOR OLDER PEOPLE

National Assistance Act 1948 section 21

Under this section, local authorities are empowered to provide accommodation for people over 18 years who are disabled or ill or are in need of care purely as a result of age. In 1993 this was converted from a power to a duty. It directed the local authorities to provide temporary accommodation for those who have no alternative accommodation; those who are in urgent need because they have a mental disorder; or to prevent mental disorder.

National Assistance Act 1948 section 29

Under this section, local authorities are empowered to provide a social work service and to make arrangements for promoting the welfare of disabled persons (i.e. those who are deaf, blind, dumb or suffer from a mental disorder of any description or are handicapped as a result of illness, injury or other disabilities).

Chronically Sick and Disabled Persons Act 1970 section 2

The services provided under this section include practical assistance in the home, home adaptations, transport for a person to use services, meals and telephones.

Health Services and Public Health Act 1968 section 45

This empowers the local authority to provide a wide range of services for elderly people in order to promote their welfare. These services may include meals, day centres, home helps, home adaptations and social work support.

The National Health Service and Community Care Act 1990

Section 47 of this Act placed the responsibility on the local authorities for planning, financing, delivery and regulation of community care services to vulnerable groups, including elderly people and those who are mentally ill.

The Carers (Recognition and Services) Act 1995

This Act enabled local authorities to assess the needs of carers and individuals in need of community care services. (It does not apply in Northern Ireland.)

The Social Work (Scotland) Act 1968

Under this Act, social work departments must provide guidance, advice and assistance to people in need of care because of age, infirmity or because they have a physical illness or mental disorder.

LEGISLATION PROVIDING FINANCIAL PROTECTION FOR ELDERLY PEOPLE

Power of Attorney

Elderly people may become unable to manage their financial affairs because of physical illness, mental illness, or both. Those who are physically disabled and have a reasonable grasp of their financial affairs can give authority to an individual (an attorney, who is usually a relative or close friend), to undertake financial transactions, such as going to the bank to get money or paying bills.

Enduring Power of Attorney

This is given by an individual who still has mental capacity and (unlike Power of Attorney) continues even when that individual becomes incapable of managing their financial affairs. It is commonly used by those in the early stages of dementia. The attorney (an individual with the Enduring Power of Attorney) has unfettered and unchecked access to the financial assets of the person who has made the power, and has the authority to sign cheques, withdraw money from savings accounts, buy or sell houses. It is also the attorney's responsibility to register this with the Court of Protection in England and Wales (or the High Court in Northern Ireland) when an individual loses mental capacity. Before registration, the attorney must inform the donor and certain relatives.

The Court of Protection

When people lose the capacity to manage their affairs, their spouses, friends or other relatives can apply to the Court of Protection. The application can also be made by a solicitor. A doctor has to complete a certificate confirming that the individual does not have the necessary capacity. The court will usually appoint someone as 'Receiver', whose duty is to act as the patient's agent (Receivers cannot just dispose of assets for their own benefit).

Assessment of testamentary capacity

People have capacity to make a will if they:

- Know the nature of action involved in making a will
- Have a reasonable grasp of the extent of their assets
- Know the person or people to whom they are leaving their property and money
- Are free of delusions, which might distort judgement

RECENT AND FUTURE DEVELOPMENTS IN LEGAL PROTECTION

Reform of the Mental Health Act

In 1999 the Government presented proposals for consultation to Parliament. These were expected to form the basis of a new Mental Health Act. Following a protracted national debate, which revealed considerable opposition to the proposals from professional and charitable organizations, the Government recently revised its plans for a new Mental Health Act. In place of the plans for a new Act, the Department of Health has now announced that an 'amending Bill' will be presented to Parliament, to amend the existing Mental Health Act. The amendments will include changes in six key areas:

- Supervised community treatment
- Definition of mental disorder
- Criteria for detention
- Mental Health Review Tribunal
- Professional roles and the responsibilities of the nearest relative
- When to use the provisions of the Mental Health Act, and when to apply the new Mental Capacity Act

Mental Capacity Act 2005

See the section below on mental capacity (competence).

The Human Rights Act 1998

This became law in the UK in 2000, and will make it unlawful for either public bodies or courts to act in a way that is incompatible with human rights (as defined by the European Convention of 1953). Of the rights included in the Act, the ones that are likely to apply to the practice of elderly medicine include:

- The right to life (article 2). This could affect the management of persistent vegetative state patients, or the management of patients requiring artificial feeding, refusal of treatment on grounds of cost, do-not-resuscitate orders, etc.
- The right not to be subjected to inhuman or degrading treatment (article 3). This could affect end-of-life care, do-not-resuscitate decision-making and the use of physical restraint
- The right to liberty and security. This may conflict with the amended Mental Health Act
- The right to respect for private and family life (article 8), which incorporates the right to protect the physical integrity of a person. This could have an impact on treatment given or provided against an individual's wishes
- The right to a fair trial. This may include disciplinary proceedings, such as those of the General Medical Council (GMC)

ETHICAL THEORY IN THE CARE OF OLDER PEOPLE

Some of the most difficult and complex decisions that a geriatrician has to make will not be about clinical issues, but about the ethical dilemmas that arise as a result of them. Deciding to withhold or withdraw treatment can be more challenging than simply continuing with full active management. This is a scenario that all doctors will encounter, although decision-making is often more complex and required more frequently with older people. Frail elderly patients are more likely to have multiple complex co-morbidities or be less able to participate in decision-making due to lack of mental capacity.

A clear understanding of simple legal and ethical principles can guide practice and provide a framework to help make complex decisions.

In this chapter we will first set out one basic ethical framework, and then discuss in more detail:

1. Mental capacity
2. Resuscitation decisions
3. Advance directives
4. Artificial feeding and fluids

In each case we will describe the current legal position, and try to summarize any guidelines that exist.

MEDICAL ETHICS

Medical ethicists continue to debate the most effective framework for ethical decision-making. One of the most widely used proposes four 'pillars' or principles to make decisions: autonomy, justice, beneficence, and non-maleficence.

Autonomy

A person's autonomy is defined by the extent to which that individual can control his or her life. In a clinical setting autonomy is the facilitation of a patient's own decision-making, and subsequently respect for that decision.

This respect for a patient's autonomy is enshrined within the GMC's 'duties of a doctor':

■ Respect a patient's dignity and privacy
■ Listen to patients and respect their views
■ Give information in a way patients can understand
■ Respect the rights of patients to be fully involved in decisions about their care
■ Make sure your personal beliefs do not prejudice your patients' care

Problems arise when patients are unable to understand or communicate their wishes or if they choose not to be involved in decision-making.

Justice

Justice ensures the equal provision of care/services to all who need it. This concept can be determined at various levels, most fundamentally in terms of individual practice to ensure no discrimination against individuals or groups, but equally at regional, national, or even international levels.

Beneficence and non-maleficence

The final two principles of biomedical ethics in essence state: 'do the best for the individual to promote health and welfare, and in turn do nothing that causes harm'. All therapies have beneficial and detrimental effects and even to fail to act can have both beneficial and detrimental effects, therefore clearly these concepts are also in conflict.

In the past it was acceptable, even expected, that a doctor would make a clinical decision by weighing the locally available options (limited by social justice), and make decisions based on personal values of the relative benefits and burdens to the patient (beneficence and non-maleficence), and then inform the patient of the decision. This approach is now seen as too paternalistic and personal autonomy has become the predominant consideration above justice, beneficence and non-maleficence. There will always be conflict between the four principles, and often in practice a degree of partial autonomy is all that is ever achieved.

MENTAL CAPACITY (COMPETENCE)

In English law, in order to consent to treatment, patients must be deemed to have mental capacity (or competence). The legal basis for determining mental capacity has evolved over many years on a case-by-case basis, and this has recently been clarified by the Mental Capacity Act 2005 (due for full implementation in 2007). The intention of the legislation is primarily to protect vulnerable people unable to make decisions for themselves, but also to prevent litigation against those who are acting in what they believe to be a patient's best interests. The Act sets out five key principles:

1. Every adult is presumed to have capacity unless proven otherwise
2. Individuals must be given all appropriate help to make a decision, before it is concluded that they are unable to make a decision
3. An individual's right to make an unwise or eccentric decision must be honoured
4. Anything done on behalf of a person without capacity must be in their best interests
5. Anything done on behalf of people without capacity should be the least restrictive of their basic rights and freedoms

A person is determined as lacking in capacity if they are unable to:

1. Understand the information relevant to a decision
2. Retain the information for sufficient time to be able to make a decision
3. Use or weigh-up the information, such that they can determine the consequences of different options, or indeed the consequence of not making a decision at all
4. Communicate that decision (by whatever means)

An assessment of capacity is for a given time, and relates only to a specific decision. A person may lack capacity as a result of a condition that is unlikely to improve (such as dementia) or through a temporary alteration in mental state (e.g. delirium). Capacity may also be affected by severe physical illness (e.g. if a patient is very dyspnoeic or in severe pain). Once somebody has been deemed to lack capacity, the person acting on their behalf must then decide what would be in their best interests and The Mental Capacity Act proposes a checklist for determining 'best interests':

■ The likelihood of the individual regaining capacity in the future should be assessed
  – If this is likely, then the chance of that person participating in the decision should be optimized

  – If this is unlikely, then their past and present wishes, and their beliefs and values should be taken into account. (This may have been made clear to next of kin or there may be a written statement made while they still possessed capacity.)
■ Those close to the individual should then be consulted and their view of the patient's best interest taken into account

If these conditions are complied with then one can be deemed to be acting in the patient's best interests.

A major change in English law is included in the legislation which, for the first time, allows for the appointment of a proxy decision-maker on behalf of incompetent patients (similar provisions have existed in Scotland for some years).

Those granted Lasting Power of Attorney (LPA) will not only have decision-making authority over financial matters (as in the current Enduring Power of Attorney) but also over health and welfare decisions, including decisions about life-sustaining treatments. This will be conferred while the individual retains capacity, granting decision-making authority to the attorney for a time in the future when capacity has been lost.

If no LPA was conferred before a person loses capacity (experience in other jurisdiction indicates that this often occurs), the Court of Protection will be able to appoint a deputy with the same powers as an LPA, except that they would not be able to give or refuse consent to life-sustaining treatments. Other health and welfare decisions would not be limited.

A new office of Independent Mental Capacity Advocates (IMCA) will be set up. Although their exact role remains to be determined, in essence they will be available to support a person who lacks capacity but has no one to speak for them. The IMCA would make representations about the person's wishes, feelings, beliefs and values and bring any relevant factors to the attention of the decision-maker or challenge them.

Most decisions about capacity do not require specialist psychiatric assessment and can be made by the treating doctor. In cases of doubt, or where consensus within the team and those close to the individual is not achieved, psychiatric advice should be sought.

CARDIOPULMONARY RESUSCITATION

There are times where attempts at cardiopulmonary resuscitation (CPR) are not appropriate but the decision-making process around this has been controversial. In recognition of this, guidelines for UK professionals have been produced by joint committees of the Royal College of Nursing, the British Medical Association and the Resuscitation Council. The General Medical Council has also produced guidance on withdrawing and withholding life-prolonging treatments with specific mention of CPR.

The recent guidelines have taken into account the provisions of the Human Rights Act and increasing public concern in the UK about medical decision-making in general and end-of-life issues in particular. Specific reference is made to the fact that relatives and those close to patients have often felt excluded by doctors from the decision-making process. Likewise, discussion of decisions with competent patients should be the norm as there is little evidence to support the previous practice of avoiding discussions for fear of causing unnecessary distress to patients.

The principles behind the resuscitation guidelines are:

1. Each decision must be specific to an individual
2. A presumption that, for people in whom no advance wishes have been made clear, CPR should be performed
3. For patients in whom there is a foreseeable risk of cardiac arrest, a decision should be made in advance if possible
4. Patients who retain capacity should be involved in decision-making if they wish, but information should not be forced on unwilling recipients
5. If a competent patient understands and refuses resuscitation attempts, this decision should be honoured
6. For incompetent patients, doctors are obliged to act in their best interests. This will usually involve discussions with those close to the patient to ascertain their previously expressed wishes or beliefs

The guidelines give some broad definitions of areas where it would be appropriate not to attempt CPR:

1. If the healthcare team is as certain as possible that CPR would not restart a patient's heart and breathing. Consensus within the team should be the aim
2. Where there is no benefit to be gained from restarting the heart or breathing, for example if only a brief extension of life would be achieved and that co-morbidity is such that death cannot be averted. Also that if the patient never regains the ability to interact, they would be unable to experience benefit
3. Where the expected burdens outweigh the benefits

There are some foreseeable practical difficulties with implementation of the guidelines. The circumstances of cardiac arrest may be difficult to predict for many patients so it could be difficult to accurately discuss the pros and cons of the treatment. Likewise, although most patients suffering cardiac arrest in hospital do not survive, it is extremely difficult to accurately predict chances of survival for individual patients.

When patients are clearly very close to death in the advanced stages of a terminal illness then decision-making is usually straightforward. In these circumstances most patients and relatives, and most healthcare professionals, would agree that CPR attempts are inappropriate. The healthcare team would usually be as certain as they could be that CPR would not succeed and, indeed, could hinder the provision of good palliative care. If families have difficulty agreeing with this, then discussion with professionals should aim to achieve an understanding of the reality of the clinical circumstances.

More often, geriatricians will face situations where it is likely, but not inevitable, that patients will face clinical deterioration and cardiopulmonary arrest in the near future. Frequently they will be able to predict that CPR attempts would have a very low, but recognizable, chance of success. Difficulties may then arise if competent patients, having been fully informed of the likely clinical situation, insist on having CPR attempts. The guidelines state that in these circumstances doctors should not make DNAR ('do not attempt resuscitation') orders, so decisions about advisability of beginning or continuing CPR attempts have to be made at the time of cardiac arrest. The guidelines do not explicitly address issues arising should relatives of incompetent patients make similar requests, although the implementation of the Mental Capacity Act may help clarify this.

Despite the practical difficulties, geriatricians need to be conscious of the need to act within the guidelines (unless there are compelling reasons for not doing so) and within the constraints of the law, including the Human Rights Act. Discussions with competent patients, and the relatives of incompetent ones, are usually best within a general discussion of the illness, its prognosis and the advisability of a range of treatments, including CPR. Doctors should try and give a realistic estimate of the possibility of survival and likely risks and benefits of CPR; it will often be sensible to convey the difficulties that exist in accurately predicting the chances of successful CPR. (Evidence suggests that patients and professionals overestimate the chances of CPR succeeding and that patient preference for CPR diminishes if they are aware of the true prognosis.)

The aim of discussion should be to achieve consensus between the healthcare team and the competent patient, or the relatives of incompetent ones. In the case of disputes, a second clinical opinion or perhaps the opinion of a clinical ethics team should be obtained. If there is still disagreement at this stage then medico-legal advice should be sought.

ADVANCE DIRECTIVES

A competent adult patient has the right to withhold consent to treatment. It is established in English case law that this principle can be extended to decisions made in advance, so that a competent adult can refuse to consent in advance to treatment which might be considered at some stage in the future when he might have become incompetent. After 2007 the principles established in case law will be governed by legislation as part of the Mental Capacity Act.

In order to be valid such advance directives (or perhaps more correctly, advance refusals) must meet certain criteria. It must be clear that the patient was competent at the time that the decision was made, was not acting under duress and was able to envisage in advance the clinical circumstances that subsequently arose. Patients do not have a right to make requests in advance for treatments that are not clinically indicated, nor are they permitted to request actions which might be illegal (e.g. euthanasia). Under the Mental Capacity Act, a directive will not be valid if the treatment is not specified, if the circumstances specified are absent, or if there are reasonable grounds to believe that circumstances exist which the person did not anticipate at the time the advance decision was made. An advance decision will not be applicable to life-sustaining treatments unless the statement specifically acknowledges this. The statement will have to be in writing, signed and witnessed. The directive can be invalidated if the patient has subsequently conferred authority to an LPA to give or refuse consent to treatment to which the advance decision relates.

If doctors are asked to witness an advance directive being drafted then they should satisfy themselves that the patient is competent, is not acting under duress and is able to understand likely future clinical circumstances (taking account of the possibility of medical advances). Careful documentation in the directive itself and of any discussions around it will help aid clear decision-making in the future.

If presented with an advance directive by the representative of a patient whom they are treating, doctors should satisfy themselves that the document is valid, that it was made when the patient was competent and that the circumstances that have arisen are as envisaged when it was drafted. They should, if possible, have a discussion with the person who witnessed the directive and the patient's family or next of kin and any other medical attendants (e.g. the GP). If the document appears to be valid then they should act in accordance with it.

If uncertainties exists about the validity of an advance directive then doctors are obliged to continue to actively treat patients while enquiries are made to resolve the uncertainties.

ARTIFICIAL NUTRITION AND HYDRATION (ANH)

The law regards enteral feeding (via nasogastric/percutaneous endoscopic gastrostomy tube), parenteral feeding and intravenous or subcutaneous fluid administration as medical treatments and therefore as artificial methods of delivering nutrition and hydration. There also is no legal distinction between withholding a treatment and withdrawing one which has already been initiated (although it is acknowledged that, in practice, many clinicians find it easier to withhold treatment than to withdraw it). The BMA and the GMC have both issued guidance to help with decisions about ANH and the judgements in the case of Burke v GMC (2005) have helped clarify the situation. It is clear from the outcome of this ruling that the BMA and GMC both support a patient's right to request, but not demand, in advance that they continue to receive ANH if they become incompetent. The BMA's handbook, *Medical Ethics Today* states:

> 'If the patient is known to have held the view that there is intrinsic value in being alive, then life-prolonging treatment would, in virtually all cases, provide a net benefit for that particular individual.'

The GMC acknowledges the difficulty of decision-making in this area, not least because the benefits and burdens may not be well known, some patients with progressive conditions may increasingly lose interest in food as a part of the disease process and personal beliefs differ widely.

The relative risks and burdens of the treatment should be determined as far as this is possible and then discussed with the individual if competent. If the patient is not competent the doctor has a duty to act in the patient's best interests, which will usually involve discussions with those close to the patient. An assessment of the patient should be made for the presence of distressing symptoms and these alleviated appropriately.

When the patient is clearly very close to death then it is accepted that it is usually not appropriate to begin ANH as any benefit is unlikely to be realized in such a short time. When it cannot necessarily be predicted that death is imminent it will usually be appropriate to provide ANH.

There may be some situations where the patient's condition is so severe or the prognosis so poor that burdens would outweigh benefits; in these circumstances, as well as consulting the other members of the team and those closest to the patient, a second opinion should be sought. Where a reasonable degree of uncertainty about the likely

benefits and burdens for an individual remains, then a trial period of ANH for further assessment would be appropriate. If significant conflict between those involved remains, which cannot be resolved after second opinions and independent review, it may be necessary to seek legal advice and approach the court for a ruling.

In the case of patients with permanent vegetative state or conditions closely resembling it, in order to withdraw ANH in England, Wales and Northern Ireland it is necessary to ask the courts for a ruling; in Scotland this is not specified but legal advice for each individual case may be helpful.

CASES

ALBERT, AGED 76

Albert is admitted to the coronary care unit (CCU) with an acute myocardial infarction. He was previously very active but has been tired for a while. He is given thrombolysis. His routine blood count result is telephoned to the CCU as it has shown a marked pancytopenia with some suspicious looking cells, possibly blasts. The haematologist thinks that this is an acute myeloid leukaemia and that his cardiac condition is being compromised by the anaemia. He advises urgent bone marrow biopsy to confirm the diagnosis, transfusion to correct anaemia and barrier nursing because of neutropenia.

The cardiologist and haematologist see Albert together that day and explain the situation in detail. The haematologist thinks that the prognosis could be as short as a few weeks without treatment but could be up to a year with chemotherapy. The cardiologist wants immediate transfusion to reduce the risk of further ischaemic damage.

Albert seems comfortable, clear thinking and not unduly distressed. He seems to understand the seriousness of his condition, the likely prognosis and what would happen if he did not have treatment. After a long discussion he states clearly that he does not want further investigation or treatment of the leukaemia, nor does he want transfusion or barrier nursing as he thinks his 'time has come'. He does, however, wish to remain 'for resuscitation' until such time as his daughter returns from holiday the following day.

Neither the cardiologist nor the CCU nurses are happy; they say that he should either decide that he wants palliative treatment or full active treatment but that he cannot pick and choose elements of this. They want him transferred off the CCU. The haematologist thinks that he must be incompetent because of his recent heart attack.

Comment

The patient appears to have been competent and fully informed about the options; he understood that refusal of treatment meant that he would die soon. He was presumably considered competent to consent to thrombolysis earlier that day. Staff should ensure that drugs which might hamper his decision-making capacity have not recently been administered.

He is entitled to make decisions with which the clinical team disagree and to choose which treatments he wants (CPR) and which he does not (all the rest). It would be worth ensuring that he understands that his refusal of other treatment may make it less likely that CPR will be effective. It is unreasonable to offer him a lower standard of cardiac care just because he has refused some of the other treatment.

It would be sensible for the treating team to ask his permission to share information with family members, close friends or spiritual advisors. All decisions should be carefully documented and reviewed at least daily and his understanding of the situation checked frequently. When he deteriorates to the extent that he is incompetent, then his previously expressed wishes should still be respected.

TOM, AGED 68

Tom is a retired merchant seaman and a heavy drinker. He is brought to A&E one lunchtime after collapsing in the pub. Staff are worried about his cough and bloodstained sputum and organize a chest X-ray. The radiographer thinks the appearances suggest tuberculosis (TB), and the medical registrar advises that sputum be sent urgently for ZN staining. Microbiology advise that acid fast bacilli have been detected in the sample and that, since he has 'open TB', he should be isolated and treatment with anti-tuberculous drugs started immediately.

By this time Tom is sober and determined to leave hospital. He seems to understand what he is being told and the health consequences of not having treatment, but he is adamant that he is not prepared to take the drugs. His neighbour, a retired social worker, has turned up and is accusing the hospital staff of infringing Tom's human rights.

Comment

There is a conflict here between the principles of beneficence (what is good for Tom's health) and his personal autonomy (what he wants to do). Usually, respect for autonomy outweighs concerns about beneficence. Tom appears to be competent and appears to understand what might happen to him if he does not have treatment.

However, an individual's right to exercise their autonomy is not absolute if, in doing so, they are likely seriously to endanger others. In this instance, if Tom is not treated then it is highly likely that he will remain infectious to others with whom he comes into contact, and he therefore represents a serious public health risk. In such circumstances it may be ethically legitimate to override his competently expressed autonomous decision and treat him against his will. Before doing so, however, staff would be well advised to ensure that they had received a second senior clinical opinion about the case, and had received specific advice from their organization's legal department. Any restriction of Tom's rights should be at the minimum level which is necessary to ensure the safe treatment of his condition. In practice, the long-term success of Tom's treatment would require his cooperation, so it would be in both his and the public interest to work towards this from the outset.

ALICE, AGED 82

Alice has advanced cancer with cerebral metastases. Chemotherapy has now been stopped and she is on high dose dexamethasone, although even this has been failing to control her symptoms. She and her family (several of whom are doctors) are aware that she is in the terminal stage of her illness.

She is admitted with increasing drowsiness and probable bronchopneumonia. She is too ill to participate in discussions but her family approach the oncology team and tell the team that she would have wanted IV antibiotics and to have CPR attempts should they be required. On further discussion it becomes clear that Alice has decided that she wanted all the family to be present when she died; one daughter is a paediatrician in Sydney and it would take several days for her to reach the UK, hence the request for her to be kept alive until this time. The consultant agrees to their request, although the nurses and the junior staff strongly disagree with him.

Comment

The family seem to be articulating the decisions which Alice had reached when she was competent and this appears to be a request for treatment which many would consider 'futile'. Sometimes such requests are made by those who have not come to terms with the inevitability of death, although this appears not to have been the case here. Most individuals would not consider prolongation of life for a few days in an unconscious or semiconscious state to be of any benefit but, in this patient's opinion, there was value attached to being kept alive until her daughter was able to see her.

The CPR guidelines state that although doctors are not obliged to offer treatment which is of no benefit they must consider 'benefit' in the patient's terms, not their own. If it is technically possible to prolong life by CPR attempts (it probably would be) and the patient regards this prolongation as useful (she obviously did) then they should be prepared to carry it out.

A patient's right to autonomous decision-making, although important, is not absolute. Under the principle of distributive justice a patient's request for treatment with minimal benefit must be considered in the light of resource implications for others. If treating Alice meant that others would be denied access to scarce resources, then it would be unlikely to be justified.

In this case it seems reasonable to accept her request for antibiotics and for initiation of CPR attempts in the event of cardiorespiratory arrest; the resources used would be unlikely to seriously disadvantage others. However, it would almost certainly not be justified to admit her to the intensive care unit post-arrest or to engage in prolonged or repeated CPR attempts because the resources then used could arguably give much greater benefit to many other patients.

MARY, AGED 86

Mary suffers a severe stroke and CT shows a left total anterior circulation infarct. After 2 weeks she still has a dense right hemiparesis and profound expressive and receptive dysphasia. Her swallow is very weak. Both the speech and language therapist and the consultant feel that she has very limited understanding of her situation but she is awake and appears comfortable. The nurses are concerned by her poor nutritional intake and are pressing the consultant to institute tube feeding ('you can't just let her starve to death').

She has no family but is visited twice daily by friends from her religious community. The consultant meets them to discuss her future care. He tells them that her chances of any sort of independent recovery are very low and that if she survives she will almost certainly require full nursing care. They explain that she has been a very active member of their church for many years and that her beliefs were that life should be sustained at all costs even if quality seemed poor. She would want all possible measures to keep her alive. They have been told about percutaneous endoscopic gastrostomy feeding by the nursing staff and insist that it is started as soon as possible.

Comment

The patient is almost certainly incompetent, but her friends seem to be articulating a previously strongly held view. BMA advice is that in these circumstances, if the patient is known to have attached an intrinsic value to being alive, then life-prolonging treatment (including tube feeding) should usually be given.

Possible exceptions to this general rule might arise if such treatment was itself associated with a very high risk to the patient (e.g. a feeding tube which required a general anaesthetic for insertion) or would be likely to have a high resource requirement to the detriment of others (prolonged ITU treatment).

REFERENCE

Burke v General Medical Council (GMC) 2005 (Official Solicitors and Ors intervening) EWCA Civ 1003, Case No: C1/2204/2086

RECOMMENDED READING

*** *Essential reading;* ** *recommended reading;* * *interesting but not vital*

British Medical Association 2000 The impact of the Human Rights Act 1998 on medical decision making. British Medical Association, London **

British Medical Association 2002 Decisions relating to cardiopulmonary resuscitation. A joint statement from the British Medical Association, the Resuscitation Council and the Royal College of Nursing. British Medical Association, London **

British Medical Association 2004 Medical ethics today, 2nd edn. British Medical Association, London ***

Coni N 1999 Achieving a good death. In: Rai G S (ed.) Medical ethics and the elderly. Harwood, Amsterdam ***

Department for Constitutional Affairs 2006 Mental Capacity Act. Online. Available: http://www.dca.gov.uk ***

Department of Health 1983 Mental health bill: plans to amend the Mental Health Act. Online. Available: http://www.dh.gov.uk **

Department of Health 1999 Revised Code of Practice (Mental Health Act 1983). Stationery Office, London *

General Medical Council 1995 The duties of a doctor. General Medical Council, London ***

General Medical Council 2001 Good medical practice. General Medical Council, London ***

General Medical Council 2002 Withholding and withdrawing life-sustaining treatments: good practice in decision-making. General Medical Council, London ***

Gillon R 1986 Philosophical medical ethics. Wiley, Chichester **

Grimley Evans J 1997 Rationing healthcare by age. The case against. British Medical Journal 314:822 ***

Harris J 1985 The value of life. Routledge, London **

Harris J 1988 More and better justice. In: Bell J M, Mendus S (eds) Philosophy and medical welfare. Cambridge University Press, Cambridge *

National Health Service 1990 A guide to consent for examination or treatment. NHS Management Executive, London ***

Rivlin M 1999 Should age based rationing of health care be illegal? British Medical Journal 319:1379 ***

UK Clinical Ethics Network. Online. Available: http://www.ethics-network.org.uk ***

SELF-ASSESSMENT QUESTIONS

Are the following statements true or false?

1. An 85-year-old man with delirium is refusing to allow his general practitioner to come into his house to examine him. The social worker decides to use the Mental Health Act 1983. Which section would be most appropriate for him to apply for?
   a. Section 2
   b. Section 3
   c. Section 4
   d. Section 5
   e. Section 7

2. When applying for the National Assistance Act 1948 section 47, the patient:
   a. Must have a mental impairment
   b. Should have reversible mental illness
   c. Should be physically incapacitated
   d. Requires financial protection

Chapter 8

Prevention and health promotion

Christopher Patterson and John W. Feightner

This chapter has three goals:

1. To present the *rationale* for preventive healthcare
2. To outline recommendations for *specific manoeuvres (actions)* based upon evidence (manoeuvres which are recommended by the UK Department of Health are indicated with an asterisk*)
3. To discuss challenges to *implementation*

THE RATIONALE FOR PREVENTION IN LATER LIFE

DEFINITIONS

Health promotion is a process of enabling people to increase control over, and to improve, their health (WHO 1986). *Screening* is a population approach, which aims to reach all individuals at risk for a specific condition. *Case finding* identifies individuals at risk for, or having, asymptomatic disease during specific or opportunistic encounters.

Issues to address when considering preventive health in older people include:

- Life expectancy: (Table 8.1) it is unrealistic to offer a manoeuvre whose benefit will not be realized within an individual's life expectancy
- Co-morbidities: may shorten expected lifespan or affect quality of life (e.g. decreased mobility or poor cognitive function)
- Patients' beliefs and values: some may choose to decline certain recommendations, even if well informed

Table 8.1 Life expectancy at different ages, United Kingdom 2001		
Age (years)	Women	Men
65–69	18.6	15.4
70–74	14.8	12.0
75–79	11.5	9.2
80–84	8.6	6.9
85–89	6.3	5.1
90–94	4.4	3.6
95–99	3.0	2.6

Source: World Health Organization life tables

Prevention may be conceptualized as: delay or prevention of premature death from preventable diseases; improvements in quality of life by reducing disabling diseases; reduction of hazardous lifestyles; and improving self-perceived health (Patterson & Feightner 1997). While much preventive healthcare is rightfully in the primary care domain (family physicians/general practitioners and health visitors or practice nurses), specialist geriatricians need to have an understanding of preventive healthcare for a number of reasons which are outlined in Box 8.1.

The history of prevention is long. One of the best-known examples of an early controlled trial of prevention is that of James Lind, the captain of HMS Salisbury, who proved in 1747 that the consumption of lime juice prevented scurvy on lengthy sea voyages. Modern preventive health-

Box 8.1   Prevention: roles of the specialist geriatrician

- Initiator of preventive health manoeuvres
- Educator of other physicians, students, healthcare workers
- Source of information for patients, relatives, senior citizens, groups
- Resource for healthcare planners
- Advocate for better living conditions for older people
- Role model for healthy behaviours

care has its origins in the annual physical examination, a reaction to physicians expressing the sentiment 'Why didn't you come sooner?' The North American insurance industry seized upon the concept of the annual physical examination, which was widely adopted in practice by general practitioners/family doctors, especially in North America. It culminated in the 'executive' physical examination, an untargeted (and ineffective) array of multiple diagnostic tests. In response to this phenomenon, a more rational approach to preventive healthcare developed. Beginning in the 1970s, organizations such as the Canadian Task Force on Preventive Health Care, the United States Preventive Services Task Force, and initiatives in the United Kingdom National Health Service, led to the development of a rational framework for the assessment of preventive healthcare manoeuvres, based upon best available evidence. The central concept of this approach is the *targeting* of a manoeuvre (action) towards a *specific* condition.

Evaluating *primary prevention* (which prevents disease before it occurs, by lifestyle counselling or inoculations) involves scrutiny of the following for each condition:

- Burden of illness (e.g. is the condition common, serious, disabling?)
- Cause of the condition (is the cause known, or are there only risk factors?)
- Efficacy of the manoeuvre (proportion prevented?)
- Adverse effects and costs of the manoeuvre

Secondary prevention has two definitions: (a) early detection of pre-clinical disease by screening

or case finding, and (b) prevention of recurrent disease (e.g. stroke, myocardial infarction) by lifestyle modification or medications. This chapter will concentrate on screening. Before a screening manoeuvre is adopted, it is necessary to determine whether it produces more good than harm by examining the following factors:

- Burden of illness
- Natural history of the condition (is there a preclinical phase?)
- Whether treatment in the asymptomatic stage changes the natural history
- Availability of an appropriate screening test with acceptable characteristics (high sensitivity and relatively high specificity)
- Potential adverse affects of screening (e.g. labelling, potential side-effects of the investigative cascade)
- Potential side-effects of treatment
- Patient acceptability
- Feasibility
- Resource requirements (i.e. policy implications)

Prevention is not cheap. Cost-effectiveness estimates are complex, and may vary widely depending upon the assumptions made (Saha et al 2001). They usually contradict the notion that 'an ounce of prevention is worth a pound of cure' (De Bracton 1240) as screening costs must be added to those of investigation and managing the newly discovered condition. In a single payer system, when total expenditures are fixed, the introduction of a new procedure may need to be funded by reduced costs elsewhere, which may require the deletion of other services. Some cost-effectiveness estimates are shown in Table 8.2.

Before any preventive health manoeuvre is adopted, evidence must affirm that more good than harm will be done. Only when all the evidence has been gathered, appraised and synthesized can a rational recommendation be formulated. There is an ethical duty for physicians and healthcare planners to hold such manoeuvres to the same rigorous standards of efficacy that we employ for therapeutic actions. This being said, it is not always possible to obtain evidence from randomized controlled trials (RCTs) of the *entire* screening/diagnosis/intervention/effect on burden of illness/cycle, and alternative approaches

Table 8.2   Examples of cost–effectiveness of preventive health manoeuvres: cost of 1 additional year of life gained

Reference	Target condition	Manoeuvre	Lower limit of cost	Upper limit of cost	Currency
Messionier 1999	Tobacco-related illnesses	Counselling against tobacco	705 1204	988 (men) 2058 (women)	$US (1984)
Messionier 1999	Pneumococcal pneumonia	Inoculation	−141	6154	$US (1986) $US (1983)
Wanhainen et al 2005	Abdominal aortic aneurysm	Single ultrasound in 65-year-old men	8309	14 084	$US (2004)
Pignone et al 2002b	Colorectal cancer	Fecal occult blood tests plus endoscopy for ages 50 and above	10 000	25 000	$US (2002)
Mandelblatt et al 2003	Breast cancer	Mammography for ages 65–75 or 80	34 000	88 000	$US (2002)

must be employed. The causal pathway or analytical framework deconstructs the cycle into its constituent parts, and gathers evidence for each step (Harris et al 2001). The strength of recommendation should be related to the quality and magnitude of the evidence, and most organizations define a hierarchy of evidence, with systematic reviews of RCTs as the highest, and expert opinion being the lowest levels of evidence. In many situations a letter or numerical grade is used to signify the strength of recommendation (e.g. the Canadian Task Force on Preventive Health Care [2003] classifies good or fair evidence to include a manoeuvre in the periodic health examination as A or B recommendations, D or E when there is fair or good evidence to exclude it, and I or C where the evidence is insufficient or ambiguous).

One caution is worthy of mention here: screening inevitably uncovers cases of disease which may never have affected the quality or quantity of life of the individual. Unless a study is designed to rule out lead-time bias, and examine health outcomes (e.g. stroke, loss of independence, admission to a nursing home, death), there is a danger of simply making an earlier diagnosis, which appears to prolong life, but in reality has no effect on the illness. As diagnostic procedures become more sensitive, one must be alert to this phenomenon, as simply detecting a disease earlier does not guarantee benefit.

THE MANOEUVRES

PRIMARY PREVENTION

Box 8.2 lists counselling procedures for which the evidence is good or fair. Counselling about safe driving involves a discussion of avoiding alcohol and wearing seatbelts. The health risks of tobacco are well known. Simple advice and short-term counselling are modestly effective, but combined with nicotine replacement therapy are considerably more effective, as long-term cessation rates approach 30%.

Unhealthy diets are associated with overweight, obesity, vascular diseases and certain malignancies. Advice concerning prudent diet involves avoiding excessive caloric intake and limiting fat to less than 30% of total energy; daily consumption of between five and ten portions of fruit or

---

Box 8.2   Primary prevention: examples of effective counselling manoeuvres

- Safe driving (use seatbelts, don't use alcohol)
- Tobacco cessation*
- Prudent diet*
- Regular aerobic exercise*
- Household injuries (scatter rugs, electrical extension cords, water temperature not to exceed 120° F, smoke alarms)

vegetables; dietary fibre to exceed 20 g if possible; sufficient amounts of calcium (1500 mg elemental equivalent for a post-menopausal woman) and adequate vitamin D – 5 µg or 800 units each day.

Regular exercise is associated with improved aerobic fitness, improved well-being and lower mortality. Promotion of regular exercise is more likely to be successful if the exercise is of moderate intensity, home based, unsupervised but with frequent professional contact (Hillsdon & Thorogood 1996). Walking is the preferred activity.

Counselling about alcohol consumption is a potential dilemma (Marmot & Brunner 1991). Consuming small amounts of alcohol reduces cardiovascular risk, and possibly dementia risk. Larger doses increase the risk of domestic and motor vehicle accidents in the short term, and the long-term risks of alcohol are well known.

Simple advice about injury prevention involves regulation of domestic water temperature, maximum 120° F, using smoke detectors and avoiding environmental hazards (e.g. scatter rugs and electrical extension cords).

Effective inoculations are listed in Box 8.3.

SECONDARY PREVENTION (Table 8.3)

Screening for cardiovascular conditions

Blood pressure should be checked at every visit. The risks of both systolic and diastolic hypertension are well recognized, with population studies firmly indicating an exponential relationship between systolic blood pressure and cardiovascular outcomes such as a stroke and myocardial infarction. There is also very clear evidence that treatment of hypertension in older individuals reduces the risk of congestive heart failure and probably dementia (Forette et al 1998). Importantly, as the cardiovascular outcome event rate increases with age, the numbers needed to treat to avoid one outcome is less in older than younger people, and the idea that older people 'tolerate' hypertension must be dismissed once and for all. A target level of 140/85 should be attempted, but is not always possible.

Atrial fibrillation, the most common arrhythmia in older people, carries a significant risk of cerebral and peripheral embolization, approximately 5% per year, and 10–12% with additional risk factors (Atrial Fibrillation Investigators 1994). There is good evidence that in younger (less than 75 years) patients without evidence of additional

Table 8.3 Secondary prevention: effective screening manoeuvres	
Conditions to be prevented	Manoeuvre
Stroke, myocardial infarction	Screening for hypertension*
Stroke, peripheral embolism	Detection of atrial fibrillation
Ruptured abdominal aortic aneurysm	Abdominal ultrasound
Breast cancer	Physical examination by physician, mammogram*
Carcinoma of cervix	Papanicolau smear*
Colorectal carcinoma	Faecal occult blood testing* or colonoscopy
Fractures	Bone mineral density
Depression	Single item or short questionnaire
Increasing disability, premature institutionalization	Screening for frailty
Falls	Simple gait assessment, other assessments and referrals as required*
Hearing loss	Whisper test or audioscope
Visual loss	Snellen type sight card

*manoeuvres recommended by UK Department of Health

risk factors (diabetes, cardiac failure, hypertension, previous transient ischaemic attack [TIA] or stroke) acetyl salicyclic acid (ASA) is an adequate prophylaxis against stroke, and for older patients and those with additional risk factors, long-term anticoagulation is highly effective for preventing strokes (Gage et al 2004). Thus, a reasonable case can be made for screening older people for atrial fibrillation. The prevalence of abdominal aortic aneurysm rises sharply with age, reaching 7% in male smokers between 65 and 75 years (see Ch. 26). The growth period is long, and rupture is almost always fatal without immediate surgery. Screening with abdominal ultrasound is justifiable in this target group (US Preventive Services Task Force 2005).

Screening for malignant diseases

Breast cancer remains a serious cause of morbidity and mortality in older women. Annual clinical breast examination and mammography every second year until the age of 69 years are accepted procedures. Routine *teaching* of breast self-examination does not reduce morbidity or mortality from cancer (Baxter 2001). The majority of invasive carcinomas of the cervix appear in older women, thus Papanicolau screening is recommended until the age of 65 or 70 years in women who have ever been sexually active. Carcinoma of the colon is increasingly prevalent with age in older men and women. Screening with faecal occult blood or endoscopy is now recommended (Pignone et al 2002a) although the recommended frequency and exact procedures differ among various authorities.

Screening of special senses

Simple vision screening tests (e.g. Snellen type sight card) should be incorporated into the periodic examination. Similarly, screening for hearing impairment using the whisper test or an audioscope is recommended.

Screening for frailty

Geriatricians are extremely familiar with the clinical condition of frailty. Although hard to define, it is generally accepted as a syndrome which leads to increasing disability, admission to long-term

care and death (Hogan et al 2003). A variety of manoeuvres, usually involving some version of comprehensive geriatric assessment, can prevent or delay these outcomes in frail individuals (Elkan et al 2001, Ploeg et al 2005, Stuck et al 2002). There is fair evidence to include screening for frailty in the periodic health examination of older people. A checklist of items for use in community settings can identify individuals at increased risk, signalling the need for complete assessment and appropriate interventions (Pathy et al 1992).

Screening for depression

Depression is common among senior citizens, frequently accompanies chronic diseases and is readily detectable using simple instruments. Screening is recommended where there are facilities for close follow-up and treatment (MacMillan et al 2005).

Prevention of falls and fractures (see Ch. 14)

In addition to counselling about household injuries, the association of sedative medications with falls (Tinetti et al 1988) and motor vehicle collisions (Hemmelgarn et al 1997) in older people supports a recommendation to review prescription medications at least annually, and at least 6 monthly when sedatives have been prescribed (DoH 2001).* Gait assessment with a simple tool such as the 'timed up and go test' with more detailed assessment and referral to community agencies as indicated is recommended for all older people (American Geriatrics Society et al 2001). Given effective treatments for osteoporosis, evidence supports screening for bone mineral density in all women at menopause or, in the event that this has not occurred, at the age of 65 years (Chung et al 2004). Such strategies may reduce the significant morbidity and mortality resulting from fractures in older people (see Ch. 36 on osteoporosis).

Prevention of recurrent illness

The other type of secondary prevention is to reduce the likelihood of downstream recurrence or complications in a wide variety of chronic diseases. These issues are dealt with under the *management* of each disease in Part 3.

CONTROVERSIAL MANOEUVRES

The relationship between elevated serum cholesterol levels and cardiovascular disease appears to weaken with age, and screening for lipid disorders may be reasonably restricted to those with established coronary artery disease, cerebrovascular disease and those with a high risk (e.g. more than 30% in 10 years) of developing these conditions, e.g. hypertensives, smokers, diabetics (Patterson & Grymonpre 2004). There is insufficient evidence at present to recommend screening in primary care for dementia (US Preventive Services Task Force 2003) or elder abuse (Patterson 1994) although physicians should remain alert for signs and symptoms of these conditions. Screening for diabetes is recommended only in the presence of additional risk factors for cardiovascular disease (Harris et al 2003). Although carcinoma of the prostate is extremely common in older men, there is as yet no clear evidence that screening with digital rectal examination or prostate-specific antigen (PSA) leads to improved life expectancy or quality of life (Harris & Lohr 2002). Several ongoing large randomized controlled trials will determine whether this procedure should be incorporated into the periodic health examination.

CHALLENGES TO IMPLEMENTATION

Numerous studies have indicated that the performance of efficacious preventive health manoeuvres falls far below the ideal level of implementation. Reasons include physician factors, patient factors and contextural factors. The National Service Framework for Older People (DoH 2001) proposed targeting three priority areas; smoking cessation, influenza inoculation and blood pressure (BP) control. While each has met with some success, reasons for poor adherence are many.

PHYSICIAN FACTORS

Most preventive health recommendations are made in the form of clinical practice guidelines (CPGs). While designed to help the physician and patient by translating evidence (often huge volumes of evidence) into practical advice, they are not always accepted. Physicians are a difficult group to influence, and behaviour change is needed to improve adherence. Physicians are often suspicious of guidelines introduced by governments (or insurance agencies) but are more likely to follow them (Hayward et al 1997) if they agree with them, and the guidelines are:

- Endorsed by respected colleagues (local opinion leaders)
- Endorsed by major professional organizations
- User friendly

Some of these reasons may be responsible for only an estimated 10% of older hypertensives achieving adequate BP control (to 140/85 or below) in 2002 (Philp 2004). Standard continuing medical education programmes do little to change physician behaviour. Research has shown that, to be effective, continuing medical education requires three components (Mazmanian & Davis 2002):

- Educational needs must be defined by learners, not presenters
- Interaction is necessary (e.g. case discussions, role play, hands-on, audit and feedback, academic detailing)
- Sequenced, multifaceted interventions (e.g. work-learn-work, opinion leaders, follow-up)

Addressing these aspects of continuing education is likely to result in greater implementation of CPGs.

PATIENT FACTORS

Many factors influence patient behaviour. (Note: it is now fashionable to refer to patients as care recipients or consumers of healthcare!) The personality, in terms of risk tolerance or avoidance, beliefs, gender (women are generally more accepting of recommendations than men) and culture, all play a part. Fear of consequences or discomfort, inconvenience, costs and forgetting are other possible reasons.

Over the age of 60 years, smoking cessation programmes in the UK claimed a 67% success rate at 1 month, significantly higher than for younger age groups (Philp 2004). This may suggest that older people are more open to change than they are often assumed to be. Strategies that have been shown to improve patient acceptance of manoeuvres include:

- Individual planning and counseling (Fox et al 1997)
- Telephone follow-up (this is surprisingly more effective when office staff rather than physicians do the calling!) (Mohler 1995)
- Regular group visits (groups of patients with chronic diseases gathering monthly) (Beck et al 1997)

In contrast, reminder letters are probably not effective. In one study, 50% of patients had no recollection of the letter, 25% recalled the letter but not the contents, and only 25% remembered the letter and contents (Ornstein et al 1993).

CONTEXTUAL FACTORS

The physical environment (e.g. how often you bump into colleagues in the corridors) and social environment (do colleagues from different disciplines dine together?) have a definite influence on the diffusion of knowledge and technology (Berwick 2003). The most influential contextual factor may be the management environment. If a practice manager and colleagues embrace a new procedure it is far more likely to succeed than if the manager is not open to change. In the UK, coverage for influenza inoculation for people over aged 60 years reached 71% (the planned target) in 2003/2004 (Philp 2004). Practice outreach activities are effective for increasing these rates (Jacobson & Szilagyi 2005) and should be considered if higher rates are to be achieved. Another contextual factor is the role of legislation. Seatbelt use rises significantly in societies *only* when it is mandated by law. Contextual factors are also important in changing lifestyles: while it is gratifying to see smoking banned in restaurants and enclosed public spaces, blatant cigarette advertising removed from the media, and far less smoking seen in film and television (remember Humphrey Bogart in Casablanca – everyone smoked!), governments still pay subsidies to tobacco growers, and collect vast revenues from tobacco sales. It is hard to see a time in the near future when this most preventable of noxious substances will disappear from our daily lives.

CONCLUSION

Older age is not incompatible with prevention! There are many important preventive actions of proven benefit that we can offer our older patients. Many of these preventive actions are relatively easy to provide and most carry little downstream risk. As physicians, we must know which actions will confer benefit, and commit to strategies to ensure that they are implemented. Equally, by knowing which actions are not of benefit we can avoid wasting time and other precious resources on ineffective care.

REFERENCES

American Geriatrics Society, British Geriatrics Society, American Academy of Orthopedic Surgeons 2001 Guidelines for the prevention of falls in older persons. Journal of the American Geriatrics Society 49:664–672

Atrial Fibrillation Investigators 1994 Risk factors for stroke and efficacy of antithrombotic therapy in atrial fibrillation: analysis of pooled data from five randomized controlled trials. Archives of Internal Medicine 154:1449–1457

Baxter N, with the Canadian Task Force on Preventive Health Care 2001 Preventive health care, 2001 update: Should women be routinely taught breast self-examination to screen for breast cancer? Canadian Medical Association Journal 164:1837–1846

Beck A, Scott J, Williams P et al 1997 A randomized trial of group outpatient visits for chronically ill older HMO members: the Cooperative Health Care Clinic. Journal of the American Geriatrics Society 45:543–549

Berwick D M 2003 Disseminating innovations in health care. Journal of the American Medical Association 289:1969–1975.

Canadian Task Force on Preventive Health Care 2003 New grades for recommendations from the Canadian Task Force on Preventive Health Care. Canadian Medical Association Journal 169:207–208

Chung A M, Feig D S, Kapral M et al 2004 Prevention of osteoporosis and osteoporotic fractures in postmenopausal women: recommendation statement from the Canadian Task Force on Preventive Health Care. Canadian Medical Association Journal 170:1665–1667

De Bracton H 1240 De legibus. (out of print)

Department of Health 2001 National Service Framework for Older People. DoH, London

Elkan R, Kendrick D, Dewey M et al 2001 Effectiveness of home based support for older people: systematic review and meta-analysis. British Medical Journal 323:719–725

Forette F, Seux M L, Staessen J A et al 1998 Prevention of dementia in randomized double-blind placebo-controlled systolic hypertension in Europe (Syst-Eur) trial. Lancet 352:1347–1351

Fox P J, Breuer W, Wright J A 1997 Effects of a health promotion program on sustaining health behaviors in older adults. American Journal of Preventive Medicine 13:257–264

Gage B F, van Walraven C, Pearce L et al 2004 Selecting patients with atrial fibrillation for anticoagulation: stroke risk stratification in patients taking aspirin. Circulation 110:2287–2292

Harris R, Lohr K N 2002 Screening for prostate cancer: an update of the evidence for the US Preventive Services Task Force. Annals of Internal Medicine 137:917–929

Harris R P, Helfand M, Woolf S H et al 2001 Current methods of the US Preventive Services Task Force: a review of the process. American Journal of Preventive Medicine 20(3S):21–35

Harris R, Donahue K, Rathore S S et al 2003 Screening adults for type 2 diabetes: a review of the evidence for the US Preventive Services Task Force. Annals of Internal Medicine 138:215–229

Hayward R S A, Guyatt G H, Moore K-A et al 1997 Canadian physicians' attitudes about and preferences regarding clinical practice guidelines. Canadian Medical Association Journal 156:1715–1723

Hemmelgarn B, Suissa S, Huang A et al 1997 Benzodiazepine use and the risk of motor vehicle crash in the elderly. Journal of the American Medical Association 278:27–31

Hillsdon M, Thorogood M 1996 A systematic review of exercise promotion strategies. British Journal of Sports Medicine 30:84–89

Hogan D B, MacKnight C, Bergman H et al 2003 Models, definitions and criteria of frailty. Aging Clinical and Experimental Research 15(Suppl to No. 3):3–29

Jacobson V, Szilagyi P 2005 Patient reminder and patient recall systems for improving immunization rates. Cochrane Database of Systematic Reviews 4. Art. No.: CD003941. DOI: 10.1002/14651858.CD003941

MacMillan H L, Patterson C, Wathen C N et al 2005 Screening for depression in primary care: recommendation statement from the Canadian Task Force on Preventive Health Care. Canadian Medical Association Journal 172:33–35

Mandelblatt J, Saha S, Teutsch S et al 2003 The cost-effectiveness of screening mammography beyond age 65 years: a systematic review for the US Pre-ventive Services Task Force. Annals of Internal Medicine 139:835–842

Marmot M, Brunner E 1991 Alcohol and cardiovascular disease: the status of the U shaped curve. British Medical Journal 303:565–568

Mazmanian P E, Davis D A 2002 Continuing medical education and the physician as a learner: guide to the evidence. Journal of the American Medical Association 288:1057–1060

Messionier M L, Corso P S, Teutsch S M et al 1999 An ounce of prevention ...what are the returns? 2nd edn. American Journal of Preventive Medicine 16:248–263

Mohler P J 1995 Enhancing compliance with screening mammography recommendations: a clinical trial in a primary care office. Family Medicine 27:117–121

Ornstein S M, Musham C, Reid A et al 1993 Barriers to adherence to preventive services reminder letters: the patient's perspective. The Journal of Family Practice 36:195–200

Pathy M S, Bayer A, Harding K et al 1992 Randomized trial of case finding and surveillance of elderly people at home. Lancet 340:890–893

Patterson C 1994 Secondary prevention of elder abuse. In: Goldbloom R (ed.) The Canadian guide to clinical preventive health care. Canada Communications Group, Ottawa, p 922–929

Patterson C, Feightner J W 1997 Promoting the health of senior citizens. Canadian Medical Association Journal 157:1107–1113

Patterson C, Grymonpre R 2004 Primary prevention of cardiovascular events in older individuals. In: Turpie I, Heckman G (eds) Aging issues for cardiologists. Kluwer Academic, Norwell, MA

Philp I 2004 Better health in old age. Department of Health, Gateway reference 4018, London

Pignone M P, Rich S, Teutsch S M et al 2002a Screening for colorectal cancer in adults at average risk: a summary of the evidence for the US Preventive Services Task Force. Annals of Internal Medicine 137:132–141

Pignone M, Saha S, Hoerger T et al 2002b Cost-effectiveness of colorectal cancer screening: a systematic review for the US Preventive Services Task Force. Annals of Internal Medicine 137:96–104

Ploeg J, Feightner J, Hutchison B et al 2005 Effectiveness of preventive primary care outreach interventions aimed at older people: meta-analysis of randomized controlled trials. Canadian Family Physician 51:1244–1245

Saha S, Hoerger T J, Pignone M P et al 2001 The art and science of incorporating cost effectiveness into evidence-based recommendations for clinical preventive services. American Journal of Preventive Medicine 20(3S):36–43

Stuck A E, Egger M, Hammer A et al 2002 Home visits to prevent nursing home admission and functional decline in elderly people: systematic review and meta-regression analysis. Journal of the American Medical Association 287:1022–1028

Tinetti M E, Speechley M, Ginter S F 1988 Risk factors for falls among elderly persons living in the community. New England Journal of Medicine 319: 1701–1707

US Preventive Services Task Force 2003 Screening for dementia: recommendation and rationale. Annals of Internal Medicine 138:925–926

US Preventive Services Task Force 2005 Screening for abdominal aortic aneurysm: recommendation statement. Annals of Internal Medicine 142:198–202

Wanhainen A, Lundkvist J, Bergqvist D et al 2005 Cost-effectiveness of different screening strategies for abdominal aortic aneurysm. Journal of Vascular Surgery 41:741–751

World Health Organization 1986 Ottawa charter for health promotion. WHO, Geneva

RECOMMENDED READING

*** *Essential reading; ** recommended reading*

Canadian Task Force on Preventive Health Care: http://www.ctfphc.org ***
This is an excellent source with many useful links.

Harris R P, Helfand M, Woolf S H et al 2001 Current methods of the US Preventive Services Task Force: a review of the process. American Journal of Preventive Medicine 20(3S):21–35 **

United Kingdom Department of Health (National Health Service): http://www.dh.gov.uk/en/Policy AndGuidance/ ***
This is a mine of useful information about all aspects of the NHS; it is sometimes hard to find information about health promotion and disease prevention, but generally worth the effort.

SELF-ASSESSMENT QUESTIONS

1. A colleague asks you: 'What are the appropriate preventive health manoeuvres for my mother, aged 78, who is in good health?' Your answer is:
   a. She is too old to worry about prevention
   b. Check for hypertension, diabetes, cognitive impairment, and hearing
   c. Check for hypertension, cognitive impairment, lipid disorders and driving safety
   d. None of the above

2. Should you recommend screening for prostate cancer in a healthy, asymptomatic 65-year-old executive?
   a. Yes, with rectal examination and PSA
   b. Yes, with PSA only
   c. Only if, after explaining all the potential risks and benefits, he is eager to proceed with testing
   d. Only if he has a first order relative with invasive carcinoma

Chapter **9**

Overview of complexity/ co-morbidity

Kenneth Rockwood

WHY GERIATRIC MEDICINE?

Many readers of this book will be students or practitioners of geriatric medicine who know what they are about, but it is still worth considering at a broad level what geriatricians do and why they do it. The range of what a geriatrician does in a typical week is so broad that no one answer entirely suffices, but we will make a good start by recognizing that geriatricians chiefly care for elderly people who are frail. Frailty is a state of vulnerability: it arises from the complex interaction of multiple medical and social problems.

FRAILTY AND COMPLEXITY

The complexity of frailty motivates and animates geriatric medicine; it is our burden and our glory. Complexity poses conceptual and pragmatic problems, the solutions of which are personally rewarding, intellectually stimulating and contribute to considerable societal good. How to deal with the complex problems of elderly people who are frail has in general been well worked out, and the specific techniques for particular problems constitute the bulk of this book (which of course is subject to ongoing refinement).

However, the techniques that are used to manage the complex problems of elderly people who are frail were not always developed in full appreciation of the nature of complexity, so that not all of our practice is coherent. Indeed, in some places, geriatric medicine appears to be practiced chiefly as the internal medicine of old age, although with perhaps more specific documentation of function and social relationships than would be usual for routine medical care. Such an approach attempts to simplify the complexity of patients and their needs.

The results of trying to do geriatric medicine in this way are often desultory: believing that a complex problem can best be dealt with by breaking it down into its simple parts, and addressing them one at a time, physicians and teams behave as though in competition to develop the longest problem list. Team meetings can become similarly dispirited affairs, with too much time spent on the first patients to be reviewed, and thus too little time on the last. 'Assessment' of problems may take precedence over treatment of problems. Without a coherent focus on overall patient outcomes, and with discipline-specific problems making up the list, team members often compete for others' attention, and many problems may become refracted through the personalities of individual team members. With an emphasis on single items in isolation and with a struggle between disciplines for dominance, information that should be fully known by all team members may be jealously guarded. Even though the case conference seems too long, small groupings of team members are seen in the corridors afterwards, as they try and get to grips with particular issues which were put off during the team meeting itself. Discharge plans run foul of delays, as patients wait for multiple consultations, or for administrative assessments to address how care needs conform to service availability.

If that dismal picture is the face of the 'one-problem-at-a-time' approach to the complex needs of frail elderly people, what is the alternative? In short, it is this: if complexity is not to be simplified, then it must be embraced. But how do we embrace complexity, and what are the consequences of our so doing?

COMPLEX SYSTEMS

Embracing the complexity of frailty begins with conceptualization. If frailty in an individual can be conceptualized as a complex problem, then it should share characteristics with problems in other complex systems. Three characteristics will have particular clinical consequences. In complex systems, there are multiple components that interact, and that change as a result of their interaction. In short, complex systems are dynamic, and change must be expected, and if it cannot be accommodated, it must at least be delimited. ('We can only get Mr Smith home if his daughter-in-law's day care re-opens, otherwise we will need an assisted living option.') In addition, their interacting components mean that they are unlikely to be susceptible to single interventions: with complex systems, you cannot do just one thing at once. These first two pieces are well known and widely accepted. There is a third consequence, which our group has particularly explored, and which, it seems to me, allows some useful insights: complex systems will also have characteristics that, while dependent on the component parts, arise at the level of the whole system. In other words, complex systems will give rise to state variables, and measuring these state variables can give us insights into how our patients are doing. For example, an automobile has a great many parts that interact, and while the functioning of each can be tested individually, the function of the system can be parsimoniously described

through a variable such as speed, or on-time performance. Such state variables can be found for our patients.

FRAILTY AND THE GERIATRIC GIANTS

From this way of thinking about the complexity of frailty, several standards of practices in geriatric medicine can be evaluated. Beginning with the patient encounter, the idea that we must understand and manage complexity allows us to re-evaluate the usual teaching about how illness presents. As is well known, many elderly people have an 'atypical' presentation of their acute illnesses, such as delirium, falls, or taking to bed. When I first learned about geriatric medicine, I was told that such signs were 'geriatric giants', and that they gained this stature because they were 'sensitive but non-specific signs of illness'. While it is true that delirium, functional decline, falls and taking to bed are sensitive but non-specific signs, it does not follow that they should be 'geriatric giants' simply on the basis of their relative sensitivity and specificity. Many elderly people do indeed present with delirium, falls and non-specific functional decline, but few *fit* elderly people have such a presentation, unless there is a focal cause (e.g. delirium with encephalitis), or unless they are very ill (Jarrett et al 1995).

By contrast, many (in some series most) elderly people who are *frail* do present this way. Apart from the illogicality ('atypical' diseases are in fact typical among those who are frail), the formulation of relative sensitivity and specificity sheds no insight on why we should give the privilege of geriatric giant-hood to delirium, falls, immobility and functional decline. It cannot just be that these signs are sensitive but not specific, as medicine is replete with such signs: chest pain, red skin, diarrhoea and dyspnoea are a few. There must be something else about delirium, falls, immobility and functional decline to account for their prominence in our field.

Here is an alternative account of the 'atypical' illness presentation. When complex systems fail, they fail with their highest order functions first. From an evolutionary standpoint, high-order function in humans arises from upright bipedal ambulation, opposable thumbs and higher order cognitive processes, starting with divided attention. Against this background, it is easy to appreciate why the systems failure presentations should be falls/immobility, functional decline and delirium. These are the highest order functions of the complex system that is an elderly person who is frail. When that person is at the edge of failure, just about any insult will tip the person into 'system failure'. The fact that the elderly person is often on the brink of failure accounts for both the sensitivity of the geriatric giants (illness results in system failure) and for their non-specificity – any insult will push the system over the edge.

Why some people's complex system failure presents as delirium, whereas others present with falls, is not always clear. While it is tempting to think that there is some system specificity (e.g. that people with delirium are more likely to have an underlying dementia) and while to some extent this is true, the identification of the presentation with the system is a snare. It is a snare which traps many elderly people whose non-syncopal falls may be routinely investigated with neuroimaging, electroencephalography and Holter monitoring, and who then wind up in a cascade of investigation and treatment of findings that would otherwise be judged incidental.

HIERARCHICAL ASSESSMENTS

Failure of mobility, cognition and function, of course, are not 'all or one'. A person whose mobility becomes impaired does not just become immobile – rather, there are grades of mobility and balance, and of cognition and of function. These grades can be defined hierarchically. Hierarchical assessments offer many advantages, including the possibility to define the intervals precisely, and efficiency (e.g. if a frail elderly patient requires the minimal hands-on assistance of one person, they will not be independent in their transfer, nor will they require a hoist and two people). Hierarchical assessments of mobility and of function are particularly well suited to single-line, plain language descriptions of their levels (e.g. again, independent transfer, minimal hands-on assistance, total lift). These properties of scaling and plain language allow them to be used to good effect in

everyday practice (MacKnight et al 2002). Using this plain language, we can empower healthcare practitioners to specify how their patients' health is changing. This can be done precisely, and without the curiously moral language that otherwise becomes routine:

'How is Mrs Jones?'
'She is very good. In fact, I think she is better than she was yesterday.'
'And Mr. Smith?'
'I am worried about him. He was bad yesterday, but now he is worse.'

By contrast, a similar conversation might proceed, with greater precision and without the burden of apparently spiritual judgments, as follows:

'How is Mrs Jones?'
'She is showing progress. Today, she can walk with only standby assistance, whereas yesterday, she required hands-on help.'
'And Mr Smith?'
'I am worried about him. Yesterday, he could sit up in bed, and feed himself once the tray was set up. Today, he needs help to position himself in his bed, and I had to help him with his utensils.'

The well-defined and readily observed differences in impairment in mobility and balance, or in function, allow subtle changes in the state of the patient to be communicated efficiently. The conversation employs an appropriate level of precision, which can be understood by all team members (and learned by many patients and most families) and which is readily verifiable by them – and by patients and family members. By contrast, elaborate descriptions of, for example, the degree of external rotation of the hip not only can be speciously precise, but also often do not convey more essential information, such as whether the patient with 22 degrees of external rotation can actually get out of bed.

Plain language is not always a virtue, however. Sometimes, what a geriatrician has to say seems so reasonable – even obvious – that learners can listen to it and conclude that they were taught 'nothing at all; it's just common sense'. A useful corrective, in an academic teaching session, is to spend a few minutes at the outset exploring with the listeners the full spectrum of their own ignorance about how to proceed with the facts at hand. Such a setting is often a way to encourage them to consider whether the response – which is sadly not rare – of dealing with the problem by calling the patients names ('bed blocker', 'social admission' or 'poor historian') is in fact the most useful starting point for elaborating a diagnostic and management plan.

As it turns out, however, there appears to be a strong mathematical basis for the intuition of the geriatrician, and this can be appealed to in order to demonstrate that complexity need not just be a metaphor in geriatric medicine. It can also be the basis for systematic inquiry using advanced computational techniques (e.g. Mitnitski & Rockwood 2006). If the mathematics of complexity in relation to frailty seems a little recherché, it is also possible to consider some of the epidemiological and statistical issues needed to evaluate the multicomponent interventions that are essential in geriatric medicine (Allore et al 2005). A rehearsal of the issues of selection of modifiable risk factors, of intervention components and their assignment in an intervention, or of the thorny issues of blinding educational interventions in usual care, or of estimation of component effects well illustrates the subtleties that apparently underlie the common sense of geriatric medicine.

GERIATRIC INTERVENTIONS

The idea of geriatric medicine as the complex care of frail elderly people is not new (Cape 1978), although calling our patients frail and not 'at risk' or some occasionally less polite euphemism – even in textbooks of geriatric medicine – is a subtlety of more recent usage. Good clinical geriatricians have always understood the idea of complexity, and the consequences that follow from it. The very idea of the multidimensional, multicomponent intervention that is a comprehensive geriatric assessment is, at its heart, recognition of patients' complexity: a complex patient requires a complex response. But, as might be inferred from the comments about the not uncommon failing of the multidisciplinary team conference, the application of a multidimensional intervention to a multidimensional problem is not an automatic remedy. This has perhaps best been seen in geri-

atric medicine in the choice of outcomes for the formal evaluation of comprehensive geriatric assessment programmes.

An early consensus emphasized the importance of improved function as best illustrating the merit of a specialized geriatric intervention. For many patients this is true, and one of the clearer benefits of management by geriatricians and multidisciplinary teams, compared with usual care, is an emphasis on patient function that results in better function at the end of the intervention. On the other hand, geriatricians can often achieve persuasively beneficial results that do not change a patient's function. For example, particularly where palliative care teams have either not been established or are devoted to the care of patients dying of cancer, a specialist geriatric intervention can help provide a peaceful death. Such a death is appropriate and desirable, but it would not be reflected in improved patient function, and any evaluative clinical trial that made patient function its primary outcome would be blind to the benefits achieved in palliative care.

In addition, there is reason to be skeptical about many of the functional assessment tools that have routinely been employed. While they can well stratify patients' overall function, and while they are reliable, many are demonstrably insensitive to clinically important change (Rockwood et al 2003). Similarly, it is often the case that the care of the frail elderly patient by the multidisciplinary geriatric team will result in a lower rate of institutionalization. On the other hand, there will be patients for whom institutionalization is clearly the best option for both the patient and the family. In such a circumstance, the geriatrician must either work against the best interest of the evaluation or against the best interest of the patient. An alternative to these measures is an individualized patient outcome approach, such as Goal Attainment Scaling (Kiresuk & Sherman 1968, Stolee et al 1999). Such a technique measures the attainment of goals in general, but leaves the choice of goals to the individual. While it is demonstrably more responsive to change than many other measures, its rejection of the standard psychometric approach – in which standardization is prized of all else, individualization is not possible – has meant that it has not been widely embraced.

THE SATISFACTION OF THE GERIATRIC PATIENT

The failure to articulate persuasively enough the challenge of complexity, and the scientific basis of how it is approached, has been a problem. This idea of seeing geriatric medicine as a highly specialized set of skills replaces the idea of viewing the specialty as a backwater. Like other disciplines that require particular skills, geriatric medicine is not for everyone.

Physicians disposed to being able to handle uncertainty seem particularly well suited to becoming geriatricians (Ghosk 2004). Being able to tolerate uncertainty means not requiring to know every answer to every abnormality, but being able to prioritize, and to act judiciously, not algorithmically. This focus on the state of the whole patient, and not on the chasing of abnormal results, is often a relief to frail elderly patients and their families, who welcome someone aiming to have them walk better, function better, not fall, not be so confused, live at home and/or to be reconciled with their families. There is much that can be achieved for our patients and it feels good to know how to do it, and to help guide a team towards those ends. Perhaps this accounts for why geriatricians report the highest life satisfaction (Leigh et al 2002).

Even the satisfaction of its practitioners has not been enough to attract large numbers of people into the specialty so that, particularly outside the UK and in Australia, the future of geriatric medicine is felt not to be entirely secure, despite an anticipated growth in demand which can only be described as immense (Besdine et al 2005). This is a problem for many reasons, not the least of which is that practitioners of general internal medicine – who, especially in North America, both provide the great majority of care to elderly people and spend most of their time providing such care – find care of the elderly patients to be particularly frustrating (Tanner et al 2006). Even in the UK, the home of the specialty, there are clouds. A recent editorial characterized the worry like this: in an era of patient choice, will people choose a geriatrician or will they instead opt for 'the relative benefits as perceived by the patient, of (a) treatment of the main morbidity by a specialist in the particular condition, hoping that co-morbidity would be managed adequately ...' In short, the idea of being treated by a specialist in the major disease of the moment would be traded off for option and 'treatment of the patient holistically by the geriatrician' (Metz & Labrooy 2005). For the patient of any age with only one thing wrong, it is easy to see the merit of being cared for by a physician (and team) who specialize in that malady, but the merit of hoping that co-morbidity would be managed adequately diminishes as co-morbidities mount. As they do, the 'most responsible diagnosis' of the 'one-thing-wrong-at-once' approach becomes increasingly metaphorical. For the patient with many things wrong all at once (some 'medical' and some 'social'), the specialist that is needed is a specialist in complexity. As this becomes understood, the answer to the question 'Why geriatric medicine?' will become obvious.

> ### Key points
>
> - Geriatric medicine, viewed chiefly as the care of elderly people who are frail, is a specialty that must deal with complexity.
> - The multiple needs of our patients require a multidimensional approach (comprehensive geriatric assessment) and a multicomponent intervention (the multidimensional team).
> - The field has probably not adequately got to grips with multidimensional outcome measurement.
> - Recent work in mathematical gerontology suggests that the complexity of frailty can be understood not just metaphorically, but quantitatively.

REFERENCES

Allore H G, Tinetti M E, Gill T M et al 2005 Experimental designs for multicomponent interventions among persons with multifactorial geriatric syndromes. Clinical Trials: Journal of the Society for Clinical Trials 2:13–21

Besdine R, Boult C, Brangman S et al 2005 Caring for older Americans: the future of geriatric medicine. Journal of the American Geriatrics Society 5(6 Suppl):S245–256

Cape R 1978 Aging: its complex management. Harper Row, New York

Ghosk A K 2004 Understanding medical uncertainty: a primer for physicians. Journal of the Association of Physicians of India 52:739–742

Jarrett P G, Rockwood K, Carver D et al 1995 Illness presentation in elderly patients. Archives of Internal Medicine 155:1060–1064

Leigh J P, Kravitz R L, Schembri M 2002 Physician career satisfaction across specialties. Archives of Internal Medicine 162:1577–1584

Kiresuk T, Sherman R 1968 Goal attainment scaling: a general method for evaluating community mental health programs. Community Mental Health Journal 4:443–453

MacKnight C, Sibley A, Rockwood K 2002 The sensibility of bedside tests of balance and mobility. Geriatrics Today: Journal of the Canadian Geriatrics Society 5:140–144

Metz D H, Labrooy S J 2005 The future of geriatric medicine in an era of patient choice. Age and Ageing 34:553–555

Mitnitski A B, Rockwood K 2006 Decrease in the relative heterogeneity of health with age: a cross-national comparison. Mechanisms of Ageing and Development 127:70–72

Rockwood K, Howlett S, Stadnyk K et al 2003 Responsiveness of goal attainment scaling in a randomized controlled trial of comprehensive geriatric assessment. Journal of Clinical Epidemiology 56:736–743

Stolee P, Stadnyk K, Myers A M 1999 An individualized approach to outcome measurement in geriatric rehabilitation. Journals of Gerontology Series A: Biological Sciences and Medical Sciences 54:M641–647

Tanner C E, Eckstrom E, Desai S S 2006 Uncovering frustrations. A qualitative needs assessment of academic general internists as geriatric care providers and teachers. Journal of General Internal Medicine 21:51–55

Chapter 10

Driving assessment

Desmond O'Neil and Alan Martin

INTRODUCTION

Driving is increasingly the most common form of transport for older people (OECD 2001) and access to transport is a key component to social inclusion and maintenance of health (TRB 2006). In some ways, driving is the instrumental activity of daily living which has become almost an activity of daily living. Therefore, geriatricians will need some skills and knowledge in appreciating the impact of their patients' health on driving and transportation.

This occurs against a background where doctors may fail to recognize the importance and relevance of driving to their patients (MacMahon et al 1996), and they may conceive the evaluation of the older driver in either over-simplified or over-complex terms. Although it is a complex assessment which requires consideration of the behavioural and functional patterns as much (or more than) physical and cognitive skills, it is no different in this respect to many of the complex decisions made by geriatricians in other areas of patient care, e.g. in elder abuse or determining that someone can no longer live in the community. Just as in these cases, the toolkit required is: an appropriate philosophy (diagnostic/enabling rather than prosthetic), general health gerontology training, some specific skills, adequate evaluation methodology and multidisciplinary support.

Geriatricians will be supported in this by recent developments, including the very useful 2003 guide from the American Medical Association (Wang et al 2003). Those in the UK are fortunate that, not only are the general guidelines ('At A Glance' leaflets, Group DM 2005) and support from the dedicated medical section of the UK DVLA (Driver and Vehicle Licensing Agency) among the best in the world, but there is also a network of specialist driving assessment centres throughout the country (http://www.mobility-centres.org.uk). However, much of the biomedical literature is negative in tone, focusing on potential negative outcomes (e.g. risk to other drivers) rather than the patient's best interests (Ngo & O'Neill 2005) and there is still a scarcity of evidence to reinforce the decision-making process. This is against a background of negative media and popular opinion about older drivers, despite consistent evidence that they are the safest group of drivers on the road (Martin et al 2005, Tay 2006). Therefore, driving assessments are rarely standardized and geriatricians can take a lead in the development of more formalized assessment and treatment procedures. *The ultimate aim of driving assessment should be to identify areas of preserved ability and remediable disability so as to find strategies to correct them in order to keep people mobile as long as possible.*

THE BACKGROUND

The development of an appropriate philosophy of care requires that we understand (a) that older drivers are the safest group of drivers, and (b) that rehabilitation/enabling is possible. Although frequent reference is made to a high crash risk per mile driven (1.6–2.4 times higher for the over-65s), this is misleading on several counts: older drivers drive a much lower number of miles per year, so the risk exposure is less. More significantly, driving a low mileage is intrinsically risky, and when adjusted for actual miles driven the difference in crashes disappears, and there is even a trend for older drivers to have fewer accidents (OECD 1985). Thirdly, it has also been suggested that this perception of an increased crash rate per mile is also skewed by the increased injury rate among older drivers involved in relatively minor crashes, which might go unreported in a younger uninjured driver (Bedard et al 2002, Guohua et al 2002, Hakamies-Blomqvist 1998).

As with many areas of health in old age, the concept of deteriorating function as a natural consequence of ageing in driving is misleading, but clearly there are medical conditions which can affect comfort, ease and safety of driving. The cause of loss of function in older people is most commonly age-related disease, and the primary aim should be to identify the process or processes causing the impairment and attempt to resolve them in order to improve the performance of the activity in question. For example, intervention for arthritis (Jones et al 1991), cataracts (Monestam & Wachtmeister 1997) and stroke (Akinwuntan et al 2002) can improve ease, comfort and safety of driving, and with dementia, manoeuvres such as driving with a companion can make driving safer (Bedard & Meyers 2004).

However, with progressive neurodegenerative disorders such as dementia and Parkinsonism, a time will come when all patients will no longer be able to drive. This too needs to be planned for as driving cessation is associated with deterioration in social interaction and access to transport, as clearly shown after driving cessation in dementia. Other potential hazards of stopping driving include higher rates of loneliness, lower life satisfaction and lower activity levels (Berg et al 1981, Gonda 1982, Taylor & Tripodes 2001). Often, little thought goes into planning for the aftermath of driving cessation and identifying means of maintaining mobility for those no longer able to drive.

ASSESSMENT OF THE OLDER DRIVER

Those involved in the assessment of older drivers need some understanding of a model of driver behaviour. From this they will understand that a simple cognitive test battery is unlikely to answer the question as to whether an older person should drive or not. The most important advance in this area has been the understanding that a purely cognitive model of driving ability does not adequately reflect the complexity and hierarchical nature of the driving task (Ranney 1994).

Driver behaviour is complex and one of the simplest and most easily applicable models has been that of the hierarchy of Michon, which uses strategic, tactical and operational factors (Michon 1985). The strategic level is the choice of whether or not to travel; the tactical decision is whether or not to overtake; and the operational level is what to do when overtaking and faced with an oncoming car. The strategic and tactical levels are probably more important in terms of driving safety than the operational level: remember, a good guide to operational skills is reaction time – 15- to 25-year-olds have the quickest reaction times and the highest crash rates! This model is very helpful in clinical practice and has been operationalized for research and clinical use (de Raedt & Ponjaert-Kristoffersen 2001).

Those involved with driving assessment also need access to supportive assessments, often from an occupational therapist, possibly from a neuropsychologist, but a sine qua non is access to a specialist driving assessor. Much effort has been expended in recent years in the pursuit of a simple test or series of tests that may assist the physician in assessing fitness to drive in the older person. This has varied from questionnaires such as the Mini-Mental State Examination (MMSE), to visuospatial tests (e.g. the maze-drawing test) and has more recently begun to include sophisticated driving simulators (Rizzo et al 1997). It is hard to see how any simple test can do justice to the complex set of behavioural, motor and cognitive skills required for the driving task. The end result of the multidisciplinary assessment is to give an overview of the patient, suggest areas of remediation, and with this overall view it may be clear that the patient is fit or not fit to drive (Carr et al 1991).

However, there will always be a considerable proportion for whom this decision is not clear, and they require an on-road test from a specialized driving assessor. This assessment is not just for fitness to drive but also to gauge the potential for remedial driving rehabilitation. In the UK, the NHS is fortunate in that there is a network of specialist driver assessment centres, the Forum, who will undertake on-road testing and may also provide rehabilitative driving lessons (http://www.mobility-centres.org.uk).

Geriatricians should make themselves familiar with DVLA regulations on fitness to drive and of their obligations to inform patients of their requirements to disclose relevant illnesses to both the DVLA and their insurance company/broker. Although in legal terms it is the DVLA which makes the decision whether one is fit to drive or not, in practice there is a need for clinicians to inform themselves of various aspects of health and driving. The DVLA will write to clinicians looking for advice, and geriatricians may have to give on-the-spot advice for immediate driving cessation for some patients, on the basis of duty of care and ahead of a formal DVLA decision.

THE ASSESSMENT

A simple, but often neglected, initial step is the taking of a brief driving/transport history. After the usual comprehensive geriatric assessment, some attention should be given to any recent change in driving behaviour, near misses or accidents. A witness history is important for those with cognitive impairment, with due consideration for bias if the informant is a non-driving spouse whose transport options will be severely curtailed if the patient can no longer drive.

Medical conditions that may affect driving performance should be catalogued: stroke, epilepsy, syncope, dementia, delirium, arthritis, etc. There has been an unduly negative approach in the literature on medications and driving, with scant attention to the fact that many medications (anti-Parkinsonians, antiinflammatories, antidepressants) probably render driving safer and more comfortable. Medications and drugs that may impair performance also need to be considered, in particular alcohol and other recreational drugs; for those on neuroleptics, it is probably the degree of the illness rather than the medication that is the problem. Long-acting benzodiazepines are almost the only medication group which can be clearly identified as a problem in their own right (O'Neill 1998).

Physical examination should include visual acuity and visual fields. Visual acuity should be above the limits set by the local driving authority. Mobility of neck, arms, hands and legs should be sufficient to allow the patient to see mirrors, look over their shoulders and operate the steering, gears and pedals. Cognition should be tested using the MMSE, though there is no evidence-based cut-off point. There is a 'near-consensus' that those with an MMSE of less than 17 require formal assessment of driving skills (Johansson & Lundberg 1997), a testament to the inappropriateness of relying overly on brief cognitive screens for assessing driving ability.

The focus should not be to identify impairments that disqualify a patient from further driving but rather on finding the cause of any deterioration in their driving performance. If impairments exist that hamper the subject's ability to drive, interventions that may remove or improve these impairments should be sought (i.e. rationalization of medications, physiotherapy, car modification). The subject should then be reassessed to evaluate the impact of these interventions.

The first decision the geriatrician must make is a risk assessment as to whether the older individual should stop driving during the assessment process. There probably should be a low threshold for asking for a temporary cessation. The on-road driving evaluation, which is the standard, is in general the final arbiter and may also be helpful for the patient's dignity and self-esteem, particularly for patients who have difficulty in accepting that their driving is dangerous. This may be difficult if you live in an area that is distant from a Forum centre, and it is possible that a local driving assessor in a remote area may take on this task.

For those who are considered fit to drive but suffer from chronic, progressive illnesses as in the case of a dementing disorder, it is important to stress that their continued driving is conditional on maintained performance and that, at a certain agreed level of disability, permission to continue driving will be withdrawn; a modified Ulysses contract (Robinson & O'Neill 2004) (Box 10.1). For those who fail the driving assessment, alternative forms of transport should be sought and efforts should be made to maintain the patient's social contacts and interests. Counselling and advice from a social worker may be helpful at this point.

ACTION

Depending on the illnesses present, there is potentially a wide range of interventions that we can undertake (Box 10.2). Adaptation of the car, following advice from the occupational therapist, physiotherapist, or specialist driving assessor can improve driving comfort and safety. Follow-up review should be organized for those with progressive illness, such as dementia and Parkinson-

> **Box 10.1   The modified Ulysses contract**
>
> This contract is named after the hero who made his crew tie him to the mast of the ship on the condition that they did not heed his entreaties to be released when he was seduced by the song of the sirens. This translates as the concept of discussing driving and transport as early as possible with the person with dementia, emphasizing that while driving may be facilitated through appropriate assessment and review, eventually the dementia will progress and that the patient will have to cease driving.

ism. A review period of 6–12 months would seem to be reasonable with dementia (Duchek et al 2003) but patients and carers should be asked to seek earlier review if they perceive a significant decline in the status of the dementia or in driving

Box 10.2   Sample diseases for which appropriate assessment and remediation may be of benefit

Neuropsychiatric
Stroke — Driving-specific rehabilitation (van Zomeren et al 1987)
Parkinson's disease — Maximizing motor function, treatment of depression, assessment of cognitive function (Anonymous 1990)
Delirium — Treatment and resolution
Depression — Treatment: if antidepressant, choose one with least potential of cognitive/motor effects (Rubinsztein & Lawton 1995)
Mild dementia — Assess, treat depression, reduce/eliminate psychoactive drugs, advise not to drive alone (O'Neill 1996)

Cardiovascular
Syncope — Advise pending investigation: treat cause (O'Neill 1995)

Respiratory
Sleep apnoea — Treatment of underlying disease (Haraldsson et al 1992)

Vision
Cataract — Surgery, appropriate corrective lens and advice about glare (Monestam & Wachtmeister 1997)

Metabolic
Diabetes mellitus — Direct therapy to avoid hypoglycaemia (Frier 1992)

Musculoskeletal
All arthritides — Driving-specific rehabilitation programme (Jones et al 1991)

Iatrogenic
Polypharmacy — Rationalize medications (Ray et al 1993)
Psychoactive medication — Rationalize, minimize (Ray et al 1992)

abilities. A clear recommendation should be made to the patient and recorded in the medical record: this should include advice to inform their insurance company of relevant illnesses, as well as any statutory requirement to inform their driver licencing authority.

The actual process of breaking confidentiality in the event of evidence of hazard to other members of the public is almost universally supported by most codes of medical practice. It is important that this disclosure has some likelihood of impact and results in the least traumatic removal of the compromised older driver from the road. In such instances, the family may be able to intervene in terms of disabling the car and providing alternative modes of transport. In our own experience, we rarely have to invoke official intervention, but find that a personal communication with a senior police officer in the patient's locality may result in a sensitive visit to the patient and cessation of driving.

CONCLUSION

Geriatricians should consider driving assessment as a routine part of their clinical practice. In their focus on strategies that promote rather than restrict mobility, they should familiarize themselves with local fitness-to-drive regulations, tailor their assessments to the needs and driving patterns of their patients, and aim to identify and remediate any physical or psychological issues that may be impairing the driving performance of their patients.

> **Key points**
>
> - Driving is an important component of the health and well-being of older people.
> - The most important priority for geriatricians is to preserve the same proportionality of mobility to safety for older people as society accords to other age groups.
> - Many age-related conditions affect comfort, ability and safety of the driving task but these effects can be ameliorated by appropriate intervention.

> - The most important factors in assessing fitness to drive are likely to be measures of function and driving behaviour: cognitive testing is less clearly helpful.
> - Eventual driving cessation with progressive neurodegenerative diseases will be aided by early diagnosis disclosure and discussion of eventual driving cessation, as well as the provision of suitable alternative transportation options.

REFERENCES

Akinwuntan A E, Feys H, DeWeerdt W et al 2002 Determinants of driving after stroke. Archives of Physical Medicine and Rehabilation 83:334–341

Anonymous 1990 Driving and Parkinson's disease (editorial). Lancet 336:781

Bedard M, Meyers J R 2004 The influence of passengers on older drivers involved in fatal crashes. Experimental Aging Research 30:205–215

Bedard M, Guyatt G, Stones M J et al 2002 The independent contribution of driver, crash and vehicle characteristics to driver fatalities. Accident, Analysis and Prevention 34:717–727

Berg S, Mellstron D, Persson G 1981 Loneliness in the Swedish aged. Journal of Gerontology 36:342–349

Carr D, Schmader K, Bergman C et al 1991 A multidisciplinary approach in the evaluation of demented drivers referred to geriatric assessment centers. Journal of the American Geriatrics Society 39: 1132–1136

de Raedt R, Ponjaert-Kristoffersen I 2001 Short cognitive/neuropsychological test battery for first-tier fitness-to-drive assessment of older adults. The Clinical Neuropsychologist 15:329–336

Duchek J M, Carr D B, Hunt L et al 2003 Longitudinal driving performance in early-stage dementia of the Alzheimer type. Journal of the American Geriatrics Society 51:1342–1347

Frier B M 1992 Driving and diabetes. British Medical Journal 305:1238–1239

Gonda J 1982 Transportation, perceived control, and well-being in the elderly. Specialized Transport Planning and Practice 1:61–72

Group D M 2005 At a glance: guide to the current medical standards of fitness to drive. DVLA, Swansea

Guohua L, Braver E, Chen L 2002 Fragility versus excessive crash involvement as determinants of high death rates per vehicle-mile of travel among older drivers. Accident, Analysis and Prevention 35:227–235

Hakamies-Blomqvist L 1998 Older driver's accident risk: conceptual and methodological issues. Accident, Analysis and Prevention 30:293–297

Haraldsson P O, Carenfelt C, Tingvall C 1992 Sleep apnea syndrome symptoms and automobile driving in a general population. Journal of Clinical Epidemiology 45:821–825

Johansson K, Lundberg C 1997 The 1994 International Consensus Conference on Dementia and Driving: a brief report. Swedish National Road Administration. Alzheimer Disease and Associated Disorders 11(Suppl 1):62–69

Jones J G, McCann J, Lassere M N 1991 Driving and arthritis. British Journal of Rheumatology 30: 361–364

MacMahon M, O'Neill D, Kenny R A 1996 Syncope: driving advice is frequently overlooked. Postgraduate Medical Journal 72:561–563

Martin A, Balding L, O'Neill D 2005 Are the media running elderly drivers off the road? British Medical Journal 330:368

Michon J A 1985 A critical review of driver behaviour models: what do we know, what should we do? In: Evans L, Schwing R C (eds) Human behaviour and traffic safety. Plenum, New York, p 487–525

Monestam E, Wachtmeister L 1997 Impact of cataract surgery on car driving: a population based study in Sweden. British Journal of Ophthalmology 81: 16–22

Ngo D, O'Neill D 2005 Balancing mobility and risk in research on older traffic users: a quantative analysis. Irish Journal of Medical Science 174(Suppl 2):46

O'Neill D 1995 Syncope and driving. In: Kenny R A (ed.) Syncope. Chapman & Hall, London, p 65-68

O'Neill D 1996 Dementia and driving: screening, assessment and advice. Lancet 348:1114

O'Neill D 1998 Benzodiazepines and driver safety (comment). Lancet 352:1324–1325

Organisation for Economic Co-operation and Development 1985 Traffic safety in elderly road users. OECD, Paris

Organisation for Economic Co-operation and Development 2001 Ageing and transport: mobility needs and safety issues. OECD, Paris

Ranney T A 1994 Models of driving behaviour: a review of their evolution. Accident, Analysis and Prevention 26:733–750

Ray W A, Gurwitz J, Decker M D et al 1992 Medications and the safety of the older driver: is there a basis for concern? Human Factors 34:33–47, 49–51 (discussion)

Ray W A, Thapa P B, Shorr R I 1993 Medications and the older driver. Clinics in Geriatric Medicine 9:413–438

Rizzo M, Reinach S, McGehee D et al 1997 Simulated car crashes and crash predictors in drivers with Alzheimer disease. Archives of Neurology 54: 545–551

Robinson D, O'Neill D 2004 Ethics of driving assessment in dementia care, competence and communication. In: Rai G S (ed.) Medical ethics and the elderly, 2nd edn. Harwood, Australia, p 103–111

Rubinsztein J, Lawton C A 1995 Depression and driving in the elderly. International Journal of Geriatric Psychiatry 10:15–17

Tay R 2006 Ageing drivers: storm in a teacup? Accident, Analysis and Prevention 38:112–121

Taylor B D, Tripodes S 2001 The effects of driving cessation on the elderly with dementia and their caregivers. Accident, Analysis and Prevention 33:519–528

Transportation Research Board 2006 Cost-effectiveness of access to nonemergency medical transportation: comparison of transportation and healthcare costs and benefits. TRB, Washington, DC

van Zomeren A H, Brouwer W H, Minderhoud J M 1987 Acquired brain damage and driving: a review. Archives of Physical Medical Rehabilitation 68: 697–705

Wang C, Kosinski C, Schwartzberg J et al 2003 Physician's guide to assessing and counseling older drivers. National Highway Traffic Safety Administration, Washington, DC

USEFUL WEBSITES

American Medical Association: Physician's guide to assessing and counseling older drivers:
   http://www.ama-assn.org/ama/pub/category/10791.html
DVLA At a Glance leaflets:
   http://www.dvla.gov.uk/medical/ataglance.aspx/
Forum of Mobility Centres (specialist driver assessment):
   http://www.mobility-centres.org.uk

SELF-ASSESSMENT QUESTIONS

Are the following statements true or false?

1. An 80-year-old man with a history of stroke presents to his doctor for advice on whether to restart driving. His doctor should:
   a. Advise against further driving
   b. Take a detailed driving history
   c. Assess for residual motor, sensory and cognitive impairments
   d. Check local regulations on driving after stroke
   e. If in doubt, refer for on-road assessment

2. The following statements are true or false:
   a. Older drivers crash more often than other road users
   b. Diving cessation is safer for those with difficulty driving
   c. Older drivers need automatic reassessment to continue driving
   d. Automatic reassessment keeps older people driving longer
   e. Drivers with dementia pose a risk to other road users

Chapter 11

Carers

Rónán Collins and Rosemary Young

'FELIX RANDAL the farrier, O he is dead
   then? my duty all ended,
Who have watched his mould of man big-boned
   and hardy handsome
Pining, pining, till time when reason rambled
   in it and some
Fatal four disorders, fleshed there all
   contended?'

              (Gerard Manley Hopkins)

INTRODUCTION

Informal carers are family or friends who provide physical and emotional support to enable older people to function and exist independently at home and without whom a statutory input of care would be required (Nolan & Grant 1989). There is probably no specialty where interaction with carers is as important and rewarding yet as time-consuming and complex as in geriatric medicine. The care provided in maintaining health and independence is paramount to our patients and constructive interaction with carers can support and enhance this (Guberman et al 2003). Our reward in this (and ultimately that of our patients) is often the early alert to something being wrong, the all-important collateral history and the support framework whereby patients can be discharged from hospital in a timely fashion and continue to live where and how they would wish.

While our duty is primarily to our patients, it would be simplistic not to acknowledge a responsibility to their carers. Moreover, not to acknowledge and support their role may endanger our patients' health. Alternative models of carers as co-clients or consumers are gaining greater acceptance and are recognized in statute (DoH 1995). Indeed, many carers will be older themselves and may have need of our services. Occasionally, it is our patient who is carer to adult offspring. Carers will have often given up their independence and careers, and might face futures of poverty, isolation, stress and ill health themselves. They are therefore fully deserving of recognition and support.

DYNAMICS OF THE CARER ROLE

Informal caregiving can involve a complex relationship between the caregiver and the person receiving the care. It is often the preferred option as it can be flexible and provided by trusted persons within an individual's social milieu. The importance of the informal care network cannot be underestimated in medical and social care policy. This is emphasized in the NHS and Community Care Act (1990) and supporting literature (see Ch. 6 on community geriatric care).

The role of the carer is full of potential conflicts, however, and sensitivity and patience are often needed to explore, acknowledge and resolve these.

Satisfaction is an important coping mechanism for carers and, where this is lacking or the role is assumed because of a lack of an alternative or a sense of social expectation, then the relationship may cease to be advantageous to patients. A consequence of this can be an unintentional transformation from carer to abuser (Nolan et al 1996, Payne 1995). The term 'carer' itself may be perceived as derogatory by family members, suggesting a dependent relationship rather than a caring family role to a loved one in need, a psychological conflict between 'professional' caregiver and spouse or lover. Conversely, the social exclusion that often accompanies being a carer can lead to re-enforcement of that role:

'Carers ... can experience alienation, stigma and loss of social and financial support, and personal independence through their association with disability. Having taken the risk of becoming a carer they may seek to retain the person for whom they care in a state of dependency and this is a risky enterprise'

(Ross & Waterson 1996)

Carer does not necessarily mean 'younger': carers are frequently older themselves. Older carers can be often resilient, displaying more adaptive skills and experiencing less stress and more satisfaction than younger carers in similar roles (Seltzer & Krauss 2001). Within older couples, different needs and abilities may produce a *reciprocity* in caregiving, so each may be carer to the other in some respect, e.g. a cognitively intact person with limited mobility living with a mobile but confused partner. There may also be important gender differences both in terms of the approach adopted to the role of carer (with men generally finding it easier to set limits and see their role as professional) and also by the response of care managers to offering additional support services, with a greater expectation sometimes placed on female carers (Bywaters & Harris 1998, Twigg & Atkin 1994).

COMMUNICATION

Early patient and carer communication and agreed goal setting can improve clinical outcomes and has been identified as one of the key advantages

> ### Box 11.1   Ethics: Carer paternalism?
>
> Using dementia as an example: many carers would not want disclosure of diagnosis to a loved one, but if placed in the scenario themselves, they would wish to know their diagnosis (Maguire et al 1996).
>
> Although ethically it seems wrong to withhold information from a patient, particularly where disclosure could be advantageous in helping patients plan for the future, it is usually in the context of more advanced dementia that carers would not want disclosure (Fahy et al 2003). In this situation, it may be a good decision, as the benefit may be outweighed by unnecessary – though possibly short-lived – distress in such circumstances.
>
> It would be foolish to always choose to ignore individual insights at the expense of too rigid and simplistic an ethical position.

of stroke units, for example (Stroke Unit Trialists' Collaboration 2007). The therapeutic role of carers is also recognized in standard 5.2 of the National Service Framework for Older People which deals with effective functioning of the multidisciplinary team (DoH 2001a). Clearly, carers have an important role in initiating treatment and rehabilitation. Conversely this must not compromise our confidential relationship and duty to patients. The 'How's my mother, Doctor?' question is an all too frequent paternalistic trapdoor through which we may fall. The urge to talk over or ignore our patients while taking conspiratorial shortcuts with their carers is bad manners and unprofessional behaviour. The correct approach is often an individually-tailored one, which is cogniscent of the carer's unique insights (see Box 11.1).

INVOLVING CARERS

The last 10 years have seen a concerted effort by the Government to make the NHS and community care services more user friendly and accountable to patients' and carers' needs (DoH 1998) (indeed, Prime Minister Blair's own mother was a carer). The role of the 6 million unpaid carers in the UK saving some £34 billion annually was given statutory recognition in the 1995 Carers (Recognition and Services) Act, acknowledging carers rights to a full assessment of their needs and the impact of such assessments on future care plans (Carers National Association 1998). However, carers have traditionally felt ignored or undervalued and barriers remain to their full participation (Warner & Wexler 1998) in decisions on patient management.

Lack of communication, exclusion from the decision-making process, an unclear role within 'alien' hospital settings and processes, and uncertain relationships with nursing staff are recurrent themes (Walker & Dewar 2001). Time and staff constraints often mean it is the carer who must initiate contact with nursing staff, though it is they that are usually on unfamiliar territory and unsure of hospital processes. Family meetings may seem like *fait accomplis* conducted by disinterested clinicians in the busy hospital environment with pagers bleeping and constant interruptions.

Early focus on establishment of a key contact, explanation of ward processes, a sharing of information and planning, in a protected time-slot, would do much to empower carers in hospitals. The involvement of patients and carers in hospital discharge procedures has been at the core of NHS policy since 1989 (DoH 1989), though difficulties with inadequate or conflicting communication, assumptions that patient–carer needs are synonymous and a lack of consultation on timing of discharge are persisting causes of dissatisfaction (Godfrey & Moore 1996, Proctor et al 2001).

Rural carers: a special consideration
Rural carers are a special consideration, given that up to a million carers may be living in rural areas in England (Office of National Statistics, 2001 census).

The Carers UK website states:

'Carers in rural areas have the same needs as carers elsewhere. However, the rural setting in which they live means they face extra barriers of physical and social isolation. Additional problems include: lack of services available; lack of specialist services; lack of respite; difficulty in accessing medical support;

isolation and [lack of] companionship, lack of privacy; [lack of] information; lack of alternatives to family care; poverty and additional costs of living in a rural area; transport; employment'
(http://www.carersuk.org/policyandpractice/Ruralcarers)

The Rural White Paper, *Our Countryside: the Future*, provides an undertaking to use creative approaches to deliver services to carers in rural areas, 'using new technology, sharing buildings, using mobile units and offering appointment bookings that take account of the distance people need to travel' (DEFRA 2002).

FINANCIAL ADVICE

Those who are already carers and people taking on a carer's role will frequently be unsure about financial entitlements. While the matter is usually referred to the medical social worker, physicians in geriatric medicine should be aware of current legislation – or at least where to source it rapidly (http://www.dss.gov.uk).

In the UK, money benefits to carers are administered by the Department for Work and Pensions via the Carer's Allowance Unit. Currently, the carers' allowance is aimed at carers on low incomes who spend at least 35 hours a week caring for a disabled person who is in receipt of the attendance allowance or disability living allowance. It is means tested and excludes savings (less than £82 per week is the current threshold for paid work) and other benefits may be affected. It is not payable to those in full-time education (more than 21 hours of tuition per week) but since 2002 people over 65 years can qualify for the carers' allowance and the allowance can be paid to more than one person in a household, e.g. a couple caring for one another. The allowance may stop if a person is admitted to hospital but can continue for up to 12 weeks in some circumstances and be paid for up to 4 weeks respite in a 26-week period. (A similar allowance and a separate carers' benefit, respite care grant and dependant relative tax credit are payable in the republic of Ireland.)

- While benefits may change, the most important advice for carers is to apply early
- Asking about allowances should be a key part of the social history in geriatric medicine.

Internet resources	
http://www.carers.gov.uk	Department of Health
http://www.carers.org	Princess Royal Trust for Carers
http://www.carersireland.com	Carers Association (Republic of Ireland)
http://carersuk.org/Home	Carers support group
http://dss.gov.uk	Benefits advice (UK)
http://kingsfund.org.uk	King's Fund Carers Project
http://oasis.gov.ie	Benefits advice (Republic of Ireland)

RECOGNITION OF ETHNIC FACTORS

Independent reports commissioned by the Department of Health have recognized the failure to provide culturally sensitive care to Afro-Caribbean and Asian communities. It is only in recent years that the provision of such care to other groups in England (such as the Irish) has even been recognized (Alexander 1999). However, reducing health disadvantage and social exclusion through the promotion of culturally sensitive services in collaboration with communities is now at the core of government policy (DoH 2001b).

Offspring, particularly daughters, from some ethnic backgrounds may be under great social expectation within communities to adopt the role of carer to an older parent. Because of this, stigmatization of disability, language barriers or a cultural

suspicion of service intrusion, they may be very vulnerable in their role and unaware or unwilling to seek the statutory and voluntary support available to them (Katbamna et al 2004). Providing 'culturally sensitive' care to ethnic families must encompass respect for individuality and spirituality, create mutual understanding and maintain dignity (Clegg 2003) (see Ch. 12 on ethnic elders). In addition there must be clear presentation of information that avoids jargon. The availability of interpreter services can be very useful.

CARER LEGISLATION

There has been increasing statutory recognition of carers' rights and aspirations in recent years in line with UK government policy. While a full explanation of all the relevant legislation is beyond the remit of this chapter, the reader is directed to the following summary of relevant legislation (http://www.carersuk.org/policyand practice/CarersEqualOpportunitiesAct).

The Disabled Persons (Services, Consultation and Representation) Act 1986

Section 4 states that local authorities have a duty to assess a disabled person for services on request of that person or the carer.

Section 8 states that 'when assessing the needs of a disabled person for services ... the local authority must have regard to the ability of a carer, who is providing "a substantial amount of care on a regular basis" to continue to provide such care on a regular basis'.

The Carers (Recognition and Services) Act 1995

This Act asserts the right of all carers who provide regular and substantial care to a full and comprehensive needs assessment, in order to allow them to continue in their caring role.

The Carers Equal Opportunities Act 2004

This Act recognizes the duty of local authorities to tell carers of their right to a carer's assessment.

Section 2 ensures that in the carer's assessment, importance is attached to whether the carer works, wishes to work, is taking courses or wishes to participate in any courses and/or any other leisure activities. In addition, local authorities are provided with 'new powers to enlist the help of housing, health, education and other local authorities in providing support for carers'.

CONCLUSION

Informal care is one of the cornerstones of maintaining health and function in many older adults' and many older adults are themselves carers. Support for carers, meeting their needs and building partnership must be addressed within the holistic model of geriatric medicine. Carers are also a vital economic resource to our health service and as such should be protected with careful investment and appropriate statutory support.

REFERENCES

Alexander Z 1999 Department of Health: study of Black, Asian and ethnic minority issues. The Stationery Office, London

Bywaters P, Harris A 1998 Supporting carers: is practice still sexist? Health and Social Care in the Community 6:458–463

Carers National Association 1998 Ignored and invisible. Carers National Association, London

Clegg A 2003 Older Asian patient and carer perceptions of culturally sensitive care in a community hospital setting. Journal of Clinical Nursing 12:283–290

DEFRA 2002 Rural White Paper: Our coutryside: the future. Department for Environment, Food and Rural Affairs. Online. Available: http://www.defra.gov.uk

Department of Health 1989 Discharge of patients form hospital. HMSO, London

Department of Health 1995 The Carers (Recognition and Services) Act. HMSO, London

Department of Health 1998 A first class service: quality in the new NHS (White Paper). HMSO, London

Department of Health 2001a National Service Framework for older people: modern standards and service models. Department of Health, London

Department of Health 2001b Essence of care. The Stationery Office, London

Fahy M, Wald C, Walker Z et al 2003 Secrets and lies: the dilemma of disclosing the diagnosis to an adult with dementia. Age and Ageing 32:439–441

Godfrey M, Moore J 1996 In: Hospital discharge: user, carer and professional perspectives. The collaborative centre for priority services research, Nuffield Institute for Health, University of Leeds, Leeds

Guberman N, Nicholas E, Nolan P et al 2003 Impacts on practitioners of using research-based carer assessment tools: experiences from the UK, Canada and Sweden, with insights from Australia. Health and Social Care in the Community 11:345–355

Katbamna S, Ahmad W, Bhakta P et al 2004 Do they look after their own? Informal support for South Asian carers. Health and Social Care in the Community 12:398–406

Maguire C P, Kirby M, Coen R et al 1996 Family members' attitudes towards telling the patient with Alzheimer's disease the diagnosis. British Medical Journal 313:529–530

Nolan M R, Grant G 1989 Addressing the needs of informal carers: a neglected area of nursing practice. Journal of Advanced Nursing 14:950,961

Nolan M, Grant G, Keady J 1996 Family caregiving - the need for a multidimensional approach. In: Understanding family care: a multidimensional model of caring and coping. Open University Press, Bucks, p 3

Payne M 1995 The social work role in community care. In: Campling J (ed) Social work and community care. McMillan Press, Basingstoke, p 3

Proctor S, Wilcockson J, Pearson P et al 2001 Going home from hospital: the patient/carer dyad. Journal of Advanced Nursing 35:206–217

Ross L, Waterson J 1996 Risk for whom? Social work and people with physical disabilities. In: Kemshall H, Pritchard J (eds) Good practice in risk assessment and risk management. Jessica Kingsley, London, p 85

Seltzer M, Krauss M 2001 Quality of life of adults with mental retardation/developmental disabilities who live with family. Mental Retardation and Developmental Disabilities Research Reviews 7:105–114

Stroke Unit Trialists' Collaboration 2007 Organised inpatient (stroke unit) care for stroke (Cochrane Review). In: The Cochrane Library, Issue 4. Art. No.: CD000197. DOI: 10.1002/14651858.CD000197

Twigg J, Atkin K 1994 Carers perceived: Policy and practice in informal care. Open University Press, Bucks

Walker E, Dewar J 2001 How do we facilitate carers' involvement in decision making? Journal of Advanced Nursing 34:329–337

Warner L, Wexler S 1998 Eight hours a day and taken for granted? The Princess Royal Trust for Carers, London

SELF-ASSESSMENT QUESTION

1. Are the following statements true or false?
   a. Carers over 65 years are ineligible for the carers' allowance
   b. Communication and support for carers can improve clinical outcomes
   c. Informal care is worth £50 million annually to the UK exchequer
   d. Carers have the right to a full assessment under the 1990 National Health Service and Community Care Act
   e. Older carers generally experience more stress than younger carers

Chapter **12**

Ethnic elders

Eric White and C. P. Wilkinson

INTRODUCTION

Ethnicity as a concept may be considered to relate to skin colour, culture, belief or religion, area of origin, or behaviour (Ebrahim 1996). The Office of Population Censuses and Surveys employs a definition based upon skin colour (ONS 2005). Ethnic minorities do not form a homogeneous group. Although genetic differences such as skin colour may seem obvious, more genetic diversity exists between individuals than between races. This diversity is increased further by social and economic factors. The cultural, social, educational and religious backgrounds of ethnic minority groups differ as widely as does the history and circumstances of their migration. Ethnic elders may endure multiple disadvantages, termed by researchers as 'jeopardy', which includes old age, racism, poverty and ill health.

HISTORY AND DEMOGRAPHY

Non-white people have settled in the UK in substantial numbers from as long ago as the early 18th century. Many came to the aid of Britain during World War 2 and many settled, mostly in ports. Since the war, there has been a steady increase in Britain's ethnic minority population, initially driven by government policy to remedy post-war employment gaps. This period was heralded by the arrival of the *SS Windrush* in 1948 which brought work-seeking black Carribean migrants. The black Carribeans remained the majority migrant group up until the early 1960s. From 1955 onwards, South Asian immigration began, particularly from Sylhet in Bangladesh and from the Punjab and Gujurat in India. The 1960s saw an influx of Cypriots, followed by displaced Kenyan Asians in 1963. Political pressure caused immigration to tail off in the 1980s, though recent crises throughout the world have led to higher numbers of people seeking refuge in Britain, notably from Asia and Africa.

Only since 1991 have ethnicity data been collected as part of the UK Census (Hoong Sin 2004). In 2001, 4.6 million people (7.9% of the population) belonged to a non-white ethnic group. The largest ethnic minority group was Indian (23% of the ethnic population, 2% of the entire population), followed by the Pakistani, mixed and black Caribbean groups, each constituting about 1% of the population (ONS 2005). Immigrant groups are younger than the host population, but there are differences in age structure between the ethnic minority groups (see Table 12.1) (ONS 2005). Black Caribbeans were the oldest group, reflecting their earlier arrival in the UK. Indian Asians were the next oldest, followed by the Chinese, 'other' Asians and Pakistanis. The mixed race group was the youngest in age structure. These age structure differences are expected to diminish with time (ONS 2005). The coming two decades will see rapid ageing of established ethnic minority groups

Table 12.1 Age structures of the UK population by ethnic group in 2001 (ONS 2005)

	Under 16 years %	16–64 years %	65 years and over %	All people (thousands)
White	19	64	17	52 481
Mixed	50	47	3	674
All Asian or Asian British	29	66	5	2329
All black or black British	26	68	6	1148
Chinese	19	76	5	243
Other ethnic groups	19	78	3	229
All ethnic groups	20	64	16	57 104

in the UK, as those arriving in their twenties and thirties in the 1950s and 1960s reach older age. This fact has received relatively little attention from social researchers and policy makers, which is surprising considering the potential effect this will have on service design.

GEOGRAPHIC DISTRIBUTION

Early migrants were economically motivated, and concentrated themselves in the large conurbations of London and Birmingham. They were also drawn to metal manufacturing in the Midlands, and to textile areas in the North West and West Yorkshire (ONS 2005). In 2001, 78% of black Africans, 61% of black Caribbeans and 54% of Bangladeshis were living in London. Other ethnic groups were more dispersed: 19% of Pakistanis were living in London, 20% in Yorkshire and the Humber, and 16% were living in the North West (ONS 2005). The Chinese were the most dispersed of the ethnic minority populations (Hoong Sin 2004).

RELIGIOUS AND SOCIAL DIFFERENCES AMONG ETHNIC GROUPS

Enduring a hospital admission when unwell is a challenge regardless of ethnic group. An appreciation of differences encountered in religious and social attitudes among ethnic groups is essential in order that compassionate clinical care may be delivered. Table 12.2 summarizes the main issues

that should be borne in mind, though this focus does not consider Christianity or Judaism.

SPECIAL CONSIDERATIONS

HEALTHCARE DURING RAMADAN

Religious rules are relaxed for Muslims who are ill. The Qur'an states that those with acute or chronic conditions are not required to fast during Ramadan (Ethnicity Online 2003). The clinician should appreciate that, during this period, some out-patients may miss appointments as they may wish to spend time with family and community. Also, Muslims on daily medication may not take oral tablets during the day, which may lead to a deterioration in their condition (Ethnicity Online 2003). The effect of the fast on those with diabetes may also cause problems. The managing clinician should anticipate these problems and act with due care.

RESUSCITATION AND ISLAM

The basis of the Islamic faith is the submission to the will of Allah; only Allah can decide the timing of death. Medical staff may be regarded as instruments of His will (Ethnicity Online 2003). Muslim families may be deeply distressed by a 'do not resuscitate' order as it implies that not all life-sustaining treatment is being offered. This must be considered and handled with great care and sensitivity. The local Imam may be of help in difficult situations.

Table 12.2   Religious and social differences among ethnic groups

	Practical issues	Care of the dying	Rituals after death	Dietary restrictions
Sikhism	■ The 'five Ks' of Sikhism include uncut hair, a wooden comb, a steel bracelet, a sharp knife, and special long undergarments ■ Females should be well covered; backless hospital gowns are inappropriate ■ Physical contact between unmarried women and men is forbidden and should be avoided if possible ■ Some older Sikhs may fast during the full moon or for certain holidays	■ Families may expect to be involved with the care of their relatives ■ The dying may receive comfort from readings from the Guru Granth Sahib, read by a family member or reader from the Sikh temple	■ Remove drains and other tubes where possible ■ Use disposable gloves to avoid direct contact with the body ■ Do not remove any of the 'five Ks' ■ The family may wish to wash and dress the body ■ Cremated or buried within 24 hours wearing the 5 colours of Sikhism ■ Post-mortem is acceptable if required to determine the cause of death ■ Organ donation may be considered acceptable if it is for the good of another human life*	■ The eating of halal or kosher meat is prohibited ■ Very few eat beef, and many are vegetarian ■ Alcohol, tobacco and other narcotics are prohibited, if strict
Hinduism	■ Females should be well covered; backless hospital gowns are inappropriate ■ Men and boys wear a sacred thread ■ Preference to wash in running water ■ Some may choose to fast when ill to restore health and balance ■ Some may see illness as a punishment for previous bad conduct	■ The family need to be informed if the relative is likely to die, so that required ceremonies can be performed ■ The family may prefer their dying relative to be accompanied at all times, so allow flexible visiting ■ May receive comfort from readings from the Hindu holy books (Vedas) ■ May request a Hindu priest for holy rites	■ Guidance from the family is advised regarding touching the body after death ■ The body should not be washed by healthcare staff ■ The body should be wrapped in a plain sheet ■ Rituals required by family to prepare body need adequate space and privacy ■ Open grief is expected	■ Most are strictly vegetarian ■ Those who eat meat avoid beef, as the cow is a sacred animal ■ Alcohol is not permitted ■ Tobacco is regarded as a harmful narcotic

Table 12.2 Religious and social differences among ethnic groups (Cont'd)

	Practical issues	Care of the dying	Rituals after death	Dietary restrictions
Hinduism (Cont'd)	■ Older Hindus may fast during the full moon	■ May tie a thread (which should not be removed) around the neck or wrist ■ If no family member is available, a Hindu priest should be contacted ■ Ideally, death should take place at home	■ Post-mortem is considered disrespectful, but if legally required it should be done as soon as possible ■ Cremation is traditional ■ No specific objections to organ donation*	
Islam	■ Illness may be perceived as a test of faith to be endured ■ Older Muslims may refuse pain relief ■ May wish to pray in hospital – require privacy ■ Women should be clothed from head to foot except for the hands and face ■ Physical contact is forbidden between unmarried men and women ■ Should not be placed in mixed wards if at all possible ■ Muslims wash in running water, and require to do so before prayer ■ Avoid unnecessary physical contact whenever possible	■ Believe that time of death is predetermined by God's will, and causing or hastening death is strictly prohibited ■ A 'do not resuscitate' policy may cause distress as it implies not everything is done to sustain life. Where possible seek advice of the local Imam (see text) ■ Many visitors are common, and they may wish to assist in the care of the patient ■ May wish to turn the bed so the feet face towards Makkah (Mecca) – south east in the UK	■ The body should not be touched by non-Muslims (except with disposable gloves) ■ The head should be turned to Makkah – south east in the UK ■ The body should be covered with a white cloth ■ The body is usually washed by a family member of the same sex ■ Relatives are duty bound to visit the bereaved, so many visitors should be expected ■ The family usually carry out rites but the local mosque may help	■ No food derived from pork ■ All meat should be halal (killed according to Islamic law) ■ Fish with fins and scales acceptable ■ Alcohol, tobacco and narcotics are prohibited ■ Ramadan is the fasting period in the 9th month of the Muslim year ■ Abstinence is required between dawn and sunset ■ Ramadan prohibits the intake of anything by any route, including injections, tablets, intravenous drips and nasal sprays

Continued

Table 12.2 Religious and social differences among ethnic groups *(Cont'd)*

	Practical issues	Care of the dying	Rituals after death	Dietary restrictions
Islam *(Cont'd)*			■ Post-mortems are forbidden unless there is an overwhelming legal need (may require discussion with the family and Imam) ■ Burial within 24 hours ■ Organ donation is much debated by Islamic scholars, though may be permitted if stated in the Will, and if intended for another Muslim*	■ Muslims who are acutely ill or have a chronic condition are permitted not to fast
Buddhism	■ A private area may be appreciated for meditation	■ Privacy for prayer and mantras should be offered ■ Believe that dying is an ongoing natural cycle	■ Belief that it may take up to 3 days for the consciousness to leave the body ■ The body should be moved to an empty room, where mantras can be chanted and prayers read ■ Cremation may be arranged by monks ■ No fundamental objection to post-mortem examination ■ Organ donation is still under debate	■ Buddhists should not be responsible for the death of any living organism, therefore offer vegetarian meals ■ No strict prohibition of alcohol

*The NHS Transplant Agency has a series of leaflets for religious groups on organ donation

PHYSICAL HEALTH OF ETHNIC MINORITIES

The 1999 Health Survey for England (DoH 2001) focused on the health of minority ethnic groups. This survey combined questionnaire-based interviews with physical measurements and blood sample analysis. It provides an extensive insight into the health of minority ethnic groups. Ethnic minorities were more likely to rate their health as 'bad' or as 'very bad' compared with the general population, except for Chinese people who reported lower levels of poor health. Higher rates of GP contact were observed in ethnic minority groups, again with the exception of the Chinese group who had lower rates.

Physical activity was lower in Asian and black Caribbean groups than in the general population, and although obesity (as measured by body mass index) was generally lower, central obesity (as measured by waist–hip ratio) was higher in South Asians.

Compared with the general population, smoking was more common in Bangladeshi and black Caribbean men. There were similar smoking rates among Pakistani and Indian men, and lower rates among women. South Asians and black Caribbeans were less likely to drink alcohol, with very few South Asian women exceeding the recommended intake.

CARDIOVASCULAR DISEASE, DIABETES MELLITUS AND OBESITY

Striking differences exist in the prevalence of cardiovascular disease, both between ethnic minority groups and the general population, and within the ethnic minority population itself (Chaturvedi 2003). Morbidity and mortality from coronary heart disease is increased in South Asians, but is lower in African Caribbeans. Stroke is more common in South Asians and African Caribbeans. There is no evidence of delayed presentation or of poorer understanding of the significance of symptoms in South Asians, but treatment may be delayed due to communication difficulties. The observed increase in coronary heart disease in South Asians is not fully explained by classic risk factors such as smoking, hypercholesterolaemia and hypertension. It is likely that insulin resistance, characterized by glucose intolerance, abnormal lipid profile and central obesity is important. Prevention should still focus on the conventional risk factors of smoking cessation, the early detection and management of diabetes, control of cholesterol, blood pressure, obesity, and by the encouragement of physical exercise. Obesity is an increasing problem in all groups, and dietary advice must be relevant to the group concerned. Facilities for female-only exercise will be important for some groups. The possibility that certain drugs may be more or less effective in different ethnic groups needs further work. Anti-hypertensive therapy may show differing efficacy in different ethnic groups but this does not affect the choice of therapy in the elderly (NIHCE 2006).

MENTAL HEALTH OF ETHNIC MINORITIES

The prevalence of dementia is raised in African Caribbeans, possibly related to vascular disease. The prevalence of depression in ethnic elders is less clear. Somatization may be more common in South Asians but the evidence for this is inconclusive (Hussian & Cochrane 2004). Language and cultural barriers can lead to misinterpretation of symptoms causing diagnostic errors, particularly where untrained interpreters are used. Standard screening tools for dementia such as the Mini Mental State Examination (MMSE) may also be subject to educational and cultural bias, though the MMSE has been adapted for use in a number of South Asian groups. The clock drawing test does appear not to have cultural or literacy bias (Parker & Philp 2004). Screening tools such as the Hospital Anxiety and Depression Score and the Geriatric Depression Score have also been adapted for use with specific ethnic groups.

There have been calls for the development of separate psychiatric services for ethnic minority groups, but the Royal College of Psychiatrists advocates that acute services remain within mainstream psychiatric services. The College does recommend that services providing continuing care in the community should be developed for the appropriate user group (Royal College of Psychiatrists 2001).

LONG-TERM AND PALLIATIVE CARE

There is a common belief that ethnic minority elders are cared for within the extended family network. While this may be true in many cases, 38% of black Caribbean households contain only one person, a similar proportion to the white British population. By contrast, only 9% of Bangladeshi households contain one person. One in ten people from a white British background provide informal care. A similar proportion of people do so from an Indian background, though slightly less Pakistanis and Bangladeshis do so. Minority ethnic groups are younger in age than the general population: after allowing for this, the South Asians – particularly Bangladeshis and Pakistanis – are twice as likely to provide informal care. Relatively few South Asians reside in care homes. Social services and care homes face similar challenges as hospitals in both ensuring the delivery of best quality care and the provision of support to ethnic elders and their carers that meet their linguistic, cultural and religious needs.

In the past, palliative care services have largely been centred on care for patients with cancer. In common with the general older population, most ethnic elders will die from non-malignant diseases such as cardiac and renal failure. There is often a poor understanding of what is important in allowing a 'good death' among different ethnic groups, with health and social care staff being insensitive to their religious and cultural needs.

THE WAY FORWARD

A greater understanding of the linguistic, cultural and religious needs of ethnic elders should ensure improved delivery of care. Hospitals must provide adequate interpreter services to avoid reliance on family members, particularly children. Future trends in the ethnic composition of medical staff should improve their level of understanding. (In 2003, 30% of medical and dental students came from an ethnic minority background, two-thirds being of Asian origin.) The uneven geographic distribution of ethnic groups places a responsibility on health and social services to understand their local population and to engage with them to identify what kind of services are required and how they are best provided.

Key points

- Ethnic minority groups living in the UK are a diverse population in terms of their migratory history, religion, culture, language, social outlook, age structure and geographic distribution.
- The coming two decades will see rapid ageing of established ethnic minority groups in the UK.
- Disease patterns differ between the ethnic groups but the presentation of disease in individuals is usually similar once language and cultural factors have been considered.
- Healthcare and social service provision for ageing ethnic minority groups are increasingly important, and should be designed to serve populations at local level.

REFERENCES

Chaturvedi N 2003 Ethnic differences in cardiovascular disease. Heart 89:681–686

Department of Health 2001 Health survey for England: the health of ethnic groups 1999. HMSO, London. Online. Available: http://www.doh.gov.uk

Ebrahim S 1996 Caring for older people: ethnic elders. British Medical Journal 313:610–613

Ethnicity Online 2003 Introduction to Islam. Norfolk, Suffolk and Cambridgeshire NHS Workforce Development Confederation. Online. Available: http://www.ethnicityonline.net/islam.htm

Hoong Sin C 2004 Sampling minority ethnic older people in Britain. Ageing and Society 24:257–277

Hussian F, Cochrane R 2004 Depression in South Asian women living in the UK: a review of the literature with implications for service provision. Transcultural Psychiatry 41:253–270

National Institute for Health and Clinical Excellence 2006 Hypertension – management of hypertension in adults in primary care. NIHCE, London. Online. Available: http://www.nice.org.uk

Office for National Statistics 2005 Social trends 35. ONS, London. Online. Available: http://www.statistics.gov.uk

Parker C, Philp I 2004 Screening for cognitive impairment among older people in black and minority ethnic groups. Age and Ageing 33:447–452

Royal College of Psychiatrists 2001 Psychiatric services for Black and minority ethnic elders (Council Report CR103). Royal College of Psychiatrists, London

SELF-ASSESSMENT QUESTIONS

1. Are the following true or false?
   a. The British government actively encouraged immigration in post-war Britain
   b. The largest ethnic minority group in 2001 was the black Caribbean one
   c. Ethnic minority groups tend to be younger than the general population and all have similar age structures
   d. Ethnic minority groups are evenly distributed throughout the country

2. Are the following true or false?
   a. Mixed sex wards are acceptable to most groups
   b. Healthcare staff should wash before direct contact with a deceased Sikh patient's body
   c. The direction of Mecca in the UK is south east
   d. The Mini Mental State Examination is validated for use in older people from all ethnic minority groups

PART 2

Core topics

Chapter 13

Urinary incontinence

Shilpa Raje and Adrian Wagg

INTRODUCTION

The current definition of urinary incontinence is a demonstrable involuntary loss of urine (Abrams et al 2002). This takes no account of the severity of the complaint or gives a time frame for its occurrence. Most studies show a greater prevalence in women and an increase in association with greater age. Estimates of prevalence vary widely according to definitions used and the population surveyed (Fig. 13.1). About 24% of the over 65s (who comprise 16% of the current UK population) will have a clinically significant bladder problem. The proportion is highest in old people in care homes.

Most elderly people do not have 'normal' lower urinary tract function: data from intensive testing of asymptomatic elderly people suggest that only 18% of individuals fall into this category (Resnick et al 1995). The physiological changes leading to this observation have been well described (Wagg & Malone-Lee 1998), and are summarized in Box 13.1. Elderly people experience the same bladder problems as other adults but their ability to respond and to compensate for problems which a younger adult may find trivial is often impaired. Concomitant disease and drug therapy, in particular, may make an elderly person incontinent.

Although urinary incontinence is not life-threatening, the associated impairment of quality of life, social isolation, depression, increased urinary tract and skin infection and increased likelihood of institutionalization have been consistently reported (Brown et al 2000, Coyne et al 2003, Diefenbach et al 2005, Hu et al 2003, Steers & Lee 2001, Wagner et al 2002). However, there is much evidence of under-diagnosis and assessment and a heavy reliance upon containment as the main method of management.

RISK FACTORS

PREGNANCY AND CHILDBIRTH

Any pregnancy lasting over 20 weeks is associated with some increased risk of urinary incontinence (Viktrup et al 1992). Women who develop incontinence during pregnancy may be at increased risk of developing incontinence as they age. Childbirth is a much stronger risk factor for the development of stress incontinence and the risk increases in association with the number of deliveries. There is an association between denervation injury and the subsequent development of incontinence (Foldspang et al 1999, Mallet et al 1994, Thom & Brown 1998).

OBESITY

There is good evidence for a positive association of stress urinary incontinence (SUI) and body mass (Kolbl & Riss 1988, Mommsen & Foldspang 1994). In community surveys, more women with incontinence reported themselves as obese, or being too heavy for their height (Roe & Doll 1999). However, the evidence that weight reduction

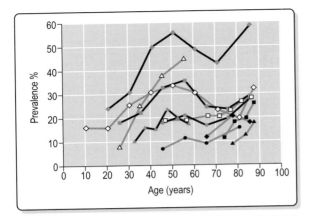

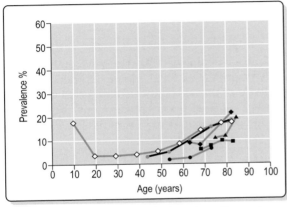

Figure 13.1 The prevalence of urinary incontinence in women and men in association with age.

<table>
<tr><th colspan="2">Box 13.1   Physiological changes in lower urinary tract function in the elderly</th></tr>
<tr><th>Decreased</th><th>Increased</th></tr>
<tr><td>Sensation of filling</td><td>Urinary frequency</td></tr>
<tr><td>Speed of contraction
of detrusor</td><td>Prevalence of post-void
residual volumes</td></tr>
<tr><td>Pelvic floor muscle
bulk and tone</td><td>Outflow tract
obstruction</td></tr>
<tr><td>Sphincteric 'resistance'</td><td></td></tr>
<tr><td>Urinary flow rate</td><td></td></tr>
<tr><td>Bladder capacity</td><td></td></tr>
</table>

might be able to correct some of this disadvantage is limited to two studies of women who had undergone surgery for their obesity with consequent massive weight reduction (Brieger & Korda 1992, Bump et al 1992, Deitel et al 1988). In women losing at least 50% of their excess weight, the prevalence of urinary incontinence was reduced by 50% (Chiarelli & Brown 1999). A recent study in 10 women has suggested that moderate weight loss may be of benefit (Subak et al 2005).

MENOPAUSE

The prevalence of SUI increases around the time of the menopause, but the role of oestrogen loss and any association with SUI is inconsistent. There are no data to suggest that oestrogen replacement leads to an improvement in the condition.

SMOKING

An association with both SUI and urge urinary incontinence (UUI) with cigarette smoking has been identified for both men and women. Smokers are 1.9 times more likely to suffer from incontinence (Kosimaki et al 1998). As with other adverse effects of smoking, this association weakened following cessation of smoking and appeared to reach baseline after 40 years of abstinence. Smoking-related cough is thought to be a precipitating factor in the development of SUI (Bump & McClish 1992). There are, however, no prospective intervention trials of smoking cessation on improving bladder symptoms. Clearly, smoking should be discouraged in view of the cardiovascular risk, regardless of its effect upon lower urinary tract function.

CONSTIPATION

One community-based study in women of 60 years and older has examined the relationship between self-reported urinary incontinence and constipation. Subjects who reported urinary incontinence were more likely to report constipation. A relationship between straining and impaired function of rectal emptying is hypothesized but there are no studies which systematically evaluate the effect of relieving constipation on urinary incontinence (Lubowski et al 1988). Faecal impaction can lead to urinary retention, and there have been conflicting reports of an association between incontinence and constipation (Diokno et al 1990, Nygaard & Lemke 1996).

CAFFEINE

Dietary advice regarding the restriction of caffeine is often given. There is evidence that theoretically supports its association with bladder overactivity (Arya et al 2000, Creighton & Stanton 1990). Clinical trials have provided conflicting evidence on which to base this practice. In trials of varying quality, most of which assessed fluid caffeine intake, no sustained clinical benefit has been found (Brown et al 1996, Bryant et al 2002, Swithinbank et al 2005, Tomlinson et al 1999). However, some patients find benefit from restricting the intake of caffeinated beverages and there is no harm in suggesting a trial of withdrawal.

DIETARY FACTORS

The Leicester MRC incontinence study has reported consistent associations between urinary incontinence (UI) and a diet poor in vegetables, fibre, white meat and high in fizzy drinks. There are no interventional studies which explore underlying hypotheses of causation (Dallosso et al 2003).

FUNCTIONAL AND COGNITIVE IMPAIRMENT

Several studies show the prevalence of UI to be higher in long-term care facilities compared to those at home, with estimates from around the world between 23% and 72%, with a median of around 55% (Aggazzotti et al 2000). This reflects the greater average age and degree of frailty of long-term care residents. The presence of UI in itself is associated with an increased likelihood of institutionalization, independent of age or other co-morbid conditions (Thom et al 1997).

Functional and cognitive impairment are associated with an increasing prevalence and severity of UI. In one study of nursing home residents, the odds ratio (OR) for incontinence increased from those requiring no help with mobility to needing support (1.8), depending on carers (5.6), and being wheelchair- or bed-bound (7.4) (Hunskaar et al 1998). Urinary incontinence may be a consequence of difficulties getting to the bathroom; there are data showing the association of increasing physical and functional impairment with UI

and also the effect of underlying systemic illness such as stroke.

Studies of nursing home residents consistently support a causative link between dementia and UI. Odds ratios of 1.2, 4.0, and 12.6 have been found for mild, moderate and severe dementia (Skelly & Flint 1995).

ASSESSMENT AND INVESTIGATION

Physical examination

For women, an examination of the perineum in order to look for vaginal atrophy and co-existing prolapse should be performed. This can be combined with a cough test, either in the supine or standing position, to look for stress-induced leakage. Both men and women should undergo a digital rectal examination, to rule out faecal loading as a cause of voiding difficulty or increased frequency and to assess prostate size in men. An abdominal examination to rule out retention of urine should also be carried out.

Urinalysis

This will identify a range of conditions that cause urinary symptoms, such as glycosuria and urinary tract infection. Conversely, infection is probably overtreated in the elderly. Asymptomatic bacteriuria may be present in up to 20% of older women. Treatment of 'infection' when in a patient with urinary incontinence who has had no worsening of symptoms will not improve the condition.

Post-micturition volume

It is common to find ineffective voiding with a post-micturition residual volume in elderly people; a volume of 200 mL is not unusual. It is important to exclude urinary retention or a significant post-void residual volume (PVR) before giving any treatment, as antimuscarinic agents can potentially worsen this (though this is rare, and the increase in PVR is seldom clinically significant). PVR of 300 mL or more is likely to require drainage; its existence will contribute to urinary frequency. In men, it is important to recognize obstructive uropathy as urinary retention can lead to renal failure, which is potentially reversible. In general, a PVR which is asymptomatic (in terms of recurrent infection) or not associated with renal impairment can safely be left alone. Treatment is by clean intermittent catheterization; if this cannot be done by the patient, an informal or formal carer may be taught how to do this.

Bladder diary or frequency–volume tick chart

Diaries can give an impression of the patient's bladder habits. They aid diagnosis but are often difficult to obtain for many frail patients. Three days' recording provides clinically useful information.

Cystometry

Whenever there is doubt about the diagnosis, or when the patient has not responded to initial therapy as expected, then multi-channel cystometry should be performed (with the exception of flow rates for men with suspected bladder outflow tract obstruction). Under current recommendations, this should also be done before surgical treatment in women.

Medication review

In the UK, people over 60 years are prescribed an average of 37.2 prescription medicines per year (DoH 2005). Most of these drugs increase the risk of incontinence through effects on fluid retention or fluid output, or as a result of increasing confusion (Box 13.2). Adjustment or removal of offending medication can result in clinical improvement.

Box 13.2   Drugs predisposing older people to urinary incontinence

- Diuretics
- Calcium channel antagonists
- Anticholinergics (including antihistamines, antipsychotics, antispasmodics, anti-parkinsonian agents)
- Alpha-adrenoreceptor antagonists
- Non-steroidal antiinflammatory drugs
- H_2 antagonists
- Benzodiazepines and neuroleptics
- SSRIs
- ACE inhibitors

INCONTINENCE COMPLEXES

Overactive bladder (OAB) syndrome

This is the commonest cause of incontinence in older people. It is a clinically defined syndrome of urinary frequency and urgency with or without urgency incontinence and frequently with nocturia (Abrams et al 2002). Other lower urinary tract pathology causing similar symptoms (infection, stones, tumour) should be excluded before making the diagnosis. In most surveys, one-third of people with the syndrome are incontinent of urine (Milsom et al 2001). The individual symptoms are:

Urinary frequency

The upper limit of 'normal' frequency of micturition is 8/24 h, but it is not until frequency reaches over 12 that impairment in quality of life can be measured. Urinary frequency varies in association with fluid intake and the influence of medications on the lower urinary tract. Some older people restrict the amount of fluids they take for fear of urinary leakage when outside and yet others adopt rigid drinking habits, which promote excessive intake. Although there is no published evidence on the effect of fluid manipulation, alteration of excesses would seem sensible. Knowledge of fluid intake and voiding habits can result in an improvement in symptoms (Griffiths et al 1993).

Nocturia

This is the complaint where the individual has to wake up at night one or more times to void. Nocturia has only relatively recently been recognized as a separate entity within the lower urinary tract symptom complex (van Kerrebroeck et al 2002). Although there are limited data on the frequency of voiding and volume voided nocturnally across all age groups, the prevalence in people at home has been measured and it is typically present in > 50% of both men and women aged > 60 years (Hennessy & Shen 1986). The prevalence increases with age such that the vast majority of any population of men and women of 80 years and over will rise at least once at night to empty their bladder. The bother associated with the symptom increases in association with the number of nocturnal voids (Lose et al 2001, Lundgren

Table 13.1 Drugs for overactive bladder syndrome		
Compound	Specific evidence of efficacy in older people	Remarks
Oxybutynin IR	Yes	Useful prn for occasional control
Oxybutynin ER	Yes	Reduced side-effects
Oxybutynin transdermal	No*	Reduced antimuscarinic side-effect Sensitivity to patch in 10%
Propiverine (tds)	No*	Has Ca^{++} blocking activity
Solifenacin	Yes	Long-acting M3 selectivity
Tolterodine IR	Yes	
Tolterodine ER	Yes	
Trospium chloride	No*	Quaternary ammonium salt – does not cross BBB

*Trials include older people, but no separate publication

2004, Sagnier et al 1994). Treatment is often difficult and depends upon the underlying cause. Because the definition of nocturia does not assign a cause, this needs to be defined and relevant medical conditions excluded before a lower urinary tract disorder is diagnosed. The use of evening diuretic, daytime recumbency and DDAVP have been shown to be effective in the management of nocturnal frequency and polyuria. Specific treatment for bladder outflow tract obstruction or OAB syndrome is of use in specific cases (Wagg et al 2005).

Urgency

This complaint of a sudden compelling desire to pass urine which is difficult to defer suggests an 'on' or 'off' phenomenon distinct from the normal sensation of urge, experienced as the bladder nears functional capacity. Urinary urgency may be the 'key' symptom of OAB (Sagnier et al 1995). In a large community survey the impact of urgency was the most bothersome symptom, outweighing frequency, incontinence and nocturia (Bertaccini et al 2001). Urgency is therefore the driving symptom of OAB syndrome which influences behavioral changes in patients with the problem.

TREATMENT

Following an assessment which leads to OAB being the most likely diagnosis, behavioural and lifestyle techniques (either alone or in combination with pharmacological therapy) may be beneficial for this complaint.

A combination of fluid management (including caffeine restriction if this is felt to be a trigger factor), bladder retraining and pelvic floor exercises (a pelvic floor contraction negatively inhibits detrusor contraction) are of benefit, even in frail older people (Burgio et al 1998, 2000, Jeffcoate & Francis 1966). Timed voiding, prompted voiding or regular toileting have been used for the management of incontinence in older frailer people (Schnelle et al 2002). These can be beneficial as a sole intervention and as an adjunct to other treatment. They are labour-intensive techniques and are difficult to maintain outside a clinical study.

Antimuscarinic medication is the current mainstay of drug therapy for the complaint. Each drug has relative benefits or disadvantages in some individuals, e.g. immediate release oxybutynin may be associated with cognitive dysfunction (Katz et al 1998) and should be avoided in those with impaired cognition. These drugs are effective in treating the symptoms of OAB, and the more modern drugs are better tolerated. However, whereas withdrawals occurring in trials are around 3–4%, the median duration of therapy in the community as monitored by repeat prescription is only 3 months, suggesting a more complex relationship between therapy and the disease. Currently available compounds are shown in Table 13.1.

For those more physically or cognitively disabled, there are few data upon which to base treatment recommendations. All drug therapy has

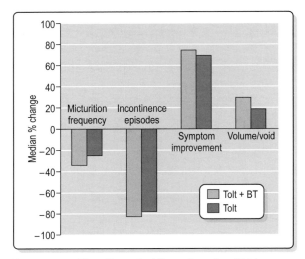

Figure 13.2 The effect of adding tolterodine (Tolt) to bladder retraining (BT) as treatment for the overactive bladder syndrome.

been shown to be effective in the absence of behavioural or lifestyle measures but should be used with caution (Chapple et al 2005). Prompted voiding regimens are effective in nursing homes but the addition of oxybutynin does not reduce the amount of input into continence care that residents require (Ouslander et al 1995). The effect of adding bladder retraining to tolterodine therapy (Mattiasson et al 2003) is shown in Figure 13.2.

Cognitively impaired individuals receiving cholinesterase inhibitors are more likely to receive antimuscarinic therapy for their incontinence. These drugs may still provide benefit for the incontinence without further impairing cognition but should be used with care (Gill et al 2005, Siegler & Reidenberg 2004).

STRESS URINARY INCONTINENCE

The involuntary loss of urine as a result of exertion is more common in women, where there appears to be a peak incidence after the menopause. Stress incontinence in men is usually as a result of prostatic surgery, the risk being highest following radical prostatectomy (Carlson & Nitti 2001). Usually diagnosis does not require complex investigation. The symptoms of SUI suggest the diagnosis with reasonable reliability, but careful phrasing of

questions to elicit symptoms is required. The precipitant feeling of urinary loss when an incompetent urethral sphincter reaches its limit may be interpreted as urgency, so a careful history is required.

Conservative therapies consist of both lifestyle and behavioural measures or pelvic floor muscle training (PFMT). A recent Cochrane review showed that PFMT appeared to be effective for adult women with stress or mixed urinary incontinence. PFMT was better than no treatment or placebo treatments. 'Intensive' appeared to be better than 'standard' programmes for women with SUI. There is insufficient evidence to determine if PFMT is better or worse than other treatments, such as electrical stimulation or weighted cones, or whether adding PFMT to other treatments is effective. On the available evidence, there is no benefit of biofeedback-assisted PFMT over PFMT alone (Hay-Smith et al 2001). There is no evidence that systemic or topical hormone replacement therapy (HRT) are of value in the treatment of UI, though topical oestrogen has a place in the prophylaxis of UTI and the amelioration of symptoms due to vaginal atrophy. Drug therapy for SUI consists of duloxetine, a serotonin noradrenaline (norepinephrine) reuptake inhibitor. The drug is more efficacious than placebo and, when used in combination, is more effective than PFMT alone. Its major side-effect, nausea, causes 24% of women to withdraw from therapy after 3 months (Ghoniem et al 2005). The incidence of nausea can be minimized by slowly increasing the dose.

Surgical therapy for SUI consists of urethral injectable materials, (such as silicone microparticles, hyaluronate, hydroxyapatite) which bulk out the urethral sphincter. The benefits tend to be transitory, but they can be done under local anaesthesia and, if necessary, repeated (Corcos et al 2005). The surgical approach has been revolutionized by the introduction of mid-urethral tapes of various types. There are data on efficacy for the tension-free vaginal tape lasting up to 8 years. This procedure has supplanted the colposuspension, performed either as an open or laparoscopic procedure (Ward et al 2002). Despite the prevalence of SUI in elderly people and the potential advantages of these minimally invasive procedures, older women are less likely to receive them.

MIXED SYMPTOMS

Up to 50% of women in late life present with frequency, urgency, urgency incontinence and SUI. A careful assessment will reveal the predominant feature and the most important symptom for the patient. Anti-muscarinic treatment can improve the urge component, and in some women, reduce stress incontinence. A trial of antimuscarinic therapy should be undertaken before surgical treatment (Khullar et al 2004).

CONTAINMENT

The introduction of formal assessment and treatment of continence problems should lead to a reduction in the indiscriminate use of pads and protective garments, external urine collection devices and indwelling urinary catheters. However, there will be a group of individuals for whom other techniques are either ineffective or inapplicable, who will benefit from the careful selection of such devices to contain their incontinence. There are many devices and pads available and few trials comparing these. The Continence Foundation hosts an up-to-date products directory which can aid choice (http://www.continence-foundation.org.uk).

Catheters may be used for management of intractable retention, voiding difficulty or incontinence if regular pad changes are uncomfortable or distressing to the patient. For mobile and dextrous patients, a catheter valve may be convenient and acceptable – this may take the form of a 'flip-flow', rather like the tap on a beer keg or wine box. This allows normal voiding into a lavatory and may be very acceptable to some people. A suprapubic catheter may be preferable to a urethral one for longer-term management, but there are no studies which confirm this (though they do avoid complications such as urethral erosion, and may be easier for staff to replace).

CONCLUSION

In 2001 the National Service Framework for Older People (DoH 2001) set the requirement that service providers should establish integrated continence services for older people by April 2004. There has been only limited action toward this and provision of services remains extremely patchy (Thomas 2003). A subsequent national audit in England and Wales demonstrated a wide variation in the structure and delivery of continence care (http://www.continenceaudit.rcplondon.ac.uk).

The assessment and management of urinary incontinence can be stimulating and rewarding for both doctor and patient. With the available evidence-based treatment options, there is no excuse for the therapeutic nihilism which has previously bedevilled this subject.

Key points

- Urinary incontinence is highly prevalent in older people.
- Physiological changes in the ageing lower urinary tract conspire to predispose older people to experience greater difficulty in maintaining continence.
- Urgency incontinence/detrusor overactivity is the commonest cause of UI in the elderly.
- A combination of behavioural and lifestyle changes in combination with pharmacological therapy is effective in treating UI in homebound adults.
- The increased availability of minimally-invasive surgical techniques should mean that older people will benefit.

REFERENCES

*** Essential reading; ** recommended reading; * interesting but not vital

Abrams P, Cardozo L, Fall M et al 2002 The standardisation of terminology of lower urinary tract function: Report from the standardisation subcommittee of the International Continence Society. Neurourology and Urodynamics 21:167–178 *

Aggazzotti G, Pesce F, Grassi D et al 2000 Prevalence of urinary incontinence among institutionalized patients: a cross-sectional epidemiologic study in a midsized city in northern Italy. Urology 56: 245–249 ***

Arya L A, Myers D L, Jackson N D 2000 Dietary caffeine intake and the risk for detrusor instability: a case control study. Obstetrics and Gynaecology 96:85–89 **

Bertaccini A, Vassallo F, Martino F et al 2001 Symptoms, bothersomeness and quality of life in patients with LUTS suggestive of BPH. European Urology 40(Suppl 1):13–18 **

Brieger G, Korda A 1992 The effect of obesity on the outcome of successful surgery for genuine stress incontinence. Australian and New Zealand Journal of Obstetrics and Gynaecology 32:71–72 *

Brown J S, Seeley D G, Fong J et al 1996 Urinary incontinence in older women: who is at risk? Obstetrics and Gynecology 87:715–721 **

Brown J S, Vittinghoff E, Wyman J F et al 2000 Urinary incontinence: does it increase risk for falls and fractures? Study of Osteoporotic Fractures Research Group. Journal of the American Geriatrics Society 48:721–725 **

Bryant C M, Dowell C J, Fairbrother G 2002 Caffeine reduction education to improve urinary symptoms. British Journal of Nursing 8:560–565 *

Bump R C, McClish D K 1992 Cigarette smoking and urinary incontinence in women. American Journal of Obstetrics and Gynecology 167:1213–1218 *

Bump R C, Sugerman J H, Fantl A et al 1992 Obesity and lower urinary tract function in women: effect of surgically induced weight loss. American Journal of Obstetrics and Gynecology 167:392–398 *

Burgio K L, Locher J L, Goode P S et al 1998 Behavioural versus drug treatment for urge urinary incontinence in older women. A randomized controlled trial. Journal of the American Medical Association 280: 1995–2000 **

Burgio K, Locher J L, Goode P S 2000 Combined behavioural and drug therapy for urge incontinence in older women. Journal of the American Geriatrics Society 48:370–374 *

Carlson K V, Nitti V W 2001 Prevention and management of incontinence following radical prostatectomy. Urological Clinics of North America 28: 595–612 *

Chapple C, Khullar V, Gabriel Z et al 2005 The effects of antimuscarinic treatments in overactive bladder: A systematic review and meta-analysis. European Urology 48:5–26 ***

Chiarelli P, Brown W J 1999 Leaking urine in Australian women: prevalence and associated conditions. Women and Health 29:1–13 **

Coyne K S, Zhou Z, Bhattacharyya S K et al 2003 The prevalence of nocturia and its effect on health-related quality of life and sleep in a community sample in the USA. BJU International 92:948–954 *

Creighton S M, Stanton S L 1990 Caffeine: does it affect your bladder? British Journal of Urology 66: 613–614 *

Dallosso H M, McGrother C W, Matthews R J et al 2003 The association of diet and other lifestyle factors with overactive bladder and stress incontinence: a longitudinal study in women. BJU International 92:69–77 ***

Deitel M, Stone E, Kassam H A et al 1988 Gynecologic-obstetric changes after loss of massive excess weight following bariatric surgery. Journal of the American College of Nutrition 7:147–153 *

Department of Health 2001 National Service Framework for Older People. HMSO, London ***

Department of Health 2005 Health and Social Care Information Centre statistical bulletin 2005/02/HSCIC. Online. Available: http://www.dh.gov.uk/assetRoot/04/11/58/87/04115887.pdf

Diefenbach K, Arold G, Wollny A et al 2005 Effects on sleep of anticholinergics used for overactive bladder treatment in healthy volunteers aged > or = 50 years. BJU International 95:346–349 *

Diokno A C, Brock B M, Herzog A R et al 1990 Medical correlates of urinary incontinence in the elderly. Urology 36:129–138 **

Foldspang A, Mommsen S, Djurhuus J C 1999 Prevalent urinary incontinence as a correlate of pregnancy, vaginal childbirth, and obstetric techniques. American Journal of Public Health 89:209–212 *

Ghoniem G M, Van Leeuwen J S, Elser D M et al 2005 A randomized controlled trial of duloxetine alone, pelvic floor muscle training alone, combined treatment and no active treatment in women with stress urinary incontinence. Journal of Urology 173: 1647–1653 **

Gill S S, Mandari M, Naglie G et al 2005 A prescribing cascade involving cholinesterase inhibitors and anticholinergic drugs. Archives of Internal Medicine 165:808–813 **

Griffiths D J, McCracken P N, Harrison G M et al 1993 Relationship of fluid intake to voluntary micturition and urinary incontinence in geriatric patients. Neurourology and Urodynamics 12:1–7 **

Hay-Smith E J C, Bo K, Berghmans L C M et al 2001 Pelvic floor muscle training for urinary incontinence in women. Cochrane Database of Systematic Reviews (withdrawn) ***

Hennessy C H, Shen J K M 1986 Sources of unreliability in the multidisciplinary assessment of the elderly. Evaluation Review 10:78 *

Hu T W, Wagner T H, Bentkover J D et al 2003 Estimated economic costs of overactive bladder in the United States. Urology 61:1123–1128 *

Hunskaar S, Ostbye T, Borrie M 1998 Prevalence of urinary incontinence in elderly Canadians with special emphasis on the association with dementia, ambulatory function, and institutionalization. Norwegian Journal of Epidemiology 8:177 *

Jeffcoate T N A, Francis W J A 1966 Urgency incontinence. American Journal of Obstetrics and Gynaecology 94:604 ***

Katz I R, Sands L P, Bilker W et al 1998 Identification of medications that cause cognitive impairment in older people: the case of oxybutynin chloride. Journal of the American Geriatrics Society 46:8–13 *

Khullar V, Hill S, Laval K U et al 2004 Treatment of urge-predominant mixed urinary incontinence with tolterodine extended release: a randomized, placebo-controlled trial. Urology 64:269–274 **

Kolbl H, Riss P 1988 Obesity and stress urinary incontinence: significance of indices of relative weight. Urology International 43:7–10 *

Kosimaki J, Hakama M, Huhtala H et al 1998 Association of smoking with lower urinary tract symptoms. Journal of Urology 159:1580–1582 *

Lose G, Alling-Moller L, Jennum P 2001 Nocturia in women. American Journal of Obstetrics and Gynecology 185:514–521 *

Lubowski D Z, Swash M, Nicholls R J et al 1988 Increase in pudendal nerve terminal motor latency with defaecation straining. British Journal of Surgery 75:1095–1097 *

Lundgren R 2004 Nocturia: a new perspective on an old symptom. Scandinavian Journal of Urology and Nephrology 38:112–116 *

Mallett V, Hosker G, Smith A R B et al 1994 Neurophysiologic predictors of surgical outcome. Neurourology and Urodynamics 13:442 *

Mattiasson A, Blaakaer J, Hoye K et al 2003 Tolterodine Scandinavian Study Group. Simplified bladder training augments the effectiveness of tolterodine in patients with an overactive bladder. BJU International 91:54–60 *

Milsom I, Abrams P, Cardozo L et al 2001 How widespread are the symptoms of an overactive bladder and how are they managed? A population-based prevalence study. BJU International 87:760 ***

Mommsen S, Foldspang A 1994 Body mass index and adult female urinary incontinence. World Journal of Urology 12:319–322 **

Nygaard I E, Lemke J H 1996 Urinary incontinence in rural older women: prevalence, incidence and remission. Journal of the American Geriatrics Society 44:1049–1054 **

Ouslander J G, Schnelle J F, Uman G et al 1995 Does oxybutynin add to the effectiveness of prompted voiding for urinary incontinence among nursing home residents? A placebo controlled trial. Journal of the American Geriatrics Society 43:610–617 *

Resnick N M, Elbadawi A, Yalla S V 1995 Age and the lower urinary tract: what is normal? Neurourology and Urodynamics 14:577–579 *

Roe B, Doll H 1999 Lifestyle factors and continence status: comparison of self-report data from a postal survey in England. Journal of Wound, Ostomy and Continence Nursing 26:312–319 **

Sagnier P P, MacFarlane G, Richard F et al 1994 Results of an epidemiological survey using a modified American Urological Association symptom index for benign prostatic hyperplasia in France. Journal of Urology 151:1266–1270 *

Sagnier P P, MacFarlane G, Teillac P et al 1995 Impact of symptoms of prostatism on level of bother and quality of life of men in the French community. Journal of Urology 153:669–673 *

Schnelle J F, Alessi C A, Simmons S F et al 2002 Translating clinical research into practice: a randomized controlled trial of exercise and incontinence care with nursing home residents. Journal of the American Geriatrics Society 50:1476–1483 *

Siegler E L, Reidenberg M 2004 Treatment of urinary incontinence with anticholinergics in patients taking cholinesterase inhibitors for dementia. Clinical Pharmacology and Therapeutics 75:484–488 **

Skelly J, Flint A J 1995 Urinary incontinence associated with dementia. Journal of the American Geriatrics Society 43:286–294 *

Steers W D, Lee K S 2001 Depression and incontinence. World Journal of Urology 19:351–357 *

Subak L L, Whitcomb E, Shen H et al 2005 Weight loss: a novel and effective treatment for urinary incontinence. Journal of Urology 174:190–195

Swithinbank L, Hashim H, Abrams P 2005 The effect of fluid intake on urinary symptoms in women. Journal of Urology 174:187–189 *

Thom D H, Brown J S 1998 Reproductive and hormonal risk factors for urinary incontinence in later life: a review of clinical and epidemiologic literature. Journal of the American Geriatrics Society 46:1411–1417 *

Thom D H, Haan M N, van den Eeden S K 1997 Medically recognized urinary incontinence and risks of hospitalization, nursing home admission and mortality. Age and Ageing 26:367–374 **

Thomas S 2003 Is policy translated into action: a report by the Royal College of Nursing Continence Care Forum and the Continence Foundation. Continence Foundation, London *

Tomlinson B U, Dougherty M C, Prendergast J F et al 1999 Dietary caffeine, fluid intake and urinary incontinence in older rural women. International Urogynecology Journal and Pelvic Floor Dysfunction 10:22–28 ** van Kerrebroeck P, Abrams P, Chaikin D et al 2002 The standardization of terminology in nocturia: report from the standardization subcommittee of the International Continence Society. BJU International 90(Suppl 3):11–15 *

Viktrup L, Lose G, Rolff M et al 1992 The symptom of stress incontinence caused by pregnancy or delivery in primiparas. Obstetrics and Gynecology 79:945–949 *

Wagg A S, Malone-Lee J G 1998 Urinary incontinence in the elderly. British Journal of Urology 82(Suppl 1): 11–17 **

Wagg A, Andersson K E, Cardozo L et al 2005 Nocturia in adults. International Journal of Clinical Practice 59:938–945 ***

Wagner T H, Hu T W, Bentkover J et al 2002 Health-related consequences of overactive bladder. American Journal of Managed Care 8:S598–607 *

Ward K, Hilton P, United Kingdom and Ireland Tension-free Vaginal Tape Trial Group 2002 Prospective multicentre randomised trial of tension-free vaginal tape and colposuspension as primary treatment for stress incontinence. British Medical Journal 325:67 ***

SELF-ASSESSMENT QUESTIONS

1. In the management of the overactive bladder syndrome, are the following true or false?
   a. Pelvic floor exercises are the treatment of choice
   b. Urodynamic studies must be performed to confirm the diagnosis before starting treatment
   c. There is good evidence to suggest bladder training is effective
   d. Anterior repair is the treatment of choice

2. Are the following statements on incontinence true or false?
   a. Genuine stress incontinence is characteristically associated with the sensation of urinary urgency
   b. Detrusor overactivity is the expected bladder disorder in neurological disease
   c. Detrusor overactivity is a common cause of incontinence in a postpartum woman
   d. Mixed urinary incontinence refers to coexisting stress and urgency incontinence

3. In the investigation of patients with lower urinary tract symptoms and established neurological disease known to cause bladder dysfunction, which of the following tests is most important?
   a. Cystometry
   b. Urine cytology
   c. Post-void residual urine measurement
   d. Cystoscopy

4. Are the following statements on oral therapy in the treatment of bladder dysfunction true or false?
   a. Detrusor muscle contraction is mediated through sympathetic activation and results in calcium influx into the detrusor cell
   b. Oxybutynin acts primarily by blocking calcium channels
   c. Oxybutynin is a selective M3 receptor blocker
   d. Anticholinergic medications also assist in cases of incomplete emptying by increasing detrusor contractility
   e. M3 receptors are most important in mediating detrusor contraction

Chapter 14

Falls and instability

Jacqueline C. T. Close and Stephen R. Lord

'Old age starts with the first fall and death comes with the second'

(Gabriel Garcia Marquez in
Love in the Time of Cholera, p. 313)

INTRODUCTION

Falls are one of the 'geriatric giants', generating diagnostic and rehabilitative dilemmas, and involving many specialties and disciplines. In a specialty committed to interdisciplinary working, falls and injury prevention presents a sizeable challenge.

Falls can result in death and disability, are commonly associated with a decline in physical function and ultimately encroach on independence and autonomy. While a fall in itself is not a diagnostic category, it is often indicative of underlying problems – whether they are age-related changes in the physiological domains contributing to postural stability or specific undiagnosed or chronic pathology.

This chapter provides an overview of the epidemiology, risk factors, causes and consequences of falls. It gives a structured approach to the assessment, investigation and management of falls and highlights successful intervention/prevention strategies. Gaps in the research literature are highlighted and a recommended reading list covers many of the areas identified in the chapter. This chapter does not cover fracture prevention through the diagnosis and treatment of osteopo-

rosis (see Ch. 36). However, any strategy aimed at fracture prevention must include interventions which address both falls and bone health.

EPIDEMIOLOGY OF FALLS

One-third of the population aged 65 years and above fall each year, rising to 50% of people aged 85 years and above (Blake et al 1988, Campbell et al 1981, Prudham & Evans 1981). Older community-dwelling women experience significantly more falls than do older men, and women living alone are at greater risk of falling and sustaining an injury (Campbell 1990b). Fall rates vary from about 2% in general hospitals to 27% in the geriatric ward of an acute hospital. The incidence of falls and fall-related injuries in institutional settings has been reported in several studies with the mean fall incidence calculated from these at 1.5 falls/bed per year (Rubenstein et al 1994). The incidence is higher after relocation to a new environment where the rate of falls can double and then return to baseline levels after 3 months (Friedman et al 1995).

Most older people live in their own homes and over 60% of women and over 40% of men who fall do so within their usual residence and in the most commonly used rooms (Campbell 1990a). Most falls occur in peak activity periods and only 20% occur at night. However, the external environment with its fast moving vehicles, and soft, slippery and irregular ground surfaces can be challenging for older people and 33–50% of falls occur outside the home (Prudham & Evans 1981).

Up to 10% of falls result in serious injury, of which 5% are fractures (Gibson et al 1987, Tinetti 1987). While the proportion of falls which result in a fracture is low, the absolute number of older people who sustain a fracture is high and this places heavy demands on healthcare systems. Falls are the leading cause of injury-related hospitalization in people aged 65 years and over and account for 14% of emergency admissions and 4% of all hospital admissions in this age group (Close et al 1999). People aged 75 years and over spend an average of 18 days in hospital if admitted after an 'accident' at home, the commonest category of which is a fall. Falls can also result in disability, restriction of activity and fear of falling – all of which reduce quality of life and independence. Furthermore, falls are mentioned as a contributing factor in 40% of admissions to nursing homes (Gibson et al 1987).

Falls account for 40% of injury-related deaths, and 1% of total deaths in people aged 65 years and above. Overall, the mortality associated with falls in older people is probably underestimated, but accurate estimates will remain unclear until falls are clearly characterized and recorded as clinical entities and a more pragmatic approach to death certification is identified.

PHYSIOLOGY OF BALANCE

Postural stability can be defined as the ability of an individual to maintain the position of the body, or more specifically, its centre of mass, within specific boundaries of space (referred to as stability limits). Maintaining postural stability requires the complex integration of sensory information regarding the position of the body relative to the surroundings, and the ability to generate forces to control body movement. Thus, postural stability requires the interaction of sensory and musculoskeletal systems.

The sensory components include vision, vestibular function and somatosensation which act to inform the brain of the position and movement of the body in three-dimensional space. The musculoskeletal component of postural stability encompasses the biomechanical properties of body

segments, muscles and joints. Linking these two components are higher level neurological processes enabling anticipatory mechanisms responsible for planning a movement, and adaptive mechanisms for reacting to changing demands of particular tasks.

Ageing is associated with changes in function of each of the sensory and musculoskeletal systems that contribute to postural stability. Consequently, age-related deficits in these systems may manifest as difficulty in undertaking tasks involving postural stability, such as standing, performing voluntary movements and responding to external perturbations.

RISK FACTORS FOR FALLS

Over the past three decades, much has been focused on risk factors for falling (Lord et al 2007). Numerous publications of varying quality have led to some 400 cited risk factors. In Table 14.1 we have extracted the findings of many of these studies and have rated each risk factor according to the strength of the published evidence, using the rating system:

*** Strong evidence — Consistently found in good studies

** Moderate evidence — Usually but not always found

* Weak evidence — Occasionally but not usually found

– Little or no evidence — Not found in published studies despite research to examine the issue

A history of falls is one of the most consistent predictors of future risk and should perhaps be considered a basic screening question in any medical consultation with an older person. Advancing age and impaired ability in performing activities of daily living have been found to be strong risk factors for falls. Women have also been shown to have higher rates of falls than men. The finding that living alone is a risk factor for falls is most likely confounded by gender and by age, in that older women comprise the majority of this group.

One of the strongest risk factor domains is impaired balance, and many studies have shown that tests of standing, leaning, reaching, stepping

Table 14.1 Risk factors for falls

Factor	Risk	Factor	Risk
Psychosocial and demographic		**Psychological**	
Advanced age	***	Fear of falling	***
Female gender	**	Reduced selective attention	**
Living alone	**	Risk taking	*
History of falls	***		
Inactivity	**	**Medical**	
Activities of daily living limitations	***	Impaired cognition	***
Alcohol consumption	–	Depression	**
		Abnormal neurological signs	**
Balance and mobility		Stroke	***
Impaired stability when standing	**	Incontinence	**
Impaired stability when leaning and reaching	**	Acute illness	**
Inadequate responses to external perturbations	*	Parkinson's disease	***
Slow voluntary stepping	**	Vestibular disorders	–
Impaired gait and mobility	***	Arthritis	**
Impaired ability in standing up	***	Foot problems	**
Impaired ability with transfers	***	Dizziness	*
		Orthostatic hypotension	*
Sensory and neuromuscular			
Visual acuity	**	**Medication**	
Visual contrast sensitivity	***	Psychoactive medication use	***
Visual field dependence	*	Antihypertensive use	*
Reduced peripheral sensation	***	NSAIDs	–
Reduced vestibular function	*	Use of 4+ medications	***
Reduced muscle strength	***		
Reduced muscle power	*	**Environmental**	
Reduced muscle endurance	*	Poor footwear	*
Slow reaction time	***	Inappropriate spectacles	*
		Home hazards	–
		External hazards	–

*** Strong evidence; ** Moderate evidence; * Weak evidence; – No evidence.

and walking can discriminate fallers from non-fallers. Generally speaking, the more challenging the balance tasks are the stronger the risk factors. Impaired functioning of sensory and neuromuscular systems due to age, inactivity or disease processes are also strong risk factors for falls. Measures of vision, peripheral sensation, strength and reaction time are significant and independent predictors of falls (Lord et al 1991, Lord et al 1994). There is now emerging evidence that, if measured rigorously, vestibular impairment, reduced muscle power and endurance are also important falls risk factors in older people (DiFabio et al 2002, Kristinsdottir et al 2001). Poor hearing is the only physiological risk factor found not to be a risk factor for falls despite systematic study. Physical activity can improve strength, balance and func-

tional abilities in older people and can prevent falls. However, being more physically active does not always prevent falls. This is probably because the more physically active older person takes part in activities which increase exposure to falls risk situations. Clearly, this risk should be balanced against the benefits of increased physical functioning, other health benefits and independence that exercise brings.

Fear of falling is prevalent in older people. In many cases, this fear may be excessive and lead to unnecessary restrictions in physical and social activity. Fear of falling is strongly associated with instability and falls (Lord et al 2007). Several studies have shown that with increasing age, balance tasks become more attentionally demanding and frail older people require even more attentional resources for balance control, to the extent that even simple tasks like answering questions may interfere with standing, stepping and walking. In these situations, older people with attentional limitations are at increased risk of falls. There is only preliminary evidence that risk-taking behaviours increase falls risk in older people.

Medical conditions strongly associated with falls include impaired cognition, stroke and Parkinson's disease (Lord et al 2007). However, other conditions commonly posited as falls risk factors, such as vestibular disease, dizziness, orthostatic hypotension, foot problems and arthritis require more rigorous investigation to adequately establish their contribution to falls. An acute deterioration in function associated with an infective process often presents as a fall in an older person.

Both community and institutional studies have consistently found strong associations between falls and the use of *multiple medications* and centrally acting medications (Lord et al 2007). The use of multiple medications is likely to be a surrogate marker for underlying chronic disease and medications from which older people stand to benefit should not be withheld on the basis of a simple number count (Lawlor et al 2003). The association between the use of centrally acting medications and both falls and fractures is strong and clear justification is required for the prescription of any centrally acting medication. Not only is there evidence to link centrally acting medications to falls but also evidence of the beneficial effects of withdrawing centrally acting medications on subsequent risk of falls (Campbell et al 1999, Leipzig et al 1999).

An unexpected finding is that *alcohol consumption* has not been found to be a falls risk factor. Indeed, there is some evidence that light or moderate drinkers may have fewer falls than those who abstain. This finding may be due to selection bias, in that older people who drink heavily may underreport their alcohol consumption, be ineligible or decline participation in research studies.

There is little evidence that *environmental factors* or *inappropriate footwear* in isolation play a role in falls (Lord et al 2007). Again, there are difficulties in assessing the contribution of these transient risk factors with conventional study design that assumes risk is constant during a follow-up period.

Despite the common finding that environmental hazards are involved in many falls, it appears that the interaction between the person and their environment is more important than the environment itself, as the homes of people who fall are not more hazardous than those who do not fall.

ASSESSMENT OF THE OLDER PERSON WHO FALLS

Given the multiplicity of risk factors associated with falls, it follows that the clinical assessment and associated interventions should ideally be formulated by a team of professionals rather than a single profession in isolation. For a specialist falls service, access to medicine, physiotherapy and occupational therapy is essential. However, not all older fallers require this level of assessment and key to ensuring that older people get access to the appropriate level of care is the development of local care pathways. These involve both primary and secondary healthcare professionals as well as social services, leisure and housing services, etc.

HISTORY

When trying to establish the cause of a fall/s, it is important to remember that most falls occur as a result of an interaction between intrinsic and extrinsic factors and that multiple risk factors increase the likelihood of falls. A detailed history of the events surrounding a fall is essential. Corroborative information should be sought when the patient has limited recollection of the incident. In addition there is a significant overlap between syncope and falls with many older people having amnesia for the event.

Points to consider in the history include:

1. Does the individual have amnesia for the event?
   Reason – possible syncopal, cardiac or neurological problem.
2. Where and at what time did the fall happen?
   Reason – postural hypotension in proximity to change in posture, falls occurring in relation to medication ingestion, slips and trips at night with poor lighting, etc.

3. What was the individual doing at the time of the fall – getting up from chair/bed, turning head, reaching up or bending down?

Reason – certain conditions are related to specific actions, e.g. postural hypotension on standing or carotid sinus syndrome related to turning of the head.

4. Was the fall preceded by any dizziness or palpitations?

Reason – possible neurocardiogenic syncope, cardiac arrhythmia, vestibular problem.

5. Was the individual able to get off the floor after the fall?

Reason – predictor of further falls as well as identifying a care need linked to interventions, i.e. training in how to get up from the floor, alarms, increased care levels.

6. Does the pattern of injury described and/or visualized fit with the details of the fall – did the individual manage to break the fall or were there facial/head injuries?

Reason – in syncopal episodes, the individual is rarely able to break the fall and more likely to sustain injuries, including facial injuries.

7. What injuries were sustained as a result of the fall?

Reason – low trauma fractures should trigger an assessment of bone health.

8. How often has the person fallen in the last year?

Reason – one of the strongest predictors of falling again.

In addition to a detailed falls history, an accurate medical and drug history is required, including over-the-counter medications and herbal remedies.

EXAMINATION

In a specialist clinic the patient should have a comprehensive medical examination including a full neurological examination. However, where time constraints would limit this practice, the clinical examination should be tailored to the history obtained from the patient and the carers, if relevant. Box 14.1 highlights some of the medical examination findings which may be actively contributing to a person's overall risk of falling.

Box 14. 1   Examination findings which might contribute to an individual's risk of falling

General
'Stops walking when talking'
Impaired visual acuity
Inappropriate use of walking aids
Poor nutritional status
Poor footwear and footcare

Neurological
Abnormal gait
Impaired visual fields
Cataract formation or macular degeneration
Altered tone (cog-wheeling, clasp knife, etc)
Deficits in power
Peripheral neuropathy
Proximal myopathy

Cardiovascular
Brady- or tachyarrhythmias
Postural hypotension
Unexplained murmurs
Carotid bruits

Musculoskeletal
Reduced range of movement
Unstable knee joints
Pain in joints on movement

Cognition and affect
Impaired cognition
Low mood

Assessment of postural stability

Gait and balance problems are potentially modifiable with strength and balance training conducted by appropriately trained practitioners. Assessment of postural stability is therefore a key area in the management of an older person at risk of falling. The AGS/BGS/AAOS (2001) guideline recommends the Timed Up and Go Test (TUGT) as a simple screening tool to identify people who require more detailed assessment of gait and balance. It involves measuring the time taken for a person to rise from a chair, walk 3 metres at normal pace and with usual assistive device, turn, return to the chair and sit down. Three retrospective studies have shown that TUGT performance can discriminate between fallers and non-fallers and that a time of 15 or more seconds to complete the tests indicates impaired functioning.

The Tinetti Performance Oriented Mobility Assessment, the Berg Balance Scale, the Modified Gait Abnormality Rating Scale and the Elderly Fall Screening Test are other useful falls risk assessment screens. However, while useful as screening tools, they do not provide detailed information on the impairments in physiological domains that contribute to falls risk and therefore provide limited information about how to target intervention strategies.

A recently developed comprehensive assessment tool, the Physiological Profile Assessment (PPA), takes a physiological approach to evaluating falls risk factors (Lord et al 2003a). This involves assessment of sensorimotor factors that contribute to postural stability, including vision (visual acuity, contrast sensitivity and depth perception), peripheral sensation (tactile sensitivity, vibration sense and proprioception), strength (ankle dorsiflexion and knee flexion and extension), reaction time (hand and foot), postural sway (on a firm surface and foam rubber mat) and leaning balance (maximal balance range and coordinated stability). In a series of large prospective studies, this combination of tests discriminates between fallers and non-fallers with an accuracy of 75%, with a similar sensitivity and specificity. A web-based software programme has been developed to assess an individual's performance in relation to a normative database, which enables the calculation of an overall falls risk score – a single index score derived from a discriminant functional analysis of large-scale prospective studies. The programme also generates a profile of individual test performances (using z-scores) to identify physiological strengths and weaknesses and allows for tailored intervention based on the deficits identified (Fig. 14 1).

Assessment of the unexplained faller

Where the cause of a fall is unclear or there is associated dizziness, palpitations or loss of consciousness, then further cardiovascular and possible neurological investigation are warranted. A

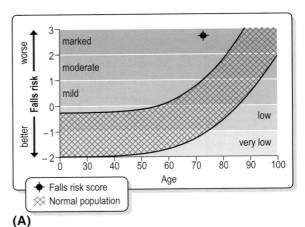

(A)

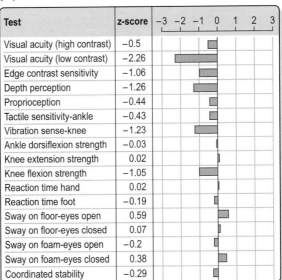

Test	z-score	-3	-2	-1	0	1	2	3
Visual acuity (high contrast)	-0.5							
Visual acuity (low contrast)	-2.26							
Edge contrast sensitivity	-1.06							
Depth perception	-1.26							
Proprioception	-0.44							
Tactile sensitivity-ankle	-0.43							
Vibration sense-knee	-1.23							
Ankle dorsiflexion strength	-0.03							
Knee extension strength	0.02							
Knee flexion strength	-1.05							
Reaction time hand	0.02							
Reaction time foot	-0.19							
Sway on floor-eyes open	0.59							
Sway on floor-eyes closed	0.07							
Sway on foam-eyes open	-0.2							
Sway on foam-eyes closed	0.38							
Coordinated stability	-0.29							

(B)

Figure 14.1 (A) Example of a falls risk score graph. (B) Example of a subject's test performance profile graph. (Reprinted from Close J C, Lord S L, Menz H B, Sherrington C 2005 What is the role of falls? Best Practice and Research. Clinical Rheumatology 19(6):913–935, with permission from Elsevier.)

routine electrocardiogram (ECG) should be undertaken in the first instance. A 24-hour ECG is a largely unhelpful investigation in the unexplained faller despite the fact that it is a regularly-requested test. The European Society of Cardiology has produced a useful clinical algorithm for the investigation of the unexplained faller (Brignole et al 2001).

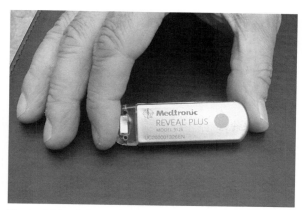

Figure 14.2 A Reveal® Plus Insertable Loop Recorder (ILR) used in the diagnosis of infrequent syncopal events. The ILR is inserted subcutaneously in a similar manner to a permanent pacemaker except no lead(s) is required. The ILR allows continuous ECG/heart monitoring for up to 14 months. (With kind permission of Medtronic Reveal Plus.)

Over the last decade, tilt table testing with carotid sinus massage has been added to the clinician's armamentarium and should be considered in those for whom the cause of a fall is unclear or associated with dizziness or syncope. In addition to looking for carotid sinus hypersensitivity and syndrome, it can also be used to diagnose postural changes in blood pressure and vasovagal/neurocardiogenic syncope. The Newcastle protocol is a recommended approach to testing for carotid sinus hypersensitivity (Kenny et al 2000) (see Ch. 23).

Carotid sinus syndrome can be defined as an abnormal haemodynamic response to massage of the carotid sinus (Kenny 2003). It is seen more commonly in old age and is characterized clinically by unexplained dizziness and/or syncope. There are three subtypes of the carotid sinus syndrome – cardioinhibitory, vasodepressor and mixed. The pathophysiology of the carotid sinus syndrome remains poorly described. The cardio-inhibitory response is characterized by a period of more than 3 seconds of asystole following carotid sinus massage. The vasodepressor response is identified by a fall in systolic blood pressure of greater than 50 mmHg in the absence of significant bradycardia. The mixed type is a combination of both responses. The drop in blood pressure is seen within seconds of massage and as such is

virtually impossible to detect without the use of continuous non-invasive blood pressure monitoring. Symptomatic carotid sinus syndrome of the cardioinhibitory subtype is treated with dual chamber pacing. Treatment of the vasodepressor response is more challenging and almost certainly reflects a limited understanding of the underlying mechanisms producing the response.

For those who experience sudden but infrequent episodes of collapse, insertion of an implantable loop recorder (ILR) may be warranted (Fig. 14.2). ILRs are inserted subcutaneously in a similar manner to a permanent pacemaker and allow for continuous monitoring of the heart rate. They have the ability to be interrogated retrospectively in the event of patient collapse and can aid in the diagnosis and subsequent management of intermittent arrhythmias.

SUCCESSFUL APPROACHES TO PREVENTING FALLS

There have been about 25 published randomized controlled trials that have shown benefit in preventing falls in older people. Box 14.2 presents these trials and the associated references are listed at the end of the chapter. Most of the evidence relates to people at home where both single and multifaceted interventions have been shown to be effective. *Exercise in the form of balance training with a strength component is the single most effective approach to preventing falls* (Barnett et al 2003, Campbell et al 1997, Lord et al 2003b, Robertson et al 2001, Skelton et al 2005, Wolf et al 1996). Exercises need to be weight bearing, tailored to the individual, progressed over time and preferably focused on functional tasks. Exercise programmes have largely been delivered by physiotherapists in the published trials, though one trial has shown benefit in training nurses to deliver exercise programmes.

Other successful approaches to prevention in older people living at home include expedited cataract extraction (Harwood et al 2005), occupational therapy home assessment in those with severe visual impairment (Campbell et al 2005) or recently discharged from hospital (Cumming et al 1999, Nikolaus & Bach 2003) and withdrawal of centrally acting medications (Campbell et al 1999).

> **Box 14.2 Randomized controlled trials that have shown the benefits of intervention in preventing falls**
>
> **Community–dwelling populations**
> *Single interventions*
> Barnett et al 2003
> Campbell et al 1997
> Campbell et al 1999
> Campbell et al 2005
> Cumming et al 1999
> Harwood et al 2005
> Li et al 2005
> Lord et al 2003b
> Nikolaus & Bach 2003
> Robertson et al 2001
> Skelton et al 2005
>
> *Multifaceted interventions*
> Day et al 2002
> Hornbrook et al 1994
> Tinetti et al 1994
> Wagner et al 1994
>
> **Emergency department attendees**
> *Single interventions*
> Kenny et al 2001
>
> *Multifaceted interventions*
> Close et al 1999
> Davison et al 2005
>
> **Hospital in–patients**
> *Single interventions*
> None
>
> *Multifaceted interventions*
> Haines et al 2004
> Healey et al 2004
>
> **Care home residents**
> *Single interventions*
> None
>
> *Multifaceted interventions*
> Becker et al 2003
> Jensen et al 2002
> Ray et al 1997

Multifactorial interventions in the community involving a variable combination of doctors, nurses, physiotherapists and occupational therapists have been consistently shown to be effective (Clemson et al 2002, Day et al 2002, Hornbrook et al 1994, Tinetti et al 1994, Wagner et al 1994).

The emergency department (ED) is an ideal place to identify a high-risk population of fallers. Three trials have shown the benefits of intervening in this population and it is important to note that assessment and intervention occurs outside of the ED (Close et al 1999, Davison et al 2005, Kenny et al 2001). The ED merely serves as a convenient mechanism by which a high-risk population can be identified.

Residents in hospitals and care homes tend to represent the frailer end of the older population. Single approaches to intervention have not been shown to be effective in these populations (Becker et al 2003, Jensen et al 2002, Ray et al 1997).

CALCIUM AND VITAMIN D SUPPLEMENTATION

Calcium and vitamin D are essential components of bone health and over the last 13 years a number of published studies have shown the benefits of calcium and vitamin D supplementation in the prevention of fractures in high-risk populations. The role of calcium in the prevention of fractures seems to be largely through the bone mechanism but for vitamin D the story is different, although still to be fully understood. There are vitamin D receptors on both muscle and nervous tissue and studies have shown that vitamin D replacement can lead to improvements in postural stability and psychomotor function. There is also an increasing body of evidence, largely through meta-analysis, that vitamin D supplementation can prevent falls (Bischoff-Ferrari et al 2004).

Several question arise: who requires supplementation? In whom do we need to check levels?

What doses and formulations of calcium and vitamin D should we be using? There are no hard and fast answers to any of these questions but the evidence would support routine supplementation of the diet in older populations living in care homes or those who are largely housebound. For younger post-menopausal women with or without fracture who do not have a diagnosis of osteoporosis, the question of supplementation becomes less clear and it is this population in whom one might consider checking vitamin D levels before prescribing any form of supplementation.

The dose of both calcium and vitamin D also generates debate but most would agree that 800 mg of calcium and 800 IU cholecalciferol daily would constitute adequate doses for replacement in the older adult. Vitamin D toxicity at this dose is extremely unlikely. Occasionally, the calcium supplementation may lead to the unmasking of an underlying myeloma or hyperparathyroidism but this is not sufficient justification for not treating with calcium and, given the relatively small numbers of cases, would not be sufficient to justify routine checking of calcium and vitamin D levels in all patients prescribed supplementation.

Failure to ensure older adults are vitamin D replete has wider reaching consequences than just the effects on the musculoskeletal system, with evidence showing increased vascular risk in those with low levels of vitamin D and the positive effects of vitamin D on the immune system and as a protective agent for certain cancers.

The role of homocysteine in the fall/fracture circle is emerging with an association between high levels of homocysteine in select populations and fracture risk. A direct causal link is yet to be described, but there are preliminary data to show that interventions with folate and vitamin B12 can reduce fracture rates.

FALLS IN HOSPITALS – LEGAL ASPECTS

The prevention of falls in hospital is difficult both from the clinical and legal viewpoint. Acutely ill and confused patients are at high risk of falling and require a level of supervision that is not always possible on a general ward. Physical and chemical restraints should be avoided; in the USA, the removal of physical and chemical restraints has not led to a substantial increase in the number of falls either in hospitals or institutions. Side rails increase the risk of injury by adding extra height to a fall – particularly if used with an overlay mattress.

It is possible to identify in-patients at increased risk of falling using a validated risk assessment tool. STRATIFY represents one such validated risk assessment tool (Oliver et al 1997). However, assessment is of limited value unless linked to intervention.

There have now been two published trials demonstrating that falls can be prevented in hospital (Haines et al 2004, Healey et al 2004). One study was undertaken in rehabilitation/intermediate care and, while multifactorial, it seems that the benefit of the approach was probably through the exercise component, as a reduction in falls was not seen until more than 40 days into the intervention. On the other hand, a UK-based study (which included a mix of aged care acute and rehabilitation wards) showed benefits from a multifactorial intervention which included a significant medical component (including infection screen, lying and standing blood pressure measurement and medication review, etc.).

More research is required, particularly with respect to linking appropriately validated tools to identify at-risk fallers with evidence-based approaches to intervention. The role of telehealth monitoring systems and bed and chair alarms warrant further evaluation. However, we are now at a point in time where hospital falls policies can at last be evidence based within the caveats of the existing populations studied.

HIP PROTECTORS

Hip protectors are designed to reduce the chance of a hip fracture in the event of an impact onto the greater trochanter (Fig. 14.3). While energy absorption and inflatable airbags have been considered, it is the energy-shunting pad that has undergone the most extensive development and appears to offer the most in terms of fracture reduction.

Energy-shunting systems function by increasing impact area and reducing peak forces, thereby leading energy away from the greater trochanter.

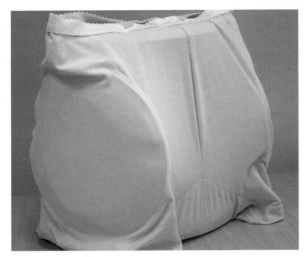

Figure 14.3   Hip protectors.

In addition, they have an energy absorption capacity. Hip protectors consist of a polymer cup surrounded by a polymer foam that is anatomically shaped to fit the shape of the greater trochanter. The pad is then fixed in to an undergarment.

There is some evidence from randomized controlled trials that hip protectors are effective in reducing hip fractures in nursing homes (Parker et al 2004). From a purely biomechanical aspect, hip protectors have the requisite properties to reduce fracture risk. The limiting factor in the success of hip protectors is whether people will wear them. Problems influencing compliance include poor fitting, weight of the protectors and difficulty toileting. Given the problems with compliance, it is necessary to target this intervention to those most likely to benefit from them or those in whom other interventions are unlikely to work. Such groups include those with Parkinson's disease and dementia, particularly those with a tendency to wander.

GAPS IN OUR KNOWLEDGE

Preventing falls in the cognitively impaired older adult remains a major challenge with more research required both in understanding the nature of the risk as well as in employing innovative approaches to prevention. However, while we do not know reliably how to prevent falls in this population, we do know how to prevent fractures through the diagnosis and treatment of osteoporosis and the use of hip protectors. At present, the cognitively-impaired population are not routinely assessed for fracture risk and there are those who would argue that drug compliance might be problematic. However, with the emergence of bone-strengthening agents which can be prescribed monthly and even yearly, poor medication compliance will no longer be justification for non-prescription of evidence-based treatment to a high fracture-risk population.

The question remains as to whether specific disease processes require disease-specific approaches to the prevention of both falls and fracture risk or whether, by taking a physiological approach to prevention, we can devise programmes that are tailored to physiological deficits (as opposed to specific pathologies). This is of particular relevance to those with multiple chronic diseases who run the risk of having to attend several different generic exercise programmes, each believed to be disease-specific, as opposed to individually tailored programmes based on objective measures of assessment.

Cost-effectiveness models are lacking in falls prevention and more research is required to help define and refine models of care which offer both clinical efficacy and cost-effectiveness in the long term. Integral to this will be an improved understanding of the barriers and motivators that determine the uptake of programmes known to prevent falls.

CONCLUSION

Falls have long been accepted as a normal accompaniment of old age both by older people and those responsible for their care. Such fatalistic attitudes need to be countered. We now know what constitutes risk and how to identify high-risk populations. A limited number of validated screening and assessment tools can help in the identification of these populations. We also have a substantial body of evidence to guide us in applying strategies to prevent falls.

Geriatricians should be actively involved in developing services locally. Models of care will vary and a 'one size fits all' approach is unlikely to work. Services should not be defined by artificial demarcation of healthcare boundaries as this generates inefficiencies and fragmentation of care, as well as frustration and confusion for the recipients of care. Open and constructive dialogue with local service managers can often ensure that resources are invested appropriately. It should not be assumed that service managers know the evidence base for falls prevention – it is necessary to work with them to ensure that resources are channelled appropriately.

Professional boundaries are now being challenged with the emergence of the role of the specialist practitioner and the nurse and therapist consultant. Given the size of the problem of falls in older people and the increasing number of successful approaches to preventing falls, this is a welcome development – as long as individuals receive the appropriate training to undertake the specified role.

Through the systematic identification and assessment of at-risk populations and the application of evidence-based approaches to prevention, it is possible to prevent many falls and injuries in our older population.

CLINICAL CASES

CASE 1

A 75-year-old woman (Mrs A) presents to the accident and emergency department with a left distal forearm fracture following a trip while coming down some steps. On further questioning, this is her third fall in the last year. The two earlier falls were also trips which occurred outdoors and as a result she has significantly reduced the frequency with which she goes out.

Immediate management

Her fractured forearm is reduced and placed in a back slab pending a review by the orthopaedic surgeon in the fracture clinic the following morning. She is discharged home from the accident and emergency department with support arranged to help with domestic and personal care during the period in which her arm will be in a cast.

Longer-term management

A distal forearm fracture is a risk factor for further fracture, including hip fracture. It is therefore important that future preventative strategies are considered. To minimize future fracture risk, both bone health and falls risk must be considered.

Bone health

Mrs A has limited exposure to the sun and even when outdoors is largely covered by clothing or sunscreen. In addition her diet is low in calcium as she drinks very little milk, though she does consume green vegetables. She is offered calcium and vitamin D supplementation of her diet.

A DEXA scan will provide data on whether this lady has a diagnosis of osteoporosis and therefore whether a bisphosphonate is warranted. Mrs A has a T score of -2.8 at her hip and -2.4 at her spine. Her hip T score confirms a diagnosis of osteoporosis and she is offered a weekly bisphosphonate preparation with clear instructions on how to take the drug.

Falls risk

Mrs A is also assessed for her risk of future falls. She is assessed using the physiological profile assessment and found to have deficits in strength and balance. An exercise programme tailored to her deficits is required. She does not relish the idea of exercising in a group setting and so a physiotherapist prescribes her exercises for the home environment and visits her on four occasions to make sure she is exercising safely and to guide the progress of the exercises.

CASE 2

A 78-year-old man (Mr B) presents to his GP with a history of four syncopal events over the last 6 months. Mr B denies blacking out but his wife has witnessed two of the events and is clear that he suffers a momentary loss in consciousness and recovers immediately. No epileptiform features are associated with the collapses. To date he has not sustained any fractures or serious injury but has had several black eyes from these events. Clinical examination does not reveal any obvious cardiac dysrhythmia, murmur or bruit. His ECG shows him to be in sinus rhythm with no ischaemic changes.

Management

In view of the nature and frequency of these events, Mr B is referred to the cardiology department of his local hospital for further investigation. There is understandably some debate as to which test/s to undertake in order to try and get a diagnosis. In the absence of any local guidelines, the cardiologist elects to follow the recommendations of the European Society of Cardiology and undertakes tilt table testing and carotid sinus massage. Right carotid sinus massage with 70° head-up tilt produces a 3-second period of asystole and associated presyncopal symptoms. A dual chamber pacemaker is inserted and his syncopal events cease.

CASE 3

An 82-year-old woman (Mrs C) presents to her GP with a painful left knee following a fall a few days previously. Over the previous 4 months, Mrs C has had an increasing number of falls mainly related to pain in the left knee and the knee giving way. As a result of the falls, she is now too scared to go out alone and her level of physical activity has been declining. Her mood has declined and her sleep pattern has been altered by her change in activity level with a tendency now to sleep for prolonged periods in the afternoon. On her last visit to the surgery she was prescribed a benzodiazepine for night sedation.

Mrs C has recently developed some bilateral leg oedema. Two weeks ago she was prescribed a diuretic for the oedema but has since developed urinary incontinence because she cannot get to the toilet in time.

Clinical examination reveals Mrs C to have a small effusion of the left knee with associated swelling and bruising. There is also evidence of some mediolateral instability, almost certainly secondary to degenerative joint disease. However, the joint is not hot and Mrs C is not systemically unwell. A recent X-ray of her knee confirms severe degenerative changes.

Management

A referral is made to the orthopaedic surgeon for consideration of a joint replacement. However, in the interim it is essential to minimize Mrs C's chances of further falls and functional decline.

Her knee pain is managed with oral analgesics, starting with paracetamol. The unstable knee is reviewed by a physiotherapist who recommends a knee brace. However, Mrs C is unable to manage the brace and so, in negotiation with Mrs C, the physiotherapist provides Mrs C with a 4-wheel walker as a temporary arrangement until her knee is replaced, and the physiotherapist practises indoor and outdoor mobility with Mrs C. At the same time, Mrs C is given specific knee-strengthening exercises.

The need for a benzodiazepine is reviewed, particularly given the association of benzodiazepines with falls and fractures. As she has only been taking it for a few weeks, the drug is discontinued and Mrs C agrees to avoid prolonged naps in the afternoon. The leg oedema is dependent oedema secondary to her reduced mobility but, with advice on elevation of the legs while sitting as well as her leg exercises and improved mobility with the 4-wheel walker, it is possible to stop the diuretic and therefore the urinary incontinence.

A home assessment undertaken by the occupational therapist leads to the provision of a raised toilet seat, bath board for bathing and a perching stool for the kitchen.

Mrs C's falls risk has therefore been minimized and her functional status maximized while awaiting surgery on her knee.

REFERENCES

American Geriatrics Society, British Geriatrics Society, American Academy of Orthopaedic Surgeons Panel on Falls Prevention 2001 Guideline for the prevention of falls in older persons. Journal of the American Geriatrics Society 49:664–672

Barnett A, Smith B, Lord S R et al 2003 Community-based group exercise improves balance and reduces falls in at-risk older people: a randomised controlled trial. Age and Ageing 32:407–414

Becker C, Kron M, Lindemann U et al 2003 Effectiveness of a multifaceted intervention on falls in nursing home residents. Journal of the American Geriatrics Society 51:306–313

Bischoff-Ferrari H A, Dawson-Hughes B, Willett W C et al 2004 Effect of vitamin D on falls: a meta-analysis. Journal of the American Medical Association 291:1999–2006

Blake A, Morgan K, Bendall M J et al 1988 Falls by elderly people at home – prevalence and associated factors. Age and Ageing 17:365–372

Brignole M, Alboni P, Benditt D et al 2001 Guidelines on management (diagnosis and treatment) of syncope. European Heart Journal 22:1256–1306

Campbell, A J, Reinken J, Allan B C et al 1981 Falls in old age: a study of frequency and related clinical factors. Age and Ageing 10:264–270

Campbell A J, Borrie M J, Spears G F et al 1990a Circumstances and consequences of falls experienced by a community population 70 years and over during a prospective study. Age and Ageing 19:136–141

Campbell A J, Spears G F, Borrie M J et al 1990b Examination by logistic regression modelling of the variables which increase the relative risk of elderly women falling compared to elderly men. Journal of Clinical Epidemiology 43:1415–1420

Campbell A J, Robertson M C, Gardner M M et al 1997 Randomised controlled trial of a general practice programme of home based exercise to prevent falls in elderly women. British Medical Journal 315:1065–1069

Campbell A J, Robertson M C, Gardner M M et al 1999 Psychotropic medication withdrawal and a home-based exercise program to prevent falls: a randomized, controlled trial. Journal of the American Geriatrics Society 47:850–853

Campbell A J, Robertson M C, Grow S J L et al 2005 Randomised controlled trial of prevention of falls in people aged 75 with severe visual impairment: the VIP trial. British Medical Journal 331:817–820

Clemson L, Cumming R G, Kendig H et al 2002 The effectiveness of a community-based program for reducing the incidence of falls in the elderly: a randomized trial. Journal of the American Geriatrics Society 52:1487–1494

Close J, Ellis M, Hooper R et al 1999 Prevention of falls in the elderly trial (PROFET): a randomised controlled trial. Lancet 353:93–97

Cumming R G, Thomas M, Szonyi G et al 1999 Home visits by an occupational therapist for assessment and modification of environmental hazards: a randomized trial of falls prevention. Journal of the American Geriatrics Society 47:1397–1402

Davison J, Bond J, Dawson P et al 2005 Patients with recurrent falls attending Accident & Emergency benefit from multifactorial intervention – a randomised controlled trial. Age and Ageing 34:162–168

Day L, Fildes B, Gordon I et al 2002 A randomized factorial trial of falls prevention among older people living in their own homes. British Medical Journal 325:128–133

DiFabio R P, Greany J F, Emasithi A et al 2002 Eye-head coordination during postural perturbation as a predictor of falls in community-dwelling elderly women. Archives of Physical Medicine and Rehabilitation 83:942–951

Friedman S M, Williamson J D, Lee B H et al 1995 Increased fall rates in nursing home residents after relocation to a new facility. Journal of the American Geriatrics Society 43:1237–1242

Gibson M J, Andres R O, Issacs B et al 1987 The prevention of falls in later life. Danish Medical Bulletin 34(Suppl 4):1–24

Haines T P, Bennell K L, Osborne R H et al 2004 Effectiveness of targeted falls prevention programme in subacute hospital setting: randomised controlled trial. British Medical Journal 328:676

Harwood R H, Foss A J E, Osborn F et al 2005 Falls and health status in elderly women following first eye cataract surgery: a randomised controlled trial. British Journal of Ophthalmology 89:53–59

Healey F, Monro A, Cockram A et al 2004 Using targeted risk factor reduction to prevent falls in older in-patients: a randomised controlled trial. Age and Ageing 33:390–395

Hornbrook M C, Stephens V J, Wingfield D J et al 1994 Preventing falls among community-dwelling older persons: results from a randomized trial. The Gerontologist 34:16–23

Jensen J, Lundin-Olsson L, Nyberg L et al 2002 Fall and injury prevention in older people living in residential care facilities: a cluster randomised trial. Annals of Internal Medicine 136:733–741

Kenny R A 2003 Syncope in the elderly: diagnosis, evaluation, and treatment. Journal of Cardiovascular Electrophysiology 14(Suppl 9):S74–77

Kenny R, O'Shea D, Parry S W et al 2000 The Newcastle protocols for head-up tilt table testing in the diagnosis of vasovagal syncope, carotid sinus hypersensitivity, and related disorders. Heart 83:564–569

Kenny R A M, Richardson D A, Steen N et al 2001 Carotid sinus syndrome: a modifiable risk factor for nonaccidental falls in older adults (SAFE PACE). Journal of the American College of Cardiology 38:1491–1496

Kristinsdottir E K, Nordell E, Jarnlo G B et al 2001 Observation of vestibular asymmetry in a majority of patients over 50 years with fall-related wrist fractures. Acta Otolaryngologica 121:481–485

Lawlor D A, Patel R, Ebrahim S et al 2003 Association between falls in elderly women and chronic diseases and drug use: cross sectional study. British Medical Journal 327:712–717

Leipzig R M, Cumming R G, Tinetti M E et al 1999 Drugs and falls in older people: a systematic review and meta-analysis. I. Psychotropic drugs. Journal of the American Geriatrics Society 47:30–39

Li F, Harmer P, Fisher K J et al 2005 Tai Chi and fall reductions in older adults: a randomized controlled trial. Journal of Gerontology 60A:187–194

Lord S R, Clark R D, Webster I W et al 1991 Physiological factors associated with falls in an elderly population. Journal of the American Geriatrics Society 39:1194–1200

Lord S R, Sambrook P N, Gilbert C et al 1994 Postural stability, falls and fractures in the elderly: results from the Dubbo Osteoporosis Epidemiology Study. Medical Journal of Australia 160:684–691

Lord S R, Menz H B, Tiedemann A et al 2003a A physiological profile approach to falls risk assessment and prevention. Physical Therapy 83:237–252

Lord S R, Castell S, Corcoran J et al 2003b The effect of group exercise on physical functioning and falls in frail older people living in retirement villages: a randomized, controlled trial. Journal of the American Geriatrics Society 51:1685–1692

Lord S R, Sherrington C, Menz H B 2007 Falls in older people: risk factors and strategies for prevention. Cambridge University Press, Cambridge

Nikolaus T, Bach M 2003 Preventing falls in community-dwelling frail older people using a home intervention team (HIT): Results from the randomised falls-HIT trial. Journal of the American Geriatrics Society 51:300–305

Oliver D, Britton M, Seed P et al 1997 Development and evaluation of an evidence based falls risk assessment tool (STRATIFY) to predict which elderly inpatients will fall: case-control and cohort studies. British Medical Journal 315:1049–1053

Parker M J, Gillespie W J, Gillespie L D et al 2004 Hip protectors for preventing hip fractures in older people. Cochrane Database of Systematic Reviews issue 3. Art. No.: CD001255. DOI: 10.1002/14651858. CD001255

Prudham D, Evans J G 1981 Factors associated with falls in the elderly: a community study. Age and Ageing 10:141–146

Ray W A, Taylor J A, Meador K G et al 1997 A randomized trial of a consultation service to reduce falls in nursing homes. Journal of the American Medical Association 278:557–562

Robertson M C, Devlin N, Gardner M M et al 2001 Effectiveness and economic evaluation of a nurse delivered home exercise programme to prevent falls. 1: randomised controlled trial. British Medical Journal 322:697–701

Rubenstein L Z, Josephson K R, Robbins A S et al 1994 Falls in the nursing home. Annals of Internal Medicine 121:442–451

Skelton D, Dinan S, Campbell M et al 2005 Tailored group exercise (Falls Management Exercise – FaME) reduces falls in community-dwelling older frequent fallers (an RCT). Age and Ageing 34:636–639

Tinetti M E 1987 Factors associated with serious injury during falls by ambulatory nursing home residents. Journal of the American Geriatrics Society 35: 644–648

Tinetti M E, Baker D I, McAvay G et al 1994 A multifactorial intervention to reduce the risk of falling among elderly people living in the community. New England Journal of Medicine 331:821–827

Wagner E H, LaCroix A Z, Grothaus L et al 1994 Preventing disability and falls in older adults: a population-based randomized trial. American Journal of Public Health 84:1800–1806

Wolf S L, Barnhardt H X, Kutner N G et al 1996 Reducing frailty and falls in older persons: an investigation of Tai Chi and computerized balance training. Atlanta FICSIT Group. Frailty and Injuries: Cooperative Studies of Intervention Techniques. Journal of the American Geriatrics Society 44:489–497

RECOMMENDED READING

Books

Kenny R A (ed) 1996 Syncope in the older patient; causes, investigations and consequences of syncope and falls. Chapman & Hall Medical, London

Lord S R, Sherrington C, Menz H et al 2007 Falls in older people: risk factors and strategies for prevention. Cambridge University Press, Cambridge

Guidelines

American Geriatrics Society, British Geriatrics Society, American Academy of Orthopaedic Surgeons Panel on Falls Prevention 2001 Guideline for the prevention of falls in older persons. Journal of the American Geriatrics Society 49:664–672

National Institute for Health and Clinical Excellence 2005 The assessment and prevention of falls in older people. Online. Available: http://www.nice.org.uk

Cochrane review

Gillespie L D, Gillespie W J, Robertson M C et al 2003 Interventions for preventing falls in elderly people (Cochrane Review). The Cochrane Library, vol 2. John Wiley & Sons, Chichester

SELF-ASSESSMENT QUESTIONS

Are the following true or false?

1. The following risk factors have been consistently shown to be associated with a high risk of falling:
   a. Centrally acting medications
   b. Parkinson's disease
   c. Poor footwear and foot care
   d. Impaired balance
   e. Alcohol

2. The following approaches to intervention have been shown to be effective in preventing falls:
   a. Exercise as a single intervention in the nursing home setting
   b. Multidisciplinary assessment in patients with Alzheimer's disease
   c. A dual chamber pacemaker for vasodepressor carotid sinus syndrome
   d. Withdrawal of centrally acting medication
   e. Expedited cataract extraction

Chapter 15

Orthogeriatric care

Colin Currie

INTRODUCTION

Fractures are common in elderly people, and commoner in frailer, older elderly subjects, because such patients combine key risk factors, namely osteoporosis and a tendency to fall. In a typical trauma orthopaedic unit older patients might account for around one-third of admissions and – because of their greater length of stay – a much higher proportion of the unit's bed days.

Hip fracture is the dominant diagnosis, since it is both the commonest and the most serious common injury, comprising perhaps half of elderly trauma admissions. A wide range of generally lesser injuries accounts for the rest.

A high proportion of elderly trauma patients are frail. Many have pre-existing medical problems and some will have fallen and sustained a fracture as a result of acute illness. Intercurrent medical problems may complicate the pre- and post-operative management of elderly trauma cases.

Most elderly fracture patients admitted to an orthopaedic unit will undergo surgery. Modern surgery for trauma in the elderly patient focuses on techniques which allow the patient to use the affected limb as soon as possible, thus minimizing the loss of function associated with prolonged disuse and allowing as early as possible a start on the serious business of rehabilitation. Such rehabilitation presents complex challenges to many agencies and clinical disciplines.

Collaboration between orthopaedic surgeons and geriatricians has become increasingly common in the UK over the past 30 years. Patterns of collaboration between care of the elderly and orthopaedic services vary greatly and continue to evolve.

The purpose of this chapter is to describe epidemiology, medical and rehabilitation management, and service organization.

Some surgical thoughts on elderly trauma patients

Professor Michael Devas FRCS, a pioneer of orthogeriatric care in Hastings in the 1960s and 1970s, was a clear thinker and a great phrase-maker. Some of his aphorisms should be very widely known:

- On the fracture: 'Fix it and forget it'
- On surgery: 'Surgery is only an incident in the rehabilitation of the elderly fracture patient'
- On bed rest: 'Bed rest is rehabilitation for the coffin'

FRACTURES IN ELDERLY PATIENTS

A woman of 50 years faces lifetime risks of 30% for a vertebral fracture, 16% for a hip fracture and 15% for a Colles' fracture. At a population level, the mass survival for frail, osteoporotic elderly subjects has resulted in a sustained increase in the incidence of fractures, most notably hip fracture.

The age-specific incidence of hip fracture has risen markedly but in a number of populations it has now ceased to rise. This is perhaps a reflection of a one-off loss of the protective effect of exercise on bone mass for women, the decline in physical exercise in women being in turn related to the effects of urbanization and industrialization.

With hip fracture numbers having doubled over the past 30 years in many areas, and with case mix tending towards older and frailer patients, various alarming projections about bed use have been published. However, over the same period, improvements in surgery have facilitated earlier mobilization, and improvements in rehabilitation and service organization have substantially reduced length of stay. Such efficiency gains are welcome, but have only partially offset the rising numbers. Resources required for hip fracture care will continue to rise for the foreseeable future.

The seriousness of hip fracture as an injury can be documented in several ways. Around one-third of patients are dead at 1 year, with excess mortality being concentrated on those who were previously frail and institutionalized and in the early post-fracture months. Around 40% of survivors lose independent mobility, and 10–20% of those admitted from home subsequently enter institutional care. Costs also are high, estimated at around £10000 per case within the NHS, with similar average downstream costs for community services and institutional care.

Most (around 80%) of hip fracture patients are female. Hip fracture is much less common among men, and male hip fracture patients frequently have poorer general health, more medical problems and are more likely to have abused alcohol.

As a common, well-defined and serious injury, hip fracture may be regarded as a 'tracer condition' that tests many specialties and agencies, including accident and emergency, surgery, care of the elderly, rehabilitation and the various community services, institutional and otherwise (Fig. 15.1).

Other fractures in elderly people are generally less serious, many not requiring hospital admission. The commonest is wrist fracture, which peaks in incidence at around 70 years (10 years before hip fracture). Fracture of the neck of

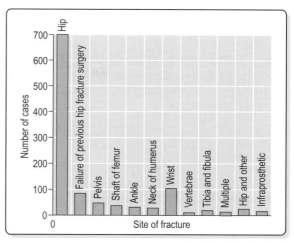

Figure 15.1 Types of fractures in patients aged over 70 years admitted to the acute orthopaedic wards at the Royal Infirmary of Edinburgh 1995. (From MacLennan W J, Currie C T 1997 Rehabilitation after minor fractures in elderly patients. Reviews in Clinical Gerontology 7:55–62, Cambridge University Press. Reprinted with kind permission of Cambridge University Press.)

humerus is another fairly common lesser fracture, also commonly managed non-surgically, as are minor ankle injuries.

Crush vertebral osteoporotic fractures are a common cause of pain and disability but only a minority are admitted to orthopaedic care. Pelvic fracture resulting from a fall is normally associated with little displacement and usually managed conservatively.

In the lower limb fractures of shaft of femur – now more commonly infraprosthetic as survivors of elective and trauma surgery at the hip increase in numbers – is a serious injury often requiring internal fixation. Displaced tibial fractures, commonly resulting from 'bumper injuries', pose considerable surgical problems, as do more complex ankle injuries.

Many minor fractures in old age may be managed satisfactorily in the accident and emergency department. In previously fit elderly subjects, discharge home may pose no particular problems. However, in the frail elderly patient, good accident and emergency care also involves evaluation of function and support, the organization of community services, good communication with primary care and, ideally, some form of follow-up, with rehabilitation continuing at home if required.

In the remainder of this chapter I will concentrate on matters relating to elderly trauma patients who require to be admitted to orthopaedic care.

THE ROLE OF GERIATRIC MEDICINE

Medical and rehabilitation skills in geriatric medicine have the potential to greatly improve both the quality and the cost-effectiveness of care for elderly trauma patients. Contributions made by geriatricians vary considerably, according to local factors such as resource availability, inter-specialty relations and the scale of the challenge. Arrangements in the regional trauma unit will differ greatly from those in a district general hospital orthopaedic unit.

Possible contributions from geriatric medicine

- Preoperative rehabilitation assessment
- Preoperative diagnosis and management of medical problems
- Care of intercurrent medical problems during acute stay
- Early rehabilitation and discharge management for previously fitter cases
- Sustained rehabilitation of patients unfit for early discharge
- Placement or terminal care, where appropriate

As in many other areas of care of the elderly, good care depends upon the existence of a broadly-based and well-functioning interdisciplinary team. In addition to surgeons and geriatricians, nurses, physiotherapists, occupational therapists and social workers should be available. Integration of their work to achieve the best possible results for the individual patient is vital. For rehabilitation purposes this is commonly achieved (as elsewhere) by means of regular multidisciplinary case conferences. However, the pace of events in trauma care may be considerable, and resource pressures, particularly those relating to the availability of beds, can result in considerable strain. To

survive and prosper as a trainee geriatrician in such circumstances requires considerable reserves of both tact and leadership (see Ch. 18 on rehabilitation).

THE SURGEON AND THE GERIATRICIAN

Many attempts to establish geriatric–orthopaedic collaboration have foundered, and poor relationships between geriatricians and orthopaedic surgeons are a common theme in such failures. Surgeons work under considerable pressure, responding to urgent events and, in the case of elderly trauma patients, having to carry out difficult procedures in frail, ill and highly vulnerable patients whose bone quality is often poor. The surgeon's core skill is obviously operative surgery, but individuals will vary greatly in their aptitude for and involvement in the medical care and rehabilitation of their elderly patients.

Similarly, their expectations of collaboration with geriatricians will vary. Some will encourage or permit close involvement by geriatricians in all but the most strictly surgical aspects of care. A few will simply demand the removal of 'bed blockers', and despair when this expectation is not or cannot be delivered. Successful collaboration depends upon surgeons and geriatricians respecting each other's skills and contributions, and facing resource issues constructively rather than adversarially.

PREOPERATIVE REHABILITATION ASSESSMENT

Though for practical reasons this is not always possible, there is much to be said for preoperative rehabilitation assessment. For many patients it will provide a reassuring view of the way ahead, up to and beyond discharge home.

Preoperative rehabilitation assessment should include the following:

- Nature of injury and likely surgery
- Previous general fitness (e.g. goes out alone; does shopping?)

- Home circumstances (living alone? Suitability of housing? Internal or external stairs?)
- Cognitive state (Abbreviated Mental Test?)
- Personal and domestic activities of daily living before injury
- Community services (Home help? District nurse? Lunch club? Day hospital?)
- Medical history
- Active medical problems
- Medication
- Dependent relatives

Such an assessment can conveniently and reliably be based on a proforma and, in the hands of an experienced multidisciplinary team, can be used to generate an early but useful impression of the likely rehabilitation needs and potential of the individual patient. In general terms, a favourable rehabilitation prognosis is associated with previous mental clarity, good previous mobility and functional independence, and favourable – or at least not adverse – home circumstances.

For example, a previously independent 75-year-old widow living alone, managing without any community services input and taking regular exercise, is likely to make rapid progress following surgery for hip fracture and will be glad to be told so. A 92-year-old with the same injury, previously house-bound, managing personal activities of daily living but dependent on domestic support from community services, is likely to require a longer period of rehabilitation but may still get home again with increased support.

A demented patient admitted from a nursing home with hip fracture will require surgery followed by a fairly brief period of postoperative care before being returned to her familiar circumstances, providing that her dependency can be managed appropriately and some physiotherapy input – mainly advice to staff – is available. The rehabilitation needs and potential of such patients are modest. Their mortality is high.

As well as allowing early planning of future care, such preoperative assessment will, for fitter patients, allow goal setting and serve to foster (where appropriate) a spirit of optimism. Informal carers and other relatives should be seen both as potential contributors to the rehabilitation assessment and allies in the effort to return patients home as soon as it is comfortable and safe to do so.

PREOPERATIVE MEDICAL ASSESSMENT AND CARE

To the experienced trainee in geriatric medicine, some aspects of life in the orthopaedic ward will be quite familiar. In many units, most patients will be old, and such patients will be in many respects similar to those seen already in the course of training as admissions to more orthodox care of the elderly settings.*

Many common chronic medical problems are associated with falls and fractures in elderly patients. These include dementia, Parkinson's disease, previous stroke, visual impairment, muscle weakness, osteoarthritis, severe anaemia, congestive cardiac failure and diabetes mellitus.

In addition, a minority of patients may present with a fracture following a fall attributable to an acute episode such as viral or bacterial infection, transient cerebral ischaemia, unstable angina, myocardial infarction or cardiac arrhythmia. In these circumstances the fracture, particularly if it is a hip fracture, dominates the clinical picture. It is important not to lose sight of a clinically important precursor event.

Sadly, for a small but important proportion of patients, the fracture is an important and painful incident in the course of a final illness. The last stages of a dementing process or a complex medical illness may be further complicated by (e.g.) a hip fracture and the related orthopaedic admission and care. A minority of hip fracture patients – perhaps around 10% – will have a prior diagnosis of a malignancy, although in only a small proportion of such cases is the fracture pathological.

In these circumstances, surgical and rehabilitation management must be tailored to the overall

---

*A medical student who assisted me on a study of dependency and sensory impairment in elderly trauma patients remarked, after about the 200th patient, 'This is not so much an orthopaedic unit as a geriatric unit that does operations'. He later went on to become an obstetrician.

context. Since surgery is the most effective form of pain relief for hip fracture, it is justified in all patients likely to survive more than a few days. Surgery, along with analgesia, should take its part in an overall strategy of good terminal care.

In a minority of elderly trauma patients active medical problems will require vigorous pre-operative management in order to render the patient fit for anaesthesia. Common examples of such problems include new or under-treated cardiac failure, diabetes mellitus in need of stabilization, bronchopneumonia and dehydration. The aim of all such treatment is to quickly optimize fitness for anaesthesia and surgery and thus minimize preoperative delay.

Sadly, not all preoperative delay occurs because patients are medically unfit for surgery. Preoperative delay not attributable to medical problems but due to administrative causes (such as lack of theatre time) is associated with poorer outcomes, including increased morbidity, mortality and length of stay. In a few unfortunate instances, repeated fasting and cancellation of surgery leads to further problems (e.g. intercurrent infection, electrolyte disturbance) leading in turn to further delay. Uncertainty, discomfort and helplessness can quickly destroy the morale essential for postoperative progress.

DELIRIUM

Acute confusional states are common in elderly trauma patients (see Ch. 17 on old age psychiatry). Contributory factors include the familiar list relating to any acute episode and hospital admission in elderly patients. However, trauma patients are at additional risk.

The distress, anxiety and situational upset of fall, fracture and admission to a busy and perhaps noisy trauma ward commonly cause decompensation in patients previously only precariously oriented. Most are in pain, which can cause restlessness and sleep deprivation. Intercurrent infection (particularly urinary tract infection and respiratory tract infection) is common. Alcohol withdrawal should be borne in mind, particularly in men. Hypoglycaemia and electrolyte disturbance caused by prolonged preoperative fasting are also risk factors.

Cerebral hypoxia is the final common path of a number of surgically-related precipitants of delirium. Hypotension during surgery correlates strongly with postoperative confusional states, which may be profound and slow to resolve. Postoperative opiate analgesia may depress respiration. In addition, intermittently low oxygen saturation may persist for some days after anaesthesia and monitoring for up to 5 days may be necessary.

In most cases delirium is multifactorial but mercifully brief, and many patients who experience even quite serious disruption for 1 or 2 days after surgery go on to regain their orientation and hence their rehabilitation impetus.

FLUID BALANCE

Many elderly trauma patients will have impaired renal function before their injury, and many will be hypovolaemic at the time of admission and subsequently. The proper management of fluid balance through preoperative, operative and early postoperative stages of care is therefore of great importance.

Fluid management has traditionally been a surgical responsibility, and one which has on occasion given rise for concern. The National Confidential Enquiry into Perioperative Deaths (NCEPOD 1999) documents more than 1000 deaths at the age of 90 years or over, 60% of which occurred in orthopaedic care, and notes that 'fluid imbalance can contribute to serious postoperative morbidity and mortality', and recommends detailed and active attention to fluid balance.

This includes the correction of preoperative hypovolaemia, particular care with spinal anaesthesia (which, by causing vasodilatation potentiates the hypotensive effect of hypovolaemia), close postoperative monitoring of fluid balance, and daily postoperative checking of serum urea, electrolytes and creatinine.

NUTRITION

Some patients admitted with hip fracture – perhaps around one-fifth – are severely undernourished. In winter, this proportion rises because of the increased vulnerability of the frailest and least well-nourished to the effects of cold weather. Such patients are at high risk of poor outcomes. There is some evidence that nutritional interventions, such as oral supplementation to increase energy and protein intake, may be beneficial.

PRESSURE DAMAGE

Pressure damage, often acquired in the hours immediately following the fracture, may take days to become apparent and then go on to require prolonged care, inhibit rehabilitation and add weeks or even months to overall length of stay (see Ch. 20 on pressure sores).

Awareness of risk, together with appropriate action, is a high priority in the care of elderly trauma patients, from the time of admission to the accident and emergency department and throughout the period of trauma-associated dependency. Detailed nursing documentation and low pressure surfaces are essential. The combination of good practice and local audit can show such interventions to be beneficial, substantially reducing the incidence of pressure damage. Prolonged bed rest is now rarely indicated for elderly trauma patients, because surgery is geared to avoid it wherever possible. A few (mainly those with major pelvic or femoral shaft fractures) may need to be immobilized for prolonged periods. Most do not. *Early mobilization and active rehabilitation are the keys to minimizing postoperative risk to pressure areas.*

INFECTION

Intercurrent infections, mainly urinary tract infection and respiratory tract infection, are common in elderly trauma patients. While sensitivities may be important, there are strong arguments for immediate treatment to minimize systemic upset, dependency and delay in rehabilitation. Cultures from material despatched before immediate treatment may be of value later, though in most cases antibiotic therapy prescribed on the basis of local protocols and clinical judgement will be effective.

Despite the routine use of preoperative antibiotic prophylaxis, wound infections – particularly in hip fracture patients – can be problematic. Most infections are superficial. The small minority of deep infections greatly increases morbidity

and dependency. The sequence of deep infection, removal of implant, an open infected wound requiring complex nursing care, etc., is a dispiriting one for the patient, surgeons and all others concerned. Morbidity and mortality are high.

The recent rise in methicillin-resistant *Staphylococcus aureus* (MRSA) infections is also a matter of great concern, with implications for operating theatre procedures, nursing care and rehabilitation. Precautions are time-consuming and not always effective. Where isolation becomes necessary, frail elderly patients do not thrive. Scope for mobilization is very limited in a single room. Self-esteem suffers. The impact on rehabilitation progress may be deleterious.

DEEP VEIN THROMBOSIS

Deep vein thrombosis with pulmonary embolus is a much-feared complication in elderly trauma patients, particularly after lower limb trauma, surgery and bed rest. Where possible, early mobilization is strongly recommended. Other thromboprophylactic measures include mechanical pumping devices and low molecular weight heparin. Where deep vein thrombosis occurs, management is determined by its extent and the overall clinical context.

Minor distal thrombosis may be managed with support stockings and continuing low molecular weight heparin. Major thrombosis other than in the frailest patients merits warfarinization. However, prolonged warfarinization, e.g. beyond a few weeks, may be hard to justify and very difficult to deliver reliably and safely in frail elderly patients who are going home.

MORALE, PAIN CONTROL AND DEPRESSION

The impact of a major fracture on the life of an elderly patient varies greatly with individual circumstances, but may be immense. For a sad minority, a hip fracture signifies the end of independent living and the loss of a loved and valued home. Many older patients, with impressions gained from what happened to their own elderly relatives many years ago, believe that hip fracture automatically means a hospital stay of months at least. *Active management of the patient's expectations and morale is an important and much under-valued part of the rehabilitation of elderly trauma patients.*

Early and positive involvement of the patient in discussions about surgery, postoperative care and rehabilitation is to be encouraged. Since hip fracture is the major clinical problem, an information sheet or booklet, outlining the main types of fracture and operation and describing the process of rehabilitation, is well worth providing. It will be appreciated by patients and, importantly, by informal carers and other relatives.

Morale can also be preserved and promoted by minimizing preoperative delay and by ensuring adequate pain control. Pain control protocols, backed up with simple pain scales (e.g. frowning face to smiling face) ensure a minimum standard of analgesia even when wards are busy and staff do not know patients well. The special problems of delirium should be remembered. Acute confusion does not protect people from pain, and poorly managed pain adds to delirium. Opiates are effective, and should be mandatory for the first few postoperative days in most cases. Good analgesia is also essential for rehabilitation, and 'pre-physio' analgesia can greatly assist in early mobilization.

The distress, discomfort and possible indignity of a sudden admission to a trauma ward should not be underestimated. A sensitive approach to the individual patient and her (and it is usually her) anxieties is essential. Explanations of events should be made in terms the patient understands. 'You *were* fasting for theatre, but there's been a multiple and now you've been cancelled' makes sense only to those of us who work in trauma wards all the time.

The patient's morale is hard to assess, hard to predict and yet vital to the rehabilitation process. Apparently robust characters may succumb to sudden despair. Aged, frail and previously disabled individuals may sail through an admission. Experienced rehabilitation staff recognize this, and know also that an approach broadly characterized as 'realistic optimism' is usually seen as both supportive and effective.

Early progress improves morale. A few steps today, a few more tomorrow and getting as far as the toilet a few days later may be hard and uncomfortable work, but the prospect of a pre-discharge home visit can be a powerful incentive, and awareness of similar patients in the ward who are a bit further along the road that leads homewards will also boost morale and in turn lead to further progress.

In the course of an acute admission for trauma it is often difficult to assess whether or not a patient is depressed. So much is going on that distress and the symptoms of possible depression are inextricably entangled. Later in the rehabilitation process the distinction may become clearer. A few patients – principally those who are disproportionately despairing or mysteriously under-performing in rehabilitation, will turn out to have treatable depression. At this stage a screening questionnaire, e.g. the Geriatric Depression Scale, may be useful. The impact on rehabilitation of successful antidepressant therapy can sometimes be dramatic.

REHABILITATION

ACUTE REHABILITATION

Trauma-related dependency is intrinsically self-limiting. Patients, though requiring considerable nursing care post-fracture and in the perioperative period, have in most cases the potential to begin rehabilitation early. To cite again the most common important injury, hip fracture patients in many units will be able to sit or even weight bear on the first postoperative day. The combination of good pain control and enthusiastic physiotherapy can maximize the early potential of the previously fitter patients.

However, many elderly trauma patients, previously frail and with limited powers of concentration, will require a more gentle approach, based on 'little and often' and seeking gradually to extend the range of comfortable mobility with a frame.

Many patients with either upper or lower limb injuries will find it difficult to begin dressing themselves, but early dressing practice under occupational therapist supervision will signify the return to normality.

For patients making satisfactory early progress, an immediate goal is the ability to mobilize to the toilet and manage independently there. This is a useful threshold at which to consider a pre-discharge home visit, usually with an occupational therapist but sometimes involving the physio-therapist too.

'HOSPITAL-AT-HOME', EARLY SUPPORTED DISCHARGE

Many such schemes have now been developed and reported. The common elements are early multidisciplinary postoperative rehabilitation in the acute unit; discharge planning and the mobilization of appropriate community or outreach rehabilitation services; and follow-up to monitor progress and ensure patient safety.

Such schemes should be properly funded, staffed and organized. Given their inevitable diversity in terms of case mix, context, staffing, outcome measures and the irreducible 'black box' element intrinsic to rehabilitation, high-quality randomized controlled trials are few, and system-atic evidence of their overall impact limited. However, there is some evidence for both the effectiveness and cost-effectiveness of early sup-ported discharge schemes (Cameron et al 2000).

What matters is service development in the local context, and what works locally. Details of arrangements concerning early supported dis-charge schemes are determined by such factors as resources, funding responsibilities, interdisci-plinary and interagency relations. Setting them up, monitoring their impact on care locally, and maintaining them are major challenges for ortho-geriatricians, but very important ones; and partic-ularly rewarding when evaluations of service improvement, falling length of stay and rising patient satisfaction emerge. When these outcomes can be achieved, they are welcome, and support the broader view that 'looking after older patients well is cheaper than looking after them badly'.

POST-ACUTE IN-PATIENT REHABILITATION

For frailer and/or more seriously injured patients who are unsuitable for the rapid rehabilitation approach described above, other arrangements have developed. Again, names and details vary from centre to centre but common elements can be identified.

Orthogeriatric units offer patients with no early prospects of home a sustained period of multi-disciplinary rehabilitation, usually under a geria-trician leadership, in order to maximize the prospects of eventual discharge home.

Patients proceeding home from orthogeriatric units may be among the frailest to be discharged from hospital. Careful discharge planning, ideally backed up by postdischarge monitoring and some continuing rehabilitation input, will be appreci-ated, and may serve to minimize the numbers readmitted.

In terms both of the aspirations of the individual patient and the overall cost-effectiveness of care, this 'last chance for home' is extremely important. Even fairly prolonged rehabilitation and relatively costly care packages to ensure adequate levels of care and safety at home can be justified. The loss of freedom and the costs associated with perma-nent institutionalization are great, and it is greatly to be regretted that, in the wake of a hip fracture, older patients may sometimes be dispatched quickly and ill advisedly to an irreversible long-term placement.

A second major function of postacute ortho-geriatric care is to achieve placement for patients unable to go home. If, after every reasonable effort has been made to maximize the patient's level of function, institutional placement is inevitable, an orthogeriatric ward provides more appropriate care pending placement than that on offer in an acute orthopaedic unit. In addition, time and expertise are available to ensure a proper process of maximizing the patient's function and thus determining the level of permanent care required: NHS long-term care, nursing home care, or resi-dential care.

A third and very important function of an orthogeriatric unit is to provide terminal care for the frailest of survivors of trauma and trauma surgery. Again, the circumstances of a postacute ward might be seen as more appropriate. The general principles of terminal care for elderly subjects apply.

Goals of postacute in-patient care for elderly trauma patients (orthogeriatric units, geriatric orthopaedic rehabilitation units, etc.)

■ Sustained rehabilitation to provide a 'last chance for home' for frailer patients
■ A placement service – following rehabilitation/ triage – for patients who cannot go home
■ Terminal care for a minority of patients

Orthogeriatric units with a non-selective approach to admitting patients from acute care (i.e. those taking all patients who cannot be discharged directly home) might expect that around half their patients will eventually return home, around 40% require placement, and the remaining 10% will die.

Orthogeriatric unit admission policies, however, vary considerably. Where the number of rehabilitation beds is very limited, there is an argument for selective admissions, restricted to those perceived on the acute ward as having 'rehabilitation potential', i.e. the previously fitter and less challenging patients. Problems, of course, result in relation to the continuing stay in acute orthopaedic care of patients with no need of the specialist services in that unit.

An alternative approach is to take from the acute unit all patients seen as facing problems and therefore more in need of prolonged specialist orthogeriatrics rehabilitation. Where resources permit, such a non-selective transfer policy is clearly preferable, both in terms of freeing acute beds and maximizing the rehabilitation potential of the frailest patients. A further important point is that selective policies rely essentially on a predictive exercise carried out on a highly unpredictable population. A non-selective transfer policy, in practice taking all patients who cannot be discharged timeously from the acute ward, has at least the merit of intellectual respectability.

SECONDARY PREVENTION

A fragility fracture, in most cases resulting from the combination of postural instability and osteoporosis, is a sentinel event which, in ideal circumstances, should trigger secondary prevention measures addressing both underlying causes. Where possible, the assessment of a fragility fracture patient should include a falls assessment, or be followed by a referral to a falls assessment clinic (see Ch. 14 on falls). With increasing evidence supporting the value of bone protection too (see Ch. 36 on osteoporosis), many patients will benefit from bisphosphonate therapy.

THE WAY AHEAD?

Growing realization of the importance of rehabilitation for elderly trauma patients has resulted in many and diverse local initiatives. Given the demographic projections – hip fractures are predicted to double by 2050 – it is likely that service pressures will continue to grow. Continuing efforts directed at improving rehabilitation will be required. However, considerable difficulties arise in evaluating evidence about effectiveness and in using such evidence to support rehabilitation developments in specific settings.

In this respect, the contrast between surgery and rehabilitation is illuminating. Surgical advances, such as the dynamic hip screw, can be evaluated and adopted for widespread use in the fairly standard conditions of the operating theatre. Advances in rehabilitation – more complex, more interdisciplinary, and much more dependent on local circumstances – are much more difficult to evaluate and replicate.

For sound logistical reasons, randomized controlled trials in trauma rehabilitation in elderly patients have been few. Again for logistical reasons, the generalization of successful approaches in different settings is much more difficult than with technical surgical advances. While ideas and procedures from successful schemes elsewhere can be incorporated into local developments, no universal formula for successful rehabilitation of elderly trauma patients exists, nor should one be expected.

The development of services depends upon a collaborative, interdisciplinary approach. Ideally this should be based on local information about existing services; the identification of definable goals for a service initiative; and a commitment both to resource and to monitor the impact of that initiative. General principles and ideas from elsewhere may help, but in the end 'all rehabilitation is local'. Local arrangements must be developed to deliver good care locally, and their effectiveness assessed at local level.

Recent interest in evidence-based guidelines on hip fracture care should be noted. Such guidelines, specifically for hip fracture care, have been developed and published both in Australia and in Scotland (March et al 1999, SIGN 2002). Based on the 'pathway of care' from the accident and emergency department, through the surgical unit and operating theatre, and on into rehabilitation and eventual discharge, these guidelines are derived from systematic scrutiny of the best available published evidence on preoperative care, surgery, anaesthesia and rehabilitation. Guidelines, which are designed to support rather than substitute for clinical judgment, appear to generate upward pressures on the quality of care, but require to be translated into protocols for local use.

Major developments in hip fracture audit, by addressing the key 'tracer condition' encountered in orthogeriatric care, offer another and perhaps complementary approach to improving care. An internationally agreed basic data set, resulting from the EU-funded SAHFE programme (Standardised Audit of Hip Fracture in Europe), has been piloted throughout Europe and is in widespread use in Scotland (www.sahfe.ort.lu.se). It offers a means of comparing case mix, process and outcome of hip fracture care both between centres and over time in individual centres. It also provides a method for monitoring case load and case mix, evaluating service pressures and developments, and, by means of optional additions to the basic data set, an approach to scrutinizing specific aspects of care such as anaesthesia, pain control and pressure area care. In a recent collaborative initiative involving the British Orthopaedic Association, the British Geriatrics Society and the Royal College of Physicians of London, a UK-wide National Hip Fracture Database – web-based, and offering continuous unit feedback and nationwide benchmarking; and covering acute care, rehabilitation and secondary prevention – has been proposed. If established, it is likely to further focus clinical, managerial and political attention on hip fracture care and its improvement – no bad thing, given the injury's current incidence importance and future projections.

There is now an urgent need to develop more systematically the training required for the subspecialty of orthogeriatric care. Centres with established services and senior expertise should take on this responsibility, perhaps with programmes analogous to those provided for trainees with a special interest in stroke care; and obviously, in view of all of the above, such training should be collaborative. In future, relationships and mutual understanding between geriatricians and trauma orthopaedic surgeons are likely to be more enjoyable and more productive if they begin their consultant careers with informed and positive attitudes about the most numerous and challenging patient group in their care.

SUMMARY AND CONCLUSION

The care of the growing numbers of elderly osteoporotic fracture patients presents a considerable challenge to surgeons, geriatricians and the interdisciplinary team. Surgery and rehabilitation have both evolved substantially over recent decades.

Collaboration in the care of elderly trauma patients has taken many forms. Schemes designed to promote early rehabilitation are being more widely adopted, and established postacute rehabilitation units continue to offer sustained multidisciplinary rehabilitation for frailer patients. Evaluation, although problematical, has been broadly encouraging, particularly for the early rehabilitation initiatives.

For the geriatrician in training, orthogeriatric care may be seen as an emerging subspecialty of elderly medicine, and one with its own challenges and satisfactions, involving both acute medical care and a particularly rewarding experience of rehabilitation. Given the projections for a continuing rise in osteoporotic fractures, the organizational challenges for the consultants of the future are likely to be just as interesting as those met in the course of the first few decades of joint working with orthopaedic services.

REFERENCES

Cameron I, Crotty M, Currie C et.al 2000 Geriatric rehabilitation following fractures in older people: a systematic review: Health Technology Assessment 4:i–iv,1–111

March L M, Chamberlain A C, Cameron I D 1999 How best to fix a broken hip? Medical Journal of Australia 170:489–494

National Confidential Enquiry into Patient Outcome and Death 1999 Extremes of age. The Report of the National Confidential Enquiry into Perioperative Deaths. NCEPOD, London. Online. Available: http://www.ncepod.org.uk/1999.htm

Scottish Intercollegiate Guidelines Network 2002 Prevention and management of hip fracture in older people – a national clinical guideline. SIGN, Edinburgh. Online. Available: http://www.sign.ac.uk

RECOMMENDED READING

*** Essential reading; ** recommended reading

Audit Commission 1995 United they stand: coordinating care for elderly patients with hip fracture. Audit Commission. HMSO, London **

British Orthopaedic Association 2007 The care of fragility fracture patients ('BOA Blue Book') BOA, London. Online. Available://www.boa.ac.uk

Heyburn G, Beringer T, Elliott J et al 2004 Orthogeriatric care in patients with fractures of the proximal femur. Clinical Orthopaedics and Related Research 425:35–43 **

Parker M, Johansen A 2006 Hip fracture. British Medical Journal 333:27–30 ***

SELF-ASSESSMENT QUESTIONS

Are the following statements true or false?

1. In hip fracture:
   a. About two-thirds of patients are admitted from home
   b. The female/male ratio is about 60:40
   c. 80% of patients regain their former mobility
   d. About 30% of patients are dead at 1 year

2. In orthogeriatric rehabilitation:
   a. Older fracture patients should only rarely be mobilized within 1 week of surgery
   b. Intercurrent infection may impede rehabilitation
   c. Cognitive impairment is a contraindication to rehabilitation
   d. The effectiveness of multidisciplinary orthogeriatric rehabilitation remains unproven

Chapter **16**

Palliative care

Suzanne Kite and Catherine O'Doherty

INTRODUCTION

'Death has dominion because it is not only the start of nothing but the end of everything, and how we think and talk about dying – the emphasis we put on dying with 'dignity' – shows how important it is that life ends appropriately, that death keeps faith with the way we want to have lived.'

(Dworkin 1993)

Patient-centred care involving complex problem solving, multiple interacting pathologies, challenging psychosocial situations and multi-professional teams are the key features shared by specialist palliative care and elderly care medicine. They require a similar approach and similar skills, and the patient groups and areas of expertise overlap.

Specialist palliative care offers geriatricians:

- *Complex symptom management*, based on a 'total symptom' perspective and using multi-professional skills
- *Experience in the care of dying patients*, including the delicate balancing of benefits and burdens at the end of life, symptom management and carer support
- *Specialist knowledge of supportive networks*, statutory and charitable, both in and outside hospital

This chapter is not an encyclopaedia of symptom control, psychosocial and spiritual care. Excellent reference texts, handbooks and symptom guides

exist (Doyle et al 2005, Fallon & O'Neill 1998, Faull et al 2005). Instead, we hope to provide helpful practical tips, to direct you to other comprehensive sources of information, and to clarify how to gain access to and use specialist palliative care services.

PALLIATIVE CARE SERVICES

DEFINITIONS

Palliative care:

- Provides relief from pain and other distressing symptoms
- Affirms life and regards dying as a normal process
- Intends neither to hasten nor postpone death
- Integrates the psychological and spiritual aspects of patient care
- Offers a support system to help patients live as actively as possible until death
- Offers a support system to help the family to cope during the patient's illness and in their own bereavement
- Uses a team approach to address the needs of patients and their families, including bereavement counselling, if indicated
- Will enhance quality of life, and may also positively influence the course of the illness
- Is applicable early in the course of illness, in conjunction with other therapies that are intended to prolong life (such as chemotherapy

or radiation therapy), and includes those investigations needed to understand better and manage distressing clinical complications (WHO 2002)

Palliative care can be either specialist or generic. Generic palliative care, or the palliative care approach, should be applied by every health professional caring for a patient nearing the end of a chronic illness, and it is an integral part of all clinical practice. Specialist palliative care is that provided in units and services with palliative care as their core specialty and where all senior members of professional staff are accredited specialists. Palliative procedures and interventions aim to improve symptom control and quality of life, e.g. radiotherapy, chemotherapy, surgery and anaesthetic techniques (NCHSPCS 1999).

FREQUENTLY ASKED QUESTIONS

Who provides palliative care?
We all do. A whole-person perspective, good communication skills, basic symptom control and multi-professional working are now expected rather than desirable.

When do I refer to specialist palliative care?
When the patient has active, progressive and advanced disease, *and* an extraordinary level of need that cannot be met by the referring team. 'Extraordinary' need is hard to quantify and will vary among patients and with the skills, experience and resources of their carers. However, this need is likely to reflect an intensity or complexity of problems across the physical, psychological, social or spiritual domains (Leeds Teaching Hospitals Trust 1999).

Who are the specialist palliative care team?
The team usually includes one or more clinical nurse specialists, with medical support from a palliative medicine doctor. Other team members may include: a social worker, counsellor, pharmacist, physiotherapist, occupational therapist, dietician, spiritual advisors, complementary therapists, volunteers and others.

How do palliative care teams operate?
Teams evolve in response to local needs and resources, with an emphasis on educating and empowering. Therefore there are differences between teams, even those on adjacent patches. Try to become familiar, and proficient, with using the palliative care services in your own area.

Specialist palliative care aims to provide a smooth service between home, secondary and tertiary care, and hospice, working alongside statutory and other specialist services.

- *Hospital support teams* act in an advisory role for referred patients and promote the palliative care approach through teaching and example. The focus is on collaborative working and shared care with referring multi-professional teams, rather than on duplicating the role of the professionals involved. Fifty-five per cent of all deaths occur in hospital.
- *In-patient hospices* are specialist palliative care units. They are neither nursing homes nor hospitals. Patients are admitted for assessment, symptom control, continuing care in the event of extraordinary need, respite and rehabilitation. The average length of stay varies between units, but is roughly 1–2 weeks, and discharge rates are often in the range of 30–50%. About 16% of all patients with cancer die in hospices. Most hospices have the facilities for some interventional procedures, e.g. blood transfusions, intravenous bisphosphonates and paracentesis. They rarely have radiological services on site, nor do they offer advanced cardiopulmonary resuscitation facilities (where relevant, this should be discussed with patients and families before transfer). Day care may also be available.
- *Community palliative care* is primarily the responsibility of the general practitioner (GP) and district nurse (DN), and referrals to the community specialist palliative care team should be discussed with them first. It is very important that the GP and DN are informed of a patient's discharge from in-patient care in advance, and that they are provided with enough information to manage the patient from the moment that they get home. In the UK less than 30% of people die in their own homes.

Why don't specialist palliative care teams take over the care of all terminally ill patients?

They do not do this, first, because there is no evidence that they need to and, second, this would de-skill other professionals in a key area.

A comprehensive and very useful list of palliative care services and resources, patient support groups and information services, and charitable organizations may be found in the *Hospice and Palliative Care Directory 2005*, published by The Hospice Information Service: http://www.hospice information.info

BENEFITS AND PALLIATIVE CARE PATIENTS OVER 65 YEARS

Attendance allowance

This is calculated at two rates. Patients with a prognosis of about 6 months or less are automatically eligible for the higher rate under 'special rules' (DS1500). In order to qualify, the patient's doctor needs to complete medical details on the DS1500 form, which is then sent directly to the relevant disability benefits unit of the Department of Social Security, or it may accompany the separate form completed by the patient, relative or social worker. The advantages to the patient of 'special rules' are:

- Higher rate: about £60 per week
- Speed: benefit usually payable within 3 weeks of application
- Easier paperwork
- The allowance does not need to be spent on anything in particular: it can be spent however the person chooses
- Application is not dependent on the presence of a carer: single people can apply
- Once attendance allowance is in place, the patient may be entitled to other benefits, such as an increase in income support and housing benefit. Carers *may* be eligible for carers allowance. However, claiming carers allowance may affect the benefits of the person being cared for, so it is always best to ring the Carers Allowance Helpline to check (01772 899 508) before submitting an application form

Macmillan Cancer Relief grants (see Useful Websites and Contacts)

- Application forms (form CR1) are considered from doctors, nurses and social workers, but not directly from patients. These must be accompanied by a very brief medical report (CR6) completed by a doctor or Macmillan clinical nurse specialist
- Grants are considered on the basis of income and savings. Income needs to be £100 or less per person in disposable income when specific outgoings have been deducted
- There must be less than £8000 savings for a couple, or less than £6000 for a single person
- It is paid quickly – within days
- It is provided for one-off purposes, e.g. travelling, heating, clothing, furnishings, care, telephones and convalescence. The average grant awarded is in the region of £370
- It is not awarded for items already purchased, or for items that should be supplied by the NHS, e.g. medical equipment and appliances

SYMPTOM MANAGEMENT

Most patients with advanced, progressive and life-limiting disease have symptoms that influence quality of life enough to require treatment (Table 16.1).

Table 16.1 Symptom prevalence in the last year of life (Cartwright 1991)		
Symptom	% cancer patients with symptom	% non-cancer patients with symptom
Pain	84	67
Loss of appetite	71	38
Nausea/vomiting	51	27
Insomnia	51	36
Trouble with breathing	47	49
Constipation	47	32
Depression	38	36
Loss of bladder control	37	33
Mental confusion	33	38
Bed sores	28	14
Loss of bowel control	25	22
Unpleasant smell	19	13

GENERAL PRINCIPLES OF SYMPTOM MANAGEMENT

These are the same as those underlying any medical problem, i.e.:

- Assessment: history, examination, appropriate investigations
- Considering underlying pathology and physiology
- Diagnosing the most likely cause/s
- Considering the context: the interaction of psychosocial and spiritual factors and the expression of symptoms
- Implementing a management plan with the patient
- Reviewing, revising

The keys to success in palliative care follow.

1. Thorough assessment

The different perspectives of the patient, carers, nurses and GP, etc., can be useful here. Notes, operation details and radiological investigations are invaluable in building up a three-dimensional anatomical/physiological image. The fourth dimension is the psychosocial and spiritual domain. In particular, establish the *significance* of the symptom to the patient – this will help to bring fears into the open and may give you the diagnosis.

You will also need to unpick the underlying and overlapping pathologies. Is the symptom problem:

- Related to the underlying disease/s?
- Related to the treatment of the disease?
- A coincidental problem (e.g. diverticular disease, scabies)?
- All of the above? Expect to find multiple causes

2. Establishment of a realistic management plan with the patient and team at the outset and revision as necessary

Is the underlying cause treatable, e.g. with disease-modifying drugs, surgery or antibiotics? If so, what is the likelihood of success? Is the treatment appropriate on the basis of the balance of risks/benefits for this individual?

Where treatment of the underlying cause is inappropriate or impossible, palliation is directed at the underlying pathological mechanism/s.

If a firm diagnosis cannot be made, treatment should be instituted on a probability basis for the most likely cause. Assessing response to this initial treatment and a further period of observation may clarify the situation.

The patient should be actively involved in symptom management, whenever possible. They need to know the likely time scale in which improvement will take place, and the degree of improvement that can be expected. They also need the reassurance that if initial treatment fails, other options will be available. Since most treatments will have some associated burdens, it is necessary to explore what is acceptable to individual patients in view of their personal goals and quality of life.

3. Routes of administration

The oral route is usually the one of choice as it is simple, many drugs are available and it is minimally invasive. Swallowing a large number of drugs, however, can be a burden. Every opportunity should be taken to rationalize drugs. *Ask patients whether they prefer tablets, capsules or suspensions, where this choice is available.* If a patient cannot swallow or absorb oral drugs then alternative routes need to be considered:

- The *rectal route* is limited by the unavailability of rectal preparations of many drugs, and the unacceptability of this method of administration to some patients. However, absorption is high, and suppositories of paracetamol, diclofenac and domperidone are available
- *Transdermal route.* Fentanyl, buprenorphine and hyoscine hydrobromide patches are useful for medium- to long-term control of stable symptoms. Because of the prolonged time to reach steady state blood levels, they are not appropriate for acute symptom control, or in rapidly changing situations
- *Transmucosal* forms of lorazepam, prochlorperazine, etc. may be useful
- The *subcutaneous route* is used widely, either for single doses or as continuous infusions delivered by a syringe driver. This permits

parenteral drug administration with minimal patient burden and has the theoretical advantage of steady plasma levels of a wide choice of drugs effective for symptom management. There are several different syringe drivers with different rate settings – seek advice if you are unsure. For problems encountered with syringe drivers, see the British National Formulary (BNF) section on 'Prescribing in palliative care'. Drugs in this context may be used beyond license. If in doubt, consult palliative care services (Dickman et al 2005, Twycross et al 2002) or ask pharmacy

> Syringe drivers are not just for use in the terminal phase. There is nothing magical or sinister about them. They are just a useful tool in any situation where oral absorption of a drug is unreliable for whatever reason. Once up, a driver can come down again. However, the need for them is greatest when a patient is dying, and the public may associate them with imminent or accelerated death. Patients and relatives may need to be reassured that there is not necessarily a causal relationship between the two.

4. Regular assessment
There should be regular reassessment, with a time interval determinant on the severity of the symptom. If the treatment is not working, reconsider your diagnosis, including the route of administration. A common error with antiemetics is to prescribe these orally for established vomiting, when absorption will be poor and a parenteral route, e.g. subcutaneously, for 24 hours could break this established pattern. Also remember that:

- Multiple causes for the same symptom may be present *sequentially,* as well as concurrently. For example, constipation that was due to hypercalcaemia may now be due to the opiates prescribed for bone pain
- Treatment of one symptom may unmask another. For example, the resolution of a severe pain may reveal other aches and pains, and a confused patient may not be able to tell you about their nausea

- The nature of the underlying disease is that it is progressive – new and evolving symptoms are to be expected
- If a drug does not work, or is no longer needed, stop it

5. Anticipate problems
Some problems can be anticipated with scope for pre-emptive management. For example, an annular carcinoma of the rectum will cause progressive constipation, and may lead to complete obstruction, so the appropriateness of a palliative colostomy should be considered early.

6. Mechanical problems need mechanical solutions
The pain of fractured bones responds poorly to analgesic drugs unless the bone is fixed or immobilized. Vomiting due to stenosis of the pylorus responds poorly to antiemetics. If a symptom has a mechanical cause, then consider a mechanical solution.

Emergencies in palliative care

Fortunately these are rare, but when they do occur they can be devastating for everybody. Often such emergencies may be foreseen, and managed more effectively with the benefit of preparation.

Overwhelming pain
Immediate management is directed at achieving sufficient comfort to permit better assessment. Find the most comfortable position for the patient and administer a strong opioid (this is likely to have some effect on most pains), e.g. morphine, remembering to use the equivalent of the 4-hourly dose if the patient is already on regular strong opioids. For bowel colic, consider hyoscine butylbromide and for biliary colic, ureteric colic, bone pain and liver capsule pain consider a nonsteroidal antiinflammatory drug (NSAID), e.g. diclofenac. Ask for expert help early if initial measures are proving ineffective.

Severe agitation
Assess for reversible causes such as pain, urinary retention, loaded rectum, drugs (e.g. opioids, corticosteroids) or withdrawal of drugs (e.g. opioids,

alcohol, nicotine) and biochemical disturbance (e.g. hypercalcaemia), and treat as appropriate. Carers and nurses may be aware of the presence of spiritual distress, heightened as death approaches (terminal agitation). Interim management with anxiolytics or neuroleptics may be needed while the treatment of the underlying cause takes effect. In terminal agitation, it may be appropriate to sedate the patient, but this is ideally a multi-professional team decision. It should be discussed with the relatives and the patient, if possible.

Hypercalcaemia

This can occur with almost any cancer, but is particularly common with myeloma, bronchial carcinoma and breast cancer. Symptoms may have developed insidiously. Treat with intravenous rehydration, followed by intravenous bisphosphonates, and further hydration as necessary. Consider longer-term management, e.g. anti-tumour therapy.

Spinal cord compression

Back pain occurs in over 90% of cases of cord compression and often predates other symptoms, i.e. sensory disturbance, motor weakness and sphincter dysfunction. Sphincter disturbance is a late feature and a poor prognostic sign for recovery. A sensory level can only be found in around half of patients. Diagnosis should ideally be confirmed by magnetic resonance imaging (MRI) scan. Management should be initiated on clinical diagnosis (do not wait for a scan!) with high dose intravenous dexamethasone, followed by maintenance oral dexamethasone (as per local oncology practice). Refer for consideration of radiotherapy or surgery as soon as the diagnosis is confirmed (and definitely within 24 hours).

Superior vena caval obstruction

Superior vena caval obstruction presents with venous distension, oedema, suffusion of the face, neck and arms, and headache. Immediate treatment is with high dose intravenous dexamethasone, followed by oral maintenance, and oncology referral for consideration of radiotherapy, chemotherapy or a superior vena caval stent.

Stridor

Stridor is fortunately rare. Reassure the patient, sit them up, and maintain a constant professional presence. Oxygen or heliox (4:1 helium:oxygen mixture) can be used if available, and an anxiolytic given. Further management, e.g. high-dose steroids, radiotherapy or stent should be considered.

Catastrophic haemorrhage

This may be a terminal event in a patient close to death, and resuscitative measures would not then be appropriate. It is a rare, but much feared and frightening event for patients, carers and staff. In reality, most patients will drop blood pressure quickly and lose consciousness. If haemorrhage is a possibility, preparations should be made. Prescribe an anxiolytic (e.g. midazolam iv/im/sc or diazepam pr/iv/im) and an analgesic (e.g. diamorphine iv/im/sc, 4-hourly equivalent dose). The intravenous, intramuscular or rectal routes are preferable in this situation as drug absorption by the subcutaneous route is slower and less predictable. Dark blankets should be readily available, carers should be forewarned and reassured and a constant professional presence should be maintained throughout the event.

Aspiration

This is more common in neurological disease than in cancer, and it is very rarely a terminal event. The distress of previous episodes leads to fear of recurrence, and an important part of management is acknowledging and addressing this fear. Speech therapy and dietetic advice should be sought. Anticholinergics (e.g. hyoscine hydrobromide) can be used to dry secretions and antitussives can be helpful. For acute episodes an 'emergency pack' of diamorphine, midazolam (or rectal diazepam) and hyoscine hydrobromide should be prescribed.

PAIN

'Pain is what the patient says hurts.'
(Twycross 1997)

Pain is both a physiological and emotional phenomenon and the management of pain needs to reflect this. Pain is moderate or severe in 40–50% of cancer patients, and very severe in 25–30% (Bonica 1990).

General principles of symptom management apply. Two-thirds of patients will have more than one pain (Grond et al 1996) and full assessment is required of *each pain*, the patient's mental and emotional state, and related symptoms.

Effective management requires a working knowledge of the pathophysiology of pain (Twycross 1994). Key *practical* aspects of management are outlined here.

Analgesics

Choice of first-line analgesic will depend on the mechanism and severity of the pain. It should be taken regularly for constant or regularly recurring pain. The patient also needs a supply of a fast-acting drug that will relieve acute exacerbations of the pain ('breakthrough analgesia') that occur in spite of the regular, background analgesia.

Through applying the World Health Organization three-step analgesic ladder, 80% of cancer pains can be controlled with regular, oral analgesics (WHO 1986):

- *Step one:* a non-opioid analgesic such as paracetamol +/– NSAID +/– an adjuvant such as a tricyclic antidepressant, as appropriate
- *Step two:* an opioid for mild–moderate pain (a 'weak' opioid), e.g. codeine +/– paracetamol +/– NSAID +/– appropriate adjuvants
- *Step three:* an opioid for moderate to severe pain (a 'strong' opioid), e.g. morphine, oxycodone, fentanyl +/– paracetamol +/– NSAID +/– appropriate adjuvants

A patient whose pain is not controlled by a trial of analgesia on one step of the ladder should progress to the next step. A patient can start on any step of the ladder according to clinical judgment.

Morphine

Morphine is usually the strong oral opioid of first choice. It has predictable therapeutic and non-therapeutic effects and is widely available in the UK. The immediate release formulation has a half-life of 2–5 hours and is given to patients regularly every 4 hours. It is also available in slow-

release preparations to aid convenience, with half-lives of 12 hours and 24 hours. Morphine is available in tablet, capsule and liquid forms. Diamorphine is generally preferred to morphine in the UK for parenteral use because of its greater solubility. The conversion rate between subcutaneous diamorphine and oral morphine is between 1:2 and 1:3 (see conversion chart in BNF). The dose of morphine and all strong opioids should be titrated to the pain.

Starting a patient on morphine

- Explain to the patient why morphine is necessary, and explore possible fears and misconceptions. Reassurance may be needed that addiction is very rarely a problem in the management of cancer pain; the use of morphine does *not* indicate that the patient is imminently terminal, and it will not speed up their death. Outline the common side-effects and how these will be managed. A patient-focused information booklet (*Controlling Cancer Pain*) is available from CancerBackup (http://www.cancerbackup.org.uk).
- A patient who is naive to opioids should be started on a low dose of regular opioid (very frail patients may only require 2.5 mg) with prn doses of breakthrough analgesia that are equivalent to the 4-hourly dose, as often as required. If the patient was previously taking a weak opioid, consider starting on 5–10 mg 4-hourly plus prn.
- Review after 24 hours, and assess for pain relief and side-effects. If the pain is still present but opiate-sensitive, adjust the dose upwards by about 30–50% with a corresponding increase in the breakthrough medication. If several prn doses are required each day, increase the dose as above. If the pain is poorly relieved and side-effects are troublesome reconsider the appropriateness of morphine for their particular pain (see Box 16.1).
- Patients often continue to require the paracetamol component of the combination analgesics which they may have been taking prior to morphine.
- Once pain is stable, convert the morphine to a sustained release preparation. Simply calculate the 24-hour morphine requirement and divide by two for the regular 12-hourly preparation,

and by six to give the breakthrough dose of immediate release morphine. For example, a patient receiving immediate release morphine 10 mg 4-hourly, receives a total of 60 mg morphine/24 hours, and will need 30 mg bd of morphine sulphate SR, with 10 mg of immediate release morphine prn.

- Most patients on opioids will become constipated and both stimulant and softener laxatives should be prescribed, e.g. codanthramer or senna + sodium docusate.
- Opioid-induced nausea is transient and affects 30–50% of patients. Prescribe antiemetics as required for a few days (e.g. cyclizine or haloperidol).
- Initial drowsiness is common but should wear off in a few days.
- Dry mouth, like constipation, affects nearly everyone and persists while opiates are being taken. Advice is required on mouth care, sips of fluid, and measures that increase saliva production, e.g. sugar-free chewing gum. Salivary substitutes may be prescribed.
- Other side-effects of morphine include vivid dreams, hallucinations, impaired consciousness, myoclonus, gastric stasis and pruritus. Treat by: reducing the dose, treating the side-effect if it is mild and the patient is not otherwise opioid-toxic (e.g. haloperidol for vivid dreams, clonazepam for myoclonic jerks), or consider changing to an alternative opioid if symptoms are significant and persistent.
- Respiratory depression is very rare if the WHO three-step ladder approach is followed and opioids are titrated appropriately.
- The four specific situations in which opioid toxicity may be a problem in palliative care are:

a patient prescribed opioid on admission to hospital who has not been taking it at home for whatever reason; inadvertent drug overdose (e.g. very rarely, faulty syringe driver); onset of organ failure resulting in reduced drug clearance (e.g. renal failure leading to reduced excretion of morphine); and improvement in underlying cause of pain, e.g. in the weeks following radiotherapy for bone pain.

Morphine in liver and renal failure

Morphine is metabolized by the liver to morphine-6-glucuronide (its active metabolite) and morphine-3-glucuronide. These water soluble conjugates are then excreted via the kidney. In patients with renal failure or severe hepatic impairment, morphine and its metabolites can accumulate. In this situation, if the patient continues to require a strong opioid, two approaches may be adopted. First, immediate release morphine can be used as required rather than regularly, as the plasma half-life will be unpredictable. Second, a drug that is not renally excreted, e.g. fentanyl, can be used regularly.

Alternative step 3 opioids

General indications for use are given in Box 16.2. Differing clinical effects of the step 3 opioids reflect their differing affinities for the different opioid receptors, and their actions at other receptors. Conversion ratios between the differing

Box 16.1

Pains that do not respond well to opioid
- Tension headache
- Muscle cramps
- Abscess

Pains that only partly respond to opioid
- Bone pain
- Neuropathic pain
- Raised intracranial pressure

Box 16.2 When should an alternative step 3 opioid be used?

1. **A different side-effect profile is required:**
   - e.g. fentanyl – may be less constipating
   - oxycodone – possible decreased incidence of vivid dreams, hallucinations and drowsiness

2. **Pain not completely morphine sensitive:**
   - e.g. methadone – may have useful action against neuropathic pain

3. **A different route of administration is required:**
   - fentanyl, buprenorphine – transdermal
   - fentanyl – oral transmucosal

opioids are highly individual, and figures where given are approximations. Seek help if unsure.

- *Oxycodone.* Immediate release (4–6 hourly), sustained release (12 hourly) and injectable forms are available. Oral oxycodone is twice as potent (milligram for milligram) as oral morphine.
- *Fentanyl.* In transdermal patch form it reaches a steady state in 36–48 hours, with minimum effective plasma concentrations being reached in 3–23 hours, so alternative analgesia will usually be required for at least the first 12 hours. Equally there is a slow decline in plasma concentration on patch removal (average 50% decline in 17 hours). A conversion chart is available from the pharmacy. Oral transmucosal fentanyl citrate (OTFC) is a rapidly absorbed short-acting preparation of fentanyl but is not used as the usual breakthrough preparation for patients on fentanyl patches; instead use morphine or oxycodone for breakthrough analgesia. OTFC can be useful for patients on any regular step 3 opioid with rapidly escalating, unpredictable breakthrough pain (e.g. incident pain) but is rarely suitable in frail patients.
- *Methadone*, an opioid agonist and an NMDA receptor antagonist. May be effective in neuropathic pain. Difficult to use because of long, variable half-life (13–100 hours, average 24 hours) with clinical need for more frequent dosing (8 to 12 hourly). Therefore, accumulation can be a problem and it is not suitable for prn use. It is best used in experienced hands.
- *Hydromorphone* (oral), *buprenorphine* (in transdermal patch form) and *alfentanil* (subcutaneously) can all be used in the management of cancer pain.
- *Pethidine.* Clinical usefulness is limited by very short half-life and the side-effects of accumulating metabolites (norpethidine causes convulsions). It is not recommended for control of cancer pain.

Neuropathic pain is usually only partially opioid sensitive and it can be a difficult pain to treat. Monitor response to an opioid but also consider:

- Adjuvants such as tricyclic antidepressants (e.g. amitriptyline, start at 10–25 mg nocte, and gradually titrate) or anticonvulsants (e.g.

sodium valproate, clonazepam, gabapentin, pregabalin)
- Corticosteroids for nerve compression syndromes

If these measures are ineffective, referral to specialist palliative care is appropriate. Other therapeutic options include:

- Other adjuvants such as antidysrhythmics (e.g. flecainide, mexiletine), ketamine and methadone – expert guidance required
- Referral to a pain anaesthetist for consideration of non-pharmacological techniques such as nerve blocks and spinal analgesia
- Transcutaneous electrical nerve stimulation (TENS) and acupuncture may help

Bone pain usually requires the use of adjuvant analgesics in addition to opioids. Paracetamol and NSAIDs are particularly effective, and the following should also be considered:

- Bisphosphonates: generally by intermittent intravenous infusion
- Referral to a clinical oncologist for consideration of external beam radiotherapy to specific sites, or hemibody irradiation or systemic radionucleotides for widespread painful bony metastases
- Corticosteroids are sometimes effective

Prescription of step 3 opioids
There are comprehensive guidelines at the front of the BNF.

NAUSEA AND VOMITING

The general principles of symptom management apply. Comprehensive guidelines are available (Twycross & Back 1998).

Reaching a diagnosis may be more difficult than with pain and a more empirical approach may be required:

- Decide on the most likely mechanism of emesis
- Choose a drug that acts at the appropriate site and prescribe regularly
- Consider the need for parenteral administration (e.g. via syringe driver) for 24 hours or so

Box 16.3   Antiemetics

Drug	Receptor/action
Cyclizine	H1, ACh:M
Haloperidol	D2
Metoclopramide	D2, prokinetic in upper gut
Domperidone	D2, prokinetic in upper gut
Levomepromazine (nozinan)	5HT2, ACh, D2, H1
Ondansetron, granisetron	5HT3
Dexamethasone	Steroid
Lorazepam	Benzodiazepine

Key: H1 histamine type 1; ACh:M muscarinic cholinergic; D2 dopamine type 2; 5HT2,3 serotonin receptors, types 2, 3 and 4.

■ Prescribe a prn antiemetic that is appropriate to the situation, but which works via a different mechanism (see Box 16.3)
■ Review, revise, etc.

Beware using metoclopramide in cases of mechanical intestinal obstruction, or in the presence of colic, as it increases peristalsis in the upper bowel.

For example, an 80-year-old woman with liver metastases from a colonic primary has just been started on morphine and diclofenac for liver capsule pain. This controls the pain, but she complains of constant nausea and vomiting after meals. Possible causes for the nausea and vomiting include:

■ *Highly probable:* the drugs, gastritis, gastric stasis
■ *Possible:* anxiety; NSAID-related renal failure
■ *Less likely:* hypercalcaemia, constipation, brain metastases, bowel obstruction

Initial treatment consisted of stopping the NSAID, prescribing metoclopramide 10 mg qds before meals, and adding regular paracetamol, with good resolution of symptoms.

BOWEL OBSTRUCTION

Bowel obstruction in palliative patients has many causes, and commonly presents insidiously with progressive constipation, vomiting and abdominal pain. Clinical differentiation from constipation can be difficult, and a plain abdominal film may be required. Few patients benefit from surgery but it should be considered in every case, particularly in fitter patients with discrete rather than multiple sites of obstruction. Most patients can be managed medically with the administration of parenteral medication:

■ Diamorphine or morphine for abdominal pain
■ Hyoscine butylbromide for colic and reduction of secretions
■ Cyclizine or haloperidol for nausea and vomiting

Some patients may also benefit from hyoscine butylbromide or octreotide to reduce the volume of intestinal secretions as well as pain from colic. Corticosteroids can sometimes be helpful.

Oral fluids and low-residue diet may be continued and parenteral fluids are often unnecessary.

High intestinal obstruction can cause intractable vomiting, and continuous nasogastric aspiration or gastrostomy drainage may be required.

CONSTIPATION

Full assessment includes a thorough history (including usual pattern, frequency, consistency, presence of strain, time since last bowel action, laxative use, mobility, diet and associated symptoms), physical examination including rectal +/- stomal examination, and, possibly, investigations such as a plain abdominal film.

The commonest causes of constipation are immobility, poor fluid and food intake, and drugs (including opioids and amitriptyline). Bowel obstruction and neurological problems also cause constipation.

Management includes attention to diet; exercise; nursing measures such as responding rapidly to requests for help, and positioning of the patient; oral laxatives, and rectal measures.

Laxatives should be chosen with consideration to the cause of the constipation, the nature of the stool and patient preference. Laxatives used in palliative care may be broadly characterized as:

- Mainly softening (e.g. docusate)
- Mainly peristalsis stimulating (e.g. senna, dantron, bisacodyl, sodium picosulphate)
- Osmotic agents (e.g. magnesium sulphate, lactulose, polyethylene glycol [Movicol])
- A combination of softener and stimulant (e.g. codanthramer, codanthrusate, licensed for use in palliative care only)

Rectal measures are indicated when constipation persists in spite of appropriate oral laxatives, or, more rarely, they may be used electively in people with paraplegia or very frail patients. Choice of rectal measures is clearly guided by rectal examination:

- Rectum full of soft faeces – bisacodyl suppository
- Rectum full of hard stools – glycerine suppositories
- Evidence of constipated stool in lower bowel – high phosphate enema
- Hard impacted stool – arachis oil retention enema (do not use arachis oil in patients with peanut allergy)

Remember:

- Associated symptoms include overflow diarrhoea, urinary retention and bowel obstruction
- Dantron in codanthramer and codanthrusate stains urine red – warn patients lest they think that this is blood! Incontinent patients need to be protected from dantron rash by using barrier cream or an alternative laxative
- Similar management applies to stomas, but stomas do not have sphincters
- Exclude hypercalcaemia, bowel obstruction and spinal cord compression

BREATHLESSNESS

Treatment of the underlying cause offers the best symptom control of breathlessness:

- Treatable causes include anaemia, infections, pleural and pericardial effusions

- Bronchial obstruction may be alleviated by radiotherapy, chemotherapy, laser therapy or stent insertion

Other palliative measures include:

- Opiates and benzodiazepines, and nebulized bronchodilators may partially relieve dyspnoea
- Oxygen may relieve dyspnoea, but in the absence of correctable hypoxia this may be due to the flow of cool air across the face. Therefore, also consider the use of fans
- Keep airways moist with humidified oxygen (if used) and saline nebulizers to aid expectoration
- Nursing and physiotherapy manouevres may be effective, including breathing exercises and relaxation techniques
- A calm and well-ventilated environment is very beneficial. Breathless patients often feel claustrophobic
- Respiratory panic is common, and responds well to benzodiazepines and the reassuring presence of a calm person. Once it has subsided, patients often respond well to the reassurance that death during such a panic is actually very rare

END OF LIFE CARE

Preparation for the last days of life needs to start as early as possible to identify the needs and wishes (both current and potential) of patients and families and to make plans around how those needs may be met, as far as possible. The recently launched End of Life Care Programme promotes three models of care that may help to enhance care at the end of life (Box 16.4).

Evidence-based guidelines for care during the last days of life are available (NCHSPCS 1997). The usual principles of palliative care apply:

1. *Recognize that death is approaching.*
   - Cancer patients experience increasing weakness and immobility, loss of interest in food and fluid, difficulty swallowing and drowsiness. These signs usually develop gradually over several weeks – if the onset is very rapid, consider a potentially reversible cause such as change in medication, hyperglycaemia, hypercalcaemia or infection.

> **Box 16.4   The End of Life Care Programme (http://www.endoflifecare.nhs.uk) promotes three tools**
>
> **Gold Standards Framework (GSF)**
> GSF was developed within primary care and embodies three processes – identification of patients nearing the end of life (months), assessment of their care needs and preferences, and development of a proactive plan of care. The framework promotes key tasks which focus on improving communication, continuity of care, advanced care planning, patient and carer support, as well as team working.
>
> **Preferred Place of Care (PPC)**
> The PPC is a patient-held record that helps patients and carers to discuss and agree the care they would like and where they would like to be cared for at the end of life. It records the patients' thoughts about their illness and the choices available to them. In particular it enables them to express what they do not want to happen. PPC provides a mechanism to record and audit.
>
> **Liverpool Care Pathway (LCP)**
> This is a clinical care pathway that outlines best practice for care of the dying irrespective of the diagnosis or location of the patient. The LCP was developed for use in hospitals but equally can be used in primary care and in care homes. Once implemented the LCP empowers generalists to care for dying patients in the last days of their life. All three tools can be used jointly to ensure that patients receive all the care they need.

2. *Encourage participation by patient, family and friends.*
   - Both in decision making and in physical care, according to their views and wishes.
3. *Continue collaborative multi-professional approach.*
   - Refer to specialist palliative care early if you anticipate problems.
4. *Assessment of the patient's needs.*
   - Focus on what the *patient* perceives as problems.
   - Tailor questions to the patient's condition, but ask specifically about likely symptoms.
   - Non-verbal clues of distress may be present.

- Examine any site of pain, the mouth, pressure areas and other areas where clinical assessment suggests that there may be a problem.
- Explore fears, misunderstandings and misapprehensions as appropriate.

5. *Treatment of the patient's symptoms.*
   - Aim to control the symptoms which are distressing the patient.
   - Stop medication which does not fulfil this aim, explaining rationale to patient and relatives.
   - Discontinue investigations and routine observations unrelated to comfort measures.
   - Medication may need to be given subcutaneously (or rectally) as swallowing deteriorates.
   - Appropriate prn medication must be prescribed for anticipated symptoms such as anxiety, agitation, pain, convulsions or noisy oropharyngeal secretions. This 'rattle' rarely distresses the patient but can be very distressing for others – consider treatment with hyoscine hydrobromide or butylbromide, or glycopyrronium.
   - Many dying patients have a dry mouth for a variety of reasons – mouth breathing, drugs and poor fluid intake. No correlation has been found between biochemical evidence of dehydration and the symptom of dry mouth, and there is the risk with parenteral hydration of peripheral and pulmonary oedema. In practice, sc or iv fluids may be used if the patient complains, or their behaviour suggests, that they are thirsty and are unable to take sufficient oral fluid. This is rare. Relatives often request discussion on this point, and careful explanation of the pros and cons of rehydration is required.
   - Mouth care is very important. Relatives can help to keep the patient's mouth clean and moist with foam stick applicators, and dry lips are eased with vaseline.
   - Skin care includes careful positioning and regular turning, gentle massage and the choice of an appropriate mattress. A urinary catheter may also be required.
   - Speak gently to the patient when you approach them, and explain what you are going to do. Even if the patient appears unconscious, hearing may persist.

6. *Assessment of relatives' needs.*
   - Time spent talking to relatives is much appreciated, to offer reassurance that the patient is comfortable and is being well cared for, and as an opportunity for relatives to ask questions that they might otherwise feel they cannot bother you with.
7. *Continued psychosocial support.*
8. *Care in different settings.*
   - Patients may be discharged to die at home. This requires careful planning, with the family and community services needing as much time as possible to prepare. Involve the GP, DN (and social services and palliative care team if appropriate) at an early stage.

When routine observations and unnecessary medication are discontinued there is the risk that the patient will be neglected. Adoption of a clinical care pathway for the dying such as the LCP (see Box 16.4) enhances care at this time.

PSYCHOSOCIAL CARE

Communicating effectively with patients and families requires sensitivity and skill. We need to be able to elicit patients' concerns, permit the expression of emotion and to clarify areas of uncertainty. We also need to be able to tailor the giving of information to the wishes and understanding of patients, particularly when this involves the imparting of bad news. Forming partnerships with patients in decision making is key, and while establishing realistic goals, we also need to take time to foster hope.

How and why should we improve our psychosocial skills? Reading books can be interesting and informative (Buckman 1993, Doyle et al 2005), but lasting change is more likely to come from active participation via a process of reflective practice or attendance at relevant courses. One of the most effective ways of improving our communication skills is to step back from everyday clinical practice and to go on a course in which active participation is mandatory. Evidence from a randomized controlled trial has shown that attendance at one such course improves the communication skills of doctors and that this change is sustained 12 months later (Fallowfield et al 2002, 2003). This 3-day, learner-focused model incorporating cognitive, behavioural and affective components has been adopted in three variants to fulfill the requirements of the National Cancer Plan (2000) for doctors to undergo training in advanced communication skills. Further information about the availability of these courses should be obtained through your local cancer network.

PSYCHOLOGICAL THERAPIES

Anything which fosters participation, independence and a sense of control and achievement is likely to foster psychosocial health. This should be the general climate of care, but specific therapies can be particularly beneficial. All professions allied to medicine have a role, and, in addition, art and music therapy may be available. Complementary therapies have an established role in palliative care in the promotion of general well-being and hope, and 'touch therapies' (such as therapeutic massage and aromatherapy) may alleviate anxiety. Some patients benefit from support groups, or from a course of counselling. Other psychotherapeutic interventions, such as cognitive-behavioural therapy, can be helpful but tend to be of limited availability.

DEPRESSION AND ANXIETY

Estimates of the incidence of depression in cancer patients vary widely, but the finding that a major depressive illness occurs in about 5–10% of patients with advanced cancer, with depressive symptoms in a further 10–20%, seems a reasonable estimate (Hopwood et al 1991). A similar incidence of depression has been reported in patients with other advanced, progressive diseases such as heart and respiratory failure. In this context, depression and anxiety can be seen to be a reaction to the multiple losses and uncertainties associated with a progressive, life-threatening illness. Both are compounded by, and aggravate, physical symptoms, which can make the diagnosis and management of all the symptoms more difficult. An added challenge is determining when appropriate natural sadness becomes depression, or when understandable anxiety becomes anxiety in need of pharmacological treatment.

Signs and symptoms, and drug treatment, of anxiety and depression are covered in Chapter 17. Counselling depressed patients can prove particularly unproductive, and it may be best to wait until antidepressants have had an opportunity to work before such discussions are resumed.

CONFUSION

It is important to clarify the difference between a hallucination and a misperception. A hallucination is the perception of something that is not there, whereas a misperception is a faulty perception, perhaps because of clouded consciousness. For example, when a patient complains of seeing little green men, she could be hallucinating, or she could be describing but not recognizing staff in theatre greens. It is a key difference because hallucinations may require treatment with antipsychotics, whereas these drugs could further befuddle a confused patient and increase their misperceptions. The treatment of someone troubled by misperceptions is to remove the cause where possible, and to provide a calm and quiet environment where sensory stimulation may be reduced.

GRIEF AND BEREAVEMENT

There are a number of different theories about the grieving process (Doyle et al 2005). The idea that in bereavement one works through a number of sequential stages is no longer in vogue. Phases of grief are recognized, but different bereaved people move backwards and forwards through phases at different times. Bereavement reactions may also be seen in patients grieving for multiple losses, including healthy body image, role, function, relationships and interests.

About one-third of bereaved spouses will develop significant physical or mental health problems, and certain 'at-risk' groups have been identified (NCHSPCS 1997).

Risk factors that predict a poor outcome include:

■ Death of a young person
■ Low levels of trust in self or others
■ Previous history of psychiatric illness
■ Perceived lack of support or understanding

■ Over-dependent relationship between bereaved people and the deceased (NCHSPCS 1997, p. 22)

It follows that good communication between health professionals and spouses and other carers can ease the bereavement reaction. When patients die unexpectedly or uncomfortably, opportunities for the bereaved family to discuss this with the healthcare team should be offered. Those at risk of a poor bereavement outcome can benefit from bereavement follow-up. Bereavement support services are usually available locally, either by statutory or charitable services, but provision varies widely across the country. Other team members or GPs may be able to direct you. It is also good practice to discuss the deaths of patients in hospital with their GP at the first available opportunity, as they may have early contact with the bereaved family.

ETHICS IN PALLIATIVE CARE

The ethics of palliative care is frequently equated with the euthanasia debate. In fact, requests for euthanasia are rare, and much more time is spent pondering the ethics of clinical decision making and team working when patients are very frail and vulnerable. The nature of informed consent, and how confidentiality should be respected in palliative care are examples of these everyday considerations (Randall & Downie 1999). The balance of benefits and burdens is as fine in ethical decisions as in clinical ones.

Geriatricians will be familiar with questions about withholding and withdrawing treatment (including GMC and BMA guidance), and discussion of the nature of futility and consent with regard to cardiopulmonary resuscitation. The implications of the Mental Capacity Act 2007 will also be highly relevant.

Very brief notes are offered here on euthanasia and the doctrine of double effect.

EUTHANASIA

The philosophical arguments around euthanasia are covered well in the literature (Dworkin 1993, Glover 1977). Personal beliefs about euthanasia tend to be polarized, focusing as they do on what makes life sacred. It is worth subjecting your own views to moral scrutiny, and to consider how you would approach the discussion of a request for euthanasia.

Specialist palliative care has traditionally opposed the legalization of euthanasia, on the following grounds:

- It is contrary to the philosophy of palliative care, which affirms life and regards death as a normal process
- Palliative care provision obviates the need for most cases of euthanasia
- It would threaten vulnerable members of society who might feel a real or imagined pressure to consider euthanasia

This said, most palliative care practitioners are aware of patients whose suffering, usually existential in nature, is not relieved by palliative care and who request euthanasia. Legally, their wish cannot be granted. Morally, a key question is how respect for the autonomy of this person should be balanced with the autonomies of all others concerned, including present and future patients, wider society and professionals. What do you think?

DOCTRINE OF DOUBLE EFFECT

'The principle of double effect permits an act which is foreseen to have both good and bad effects, provided: the act itself is good or at least indifferent; the good effect is the reason for acting; the good effect is not caused by the bad effect; a proportionate reason exists for causing the bad effect, e.g. morphine for pain may shorten life.'

(Boyd et al 1997)

Many in palliative care would dispute whether the right dose of morphine, for the right indication, need shorten life, and there is no evidence that morphine is used in this way in hospices. The doctrine of double effect is more relevant to the use of sedation at the end of life. Here there may be a fine line between the intention of effective symptom management, and the intention to end suffering by shortening life. The problem with the

doctrine is that real intention can be so difficult to establish. Motive is the critical issue.

In clinical practice it is informative to apply the test: *If a treatment came along which fulfilled the aim without the secondary effect, would you use it?*

RELIGIOUS AND CULTURAL CONSIDERATIONS

Ask patients and relatives about their cultural or religious observances and requirements before and after death, and plan accordingly (Neuberger 2004). Within stated religious affiliations, assumptions cannot be made because of varying commitment and practice. However, note that some people of Jewish or Islamic faith may wish to be buried within 24 hours of death, so the death certificate needs to be made available immediately. Ensure that there is a doctor available who can complete the certificate in the case of expected deaths. Special arrangements may need to be made with the Registrar of Births, Marriages and Deaths at weekends and on bank holidays.

Where there are language barriers, advocates may be required. Decisions regarding the most appropriate interpreter for a particular patient will need to be decided individually. Using young children in this role should generally be avoided. Family members will be the best advocates in some circumstances, but their relationship to the patient should be taken into consideration. Volunteer or paid advocates from the local community are often available, but may be unacceptable to the patient and family if the relevant community group is small and close-knit (for confidentiality reasons). 'Language lines' – three-way telephone services – may be available in certain languages: make enquiries locally.

ROLE OF THE CORONER

The coroner and death certification service has been undergoing reform since 2003, and the process gained momentum with the publication of the third report of the Shipman Enquiry. A draft Coronor's Bill was published in June 2006. The responsibility for coroners now lies with the Department of Constitutional Affairs, and up-to-date information can be accessed at http://www.dca.gov.uk (legal policy/coroners and burials). It is likely that reforms will be in line with government proposals for full-time independent coroners with legal qualifications, closely supported by medical expertise. Increased medical scrutiny of death certification is also expected.

Greater vigilance is already being applied to death certification. It is particularly important that the patient's GP be alerted to the possibility of a patient's expected and imminent death at home (if the patient is being discharged from in-patient care) so that they have the opportunity to visit the patient at home in the days/weeks before death. Where this has not proved possible, the police may need to be involved, with the possibility of attendant distress to the family.

An informative booklet is available and should be available to relatives, and is also worth reading yourself (Department for Work and Pensions 2006).

Acknowledgment

We wish to thank David McCracken, Specialist Palliative Care Social Worker, The Leeds Teaching Hospitals Trust, Leeds, for helpful advice on financial benefits.

REFERENCES

Bonica J J 1990 Cancer pain; current status and future needs. In: Bonica J J (ed) The management of pain, 2nd edn. Lea & Febiger, Philadelphia, p 400–445

Boyd K M, Higgs R, Pinching A J 1997 New dictionary of medical ethics. BMJ Publishing Group, London, p 76

Buckman R 1993 How to break bad news – a guide for health care professionals. Macmillan Medical, London

Cartwright A 1991 Changes in life and care in the year before death 1969–1987. Journal of Public Health Medicine 13:81–87

Department for Work and Pensions 2006 What to do after a death in England and Wales. HMSO, Oldham

Dickman A, Schneider J, Varga J 2005 The syringe driver: continuous subcutaneous infusions in palliative care, 2nd edn. Oxford University Press, Oxford

Doyle D, Hanks G, Cherny N et al (eds) 2005 The Oxford textbook of palliative medicine, 3rd edn. Oxford University Press, Oxford

Dworkin R 1993 Life's dominion. Harper Collins, London

Fallon M, O'Neill B (eds) 1998 ABC of palliative care. BMJ Books, London

Fallowfield L, Jenkins V, Farewell V et al 2002 Efficacy of a Cancer Research UK communication skills model: a randomised controlled trial. Lancet 359: 650–656

Fallowfield L, Jenkins V, Farewell V et al 2003 Enduring impact of communication skills training: results of a 12-month follow-up. British Journal of Cancer 89:1445–1449

Faull C, Carter Y, Daniels L (eds) 2005 Handbook of palliative care, 2nd edn. Blackwell Science, Oxford

Glover J 1977 Causing death and saving lives. Harmondsworth-Penguin, Middlesex

Grond S, Zech D, Diefenbach C et al 1996 Assessment of cancer pain: a prospective evaluation in 2266 cancer patients referred to a pain service. Pain 64:107–114

Hopwood P, Howell A, Maguire P 1991 Psychiatric morbidity in patients with advanced cancer of the breast: prevalence measured by two self-rating questionnaires. British Journal of Cancer 64: 349–352

Leeds Teaching Hospitals Trust 1999 Eligibility criteria for specialist palliative care services.

National Council for Hospice and Specialist Palliative Care Services 1997 Changing gear – guidelines for managing the last days of life in adults. NCHSPCS, London

National Council for Hospice and Specialist Palliative Care Services 1999 Palliative care 2000: Commissioning through partnership. NCHSPCS, London

Neuberger J 2004 Caring for dying people of different faiths, 3rd edn. Radcliffe, Oxford

Randall F, Downie R 1999 Palliative care ethics: a companion for all specialties, 2nd edn. Oxford Medical Publications, Oxford

Twycross R 1994 Pain relief in advanced cancer. Churchill Livingstone, Edinburgh

Twycross R 1997 Symptom management in advanced cancer. Radcliffe Medical Press, Oxon

Twycross R, Back I 1998 Nausea and vomiting in advanced cancer. European Journal of Palliative Care 5:39–45

Twycross R, Wilcock A, Charlesworth S et al 2002 Palliative care formulary, 2nd edn. Radcliffe Medical Press, Oxford

World Health Organization 1986 Cancer pain relief. WHO, Geneva

World Health Organization 2002 WHO definition of palliative care. Online. Available: http://www.who.int/cancer/palliative

RECOMMENDED READING

Doyle D, Hanks G, Cherny N et al (eds) 2005 The Oxford textbook of palliative medicine, 3rd edn, Oxford University Press, Oxford
This is an extremely informative reference book and teaching resource.

Fallon M, O'Neill B (eds) 1998 ABC of palliative care. BMJ Books, London
This is a practical and highly illustrated introduction to palliative care.

Faull C, Carter Y, Daniels L (eds) 2005 Handbook of palliative care, 2nd edn. Blackwell Science, Oxford
A comprehensive and practical guide, aimed at the generalist audience.

Neuberger J 2004 Caring for dying people of different faiths, 3rd edn. Radcliffe, Oxford
An excellent introductory text.

Twycross R 1994 Pain relief in advanced cancer. Churchill Livingstone, Edinburgh
Although the focus is on the management of cancer pain, the principles and pharmacology are readily transferable to other contexts.

Twycross R, Wilcock A, Charlesworth S et al 2002 Palliative care formulary, 2nd edn. Radcliffe Medical Press, Oxford
A comprehensive compendium of essential therapeutic information. Aimed at specialists, but a useful reference text for generalists. See also the accompanying http://www.palliativedrugs.com for drug information, a bulletin board and regular newsletter.

Several symptom management books are available and the following are recommended

Regnard C, Hockley J 2004 A guide to symptom relief in palliative care, 5th edn. Radcliffe Medical Press, Oxford
Advice on clinical decision making given on the basis of patient history. Comprehensive and pragmatic.

Twycross R, Wilcock A 2001 Symptom management in advanced cancer, 3rd edn. Radcliffe Medical Press, Oxford
Lecture notes format.

USEFUL WEBSITES AND CONTACTS

Cruse Bereavement Care:
   http://www.crusebereavementcare.org.uk
Macmillan Cancer Relief:
   England and Wales: Anchor House, 15-19 Britten Street, London SW3 3TZ. Tel: 0171 351 7811
   Scotland and Northern Ireland: 9 Castle Terrace, Edinburgh EH1 2DP. Tel: 0131 229 3276
National Association of Bereavement Services:
   http://www.stjohnshospice.org.uk
   http://www.goldstandardsframework.co.uk
   http://www.lcp-mariecurie.org.uk
   http://www.endoflifecare.nhs.uk

SELF-ASSESSMENT QUESTIONS

1. Reflect on the last three palliative patients that you have managed. What would you do differently?

2. Are the following true or false for morphine?
   a. It should not be used in patients with renal failure because of the risk of respiratory depression
   b. It causes constipation and therefore all patients should be prescribed lactulose
   c. It causes dry mouth in most patients
   d. It causes nausea and vomiting in most patients
   e. It should not be prescribed for chronic benign pain

Chapter 17

Old age psychiatry

Sube Banerjee and Lydia Chambers

WHAT IS OLD AGE PSYCHIATRY?

Old age psychiatry deals with the mental health problems of elderly people. As a discipline it is characterized by enthusiastic multidisciplinary and interagency working in response to the biological, psychological and social complexity presented by old people who are mentally ill. Old age psychiatry has a primary community focus, insisting on the importance of home-based assessment and care. The World Health Organization (WHO) consensus statement on old age psychiatry has recently affirmed that assessments should be carried out in the patient's home. Unlike many principles, these appear to be the reality of clinical practice, with nine out of ten old age psychiatric referrals seen at home rather than in out-patient clinics.

People over 65 years make up around a third of all mental health activity in the UK in terms of admissions, readmissions and community contacts. However, the profile of disorder and needs differs from younger age groups. The challenges presented by dementia and co-morbid physical illness and disability require particular professional skills, and services must deal with a complex mixture of social, psychological, physical and biological factors. The scope of old age psychiatry cannot be contained in this single chapter. This chapter is therefore selective, focusing on practical issues in the management of older adults with mental health problems.

DEPRESSION

DEFINITION

The American Psychiatric Association's diagnostic criteria for major depression require depressed mood, or loss of interest, enjoyment or pleasure with four or more of the following symptoms for 2 weeks or more, for most of the time almost every day, and this being a change from prior levels of functioning:

A. A significantly reduced level of interest or pleasure in most or all activities
B. Loss or gain of weight (e.g. 5% or more change of weight in a month when not dieting)
C. Difficulty falling or staying asleep (insomnia), or sleeping more than usual (hypersomnia)
D. Behavior that is agitated or slowed down
E. Feeling fatigued, or lowered energy
F. Thoughts of worthlessness or extreme guilt
G. Reduced ability to think, concentrate or make decisions
H. Frequent thoughts of death or suicide (with or without a specific plan), or attempt of suicide

Severity of the disorder can be determined by the number, the frequency and impact of the depressed mood and these symptoms. Clinically significant depression warranting treatment may be present without meeting the criteria for major depressive disorder.

PREVALENCE

Depression is the most common mental disorder in later life. Over the past 15 years there has been a concerted research effort to describe and quantify the burden of depression in elderly people. Using psychometrically valid and reliable instruments, the prevalence of depression requiring clinical intervention in the over-65s in the UK is between 13% and 16%. In global terms, taking all ages, in 1990 depression was calculated to be the fourth highest in rank order of disease burden as measured in Disability-Adjusted Life Years (below lower respiratory infections, diarrhoeal diseases and perinatal conditions). The projections are for this to rise to second in rank order, behind ischaemic heart disease, in 2020.

There are high-risk groups for depression. The prevalence is higher in primary care attenders and in all forms of secondary care contacts (both in- and out-patients). The prevalence of depression in recipients of local authority home care services is twice (26%) that in the community in general, including a four-fold excess of the most serious types. In residential care of all kinds there is a high proportion of dementia, but up to 50% of residents have clinically significant problems with depression.

UNDER-TREATMENT

Only between 10 and 15% of these people with depression receive any active treatment for their depression. This finding is true for those on medical and surgical wards as well as for GP attenders and community populations.

Current service activity can therefore be said to be failing older people with depression. There are discontinuities along the path from disorder to recognition to treatment in all health and social care settings. We need to understand these barriers to care better so as to formulate policy, service and clinical management plans to overcome them.

MISCONCEPTIONS ABOUT DEPRESSION

Major problems in mounting an effective response to the challenge of depression in old age are presented by the misconceptions (often sincerely and benignly held) of clinicians in primary and sec-

ondary care, social care staff, by the older people themselves and their carers and by society as a whole.

Common misconceptions concerning depression in old age are that it is:

- Not a real disorder
- Inevitable
- A normal part of ageing
- Untreatable
- Unimportant in individual, clinical or service terms

All these statements are unsupported by the evidence.

Depression in old age is a *real disorder*

Depression is a serious disorder which occurs at all ages; it is as real an illness as rheumatoid arthritis, hypertension or dementia. It is a syndrome which has somatic, cognitive and behavioural symptoms and signs. It has known predisposing, precipitating and perpetuating factors and a well-described course and outcome. There are specific treatments which can treat the disorder as successfully as most others in medicine, and a lot better than many. It is not the same as uncomplicated bereavement or normal sadness and unhappiness.

Depression in old age is not *inevitable*

Depression is a common disorder of later life but it is not inevitable. Beliefs concerning the inevitability of depression in old age are based upon ageist formulations of old age as a time of inevitable and irretrievable loss and decay, to which the only response could be profound depression. In the general population, 85% of the elderly are not depressed. Even in high-risk groups with much physical illness, disability and handicap, such as those receiving home care and those in residential care, 74% and 50% respectively do not have depressive disorders.

Depression is not a *normal part of ageing*

If this were the case then depression would increase with each 5-year age group from 65 years. This does not occur. Depression is associated with physical disorders, disability and handicap and these all rise in frequency with age. However, this does not mean that depression is a normal part of ageing, but instead suggests ways of preventing and managing depression by addressing treatment needs in these areas. Similar misconceptions include beliefs that depression is a prelude to or the same as dementia.

Depression in old age is *treatable*

The evidence clearly points to this being a treatable disorder. There is no evidence that antidepressants or psychological therapies work any less well in older compared with younger people. There is evidence of the effectiveness of intervention even in what might be considered poor prognostic groups, such as disabled elderly people at home or people with dementia.

Depression in old age is *important*

Whether the viewpoint of the individuals with depression and their carers or that of health and social services is taken, depression is important in clinical and economic terms. Depression causes a profound decrease in quality of life for people with depression and for their families and carers. Depression is also associated with suicide and, in addition to this, increased mortality (controlling for physical co-morbidity). People with depression use more health and social services than people without the disorder, even after controlling for levels of disability. The UK annual health and social care cost (not including the opportunity costs of carers) of depression in elderly people at home is about £1 billion.

DETERMINANTS OF DEPRESSION IN OLD AGE

In each individual with depression there will be an interplay of the biological (e.g. physical illness, disability, genetic predisposition), the psychological (e.g. losses of individuals, function or home) and the social (e.g. supports available, financial and housing status). While it is helpful to try to understand these factors in detail in each case, a lack of complete understanding should not be a barrier to treatment. Causes may be more or less

proximal to the onset of depression, and a factor of major importance seems to be disablement, specifically handicap. Handicap can be understood as the disadvantage imposed on a person with chronic disease as a consequence of their imperfectly organized environment. This appears to be of particular importance in depression in later life, and may suggest paths for intervention on a population and an individual level.

Factors of importance in depression in earlier life (such as being a woman and life events) appear to play a less prominent role in the aetiology of late-life depression. Other factors of importance include: pain, low social contact, loneliness (as distinct from depression) and marriage (protective for men and a risk factor for depression in women). The extent to which the disablement directly attributable to depression itself predicts movement to hospital or residential care in itself is unclear.

MANAGEMENT OF DEPRESSION IN OLD AGE

The evidence base for the treatment of depression in elderly people is growing but has large gaps, especially where evidence of effectiveness in real clinical populations is sought rather than efficacy in the highly selected groups enrolled into drug trials.

Without specific intervention, the natural history of depression in elderly people at home is bleak with only 33% of older people at home recovering in a year, and less (25% in 6 months) in disabled groups. However, in the community at large, people screened as depressed can be successfully and acceptably engaged and treated by old age psychiatric services and community nurses.

Principles for the successful management of depression

1. Vigilance for depression
2. Recognition of depression
3. Active management
4. Maximize physical function
5. Prescribe and enable concordance with antidepressants
6. Attend to social needs (often via social services)

7. Attend to psychological needs (e.g. bereavement, other losses)
8. Review

CHOICE OF ANTIDEPRESSANT

One of the difficulties in assessing the relative merits of newer antidepressants, such as the selective serotonin reuptake inhibitors (SSRIs), compared with older compounds, such as the tricyclic antidepressants (TCAs), is that frail elderly subjects and those with complex co-morbidity are systematically excluded from drug trials. This means that there are no good data with which to assess the cost:benefit equation for those who might be most affected by the adverse effects of medication (e.g. side-effects or drug interactions). However, most old age psychiatrists would use an SSRI as a first-line treatment rather than TCAs. If first-line treatment with an adequate dose of SSRI given for an adequate time (at least 6 weeks) does not work, then clinicians would tend to turn to a trial of a another non-TCA class of antidepressants such as selective noradrenergic reuptake inhibitors (SNRIs) or a noradrenaline (norepinephrine) and specific serotonergic antidepressant (NASSA).

WHEN TO SEEK SPECIALIST HELP

Just as not all older people with hypertension need to see a geriatrician, not all older people with depression need to see an old age psychiatrist. Referral may be indicated when:

- The depression is resistant to an adequate trial of antidepressants (i.e. at least 4–6 weeks at a therapeutic dose)
- There is concern about life-threatening behaviour (by extreme neglect, food refusal or suicidal ideas, plans or intent)
- There is diagnostic uncertainty
- The depression is severe (including depression with psychotic features, e.g. hallucinations and delusions)

SUICIDE AND DELIBERATE SELF-HARM

Suicide is as an intentional, self-inflicted, life-threatening act which results in death.

Box 17.1 Suicidal intent

Suicidal intent is indicated by:

- Evidence of premeditation, such as hoarding tablets
- Taking precautions to avoid discovery
- Failing to alert potential helpers after the act
- Carrying out the act in isolation
- Performing 'final acts' such as writing a note or making a will
- Violent methods (however, ignorance of lethal dosage means that intent may be high despite an apparently trivial overdose)

Incidence

About 4500 people commit suicide each year in the UK, compared with several hundred thousand acts of non-fatal deliberate self-harm. Across all age groups male suicides outnumber female suicides. The suicide rate increases with age, reaching a peak in the mid-60s for women and a decade later for men. Drug overdose accounts for half of all suicides, the remainder resulting from more violent methods.

Assessment and management of the suicidal patient

This should establish the degree of current suicidal ideas, plans and intent and evaluate the risk of completing suicide (see Box 17.1). Factors associated with an increased risk of suicide are presented in Box 17.2.

Management is directed towards treating any underlying physical and/or psychiatric disorder. This may require hospital admission. Long-term management will involve improving coping skills and attempting to resolve the personal or social problems that have led up to the act.

Prevention

Acts of deliberate harm should always be taken seriously in elderly patients. They may need to be admitted to a medical or surgical ward for treatment of the results of the act of self-harm. Risk assessment should include the risk of absconding

Box 17.2 Factors associated with increased risk of suicide

Socioeconomic factors
Sex: male
Age: over 40
Work: unemployed or retired
Marital status: divorced, widowed or separated
Social network: living alone, lack of social support

Mental and physical health
Mental disorder: current psychiatric illness
Substance abuse: especially alcohol abuse
Physical disorder: chronically disabling physical
    illness, pain
Recent loss: bereavement, divorce, retirement,
    redundancy
Family history: affective disorder, alcohol abuse,
    suicide
Past history: mental disorder or deliberate
    self-harm
Personality: antisocial personality disorder (rare in
    elderly subjects)

Mental state examination
Thoughts: suicidal ideas, plans and/or intent
Depression: biological (e.g. sleep disturbance,
    diurnal variation of mood, weight loss,
    anhedonia) and cognitive (e.g. hopelessness,
    helplessness, guilt, worthlessness) features,
    severe and psychotic depression
Abnormal perceptions: persecutory delusions,
    auditory hallucinations or delusions of control
    (especially instructing or compelling the patient
    to kill themselves)

Key messages

1. Depression in old age is common (12–15% of the whole population).
2. It is serious (associated with profound decrease in quality of life, increased all-cause mortality and suicide).
3. It increases service use (all health and social care).
4. Depression in old age is expensive (estimates of £1 billion pa attributable to depression in the community).
5. It is treatable (60–70% may recover with active treatment compared with 25–30% with normal care).
6. Depression in old age is only rarely actively treated (only 10–15% of older people with depression are being treated).
7. Changes need to be made in the delivery and organization of health and social services to enable depressed elderly people to receive active treatment.

DEMENTIA

INTRODUCTION

Dementia is essentially a clinical syndrome of later life, though it may affect younger people. It has many important associations that may influence its presentation to health services including with delirium, falls and incontinence as well as more frequent admissions and increased length of stay in hospital. In addition, it is associated with behaviours that can be difficult to manage – especially on acute medical wards – such as night-time disturbance with wandering and shouting, poor oral intake of nutrition and poor compliance with medication.

Dementia is one of the most common and serious disorders in later life with a prevalence of 5% and an incidence of 2% per year in the over-65s. In the UK dementia therefore affects 500 000 people at any time with 200 000 new cases a year. Dementia causes irreversible decline in global intellectual and physical functioning. There are profound impacts on the person with dementia, their family and carers, and also on health, social

and completion of suicide on the ward. Appropriate levels of nursing observation should be instituted and a clear management plan should be set out in the notes. *All older people completing an act of self-harm should be assessed by a psychiatric team*; the degree of urgency of this assessment will depend on the patient's medical and mental state. Prevention has been aimed at improving ways of detecting the potential victim of suicide, increasing help available to those faced with social and emotional problems, and limiting the availability of prescribed drugs frequently used in suicide attempts.

and voluntary services, in personal, social, health and economic terms. In the community, dementia has been estimated to cost £2.4 billion per year. This doubles if the costs of residential care and carer opportunity costs are added. While the economics are striking, the negative impact of dementia on people with dementia themselves, in terms of deteriorating function, and on carers in terms of high levels of stress, carer burden and mental disorder is also enormous.

The management of medical problems in patients with dementia can be more complicated because of barriers to verbal communication that mean symptoms and signs cannot be elicited directly and so screening investigations become more important to guide treatment. Collateral history from family and carers, including their expectations from services, is essential because these relationships influence how effectively the patient with dementia can be managed at all points of contact with health services. In the wider setting of health, social and voluntary services and society in general, dementia can have far reaching effects psychologically, socially and economically for patients and their carers. The cost to carers in terms of burden, stress and mental disorders is often overlooked.

DEFINITION

Dementia can be defined as a syndrome of widespread, progressive and irreversible loss of brain functions occurring in clear consciousness. It is manifested by a deterioration in memory, disorientation, decline in intellectual functions such as language and capacity to learn, as well as changes in personality, emotions and behaviour.

The ICD 10 guidance for diagnosis of dementia is summarized in Box 17.3.

EPIDEMIOLOGY

The most common causes of dementia include Alzheimer's disease (AD) responsible for up to 60% of cases, vascular dementia (VaD) which makes up about 20% of cases, Lewy body dementia (LBD) which accounts for up to 15% of cases and frontotemporal dementia (FTD) including Pick's disease which accounts for 20% of cases before age 65 years but a far lower proportion of

---

> **Box 17.3   Summary of ICD 10 criteria for dementia**
>
> 1. A syndrome due to disease of the brain, usually chronic (over 6 months duration) and progressive. Disturbance of memory and one or more other higher cortical functions (e.g. thinking, orientation, comprehension, calculation, learning, language and judgment)
> 2. No clouding of consciousness
> 3. Commonly accompanied by deterioration in emotional control, social behaviour and/or motivation
> 4. Usually interference with activities of daily living

---

those over the age of 65 years. There is no single disease entity that is responsible for any one of these categories and there is much overlap between them. The remaining much more rare and specific causes include hypothyroidism, normal pressure hydrocephalus, vitamin B12 or folate deficiency, Wernicke-Korsakoff's dementia, neurosyphilis, Huntington's disease, HIV/AIDS dementia, hypercalcaemia and Creutzfeldt-Jacob disease (CJD). There are about 17 000 people with dementia in younger age groups. The Government estimates that the total number of people with dementia in UK in 2050 will be 1.2 million.

CLINICAL PRESENTATION OF DEMENTIA

Individual cases of dementia can vary greatly in terms of their clinical presentation depending on the type and stage of dementia, the presence of behavioural and psychological symptoms, the presence of co-morbid physical illness, personality and the social context. There are, however, features that are commonly reported. Patients may complain of forgetfulness or a decline in intellectual functioning but may also report mood disturbance such as depression. However, patients may also have no concerns about themselves and so it is the carers who report changes in memory, personality and behaviour such as poor personal hygiene and deteriorating social interaction. Occasionally, both patients and their closest contacts are unaware of or unconcerned about apparent disorientation, poor memory and deterioration in function that may seem obvious to the outside observer. This may be because the changes have been gradual and are attributed to normal ageing or the result of denial of a highly anxiety-provoking problem. Some cases present with dangerous behaviour such as wandering outside with vulnerability to accidents or the weather, or the misuse of cookers and heaters with the potential for fires and explosions.

Alzheimer's disease

Alzheimer's disease is the most common dementia accounting for up to 60% of cases of dementia in the UK. It represents a group of disorders and can be divided into the rare young onset disease (before age 65 years) and common late onset disease (age 65 years and over). With young onset dementia there is commonly a family history and a proportion of cases have specific genetic mutations. AD may also present in combination with other dementias, most commonly vascular dementia, and concomitant cerebrovascular disease may unmask subclinical AD and makes AD more severe. The onset of AD is insidious with a course that is usually a progressive decline with survival rates on average between 5 and 10 years. After the exclusion of other possible causes of the presentation, the diagnosis is based on a characteristic history of decline in memory, especially in short-term memory at early stages, disorientation in time and place, language problems from word finding difficulties to aphasia, acalculia, impaired ability to carry out activities of daily living such as meal preparation and dressing, and impaired skills such as driving to apraxia and various manifestations of misidentification to agnosia. Delusions, hallucinations and depression also occur in a significant proportion of cases.

Vascular dementia

Vascular dementia is the second most common cause of dementia in the UK and may be responsible for up to 20% of cases. It results from a variety of conditions that can cause vascular damage to the brain, most commonly atherosclerotic thrombo-embolic disease. It commonly coexists with AD in that one-third of VaDs have significant AD

pathology and 60–90% of AD cases have cerebrovascular pathology. It has a fluctuating course with patchy neuropsychological deficits depending on the pattern of underlying brain tissue damage. Survival is also variable and depends on the extent of underlying disease and its response to treatment as well as the control of the familiar risk factors: hypertension, cigarette smoking, obesity, hypercholesterolaemia, diabetes mellitus and atrial fibrillation. Although VaD historically has been characterized by a stepwise progression, it may have a clinical course that is indistinguishable from AD. Features like sudden onset, emotional lability and night-time confusion may be suggestive of a vascular cause but diagnosis depends on evidence of dementia with a temporal relationship to vascular damage. Focal neurological symptoms and signs, along with evidence of cerebral damage on central nervous system (CNS) imaging can be very useful in supporting the diagnosis. History of other end-organ damage, e.g. myocardial infarction, can raise suspicions and long-standing cardiac disorders are associated with cognitive impairment.

Lewy body dementia

Lewy body dementia is a degenerative brain disorder responsible for up to 15% of dementia in the UK in some series but it is often much more rarely seen in clinical rather than in research settings. There is a great deal of overlap between LBD, Parkinson's disease and AD. Overall, there is a progressive decline in brain function but there are some characteristic features including a confusional state with clouding of consciousness (which can present very similarly to delirium), fluctuating cognitive impairment, hallucinations and delusions and parkinsonism. Treatment can be difficult as anti-parkinsonian medication will improve mobility but can worsen confusion and hallucinations. In addition, there is usually a high sensitivity to antipsychotic medication with high morbidity and mortality. *Antipsychotic agents are best avoided in these patients.* Caution must be used in an emergency situation where delirium is suspected and there is a potential diagnosis of LBD. The risks of the behaviour and the risks of the treatment must be considered. Clinical features of LBD are summarized in Box 17.4.

Box 17.4   Clinical features of Lewy body dementia

1. Pronounced fluctuating impairment of memory and higher cortical function (e.g. language, praxis, reasoning) with episodes of confusion and lucid intervals
2. Visual or auditory hallucinations often with secondary delusions; and/or spontaneous extrapyramidal symptoms or high sensitivity to antipsychotics; and/or unexplained falls ± transient clouding of consciousness
3. Clinical features persist over weeks or months and there is progressing cognitive decline overall
4. Exclusion of explanatory physical disorder
5. Exclusion of vascular aetiology

Frontotemporal dementia

Frontotemporal dementia is a group of diseases including Pick's disease, which is responsible for up to 20% of cases of dementia before 65 years and with most common onset between the ages of 45 years and 65 years. Older age of onset occurs but it is less common. The onset is insidious and progression is gradual with a mean survival of 8 years. Early features include changes in personality and behaviour, usually seen as a decline in social interpersonal skills and emotional blunting. There may be increased mental rigidity and a decline in personal hygiene with decline in memory, spatial orientation and aphasia occurring later in the illness. Other features include disinhibition, hyperorality, distractibility and stereotyped behaviour with early loss of insight. Diagnosis is by a suggestive history and can be supported by neuropsychological testing. Brain imaging may show frontal and/or temporal abnormality.

MANAGEMENT OF DEMENTIA

The first priority with a case suggestive of dementia is to exclude delirium and other potentially reversible causes of a dementia-like presentation, such as hypothyroidism, vitamin B12 deficiency and neurosyphilis. A thorough history is required for diagnosis. It is important to obtain as much of the patient's account as possible but, because of the nature of the illness, collateral history from all the available sources is essential to discern the mode of onset, time course, development and associations of the symptoms and the effect of these on the daily life of the patient. Other important features of the history include pre-existing medical and psychiatric problems, prescribed drug use, e.g. of sedative drugs or those with anticholinergic effects, alcohol use, family history of medical or psychiatric problems and current levels of social support, along with the capacity of carers to continue with their input in the context of their own physical and mental health.

Important findings on mental state examination would be to identify current evidence of depressive disorder and psychotic symptoms such as delusions or hallucinations as well as a cognitive assessment with a screening test such as the Mini-Mental State Examination (MMSE). A risk assessment of potential harm to the self either deliberately or by self-neglect or from the environment, and of harm to others or the environment, is also useful especially where dangerous behavioural problems are prominent (e.g. the unsafe use of heaters or cookers).

In addition, complete physical examination including urinalysis and BMstix can be useful initially before the results of screening blood tests (FBC, ESR, U+Es, Ca^{2+}, LFTs, TFTs, fasting blood glucose, CRP, haematinics, syphilis serology) are known. CXR and ECG may be indicated depending on the history and examination and brain imaging where there is an unusual course or rapid progression, evidence of focal damage, history of malignancy, fits, head injury or the possibility of normal pressure hydrocephalus (i.e. a triad of symptoms appearing in the order of gait disturbance, urinary incontinence, cognitive decline). EEG may be considered if seizures are suspected.

When the diagnosis of dementia is reached, including the likely subtype, then a profile of the biological, psychological and social needs should be identified that will be addressed by the management plan. This will require the mobilization of the multidisciplinary team and the close liaison with carers.

Physical health should be optimized and antidementia drugs should be considered in all eligible patients. In January 2001, the National Institute for Clinical Excellence (NICE) introduced guidelines for the treatment of mild to moderate Alzheimer's disease with the acetylcholinesterase inhibitors donepezil, galantamine and rivastigmine. This was to be done under the supervision of a specialist service and was indicated for cognitive and behavioural functioning with a MMSE score above 12. These medications have been accepted as being clinically effective. However, the recent February 2006 controversial advice from NICE restricts the use to moderate AD with MMSE scores of 10–20. In addition, memantine, which is licensed for moderate to severe AD, is recommended only for use in clinical trials. This current advice threatens the availability of these medications on the NHS and so all the relevant groups are continuing to protest against this decision. In the meantime, suitable patients with AD should be referred to specialist clinics.

Other reasons to refer to old age psychiatry and memory clinics are where further assessment is needed because the diagnosis is in doubt or the presentation is atypical, or for management of complicated cases and intractable behavioural and psychological symptoms of dementia (BPSD). Management of BPSD is dealt with later.

Nursing and social care needs can be assessed directly by the multidisciplinary team in the in-patient setting but in the community the assessment of the burden on carers is central to these needs being met. The effect of caring on the carers depends on the characteristics of the carer as well as the person with dementia. However, it is possible to identify four main sources of stress and burden:

1. *Practical* – need for help with personal care and housework
2. *Behavioural* – examples include active problems (e.g. aggression, wandering, night disturbance, incontinence) and passive problems (e.g. apathy, decreased social interaction) which may be particularly difficult to deal with
3. *Interpersonal* – difficulty in communication and change in the nature of the relationship with the person with dementia
4. *Social* – restrictions on the carer leaving the home, socializing or going to work

Voluntary services such as the Alzheimer's Society can benefit patients and carers, with services including advice, support groups and day centres.

Social services can provide home care, day centres and respite care for patients at home. There may be ambivalence about placement in residential or nursing care homes for many reasons, not least the extreme environmental poverty of most care homes and carers may feel that they have failed their loved ones.

BEHAVIOURAL AND PSYCHOLOGICAL SYMPTOMS OF DEMENTIA

Introduction

Behavioural and psychological symptoms of dementia (BPSD) represent some of the most troubling and disabling symptoms for patients and their carers and are frequently the precipitants of transition into residential care. Behavioural disturbance occurs in other disorders (delirium, affective and psychotic disorders as well as other psychiatric disorders) but generally improves with treatment of the underlying disease. In dementia, worsening of BPSD may be attributable to other reversible causes such as pain, constipation and under- or over-stimulation. Effective management of these symptoms is important.

Description

BPSD includes psychotic symptoms (delusions and hallucinations), aggression (physical and verbal), affective symptoms (depression to elation, anxiety, irritability, disinhibition, apathy, wandering, shouting, resisting care), appetite and feeding disorders, and sleep disorders. Nocturnal restlessness or 'sundowning' is reported commonly.

Management

A careful history, examination and investigation are required to identify the causes of BPSD. Treatment begins with an explanation of the problems, especially reassuring carers that the problems are not premeditated on the part of the patient. BPSD should be treated by environmental adaptation and a behavioural approach wherever possible as well as addressing the physical and psychiatric problems.

A calm, structured and secure environment that is uncluttered and kept at a comfortable temperature along with a consistently calm and respectful approach from carers (including residential care staff) is a good situation in which behavioural approaches have the best chance of efficacy. These can range from ensuring good sleep hygiene to behavioural therapy under the supervision of a qualified therapist.

For behavioural therapy to be worthwhile, carers need to be aware of the amount of record-keeping and persistence that is needed. Behavioural therapy involves behavioural analysis that involves diary keeping by the carers. This includes a detailed description of the context and triggers of behaviour, the type and frequency of the behaviour and the consequences of the behaviour. Then ideas are generated to modify the precipitants and any reinforcing reactions to the behaviour and a programme of interventions is drawn up. The effect of the intervention is assessed by further behavioural analysis. This process can be repeated several times for different interventions.

Antipsychotic medication has been used widely to treat the most severely agitated, aggressive and psychotic symptoms in dementia. In 2004, the Committee on Safety of Medicines (CSM) issued advice about the use of the atypical antipsychotics, risperidone and olanzapine, for behavioural disturbance in dementia. Data from the manufacturers showed an excess of cerebro-vascular events in older people using these medications and so the CSM advised against the use of these medications for BPSD and suggested cautious use for psychotic disorders in older people. Of note is that similar data were not available for other atypical or typical antipsychotics and so this may well be a group-wide effect. The best advice for use of these medications as a whole is to consider the potential risks and benefits of drug treatment alongside the risks of the behaviour, and to explain this to the patient and carers. After discussion, a decision about treatment can be made jointly and the reasons documented. Patients and carers who feel they have benefited from treatment with risperidone or olanzapine may choose to continue despite the risks described. Other drugs that have been suggested for treatment of the most difficult BPSDs include mood stabilizers, e.g. carbamazepine, valproic acid and antidepressants.

DELIRIUM

INTRODUCTION

Delirium is a term that encompasses acute confusional state, acute brain syndrome and toxic confusional state. It is common and associated with longer episodes in hospital as well as falls and pressure sores. It is important because delirium is a marker of increased risk in mortality and morbidity in patients independently of the underlying disease process.

DEFINITION AND CLINICAL FEATURES

Delirium may be defined as an acute onset organic mental syndrome with a fluctuating course of global deterioration in brain functioning especially in the domains of perception (leading to illusions and hallucinations), orientation, attention, concentration and short-term memory occurring with impaired consciousness. There is usually disturbance to the sleep–wake cycle with symptoms being worse at night, as well as behavioural disturbance with increased or decreased levels of activity. There may also be changes in mood and anxiety. Arriving at the diagnosis of delirium is usually straightforward provided that a clear and accurate history is obtained. However if no evidence for underlying physical illness is found, then the main differential diagnoses include functional psychosis, e.g. schizophrenia, and affective disorder, e.g. mania and dementia. Delirium and dementia frequently occur together. Delirium with hypoactivity may go unrecognized or be mistaken for depression and is therefore associated with a poorer outcome. However, delirium with hyperactive behavioural disturbance is diagnosed more readily and usually treated early, hence it has been associated with a better outcome. The ICD 10 guidance for diagnosis of delirium is summarized in Box 17.5. (For definite diagnosis, symptoms should be present in all areas.)

EPIDEMIOLOGY

Up to 30% of elderly hospitalized patients will suffer from delirium and about two-thirds of these may have a pre-existing dementia. Delirium in

---

Box 17.5   ICD 10 diagnostic guidelines for delirium

a. Impairment of consciousness and attention
b. Global disturbance of cognition (perceptual distortions, impaired comprehension, impaired memory, disorientation)
c. Psychomotor disturbances (hypo- or hyper-activity)
d. Disturbance of sleep–wake cycle
e. Emotional disturbances, e.g. depression, anxiety, euphoria, apathy, perplexity

---

the elderly postoperative patient has been estimated to occur in 10–15% of cases and this rises to between 25–65% for surgical repair of hip fracture.

AETIOLOGY

Virtually any physical insult can cause delirium in a predisposed individual. It occurs more commonly with increasing age, severe co-morbid physical illness, dementia and if there is a history of delirium. Delirium occurring in a younger age group is a marker of severe underlying physical illness and is associated with a high mortality. Box 17.6 lists some of the common causes of delirium.

MANAGEMENT

This involves identifying and treating the underlying cause as a priority and creating the optimal environment for recovery (see Box 17.7). Behavioural disturbance will begin to be alleviated by this but if there are dangerous behaviours then the risks and benefits of additional drug treatment must be weighed against the risks of such behaviours continuing. Under these circumstances treatment with lorazepam or an antipsychotic can be considered. Medication should be started at as low a dose as possible orally (e.g. lorazepam 1 mg, haloperidol 0.5 mg, risperidone 0.5 mg) titrating the dose upwards very carefully, balancing clinical response, side-effects and continued risk. Intramuscular lorazepam or haloperidol should only be used in exceptional circumstances. Antipsychotic

---

Box 17.6   Some causes of delirium

1. **Infection:** chest, UTI, surgical wound, pressure sore, meningitis, encephalitis, neurosyphilis AIDS
2. **Metabolic disorder:** acid–base or electrolyte disturbances, hypoglycaemia, hypoxaemia, hypercapnia, hypothyroidism, hyperadrenalism, hypoadrenalism, renal and hepatic failure, vitamin B deficiencies
3. **Vascular:** myocardial infarction, heart failure, cerebrovascular accident, transient ischaemic attack
4. **Neoplasia:** carcinomatosis
5. **Trauma:** burns, surgery, multiple injuries and trauma
6. **Neurological disorders:** vasculitides, subdural or subarachnoid haemorrhage, head injury, space-occupying lesion, seizures, raised intracranial pressure
7. **Drug use, illicit and prescribed:** anti-depressants, anticholinergics, antipsychotics, antihypertensives, antiarrhythmics, diuretics, NSAIDs, hypoglycaemic agents, sedatives/hypnotics, narcotics, analgesics, cimetidine, digoxin, lithium, L-dopa
8. **Drug withdrawal:** e.g. from alcohol, benzodiazepines or barbiturates

---

Box 17.7   Management of delirium

1. Treat or remove the underlying cause(s)
2. Ensure optimal nutrition, fluid and electrolyte balance, and vitamin supplementation if indicated
3. Supportive and orienting nursing care in quiet, well-lit environment
4. Allow trusted family member to stay with patient
5. Monitor mental state and behaviour closely and avoid physical restraint
6. If behavioural disturbance persists or is dangerous, consider treatment with lorazepam or an antipsychotic starting at as low a dose as possible orally and titrating upwards very carefully, balancing side-effects with continued risk

medication should be avoided if there is a history of Lewy body dementia because of the hypersensitivity to these drugs associated with morbidity and mortality.

ALCOHOL USE DISORDERS

INTRODUCTION

Alcohol use disorders are common and associated with high rates of physical and psychiatric illness. It is likely that the absolute numbers of older people using alcohol is on the increase because of the ageing population. Alcohol use disorders are coming to be accepted as a growing problem for older adults. However, it is also likely that there is under-detection of alcohol use disorders because older people are less likely to spontaneously disclose the information and health workers are less likely to ask older people about alcohol use. In addition, there may be atypical presentation (poor international normalized ratio control on warfarin) because of the co-morbid illnesses. Interventions are no less useful than in younger adults.

DEFINITION

Alcohol use disorders can be thought of as any usage of alcohol which impacts adversely on the biological, psychological (including emotional) or social life of an individual. It may be that current recommended intake limits are not as applicable to older adults because of age-related changes in physiology and pharmacokinetics, which may mean that there is more sensitivity to the effects of alcohol.

EPIDEMIOLOGY

Estimates of the prevalence of alcohol use disorder in older people vary widely. There are differing methodologies (including definitions of problems) and screening tools (which may be less sensitive in older people because they are less likely to have the social, legal and occupational consequences seen in younger age groups). There is a higher rate among hospital samples than community samples. Estimations of prevalence are: medical

> **Box 17.8 ICD 10 mental and behavioural disorders due to the use of alcohol**
>
> - Acute intoxication
> - Harmful use
> - Dependence syndrome
> - Withdrawal state
> - Withdrawal state with delirium
> - Psychotic disorder
> - Amnesic syndrome
> - Residual and late onset psychotic disorder
> - Other

in-patient 10–20%; psychiatric in-patients 23–44%; community 2–17%. Factors associated with alcohol use disorders in old age are male gender, social isolation, and being single, separated or divorced.

CLASSIFICATION

Box 17.8 lists the range of alcohol use disorders described in the ICD 10.

CLINICAL FEATURES

Alcohol use disorders usually develop over time but may arise in old age following bereavement or in illness. Sometimes alcohol is used as self-medication for sleep disorders, pain, anxiety disorders and depression. In older adults, alcohol use disorders may present with self-neglect, confusion, falls and with the complications or harmful sequelae of alcohol use. The criteria for alcohol dependence in the ICD 10 are based on the 'Alcohol Dependency Syndrome'. The features include: a stereotyped pattern of drinking behaviour; prominence of drink-seeking behaviour; increased tolerance to alcohol; repeated withdrawal symptoms; relief or avoidance of withdrawal symptoms by further drinking; subjective awareness of the compulsion to drink; and reinstatement after abstinence.

In withdrawal, which begins about 6 to 12 hours after the last drink, a patient may complain of nausea and vomiting, sweating, palpitations and anxiety and this will be supported by the physical signs including tachycardia, tachypnoea, pyrexia and tremor. Delirium tremens can develop

---

Box 17.9   Medical and neuropsychiatric complications of alcohol dependence

- Vitamin deficiencies (e.g. B and C)
- Peripheral neuropathy
- Infections
- Cancer, especially of the gastrointestinal tract
- Liver disease
- Heart disease
- Drug interactions
- Acute intoxication
- Withdrawal syndrome
- Wernicke–Korsakoff's syndrome
- Alcoholic cerebellar degeneration
- Alcoholic hallucinosis
- Morbid jealousy
- Alcoholic dementia and cortical atrophy
- Alcoholic amblyopia

Box 17.10   CAGE questions

- Have you ever felt you should **C**ut down on your drinking?
- Have you ever felt **A**nnoyed by criticism of your drinking?
- Have you ever felt **G**uilty about your drinking?
- Have you ever taken an **E**ye-opener first thing in the morning?

---

between 1 and 4 days after abstinence or sometimes after reduction in alcohol intake. Seizures may be the presenting feature and other characteristics include clouding of consciousness, confusion, hallucinations (especially tactile and visual) and autonomic overactivity.

Other important complications to be aware of during assessment are Wernicke's encephalopathy (featuring confusion, clouding of consciousness, opthalmoplegia, ataxia and peripheral neuropathy) and Korsakoff's dementia (with inability to form new memory, confabulation, peripheral neuropathy). Wernicke's encephalopathy can lead to Korsakoff's dementia but this may be prevented by prompt administration of intravenous thiamine.

COMPLICATIONS OF ALCOHOL DEPENDENCE

The effect of alcohol is pervasive. Some of the main complications of alcohol abuse are summarized in Box 17.9.

MANAGEMENT

A thorough history including current and lifetime drinking and a complete physical examination will help to clarify the nature of the alcohol use

disorder. The CAGE questions can be a useful screen (see Box 17.10). Collateral history is always useful. Symptoms of depression, psychosis and dementia should be identified from examination of the mental state.

Treatment can be divided into short term and long term.

SHORT–TERM STABILIZATION AND MANAGEMENT

1. *Stop alcohol intake.* Elective withdrawal from alcohol is best done under advice from specialist services because older people have increased sensitivity to adverse effects of benzodiazepines. Acute withdrawal on in-patient medical wards usually takes place during an admission for some other reason.

2. *Relief of withdrawal symptoms.* Longer-acting benzodiazepines such as oxazepam or chlordiazepoxide are the drugs of choice. Doses must be carefully titrated in the first 24–48 hours of withdrawal to avoid over-sedation and under-treatment. The initial dose must be estimated based on the severity of the alcohol dependence and the severity of alcohol withdrawal symptoms. Local hospital or trust policies should be consulted for recommended schedules. For chlordiazepoxide, the British National Formulary recommends initial doses between 10 and 50 mg qds with a gradual reduction over 1 to 2 weeks. An example of an average dosage schedule would be:

day 1   chlordiazepoxide 25 mg qds
day 2   chlordiazepoxide 20 mg qds
day 3   chlordiazepoxide 15 mg qds
day 4   chlordiazepoxide 10 mg qds

day 5   chlordiazepoxide 10 mg bd + 5 mg bd
        (i.e. halve middle two doses)
day 6   chlordiazepoxide 5 mg qds
day 7   chlordiazepoxide 5 mg bd
Then stop

Care must be taken in the case of hepatic impairment where a build-up of metabolites and over-sedation may be a problem. In this case, oxazepam may be preferred in conjunction with advice from local specialists. Sometimes withdrawal symptoms can be prolonged in the older adult and so a more gradual reduction may be required with additional doses as required if there is further evidence of withdrawal.

3. Restoration of fluid and electrolyte balance.
4. Administration of parenteral B vitamins.
5. Prompt treatment of seizures and delirium. *This is a medical emergency.*

LONG-TERM MANAGEMENT

After detoxification, psychoeducation, counselling and motivational interviewing can be useful to engage the patient in the work of remaining abstinent. Other family members should be involved in the process as much as possible. Four key areas have been identified that are associated with a likelihood of abstinence:

1. The time spent drinking must be replaced with substitute activities with other people that do not involve drinking. This may be in the form of self-help groups, therapy groups, voluntary or community interests.
2. Successful abstainers often find a source of increased self-esteem or hope in their lives. Some may find this in religion or the 'spiritual' concept of sobriety in Alcoholics Anonymous (AA).
3. A sustaining, rehabilitative relationship such as with a spouse, a physician, an AA sponsor or a psychotherapist produces longer abstinence.
4. There can be a role for negative reinforcers of drinking, such as the threatened loss of a driving licence, or episodes of pancreatic pain. Disulfiram is not generally recommended in elderly subjects.

RECOMMENDED READING

*** Recommended reading; * interesting but not vital*

Epidemiology
Copeland J R M, Dewey M E, Wood N et al 1987 Range of mental illness among the elderly in the community: prevalence in Liverpool using the GMS-AGECAT package. British Journal of Psychiatry 150:815–823 **
Kay D, Beamish P, Roth M 1964 Old age mental disorders in Newcastle upon Tyne. Part I: a study of prevalence. British Journal of Psychiatry 110: 146–158 *
Livingston G, Hawkins A, Graham N et al 1990 The Gospel Oak Study: prevalence rates of dementia, depression and activity limitation among elderly residents in inner London. Psychological Medicine 20:137–146 *

Dementia
Blessed G, Tomlinson B, Roth M 1968 The association between quantitative measures of dementia and of senile change in the cerebral grey matter of elderly subjects. British Medical Journal 114:797–811 *
Knapp M, Wilkinson D, Wrigglesworth R 1988 The economic consequences of Alzheimer's disease in the context of new drug developments. International Journal of Geriatric Psychiatry 13:531–543 *
McShane R, Keen J, Gedling K et al 1997 Do neuroleptic drugs hasten cognitive decline in dementia? Prospective study with necropsy follow up. British Medical Journal 314:266–270 **
Melzer D, McWilliams B, Brayne C et al 1999 Profile of disability in elderly people: estimates from a population study. British Medical Journal 318: 1108–1111 **

Depression
Anstey K, Brodaty H 1995 Antidepressants and the elderly: double blind trials 1987–1992. International Journal of Geriatric Psychiatry 10:265–279 *
Banerjee S, Dickinson E 1997 Evidence based health care in old age psychiatry. International Journal of Psychiatry in Medicine 27:283–292 *
Macdonald A J D 1986 Do general practitioners 'miss' depression in elderly patients? British Medical Journal 292:1365–1368 *
Murphy E 1982 The social origins of depression in old age. British Journal of Psychiatry 141:135–142 **
Post F 1972 The management and nature of depressive illness in late life: a follow-through study. British Journal of Psychiatry 121:393–404 *
Prince M J, Harwood R H, Thomas A et al 1998 A prospective population-based cohort study of the

effects of disablement and social milieu on the onset and maintenance of late-life depression. The Gospel Oak Project VII. Psychological Medicine 28:337–350 *

Residential care

Ames D 1991 Epidemiological studies of depression among the elderly in residential and nursing homes. International Journal of Geriatric Psychiatry 6:347–354 **

Services

Arie T 1970 The first year of the Goodmayes psychiatric service for old people. Lancet ii:1175–1182 *

Collighan G, Macdonald A, Herzberg J et al 1993 An evaluation of the multidisciplinary approach to psychiatric diagnosis in elderly people. British Medical Journal 306:821–824 **

Cooper B 1997 Principles of service provision in old age psychiatry. In: Jacoby R, Oppenheimer C (eds) Psychiatry for the elderly. Oxford University Press, Oxford, p 357–375 *

Further reading

International Journal of Geriatric Psychiatry *(journal)* **

Jacoby R, Oppenheimer C (eds) 2002 Psychiatry in the elderly, 3rd edn. Oxford University Press, Oxford **

SELF-ASSESSMENT QUESTIONS

Are the following statements true or false?

1. Depression in older adults:
   a. Is associated with being a recipient of local authority care
   b. Is a feature of the majority of people with physical illness
   c. Is associated with a suicide rate that peaks at age 85 years and above
   d. Has a poor response to drug treatment
   e. Can be mistaken for delirium in hospital in-patients

2. Dementia:
   a. Lewy body dementia is responsible for 5% of all cases of dementia
   b. People with Alzheimer's disease have a higher threshold for delirium
   c. A score of over 28/30 on MMSE effectively excludes a diagnosis of dementia
   d. Cerebral vaculitis can cause vascular dementia
   e. Pain is a cause of behavioural disturbance in patients with dementia

Chapter 18

Rehabilitation

John Young and Alison South

Rehabilitation is the most powerful intervention at your disposal to help disabled older people. However, specialist registrars often find it a difficult topic and this chapter will require your full attention. It is designed as a study guide to provide understanding rather than dry knowledge.

REHABILITATION AND GERIATRIC MEDICINE

It may come as a surprise to some specialist registrars that geriatric medicine is a relatively new specialty. Less than five decades ago society's main response to sick older people was the institution of the workhouse in which the chronic sick languished in the most miserable of circumstances. Into this arena stepped the early pioneers of our specialty. Their contributions were based on a new enthusiasm for older people, common sense and a systematic approach. They developed simple principles that we would still recognize today as the process of rehabilitation. Thus, at the inception, geriatric medicine and rehabilitation for older people were inextricably intertwined.

EFFECTIVENESS OF REHABILITATION FOR OLDER PEOPLE

THE MARJORY WARREN EXPERIMENT

Marjory Warren has been referred to as 'the Mother of Geriatrics'. She was given responsibility for the West Middlesex County Hospital (previously a workhouse) with several hundred chronically ill, bedfast older people. She developed a new and highly successful process of care: rehabilitation. A summary of her work is given in Box 18.1. These days we have become accustomed

Box 18.1	The Marjory Warren experiment
Objective	To improve the health of disabled older people
Setting	The Poor Law Infirmary of the West Middlesex Hospital in 1935 (an 'ill assorted dump ... large wards which are devoid of any signs of comfort or interest')
Subjects	714 chronic sick, bedridden 'incurables'
Design	Unblinded, uncontrolled, retrospective study
Intervention	Rehabilitation, comprising: – individual patient assessment – team working – environmental modification
Primary outcome	Hospital discharge
Outcome results	514 'incurable' patients discharged (and subsequently beds closed)
Conclusion	Rehabilitation is a powerful intervention for bedridden older people

Table 18.1 Effectiveness of comprehensive geriatric assessment	
	Hospital geriatric unit v alternative care odds ratio (95% confidence limits) at 6 months
Living at home	1.8 (1.28–2.53)
Reduced mortality	0.68 (0.45–0.91)
Improved physical function	1.63 (1.00–2.65)
Improved cognitive function	(1.13–3.55)

(From Stuck et al 1993)

Box 18.2   Zimmer frame or delta rollator to promote walking in older people

The Zimmer frame has been used for over 70 years as a walking aid for older people. However, there are several inherent disadvantages because it promotes a slow, stop/start, non-physiological gait pattern. The delta rollator, a three-wheeled walking frame, encourages a smooth, physiological striding type of gait pattern. Which of the two devices promotes optimum recovery in older people with a temporary decline in mobility is unknown.

to small treatment effects requiring large trials to demonstrate effectiveness reliably. What if a treatment is so powerful that even an inauspicious situation (bedridden incurables) and a crude outcome (hospital discharge) can be unequivocally influenced? So it was with Warren's new process of rehabilitation.

'COMPREHENSIVE GERIATRIC ASSESSMENT' (CGA)

Although geriatric medicine and rehabilitation were originally conceived and implemented nationally in the UK, much of the effectiveness evaluation has been conducted in North America. The effectiveness studies have been summarized in a systematic review and meta-analysis (Stuck et al 1993). The studies (UK n = 8; North America n = 15; Others n = 5) are diverse randomized trials but have as a common thread an evaluation of 'comprehensive geriatric assessment': a core process characterized by multidisciplinary assessment and treatment. The pooled estimates of effectiveness across a range of outcome measures were encouragingly positive. The best effects were obtained for CGA delivered by hospital-based elderly care departments in which the assessment process and subsequent interventions were integrated and when organized post-discharge follow-up was arranged (Table 18.1).

THE 'BLACK BOX' OF REHABILITATION

One report identified a staggering 35 systematic reviews for rehabilitation topics of relevance to older people. Reviews were available for back pain, neck pain, diabetes mellitus, fractured neck of femur, occupational therapy in nursing homes, chronic pulmonary disease, cardiac rehabilitation, falls and stroke. However, these reviews disguise an important general deficiency in our knowledge. They largely describe the effects of complex, multicomponent interventions; sometimes called 'packages of care'. But what item, or items, has greatest effect? The 'black box' concept has been a fashionable term to indicate our imprecise understanding of the complex process of rehabilitation. The inputs and outcomes can be quantified but the relationship between the two is opaque. What are the critical factors for successful rehabilitation? Are benefits due to specific therapeutic techniques or to better delivery and organization? How much can be attributed to the greater enthusiasm of the staff? Even apparently simple (yet important) questions await clear resolution. For example:

- Is the the most effective transitional walking aid a Zimmer frame or delta rollator? (Box 18.2)
- What is the health gain of home assessment visits?
- What is the most effective training programme for nurses in rehabilitation?
- Do multidisciplinary collaborative notes improve rehabilitation team working?
- How can we reduce falls in rehabilitation wards?

DEFINING REHABILITATION

DEFINITION OF REHABILITATION

Understandably, specialist registrars prefer compact definitions for common questions such as 'What is rehabilitation?' If only it were that simple! Let us first have a look at a definitional approach to understanding rehabilitation for older people.

Exercise 1

First consider any organ 'ology' you are particularly familiar with (e.g. cardiology). Spend a few minutes considering how you might define it for a first year medical student. Now adopt a similar approach to define rehabilitation.

Exercise 1: response

How did you get on? You probably had no trouble with an organ 'ology'. For example, cardiology is a clinical specialty of the diseases affecting the heart and circulation in terms of anatomy, physiology, pathology, epidemiology and therapeutics. Did it cross your mind, and would you have told the medical student, that most 'ologies' have a rehabilitation component (cardiac rehabilitation, pulmonary rehabilitation, rheumatological rehabilitation, etc.)? Probably not, because we have not been trained to value these programmes (although there is accumulating evidence of effectiveness). Thrombolysis in myocardial infarction is drilled into us. Yet the successful National Heart Foundation Cardiac Rehabilitation Manual is still a mystery to many.

How did you manage with rehabilitation? Was this more difficult to encapsulate succinctly? Why is this? The 'ologies' reflect organ structures – they are therefore readily *bounded* systems. The concept of a kidney can be held in your mind as a tangible discreet entity. Not so with rehabilitation. It is *unbounded* and 'fuzzy'. It relates more to the *whole system*, i.e. the person. It is therefore an antithesis to familiar and comfortable reductionist medical practice: 'find the broken part and fix it' approach.

Exercise 2

You are not alone in finding rehabilitation a difficult concept to define. There are probably as many definitions offered for rehabilitation as there are writers on the subject. A selection of these follow. Read and familiarize yourself with them, underline key words and then attempt to analyse the similarities and differences between the various definitions.

'Rehabilitation must be a continuous process, beginning with the onset of sickness or injury, and continuing throughout treatment until final re-settlement in the most suitable work and living conditions is achieved.'
(Piercy Report 1956)

'Rehabilitation comprises reablement – the acquisition of skills needed for independent life, and re-settlement, the restoration of the person to his own or to another environment.'
(Gompertz & Ebrahim 1992)

Rehabilitation is 'about the tertiary response to insult or disease'
(Goodwill & Chamberlain 1988)

'The restoration of the individual to his (or her) fullest physical, mental and social capability.'
(Mair 1972)

'The primary objective of rehabilitation involves restoration (to the maximum degree possible) of either a function (physical or mental) or a role (within the family, social network or workforce).'
(Nocan & Baldwin 1998)

'Rehabilitation is a problem solving and educational process aimed at reducing the disability and handicap experienced by someone as a result of disease, always within the limitations imposed both by the available resources and by the underlying disease'
(Wade 1992)

'An active process by which those disabled by injury/disease achieve full recovery, or if full recovery is not possible, realise their optimal physical, mental and social potential and are integrated into their most appropriate environment'
(British Geriatrics Society 2004)

Exercise 2: response

You should now appreciate the variation in rehabilitation definitions. This variation stems partly from the diversity of rehabilitation applications: childhood to old age, numerous diseases and trauma and different settings (home, hospital, healthcare, social care). Considering rehabilitation just for older people does simplify our task. With this restriction, there is probably more agreement than disagreement between the definitions. The focus is that of the *whole person* expressed variously in terms of function, abilities, independence or role. Did you notice how often 'restoration' was used? Restoration ('to bring back to a former state') is rather optimistic for an overwhelming disease (e.g. severe stroke) or progressive disease (e.g. Parkinson's disease). For older people, therefore, we might wish to distinguish between *active* and *maintenance* rehabilitation. The former implies an expectation of improvement and the latter prevention of deterioration. Moreover, we also need to address the general older age concept of *frailty* (see Ch. 9). Although difficult to quantify reliably at the bedside, frailty implies an age- and disease-related loss of physiological reserve such that minor stress events result in disproportionate functional consequences. Rehabilitation has particular relevance in these circumstances.

Beware the use of value-laden words such as 'fullest' or 'optimal'. They beg the question of from whose perspective the rehabilitation results are being judged. There is a dangerously implicit assumption of a professionally-based judgment for a process which should be patient/carer-centred. This is not inconsequential nit-picking. A patient with a fractured neck of femur may not share the notion of 'a successful home discharge' when returning to the prospect of a commode in the living room. These ambiguities in rehabilitation perspective, commonly unvoiced, can smoul-

Table 18.2   Key attributes of rehabilitation

Key rehabilitation attributes	Comment
Wholeness	The whole person rather than a part
Highly individualized	Therefore not a standard response, e.g. myocardial infarction management
Emphasis on functional abilities	Self-care, mobility and life spaces, leisure
Not time limited	Need to have a wider vision than just hospital care
Active, planned responses	Requires a creative problem-solving approach in which the patient works at the extremes of their physical and functional abilities

der and lie at the heart of disability adjustment difficulties.

Having examined these rehabilitation definitions, we hope you might now understand that rehabilitation for older people is better understood as a *healthcare concept* within which key attributes can be identified (Table 18.2).

THE IMPORTANCE OF REHABILITATION FOR OLDER PEOPLE

Why should rehabilitation be at the heart of geriatric medicine? There are two reasons. First, acute illness in older people commonly has functional consequences, especially mobility and self-care skills. Second, many disease processes, often referred to as degenerative diseases, are strongly age related. These diseases are progressive, only partially ameliorated by our medical model (drugs and surgery), and can have a major impact on daily life activities of older people.

Exercise 3

Jot down the 'Big Six' degenerative disease processes faced by older people. List alongside these their associated rehabilitation responses.

Table 18.3 The 'Big Six' degenerative diseases affecting older people and their rehabilitation responses

	Prevalence	Rehabilitation responses
Generalized osteoarthrosis	30% > 75 years	Exercise programmes
Chronic respiratory disease	30% > 65 years	Pulmonary rehabilitation programmes
Ischaemic heart disease/chronic heart failure	6–10% > 65 years	Cardiac rehabilitation programmes
Peripheral vascular disease	12–15% > 75 years	Progressive exercise for claudication
	Annual incidence per 10000	
Osteoporosis/fractured neck of femur	90 (women 75–84 years)	Mobility exercise programmes
Stroke	140 (75–84 years)	Stroke rehabilitation units

Table 18.4 Self-reporting long–term limiting conditions

	% Prevalence in > 75–year–olds living at home	Professional or service response
Mobility	82%	Physiotherapy
Hearing	55%	Audiometry department
Personal care	46%	Occupational therapy
Vision	40%	Eye department/optician
Dexterity	33%	Occupational therapy
Continence	21%	Gynaecology/urology/continence services
Communication	20%	Speech and language therapist

Exercise 3: response

See Table 18.3 for our 'Big Six' list. How does your list compare? You may, quite reasonably, have some alternatives because the question was deliberately a little ambiguous (sorry!). The exercise was designed to emphasize our medical concern for neat pathological classifications. An apparent advantage of considering the health problems of older people in terms of pathology is that the rehabilitation responses can be neatly juxtaposed. At least it looks comfortable on paper, but in real life it is more complex. Most older people have multiple pathology. What should be the rehabilitation response for an older person with a combination of osteoarthritic knees, chronic bronchitis, chronic heart failure and peripheral vascular disease?

Exercise 4

Having examined the traditional medical approach to illness and older people, let us now consider a fresh perspective – that of the older person. List the main threats to health and personal independence that older people might report, and alongside them, note the key professional and/or service best placed to respond to each problem.

Exercise 4: response

Hopefully you now have a different list. Our list (Table 18.4) is extracted from the National Disability Survey conducted by the Office of Population Censuses and Surveys (OPCS) in 1989. Note that the term *disability* has been introduced, of which more later.

A key purpose of the OPCS study was to provide 'a comprehensive estimate of the prevalence of disability by age, degree of severity, and type of disability'. This type of national information is critical for government planning of services and benefits. The estimate for the numbers of people with disabilities in the UK was 6 million adults of whom 4.3 million (70%) were over the age of 60 years – or 46% of all older people. Most (over 90%) older disabled people live in their own homes, and most (over 80%) have only 'mild' disability but many have several types of disability. A key learning point which emerges when the problem list is constructed in this way is the range of professionals and services required to respond to disabled older people. This introduces the ideas of *team working* and *coordination of care* for older people with disabilities.

THE WHO INTERNATIONAL CLASSIFICATION OF FUNCTIONING, DISABILITY AND HEALTH (ICF)

We now have two different 'truths': a pathological and a disability classification of rehabilitation need for older people. Each has something useful to offer. This formed the basis of the 1980 four-level WHO classification that enabled the 'consequences of illness' to be considered in terms of pathology; impairment; disability and handicap (ICIDH). In 2001 this system was revised to a 'components of health' classification that aimed to describe in more positive terms how people live with their health condition(s). It facilitates a multidimensional view of disablement in older people (and others) and is a useful framework within which to consider the rehabilitation process. It prompts the need to uncover the cause (pathology or impairment) when a person presents with, for example, a mobility problem; while also prompting examination of the consequences of a disease in functional terms (formerly called disability, now known as activity limitation) and in relation to the lifestyle of the individual patient (formerly handicap, now participation restriction). Thus a balanced approach is promoted between disease modification (usually drugs) and maximizing independence (physical treatments, aids and adaptations). The revised model offers more than just the substitution of more politically correct terms, with greater emphasis on the importance of contextual mediators, i.e. environmental and personal factors (such as an individual's goals and beliefs) (see Fig. 18.1).

The definitions of the ICF component items are worthy of study:

■ *Impairment:* a loss or abnormality of body structure or a physiological or psychological function

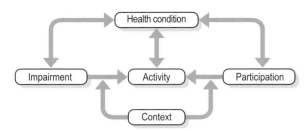

Figure 18.1   Diagrammatic representation of the WHO International Classification of Functioning (ICF).

■ *Activity:* the nature and extent of functioning at the level of the person
■ *Participation:* the nature and extent of a person's involvement in a life situation in relation to impairment, activities, health condition and contextual factors

It is easy to assume some form of proportional relationship between a pathology leading to impairment(s), activity limitation and participation restriction. However, the relationship is often frustratingly discontinuous. This is easiest to understand for participation restriction, as here the context is the individual and their particular circumstances. For example, an isolated homonymous hemianopia (impairment) has considerably greater lifestyle consequences for a car driver (loss of licence) than for a non-driver. However, the discordance between impairment and activity limitation is not so widely appreciated and is currently unexplained and requires new research. Greater impairment burdens do not necessarily imply greater activity limitation. Moreover, changes in impairments do not adequately explain the enhanced activity and participation that result from successful rehabilitation. This may simply reflect an important characteristic of rehabilitation techniques in that they largely improve function without influencing biology.

REHABILITATION IN PRACTICE

The 'six Rs' of rehabilitation, and their associated supporting processes, provide a practical clinical scheme (Fig. 18.2). Notice how primary assessment is the foundation but that it is an iterative process with regular reviews influencing the reablement process.

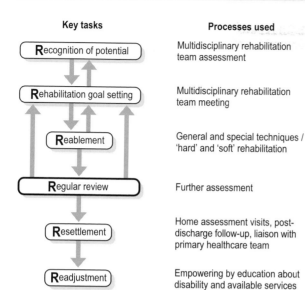

Key tasks | Processes used

Recognition of potential — Multidisciplinary rehabilitation team assessment

Rehabilitation goal setting — Multidisciplinary rehabilitation team meeting

Reablement — General and special techniques / 'hard' and 'soft' rehabilitation

Regular review — Further assessment

Resettlement — Home assessment visits, post-discharge follow-up, liaison with primary healthcare team

Readjustment — Empowering by education about disability and available services

Figure 18.2 The 'six Rs' of the clinical process of rehabilitation.

REHABILITATION ASSESSMENT

Although much is written about assessment in rehabilitation, clinical practices are largely anecdotally described rather than research based. They can be perplexing clinical skills to acquire. The medical model using the standardized history and examination with which you are familiar should give you an idea of the pathology and impairments. But beware! Doctors are poor at identifying activity limitation, and even worse with participation restriction. How can you do better? Three tips may help:

1. You need enough *time*
2. You need to *modify* your approach to the history
3. You need to maximize use of '*the telephone test*': call up anybody who knows the patient well – formal or informal carers – for background information

HOW TO MODIFY YOUR APPROACH

Hold in your mind three simple themes to be explored:

1. Who *was* my patient?
2. Who *is* my patient?
3. *How* did he get there?

Box 18.3 Key assessment questions suggested by Isaacs

Information gathering

1. Who is the patient?
2. What functional changes has he undergone? Over what period?
3. What adaptation has he made to the functional changes?
4. In what way has his occupational, social and family role altered?
5. What diseases have caused the functional changes?

Interpretation

6. What is the likely course of these diseases, given optimum medical treatment?
7. What improvement in functional level is potentially achievable?
8. If these functional improvements are attained, how will this alter this patient's potential social role?
9. How acceptable is this alteration of role to the patient?
10. What secondary effects will these functional changes in the patient have on his carers?

The trick is to get the older person (often reluctant with an authority figure) to talk discursively. This is called the *narrative approach* and is the antithesis of the more familiar rapid closed questioning (e.g. did the pain go down your arm? Yes/No).

Exercise 5

Professor Bernard Isaacs has suggested 10 key questions to use in rehabilitation assessment that we have grouped under *information gathering* and *interpretation* in Box 18.3. Have a look at the information gathering questions 1–4 and write down the form of words you might use in practice to obtain each section of information.

Exercise 5: response

1. Tell me about yourself and your life.
2. What problems do you have looking after yourself at home now?

3. How do you cope with these problems?

4 What do your family say about these problems?

Notice how they are very open-ended questions – really nothing more than prompts.

The *narrative approach* has several advantages in rehabilitation:

a. The telling of the story generates a therapeutic relationship based on shared understanding.

b. The patient's interpretation becomes dominant and the trap of 'normative' responses is avoided (see Box 18.3).

c. A more elaborate, informed and useful analysis can be made.

(Greenhalgh & Hurwitz 1999)

STANDARDIZED MEASUREMENTS

Standardized measurement instruments are structured questionnaire tools, which are used increasingly frequently in routine rehabilitation practice. The clinical assessment of disabled people is a difficult skill to acquire and specialist registrars can therefore be forgiven the apparent shortcut of using a battery of standardized measurement instruments (Box 18.4). But be warned:

1. Assessment involves *evaluation* and *interpretation* of patient problems. The standardized measurement instruments quantify components but can only inform the assessment process more reliably. Better measurement complements, but does not replace, assessment. The measurement instruments cannot determine underlying causes for activity limitation, nor can they determine the interventions that are required for individual patients.

2. *'My name is Legion for we are many'* (Mark 5:9). There are multitudes of standardized assessment instruments available. Which ones should you use?

3. Standardized assessment instruments form the backbone of quantitative evaluation in clinical trials. Therefore there is a seductive notion that what works in research (good science) should be just as valuable in clinical practice. However, most rehabilitation trials have a research worker

---

Box 18.4   Rehabilitation assessment: get at the facts

The plot:	Mrs Smith who lives with her daughter is severely disabled by knee arthritis and is admitted after a fall.
The ambush:	Angry daughter: 'Why are you *dragging* (her emphasis) my mother up and down the ward?'
The real plot:	Although chairfast for several years, she is well adapted to her activity limitation so that, with her daughter's help, she has a content lifestyle and is self-fulfilled with her family around her.
The lesson:	Avoid a routine approach. The more individualized and patient centred the better. Try to find out the *real* rather than the *apparent* problems.

---

dedicated to obtaining the measurements. Completing a battery of instruments can be extremely time consuming.

4. Many older people, particularly those with cognitive impairment, depression, poor hearing or vision – just the people for whom comprehensive assessment is critical – find questionnaire completion, even with help, beyond them. The currently popular SF36 (a global health measure) has low response rates when used by older people.

5. Remember you are part of a team. What are the views of the other members of your team about a proposed new instrument?

These negative comments are not to detract from the genuine importance of standardized assessment measures in rehabilitation, but over-reliance and an unquestioning use is an intellectually lazy attribute for a specialist registrar. It is generally more rewarding to talk to patients directly than through questionnaires. The Royal College of Physicians and the British Geriatrics Society (1992) have jointly recommended the standardized assessment instruments shown in Table 18.5 for routine use when assessing older people.

Table 18.5 Standardized assessments recommended by RCP and BGS	
Domain of interest	**Recommended scale**
Activities of daily living	Barthel Index
Vision and hearing	Lambeth Disability Screening Score
Mental impairment	Hodkinson Abbreviated Mental Test
Depression	Geriatric Depression Score
Quality of life	Philadelphia Geriatric Centre Morale Scale
Social circumstances	Social indicators checklist

Which of the scales in Table 18.5 have you seen in use? You have possibly only seen the Barthel Index and Abbreviated Mental Test. The others have not really caught on. The Philadelphia Morale Scale, in particular, has not become popular. Many older people find it frankly upsetting to complete. Moreover, quality of life is a nebulous concept and probably too subjective to be captured in a question- naire. Wade (1992) has referred to it as 'an illusion that cannot be defined or measured'.

Properties of measurement instruments

Given the mountain of scales available, it might be thought that they are simple to create. This is not so. A 'good' scale takes about 5 to 10 years to develop. What makes a 'good' scale? There are various measurement properties that need to be demonstrated in research studies using different patient groups in different settings:

Validity: does the instrument actually measure what it purports to?

Reliability: does the instrument give similar scores when used by two observers for the same patient, or when repeated on stable patients?

Sensitivity: does the instrument detect clinically important changes?

Acceptability: it should be simple and quick to apply, easy to understand (by the whole team), and easy for patients to complete (high response rate)

These instrument qualities are not independent and perfect scales do not exist. Compromises have to be achieved between, for example, sensitivity and reliability – a scale sensitive to small changes has low reliability (variation in score).

Impairment measures

Many of these will be covered in chapters dealing with specific diseases. Our purpose here is general principles.

Exercise 7

Consider the following common impairments and list the measurement instrument you might apply: poor vision, poor hearing, confusion, uncomfort- able feet, poor mobility.

Exercise 7: response

If you are still alert and reading actively, you will have been perplexed by 'poor mobility', 'confu- sion' and 'uncomfortable feet'. These are clinical problems rather than genuine impairments. The genuine impairments are, in fact, very complex. We have set down a more precise list of impair- ments with a simple clinical assessment to enable their detection and a more definitive quantitative measurement (Table 18.6). Some of the practical difficulties in using the WHO ICF model should now become more apparent to you.

'Confusion' contains several separate cognitive impairments including orientation, memory and attention deficits. We might get a clue to the pres- ence of these during our clinical assessment through a patient's apparent vagueness to our questioning (assuming that the patient is not deaf and is able to hear our questions). With 'uncom- fortable feet' we should really be considering range of motion of the ankle and subtalar joints, and at the forefoot, and deformities and distur- bances of foot stance and movement biomechan- ics. All we can easily do in the clinical setting is provide a description of our findings. Podiatrists would use standardized measures and special equipment to define more precisely the impair- ments present.

The gait impairments underlying 'poor mobil- ity' could include balance, walking speed, cadence (steps per minute), stride length and gait cycle times (support, swing and double support). Such detailed gait impairment analysis requires the facilities of a gait laboratory and an experienced technician. However, gait speed is an excellent summary measure of gait impairment. It is a per- fect example of a measure that is valid, reliable,

Table 18.6 Detection and measurement of some common impairments

Problem	Impairment	Clinical assessment	Impairment measurement
Vision	Visual acuity	Do you have difficulty: '... seeing newsprint even with glasses?' '... recognizing people across the road even with glasses?'	Snellen chart
Deafness	Loss of appreciation of sound frequencies	Do you have difficulty: '... hearing a conversation?'	Audiometry
Confusion	Orientation, memory, attention, etc.	Ability to provide clear history	Abbreviated Mental Test Score Mini-Mental State Examination Score
Uncomfortable feet	Multiple impairments	Clinical description	Foot Health Status Questionnaire Foot Morbidity Index
Poor mobility	Multiple impairments possible	Gait speed	Gait laboratory

sensitive, acceptable and useful. The patient is simply timed using a stopwatch over a measured and marked 10-metre distance. The measure correlates with other gait parameters, including balance and clinical assessment of gait pattern (see Ch. 24 on gait disorders). It should be used as part of routine practice.

Activity (disability) measurement

Activities of daily living

There are many instruments available to quantify activities of daily living (ADL) but the Barthel Index has become popular and is in widespread routine use in the UK. It is an ordinal scale (as are most rehabilitation measures) and this means that an improvement in score of, say, 5 points to 6 does not represent the same clinical improvement as a score of 10 moving to 11. The Barthel Index assesses levels of independence or dependence for ten ADL tasks with a score range of 0 (dependent) to 20 (independent):

Dressing	Bed/chair transfers
Feeding	Walking
Grooming	Stairs
Toilet	Bladder
Bathing	Bowels

The score is quick and easy to use. It can aid both systematic activity limitation assessment and also show rehabilitation progress if repeated at intervals. The measurement properties are well researched. Validity has been well demonstrated and is a key strength. Reliability is less than might be expected: a change of 4 points is required to be certain that a real difference has been measured. The main disadvantage of the Barthel Index is that the steps on the scale are fairly large – it is therefore not very sensitive to change. Also, especially for people living at home, there is a marked 'ceiling' effect in as much as patients can score a maximum of 20 points and be 'independent' but still have daily living restrictions. *Nonetheless, the Barthel Index provides a valuable tool to assess older people and its routine use has much to commend it.*

Extended activities of daily living

Extended, or instrumental, ADL scales extend the range of the Barthel Index to include important other daily tasks such as housework, shopping and trips. They are especially useful for patients at home for whom the ceiling effect with a Barthel Index is a great limitation. Examples are the Frenchay Activities Index and the Nottingham extended ADL score.

Participation (handicap) measurement

Participation restriction, the disadvantage to the individual as a result of ill health, is the critical level to effect change from the patient's point of view. It involves placing the individual in the context of their home, local environment and facilities, their relationships, motivation, mood and expectations. Unsurprisingly, the uniqueness of this context makes the development of a generic scale difficult. Some aspects of participation restriction are covered by the extended ADL measures (e.g. social activities).

The best insight into participation restriction comes from the clinical assessment process. There is no substitute for knowing the patient as an individual, supplemented by observing how they cope in their own home (home assessment visits). Helpful tips to identify participation restriction are to ask broad questions such as:

1. What would make the biggest difference to your life?
2. What do you see as your number one problem?
3. Asking patients/caregivers to describe a typical 24-hour day

Thus, we have come full circle, back to the critical importance of a skillfully obtained clinical assessment process. This is the skill you need to acquire.

TEAM WORKING

A key aspect of successful rehabilitation is that your medical assessment is only one component. Other professionals will make equally important contributions but from different perspectives. This is the concept of team working which was an essential component in Warren's early work. Surprisingly, the General Medical Council has only recently produced explicit guidance on effective medical teams (http://www.gmc-uk.org). However, rehabilitation has a special dimension in the *multiprofessional* nature of the team. Given its importance, it is remarkable how little rehabilitation research has addressed this issue (considerable opportunities for a curious specialist registrar). The best available knowledge base has to be plagiarized from management literature. The man-agement popularist, Charles Handy, has written extensively on teams (and also leadership styles). He regards teams as providing better ideas, solutions that are better evaluated and, interestingly, notes that teams are prepared to take more risky decisions than individuals.

Characteristics of effective teams (after Handy)

- Motivated by shared aims and philosophy
- Prepared to coordinate their work
- Recognize their complementary skills
- Ability to resolve conflict
- Mutual respect
- Flexible and open to ideas

'The team as the hero'

Robert Reich, writing in the Harvard Business Review, challenges the myth of the entrepreneurial hero (akin to the aloof and authoritarian doctor) who personifies freedom and independence, who creates the Big Idea, builds Big Machines and Big Organizations. He argues it was, and is, rarely so. Rather, there is a collective entrepreneurial culture in which individual skills are integrated into a group and the collective capacity becomes something greater than the sum of its parts. 'The team as the hero' is characterized by close working relationships so that, as problems are worked through, team members learn about each other's abilities and how they can help one another to perform better. Coordination and communication replace older practices of command and control.

TEAM MEMBERS AND LEADERSHIP

Who should be in the multidisciplinary rehabilitation team? 'Obviously', you would say, 'a doctor'. And you might imply the doctor as the natural team leader. However, although the doctor could (if he/she has the appropriate skills) become the team chairperson (a role of coordination), leadership of an effective team should rotate according to patient need. The care of the older patient admitted with pneumonia will initially be led by a doctor; the nursing staff will have a lead

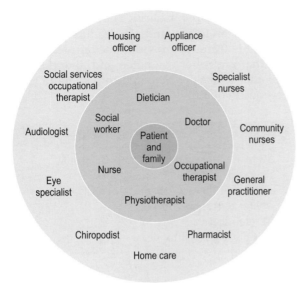

Figure 18.3 The core (inner circle) and extended (outer circle) rehabilitation team members.

role in preventing pressure sores and maintaining nutrition, continence and morale, and the therapy staff will lead in the rebuilding of independence. A doctor as a (poor) leader might say: 'Please arrange a home visit'. Better to act as a chairperson, synthesizing information within the team and allowing sufficient professional space to create a team decision about the need for a home visit. Beware the situation where:

■ The therapist proposes
■ The doctor orders
■ And the nurse executes

So far we have mentioned doctors, therapists and nurses. Who else should be in the team? The answer is, 'it depends' – it depends on the patient's problems. For example, a patient with a severe osteoarthritic hip will require a different team (perhaps orthopaedic staff) to a patient with a below-knee amputation (prosthetists). However, we can usefully consider a *core* rehabilitation team and an *extended* rehabilitation team shown diagrammatically in Figure 18.3. Imagine the circles as revolving rims to accommodate the idea of rotating leadership. Pluralistic leadership is a high-level team function and is not always easy to achieve in practice, particularly if some team members have relatively less clinical experience. Patience is needed.

TEAM FUNCTIONING

Teams need to meet regularly to generate cohesion and function effectively. There are two purposes to team meetings:

1. Patient management
   ■ share assessments
   ■ plan and agree rehabilitation goals and interventions
   ■ evaluate progress
   ■ plan discharges

2. Team building
   ■ getting to know each other
   ■ local gossip and events
   ■ proposed practice changes
   ■ concerns, grumbles and special pressures
   ■ feedback

Traditionally, multidisciplinary rehabilitation teams meet primarily to discuss patient management but, increasingly, more specialist teams (e.g. stroke units) will meet from time to time with the specific purpose of team building.

TIPS FOR SUCCESSFUL TEAM MEETINGS

1. Time management:
   There is much to do in these meetings so allocate sufficient time and arrive promptly. Some doctors have them before ward rounds, others afterwards. Try both to see what works for you and your team. Use the time available intelligently: most time for the most complex patients.

2. Summarize:
   Team assessments and information gathering need to be made manageable by an effective summary. This should be the role of the meeting chairperson, usually (but not invariably) a doctor. There are different approaches to summarizing:
   ■ Set out a short biography which describes the patient in their individual context (i.e. avoid 'an 83 year old man with a fall')
   ■ Construct a problem list or, better, list the impairments, activity limitations and participation restrictions
   ■ Create a formulation in terms of strengths and weaknesses

3. General points:
- Do not assume that you, because you are a doctor, know what needs to be done
- Listen more than talk
- Get everybody to contribute
- Someone should keep notes
- Involve community staff when necessary (they will often know the patient well)
- Involve patient and family by:
  - discussion of interim conclusions
  - considering inviting them into the meeting
  - meeting with them separately and in private (wards are public places)

REHABILITATION IN ACTION ('REST IS RUST')

Newly appointed (but *not* experienced!) specialist registrars might possibly be forgiven the idea that rehabilitation is something 'done by therapists to patients'. This statement is doubly wrong. First, as we have seen, effective rehabilitation is about team working, and you are part of that team with an important role to play. Second, rehabilitation is not passively *done* to somebody. The somebody has to be encouraged, cajoled and motivated to struggle against their disability under skillful guidance from the rehabilitation team. It is much easier to sit comfortably and passively in a chair if you have painful knees or if you are recovering from a fractured neck of femur. Even more comfortable is to stop in bed. Unfortunately, even athletes become deconditioned after a few days of rest. An older person with limited physiological reserves may very rapidly lose sufficient cardiovascular and muscle function to the extent that the slightest exercise, say standing up from a chair unaided, becomes beyond their physiological capacity.

The dangers of going to bed

Richard Asher was an inspiring medical writer and, in an article with the above title, popularized the importance of early mobilization. 'Too often a sister puts all her patients back to bed as a housewife puts all her plates back in the plate rack – to make a generally tidy appearance'. He modified a stanza from a well known hymn into:

> 'Teach us to live that we may dread
> Unnecessary time spent in bed.
> Get people up and we may save
> Our patients from an early grave.'
>
> (Asher 1947)

The dangers of sitting in a chair

Lying in bed is 'rehabilitation for the grave'. Yet, simply decanting a patient and immobilizing them in a chair does not represent huge progress. How long do your patients spend sitting in chairs? There are hazards:

Psychological (boredom!)	Enforced dependency
Tissue viability	Deep venous thrombosis
Dependent oedema	Constipation/urinary
Deconditioning	retention
Insomnia	Contractures

We should replace Asher's dread of beds with that of chairs:

> Teach us that we may be scared
> Of unnecessary time spent in chairs.
> Get people up and we may save
> Our patients from an early grave.

Exercise 8

Consider an older lady who has knee and back arthritis with associated weak muscles and who is now 24 hours post-internal fixation for a fractured neck of femur. What steps should be taken over the next ten days or so to promote independence and mobility?

Exercise 8: response

Many specialist registrars respond to this question by producing a shopping list of items such as: 'refer to physio' or 'get the patient out of bed'. However, rehabilitation is a *total* approach. So let us start with a bigger vision.

Rehabilitation culture

In this situation it is the *whole ward* that provides the platform for the rehabilitation process. The ward culture, staff skills and attitudes and the physical environment generate an atmosphere that either promotes or impedes rehabilitation. By culture we mean the pervading values, beliefs and the usual way of doing things. Ideally, the culture needs to be actively led and promoted by senior staff. Some people are better able than others to create a positive rehabilitation culture. Consider your current wards. Which provides best rehabilitation? And why? Tactfully ask your consultant trainer about the rehabilitation culture on his/her ward.

The concept of a ward rehabilitation culture leads to the controversial issue about whether to combine acute and rehabilitation care on the same ward or, alternatively, have separate rehabilitation facilities. This issue is controversial because it is an area where there is scanty research evidence and therefore people are able to express (strongly) opinion-based views. On the face of it, it could be argued that there will inevitably be a clash of cultures with resulting uncertainty of purpose. 'The urgent (= acute care) drives out the important (= rehabilitation)'. If you are interested in one answer, refer to Young et al 1998 in the References list.

Staff rehabilitation knowledge and skills (including your own) are acquired by training. Rehabilitation training for nurses is particularly poorly developed and this can be a critical detrimental factor to the whole environment approach to rehabilitation.

Nurses and rehabilitation

Nurses have considerable potential to progress (or impede) rehabilitation. They have 24-hour close contact with patients and are usually the first to be approached for information by families. However, descriptive research literature suggests considerable ambiguity concerning their rehabilitation role. There is a conflict between a doing/caring role and that of promoting/facilitating. Consider this statement obtained from a nurse during a Bradford rehabilitation project:

'(Nurses) should stimulate patients but it is hard; it is not how we are trained. It is easier to do something in 30 seconds for a patient

---

rather than standing back and watch them struggle for 5 minutes with eating, dressing, walking or transferring.'

Training programmes should be routine on rehabilitation wards. They are powerful tools to influence change:

'This last 12 months the team has really come together. We have a better understanding of each other's roles, the right staff are in the right place and they understand rehab.'

(Forster et al 1999a,b)

Rehabilitation and prevention ('Rehabilitation starts at day one')

Do not start rehabilitation for this patient *post-operatively* (or in other patients after an acute illness has resolved). She should be prepared physiologically and psychologically *preoperatively* for her recovery period. Adequate hydration, nutrition and pain control will be the minimum physical requirements to foster a prompt postoperative recovery. However, unless she is unlucky and has had a previous fractured neck of femur this will be this patient's first experience of the condition. She needs to be prepared psychologically by a simple explanation of the anticipated care pathway before her operation.

Promotion of independence

Again it is easy to shortcut to a narrow perspective of 'get the patient out of bed' – an orthopaedic surgeon's commandment, and not hopefully that of a specialist registrar in elderly care medicine. There is much to consider: How does she feel? Is there an appropriate chair? Can she reach for a drink? What walking aid is to be used? Are spectacles, hearing aid, dentures and footwear in place? One general conceptual approach which can be helpful here is to consider the rehabilitation inputs required in terms of 'hard' and 'soft' rehabilitation (Fig. 18.4). 'Hard' rehabilitation is the tangible component: the readily visible aspect of rehabilitation: the aspects that are quantified in rehabilitation process and health economic studies. 'Soft' rehabilitation is more easily over-

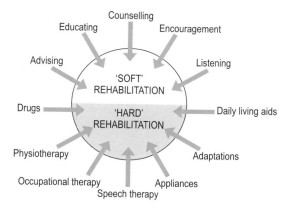

Figure 18.4   Common rehabilitation interventions.

specific interventions. This encouraging research, however, is based almost exclusively on studies of stable disability, generally in the context of outpatient work. Further work is needed to examine the process and outcome of goal setting for disabled older people.

How would you recognize a rehabilitation goal? A useful acronym is SMART:

Specific: Who will do what, under what circumstances, with what degree of success (Table 18.7)?
Measurable: Pass or fail
Achievable: Not too easy, but hard enough to be taxing
Realistic: Could the patient do it if his/her life depended on it?
Timed: When should the goal be achieved?

And finally: does rehabilitation for older people have a future?

If you have followed this chapter, it may seem unexpected to raise this question now. After all, we have argued that rehabilitation is the basis for the practice of effective geriatric medicine. But we have primarily been describing rehabilitation from a hospital perspective – the familiar working environment for most geriatricians. In a brief but provocative article, Norman Vetter, adapting a well-known catch phrase, referred to 'Hospitals, Jim, but not as we know them!' Vetter described the remorseless evolution of the general hospital to specialist, high-efficiency acute facilities. One overt manifestation of this process has been, and continues to be, the contraction of bed numbers with a compensatory reduction in lengths of stay. This has inevitably eroded the time, space and opportunity for rehabilitation (Young et al 1998). Paradoxically, rehabilitation in stroke and orthopaedic units has become more firmly established in hospitals but general rehabilitation has been

looked and is difficult to quantify yet research has shown it to be greatly valued by the patient. It involves talking, listening, understanding and counselling.

REHABILITATION GOALS

'Unplanned rehabilitation is like an unplanned holiday. You don't know where you are going until you get there, and when you get there, you don't know if that is where you want to be'
(Bernard Isaacs)

Rehabilitation goals are highly focused statements of intent that should be generated from the assessment process. Goal planning or goal setting is the process of agreeing the goals. Wade (1992), reviewing the goal-setting literature, concluded that using rehabilitation goals does lead to improved outcomes but with the proviso that significant patient involvement occurs, and that both short- and long-term goals are developed. It is clearly axiomatic that the goal planning is supported by

Table 18.7 Examples of rehabilitation goals		
	Mrs Jones	Mr Brown
Will do what?	Walk to the toilet and back	Dress his top half
Under what conditions?	Using a Zimmer frame but with no physical help	With clothes passed to him in order
With what degree of success?	At least four times each day	Each morning

Box 18.5   Definition of intermediate care

Intermediate care should be regarded as describing services that meet *all* the following criteria:

1. Services targeted at people who would otherwise face unnecessarily prolonged hospital stays or inappropriate admission to acute in-patient care, long-term residential care, or continuing NHS in-patient care.
2. Services provided on the basis of a comprehensive assessment, resulting in a structured individual care plan that involves active therapy, treatment and opportunity for recovery.
3. Services which have a planned outcome of maximizing independence and typically enabling patients/users to resume living at home.
4. Services which are time limited, normally no longer than 6 weeks, and frequently as little as 1 to 2 weeks or less.
5. Services which involve cross-professional working, with a single assessment framework, single professional records and shared protocols.

(Department of Health 2001)

increasingly squeezed out. The proposed solution is the national introduction (in England) of intermediate care services.

The purpose and expectations of intermediate care were presented in detail in the National Service Framework for older people and an official government definition of intermediate care was produced (Box 18.5). You will quickly see that points 2 and 3 incorporate the fundamental principles of rehabilitation already described in this chapter. This is reassuring and perhaps during the next several years we will see the re-emergence of rehabilitation of older people as a community-based discipline. Rapid progress has been made but many obstacles remain before intermediate care is accepted as a mainstream older people's service. A more robust evidence base, skill mix, service configurations, systems for clinical governance, including demonstration of patient safety, are just some of the critical issues that need to be addressed. One version of the future was summarized by the strap line: 'Geriatricians must move with their patients into the community' (see Young & Philp 2000).

SUMMARY

You should now appreciate that rehabilitation lies at the heart of geriatric medicine. It is a set of complex processes usually involving several professional disciplines and aimed at reducing the disability and handicap of older people facing daily living difficulties. There are three key processes:

1. A sound assessment and analysis of problems
2. Interventions to remedy or modify impairments, activity limitations and participation restrictions
3. An evaluation of progress and subsequent changes to the interventions

REFERENCES

Asher R 1947 The dangers of going to bed. British Medical Journal ii:967–968

British Geriatrics Society 2004 Compendium document 1.4. British Geriatrics Society, London

Department of Health 2001 Health service circular. Department of Health, London

Forster A, Dowswell G, Young J et al 1999a Effect of a physiotherapist-led training programme on attitudes of nurses caring for patients after stroke. Clinical Rehabilitation 13:113–122

Forster A, Dowswell G, Young J et al 1999b Effects of a physiotherapist-led stroke training programme for nurses. Age and Ageing 28:567–574

Gompertz P, Ebrahim S 1992 Organisation of rehabilitation services. Reviews in Clinical Gerontology 2:329–343

Goodwill J C, Chamberlain M A (eds) 1988 Rehabilitation of the physically disabled adult. Croom Helm, London

Greenhalgh T, Hurwitz B 1999 Narrative based medicine: why study narrative? British Medical Journal 318:661–664

Mair A 1972 Report of the sub committee of the Standing Medical Advisory Committee, Scottish Health Service Council on Medical Rehabilitation. HMSO, Edinburgh

Nocan A, Baldwin S 1998 Trends in rehabilitation policy. Audit Commission, London

Piercy Report 1956 Report of the committee of inquiry on the rehabilitation, training and resettlement of disabled persons. HMSO, London

Royal College of Physicians, British Geriatrics Society 1992 Standardised assessment scales for elderly people. Report of joint workshop of the Research

Unit of the Royal College of Physicians and the British Geriatrics Society

Stuck A E, Siu A L, Wieland G D et al 1993 Comprehensive geriatric assessment: a meta-analysis of controlled trials. Lancet 342:1032–1036

Wade D T 1992 Measurement in neurological rehabilitation. Oxford University Press, Oxford

Young J B, Philp I 2000 Future directions for geriatric medicine. British Medical Journal 320:133–134

Young J, Robinson J, Dickinson E 1998 Rehabilitation for older people. British Medical Journal 316:1108–1109

RECOMMENDED READING

Blaxter M 1976 The meaning of disability. Heinemann, London
A person-centred research report about the experience of disability.

Department of Health 2001 National Service Framework for Older People. Department of Health, London

Mulley G (ed.) 1989 Everyday aids and appliances. British Medical Journal Press, London

Mulley G (ed.) 1991 More everyday aids and appliances. British Medical Journal Press, London

Nocan A, Baldwin S 1998 Trends in rehabilitation policy. Audit Commission, London

Stuck A E, Siu A L, Wiland G D et al 1993 A comprehensive geriatric assessment: meta-analysis of controlled trials. Lancet 342:1032–1036

Wade D T 1995 Measurement in neurological rehabilitation. Oxford University Press, Oxford
A good discussion of the WHO ICIDH and an extensive listing of standardized measurement instruments.

Warren M W 1943 Care of chronic sick. A case for treating chronic sick in blocks in a general hospital. British Medical Journal ii:822–823
A classic paper.

Young J B, Philp I 2000 Future directions for geriatric medicine. British Medical Journal 320:133–134

Young J, Robinson J, Dickinson E 1998 Rehabilitation for older people. British Medical Journal 316: 1108–1109

SELF-ASSESSMENT QUESTION

1. A frail elderly man with limited mobility due to arthritis and chronic bronchitis is admitted with pneumonia. Are the following true or false?
   a. He should be encouraged to talk about his life at home.
   b. He should be referred to a physiotherapist and occupational therapist when the acute illness has settled.
   c. The doctor should set the rehabilitation goals.
   d. The main emphasis for rehydration should be on intravenous fluids.

Chapter **19**

Management of stroke

Peter Langhorne and Scott Ramsay

Stroke is one of the major public health problems in the UK where it represents the third commonest cause of death and commonest cause of acquired adult disability (Warlow et al 2001). An understanding of stroke management is an essential part of training in geriatric medicine because:

- It is largely a disease of elderly people
- Geriatricians often take the lead role in stroke service delivery in the UK
- The combination of acute medical care with more prolonged rehabilitation and social reintegration make it a good model of 'classical' geriatric medical practice

In this chapter we have approached the subject from a clinical perspective in a way which we hope will serve both as a practical guide to the management of the individual patient and an illustration of key aspects of the aetiology, epidemiology, diagnosis and management of stroke.

When faced with a patient presenting with a suspected stroke there are seven key questions you must address:

1. Is this a stroke? (Diagnosis)
2. What kind of stroke? (Classification)
3. What was the cause of the stroke? (Aetiology)
4. What problems has it caused? (Assessment)
5. What care is needed? (Management)
6. What can be done to prevent a further vascular event? (Prevention)
7. What advice should be given? (Advice)

IS THIS A STROKE?

Stroke is a clinical diagnosis characterized by an acute, focal neurological deficit of vascular origin (Box 19.1). This definition is not quite all encompassing since (a) stroke can occasionally cause a global loss of consciousness and (b) a rarer cause of stroke (subarachnoid haemorrhage) can present only with neck pain rather than focal neurological symptoms (Warlow et al 2001).

Transient ischaemic attacks (TIAs) have the same clinical definition, except the symptoms resolve within 24 hours (and in most cases within 1 hour). TIAs also include transient monocular blindness (*amaurosis fugax*).

PRESENTATION

The typical presentation of stroke is one of sudden onset, focal symptoms and signs which are 'negative' in character (e.g. loss of power or sensation) and tend to be maximal at onset (Box 19.2).

Box 19.1   Diagnosis of stroke

A clinical syndrome characterized by rapid onset focal neurological symptoms (and/or signs) lasting more than 24 hours* or leading to death, with no apparent cause other than vascular.

*Transient ischaemic attacks (TIAs) always resolve within 24 hours (usually within 1 hour)

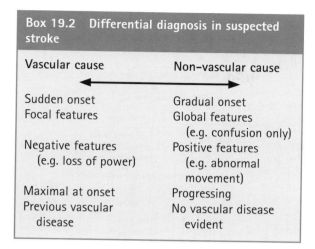

Box 19.2   Differential diagnosis in suspected stroke

Vascular cause	Non-vascular cause
←	→
Sudden onset	Gradual onset
Focal features	Global features (e.g. confusion only)
Negative features (e.g. loss of power)	Positive features (e.g. abnormal movement)
Maximal at onset	Progressing
Previous vascular disease	No vascular disease evident

Box 19.3   Pitfalls

Beware of the patient with:

- Gradual onset of symptoms (or no clear time of onset)
- Features of raised intracranial pressure (headache, drowsiness, papilloedema)
- Global symptoms (confusion)
- Low risk of vascular disease

Common examples of this include unilateral motor loss (hemiparesis), unilateral sensory loss (hemisensory loss), slurred speech (dysarthria), disorders of language (dysphasia), visual field defect (homonymous hemianopia) and unsteadiness (ataxia).

DIFFERENTIAL DIAGNOSIS

The clinical diagnosis of stroke is usually reliable where there is a clear history of rapid onset of focal neurological deficit. However, difficulties can arise where there is an inadequate history due to reduced consciousness or communication problems (or an inadequate history has been taken!). The differential diagnosis includes:

- Subdural haematoma
- Cerebral tumour or abscess
- Hypoglycaemia
- Post-seizure (Todd's) paresis
- Multiple sclerosis

Although the clinical diagnosis will be correct in the majority of cases (95%) further investigation is often required (Warlow et al 2001).

Box 19.3 outlines some features which should alert the wary clinician.

POPULAR MISDIAGNOSES

Acute confusional state: Remember to check for visuo-spatial dysfunction (such as sensory in-attention, constructional apraxia, neglect) and

dysphasia. These are often labelled as confusion when in fact they represent focal neurological signs.

Failure to cope: Remember to check for organizational problems (apraxia), gait apraxia or truncal ataxia. These may be labelled as 'confusion' or 'off feet' but again represent a focal neurological problem.

WHAT KIND OF STROKE?

WHY CLASSIFY?

The days of diagnostic and therapeutic nihilism in stroke management should be over. We need to make a proper diagnostic assessment (including classification) in order to:

- Make an accurate diagnosis
- Identify the underlying cause
- Anticipate patients' problems
- Make an accurate prognosis (for survival, recovery and stroke recurrence)

Stroke classification has often followed an aetiological model (e.g. embolic stroke, thrombotic stroke) which is of limited practical value and often based on a number of dodgy assumptions. We will focus on a more practical clinical classification (Fig. 19.1).

INFARCTION OR HAEMORRHAGE?

Distinguishing cerebral infarction from cerebral haemorrhage is a fundamental step in the management of a stroke patient. Without knowing the underlying pathology it is impossible to make an informed plan of treatment. Unfortunately,

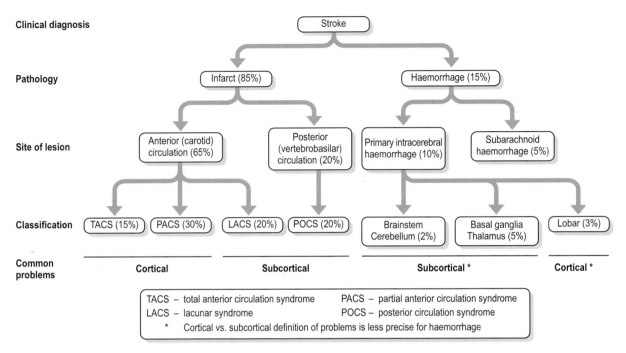

Figure 19.1 Stroke classification.

attempts to clinically distinguish cerebral infarction from primary intracranial haemorrhage, either informally or formally using scoring systems, are not sufficiently reliable to guide individual patient management (Weir et al 1994). Computed tomography (CT) scanning is essential and should be carried out within 48 hours (ideally < 24 hours) of the stroke. The high attenuation X-ray signal of blood will be lost within 14 days. Magnetic resonance imaging (MRI) can detect haemosiderin deposition and may be useful in excluding haemorrhage several weeks after the event.

Subarachnoid haemorrhage can often be distinguished clinically because of its characteristic presentation of sudden headache plus the associated features of meningism, vomiting and reduced consciousness. CT scanning and lumbar puncture are required to confirm the diagnosis and guide neurosurgical referral. Angiography is subsequently required to plan neurosurgical intervention such as clipping or coiling of aneurysms. As geriatricians, our main practical management steps are to make the diagnosis and refer to the appropriate neurosurgical service.

Cerebral vein thrombosis is a rare cause of focal neurological signs, which more commonly presents with headache, seizures, papilloedema and declining consciousness level associated with hypercoagulable states, sepsis and pregnancy (Warlow et al 2001). Cerebral vein thrombosis forms part of the differential diagnosis of benign intracranial hypertension and encephalitis. The diagnosis can be confirmed by CT or magnetic resonance venography.

STROKE SYNDROMES

Cerebral infarction

Having established the stroke is due to cerebral infarction a clinical classification can be used. (Fig. 19.1, Table 19.1). Cerebral infarction can be subdivided into four syndromes (Table 19.1). Two of these syndromes (total anterior circulation syndrome (TACS) and partial anterior circulation syndrome (PACS) are caused by occlusion of the internal carotid artery, middle cerebral artery, anterior cerebral artery or their branches (Fig. 19.2). They usually result in 'cortical' problems

Table 19.1 Clinical stroke syndromes

Syndrome	Site of lesion	Features
Total anterior circulation syndrome (TACS)	Middle cerebral artery or internal carotid artery	**All 3 of:** Hemiparesis and/or hemisensory deficit Homonymous hemianopia Higher cerebral dysfunction (e.g. dysphasia, visuo-spatial dysfunction)
Partial anterior circulation syndrome (PACS)	The middle cerebral artery or the branch of anterior cerebral artery (ACA)	**Any 2 of:** Hemiparesis and/or hemisensory deficit Homonymous hemianopia Higher cerebral dysfunction or Limited hemiparesis/hemisensory deficit (e.g. face and hand, monoparesis) or Higher cerebral function alone
Lacunar syndrome (LACS)	Deep perforating arteries	**Motor and/or sensory loss affecting any 3 of:** Face, arm, hand, leg or Ataxic hemiparesis
Posterior circulation syndrome (POCS)	Vertebral or basilar arteries	**Any of:** Cranial nerve palsy, bilateral motor/sensory loss, disorder of conjugate eye movement, cerebellar syndrome, isolated hemianopia

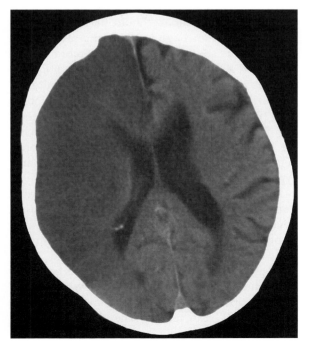

Figure 19.2 Right middle cerebral artery infarct with low attenuation, effacement of the cortical sulci and loss of grey-white matter definition. The patient presented with a right total anterior circulation syndrome (TACS). (Reproduced with kind permission of Dr Andrew Farrall, Edinburgh.)

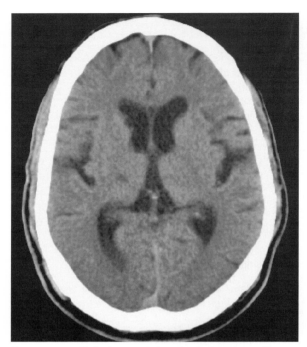

Figure 19.3 Right lacunar infarct in the basal ganglia causing a right lacunar syndrome (LACS). (Reproduced with kind permission of Dr Andrew Farrall, Edinburgh.)

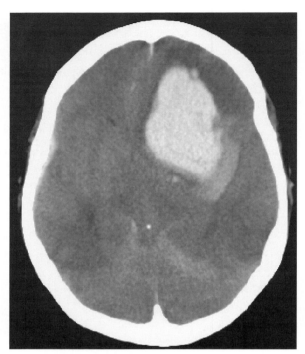

Figure 19.4 Left frontal lobar intracerebral haemorrhage with associated mass effect and compression of the ventricles. The patient presented with reduced consciousness and a left total anterior circulation syndrome (TACS). (Reproduced with kind permission of Dr Andrew Farrall, Edinburgh.)

(higher cerebral dysfunction with variable degrees of motor and sensory loss). Lacunar syndromes (LACS) also occur in the carotid artery territory, but are due to occlusion of the deep perforating arteries in the subcortical areas of the brain (Fig. 19.3). Posterior circulation syndromes (POCS) affect the vertebrobasilar territory. This classification combines all the weird eponymous brainstem syndromes in one group. Posterior circulation and lacunar syndromes typically result in 'subcortical' problems (motor loss, sensory loss, ataxia) (Warlow et al 2001). The value of this classification may not yet be apparent, but bear with us – it helps improve the understanding of the underlying stroke problem and it is fun to use the clinical classification to try and predict the CT scan result!

Cerebral haemorrhage

Cerebral haemorrhage is typically divided into primary intracerebral haemorrhage (in which the original haemorrhage occurs within the substance

of the brain) and subarachnoid haemorrhage (in which the haemorrhage occurs primarily into the subarachnoid space). Primary intracerebral haemorrhage (PICH) can be subdivided on CT scan features into lobar (affecting the white matter of the parietal, temporal, frontal and occipital lobes) (Fig. 19.4), basal ganglia/thalamus and cerebellum/brainstem (Warlow et al 2001). For simplicity, we have collected these into two groups, lobar versus the rest, to reflect the underlying cause and symptomatology of the haemorrhage.

A further type of haemorrhage, haemorrhagic transformation of an infarct, occurs when bleeding develops within an area of infarction. This is a recognized complication of cerebral infarction and some acute drug therapies.

Please note the clinical classification is based on the patient's symptoms and signs whereas the classification of intracerebral haemorrhage is based on CT scan results. The alert reader will therefore be wondering how to classify a stroke before the CT scan result is available. We suggest you still use the clinical stroke syndrome classification since as a general (and anecdotal) observation:

- Lobar haemorrhage often has clinical features of TACS or PACS
- Basal ganglia/thalamus haemorrhage has features of LACS
- Cerebellar/brainstem haemorrhage has features of POCS

WHAT IS THE CAUSE OF THIS STROKE?

This process involves both the attempts to identify the cause of the stroke and also to clarify the risk factors that put the individual at risk of further stroke and vascular disease.

RISK FACTORS

We wish to identify risk factors which are treatable. Untreatable risk factors (e.g. age, sex, race and sometimes family history) are of epidemiological interest, but of little practical value. The main treatable risk factors for both cerebral infarction and cerebral haemorrhage are outlined in Box 19.4.

Box 19.4 Major risk factors for stroke	
Cerebral infarction	**PICH**
Hypertension	Hypertension
Cigarette smoking	Coagulation disorder
High cholesterol	AVM or aneurysm
Atrial fibrillation	Cigarette smoking
Carotid artery stenosis	
Cardiac (recent MI, rheumatic heart disease)	
Haematological (e.g. polycythaemia, thrombophilias)	
Rarities (e.g. neurosyphilis, vasculitis)	

Key: PICH – Primary intracerebral haemorrhage, AVM – arteriovenous malformation, MI – myocardial infarction

Through recognition of these risk factors the common diagnostic process in stroke management is developed (Table 19.2).

Cerebral infarction

'Cortical strokes' (TACS and PACS) tend to be caused by embolism (less commonly thrombosis) affecting the carotid artery territory. Up to a quarter of these patients will have an occluded carotid artery and a smaller proportion will have a severe carotid artery stenosis which is presumably a source of embolism. Embolism due to atrial fibrillation is also common in this group.

In contrast, lacunar infarcts are more likely caused by occlusion in situ and have a much lower prevalence of carotid artery occlusion or severe carotid stenosis. Posterior circulation infarcts have a more heterogeneous aetiology, including thrombosis, embolism and dissection, but rarely have clinically significant carotid artery disease.

Primary intracerebral haemorrhage
(Table 19.3)

Younger individuals with intracerebral haemorrhage are more likely than older people to have a surgically treatable lesion, such as an arteriovenous malformation (AVM) or aneurysm. In addition, aneurysms are much less prevalent in non-lobar haemorrhage (i.e. basal ganglia, thalamus, cerebellum, brainstem). In elderly patients, cerebral haemorrhage is usually thought to be due to degenerative small vessel disease or amyloid angiopathy (look it up!) both of which are not amenable to surgical treatment. However, younger individuals, particularly those presenting with a lobar haemorrhage and no other risk factors (e.g. hypertension) should have further investigation for an underlying structural abnormality and be considered for neurosurgical intervention.

WHAT PROBLEMS HAS IT CAUSED?

The management of the stroke patient is a problem-solving process requiring detailed assessment of impairments, activity limitations and participation restrictions and an analysis of their causes.

Table 19.2 Investigations of acute stroke	
Investigation	**Indication**
Routine tests Full blood count Erythrocyte sedimentation rate Blood glucose Urea and electrolytes Blood cholesterol Chest X-ray ECG	Routine tests to identify haematological disorders, cranial arteritis, diabetes mellitus, dehydration, hyperlipidaemia, cardiac disease and arrhythmia
Cranial CT scan	Exclude cerebral haemorrhage Doubt about diagnosis Exclude obstructive hydrocephalus with cerebellar stroke
Coagulation screen	Cerebral haemorrhage
Selected tests Carotid duplex scan	Recent (< 6 months) carotid artery TIA or ischaemic stroke (hemiparesis, aphasia, monocular visual loss). Patient fit for carotid surgery Exclude carotid artery dissection
Echocardiography (± Bubble contrast)	Clinical features and routine tests raise possibility of endocarditis or structural disease of the valves or myocardium Unexplained stroke in a young person
Angiography/MRI angiography	Prelude to carotid surgery Exclude cerebral vein thrombosis Investigation of lobar haemorrhage in young person
Blood cultures Syphilis serology Antinuclear factor Anti-DNA antibodies 'Sticky blood test' (lupus anticoagulant, anti-phospholipid antibodies, anti-thrombin III, activated protein C resistance, factor V Leiden, protein S & C, sickling tests)	Unexplained stroke, especially in a young person. Associated clinical features

Table 19.3 Main causes of primary intracerebral haemorrhage (PICH)		
	Lobar PICH	PICH of basal ganglia, thalamus, cerebellum, brainstem
Age under 65 years	Arteriovenous malformation (AVM) Saccular aneurysm Small vessel degeneration (e.g. microaneurysms)	Arteriovenous malformation (AVM) Small vessel degeneration
Age over 65 years	Small vessel degeneration Amyloid angiopathy Saccular aneurysm	Small vessel degeneration Amyloid angiopathy AVM

N.B. The epidemiology of PICH is not well researched. This scheme summarizes a 'best-guess' based on current knowledge.

Table 19.4 Assessment of problems

Problem	Assessment
Pre-stroke dependency	Modified Rankin score
Swallowing	Bedside swallowing assessment
Mobility	Rivermead Mobility index, Barthel index
Activities of daily living	Barthel index
Visuo-spatial dysfunction	Star cancellation test, picture drawing
Intellectual impairment	Abbreviated Mental Test score

Box 19.5 Complications of stroke

Early (days–weeks)	Late (months–years)
Urinary tract infection	Falls
Chest infection	Depression/anxiety
Pressure sores	Pain (various)
Falls	Urinary tract infection
Pain (various)	Chest infection
Depression/anxiety	Recurrent stroke
Recurrent stroke	Seizure/blackouts
Deep vein thrombosis	

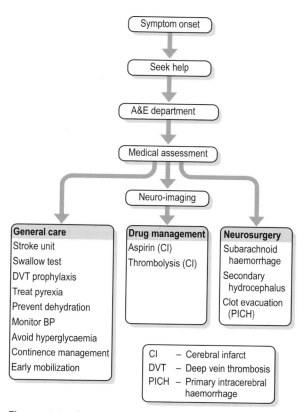

Figure 19.5 Summary of acute stroke management.

Identification and treatment of common complications of stroke and any co-morbid illness (e.g. angina, cardiac failure, arthritis, peripheral vascular disease) which may impede recovery is imperative.

In routine practice a standard proforma (and some assessment scales) can assist with patient assessment (Table 19.4) ensuring a rational future management plan.

COMPLICATIONS

A number of complications occur early after stroke which may well act as barriers to recovery. The commonest are listed in Box 19.5.

WHAT TREATMENT DOES THIS PATIENT REQUIRE?

We have deliberately combined acute care and rehabilitation in one section (see Fig. 19.5) because the arbitrary division of the two can lead to a number of problems. First, rehabilitation in the broadest sense should begin as soon as the patient is in contact with healthcare staff and to 'wait for rehabilitation' is to neglect your patient's needs. Secondly, patients being managed in a rehabilitation setting often develop acute medical problems and need 'acute care'.

THE OPTIMAL SETTING FOR STROKE CARE

There is considerable interest in identifying the best setting for managing stroke patients.

Home versus hospital

A number of clinical trials have compared the standard hospital-based care with attempts to provide stroke care within a home setting (Langhorne et al 1999). There is limited information to guide policy making but on current evidence there are no grounds to move away from the standard hospital-based care for acute stroke

patients. Earlier discharge home with more rehabilitation in the home may prove to be an effective
service model for the future (Early Supported
Discharge Trialists 2005).

Stroke unit versus general ward

There is now considerable evidence from clinical
trials to show that stroke patients managed in an
organized stroke unit are more likely to survive,
return home and regain independence than those
receiving conventional care in a general ward
(Stroke Unit Trialists' Collaboration 2001). This
then raises the question of what kind of stroke
unit is most appropriate. Although various models
of stroke unit care have been tested they all had
the following features in common:

■ Multidisciplinary team care coordinated
  through regular meetings
■ The ability to provide rehabilitation for several
  weeks if necessary
■ Staff with an interest in stroke and/or rehabilitation
■ Education programmes and training in stroke

The most researched stroke unit model is a 'comprehensive' approach combining acute care with
rehabilitation, but there is also evidence to support
stroke rehabilitation units and, to a lesser extent,
units which have provided assessment and rehabilitation for stroke patients within a mixed setting. This is of particular interest to geriatricians
who may believe (with some justification) that
their processes of care are as good in their general
rehabilitation ward as in a disease-specific stroke
unit (Pound et al 1999). Current evidence suggests
that geriatric assessment units would be better
than acute medical wards for the rehabilitation of
stroke patients, but it is not possible to say if they
are as good as a disease-specific stroke unit.

ACUTE MEDICAL TREATMENT

Aspirin

Aspirin (300 mg per day) should be prescribed
acutely to all patients in whom a cerebral haemorrhage has been excluded (Counsell & Sandercock
2003). Aspirin should be withheld in the acute
phase until a CT scan of the brain has been performed, should be delayed for 24 hours after

thrombolytic treatment and should be avoided
in cerebral haemorrhage. *If the patient is unable
to swallow, aspirin should be administered rectally.*
Although the net benefit from aspirin is small
(preventing one death or disability per 100 patients
treated), the treatment is simple, safe and usually
well tolerated. The maintenance aspirin dose is
discussed later.

Thrombolysis

Several randomized trials have been carried out
with tissue plasminogen activator (rt-PA) which
indicate that thrombolysis may improve outcomes
in carefully selected patients (Wardlaw et al 2003).
Despite a risk of haemorrhagic transformation of
the infarct and increased adverse outcomes, the
risk–benefit ratio for rt-PA is favourable if administered within 3 hours of stroke onset. rt-PA is
now licensed for use in the UK with strict inclusion criteria (in line with the NIND trial [NIND
& Stroke rt-PA Stroke Study Group 1995]) to be
administered in centres with appropriate expertise
and monitoring of outcomes.

Heparin

Several large randomized trials have shown that
there is no net benefit from the routine use of
heparin (unfractionated or low molecular weight
heparin) in stroke patients (Gubitz et al 2004).
Within these trials heparin has been relatively
safe and so can probably be used with caution in
individuals believed to be at higher embolic risk
(e.g. rheumatic heart disease). However, routine
use of heparin should be discouraged.

Antihypertensives

Blood pressure is often elevated in acute stroke,
but usually settles spontaneously over the following days. Lowering blood pressure acutely in
stroke has been associated with a poorer outcome
and may increase infarct size. If the patient is
already on an antihypertensive agent it is probably
safe to continue this if care is taken to avoid hypovolaemia. On the rare occasion when the blood
pressure is very high (> 200/120 mmHg) or there
are signs of malignant hypertension, acute left
ventricular failure, acute renal failure or aortic

dissection, lowering of blood pressure with oral ACE inhibitors, intravenous labetalol or sodium nitroprusside (not in intracerebral haemorrhage) may be indicated with careful monitoring. The angiotensin receptor blocker candesartan has been used safely in acute stroke in one recent study (ACCESS trial [Schrader et al 2003]).

Neurosurgery

Acute neurosurgical intervention is indicated for primary intracerebral haemorrhage in the posterior fossa, posing a significant risk of obstructive hydrocephalus. The recent STICH trial (Mendelow et al 2005) has shown no benefit of surgical evacuation of supratentorial intracerebral haematomas over conservative management and cannot be recommended routinely.

Following large middle cerebral artery infarcts with cerebral oedema and raised intracranial pressure, neurosurgical decompression has been used but there is insufficient randomized controlled trial evidence to recommend this routinely.

Other therapy

There have been many randomized trials of potential neuroprotective therapies (including corticosteroids and calcium antagonists), however, to date none has been proven effective in clinical practice.

GENERAL CARE

In all patients with disability, good general care is essential. Awareness of the potential complications of stroke and the steps for their prevention or treatment is paramount. Particular care should be taken with the following.

Airway/breathing

The airway must be maintained and the safety of swallowing assessed. Regular chest physiotherapy may be required in immobile patients.

Pyrexia

Raised temperature is associated with a poorer outcome following stroke. Fever should prompt a

search for evidence of infection or an alternative cause (e.g. deep vein thrombosis) and should be treated promptly with paracetamol and a cooling fan.

Fluids and nutrition

Care must be taken to avoid dehydration. If swallowing is not safe, food and fluids can be modified in consistency or may have to be provided via intravenous or nasogastric routes. Medication may need to be given as suspensions, intravenously or rectally. Hyperglycaemia poststroke appears to be associated with a poorer outcome and should be treated. The optimal strategy for hydration is not currently known, but dehydration may increase the risk of electrolyte abnormalities, vascular events and urinary tract infection. If the recovery of swallowing is likely to be delayed, insertion of a nasogastric tube provides a more convenient means of enteral feeding. Percutaneous endoscopic gastrostomy (PEG) tube insertion provides an easier route of feeding in the longer term, however, the FOOD trial (Clarke et al 2005) suggests that early insertion of a PEG tube may be associated with a poorer outcome.

Prevention of complications

Good nursing care and early mobilization may help prevent complications such as pressure sores, pneumonia, venous thromboembolism, spasticity and shoulder injuries. Good positioning and early mobilization may also prevent episodes of hypoxia. Avoidance of the use of catheters probably helps prevent urinary tract infections.

Prevention of deep vein thrombosis (DVT)

There is no net benefit in the routine use of heparin in the recovery of stroke patients. For this reason many practitioners recommend the use of physical measures (early mobilization and graduated compression stockings) for the prevention of DVT. Graduated compression stocking use post-stroke is being evaluated in the ongoing CLOTS (Clots in Legs or TED Stockings after Stroke) trial. Care must be taken with graduated compression stockings in the presence of peripheral vascular disease.

Others

Anxiety and depression are relatively common after stroke and may require antidepressant treatment, often long term. Cognitive impairment and vascular dementia can follow either recurrent or single stroke and may adversely affect rehabilitation.

GOAL PLANNING/REHABILITATION

Much of the management of stroke patients incorporates a multidisciplinary process in which the patient (and carers) may interact with a wide variety of healthcare professionals. The key members of the multidisciplinary team and their roles are outlined as follows:

■ *Doctor:* The physician must have a working knowledge of the diagnosis, prognosis, complications and co-morbidities of stroke. They are often involved in battling for resources for the stroke team and chairing the multidisciplinary meetings.

■ *Nurse:* Nurses have the central role in interdisciplinary stroke care providing for the daily needs of patients, preventing complications, providing regular reassessments of their progress and providing support for patients and family. Clinical stroke nurse specialist posts are developing and may also incorporate the role of stroke care coordinator.

■ *Physiotherapy:* The physiotherapist's role is largely the recovery of movement and involves assessing motor and sensory function, advising and managing positioning and handling issues, training in walking, the provision of aids and also the prevention of complications (particularly respiratory).

■ *Occupational therapists:* The key role of occupational therapy is the recovery of functional tasks requiring more detailed assessments of activities of daily living and other aspects of occupational performance. In particular, they assess visuo-spatial function, provide aids and appliances and assess patients' abilities within the home.

■ *Speech and language therapists:* Their key role is to aid the recovery of communication and speech through assessments of these functions

and developing strategies to overcome problems. They are increasingly involved in the more detailed assessment of swallowing problems.

■ *Social work:* Within the UK healthcare setting, medical social workers usually help access services and facilities within the community.

■ *Others:* Clinical psychologists are frequently involved in managing psychological and behavioural complications of stroke. Dieticians aid in the management of nutritional problems and dietary modification. Psychiatrists assist with the management of affective complications of stroke, ophthalmologists help manage individuals with visual problems and pharmacists advise on drug therapies and administration.

MULTIDISCIPLINARY TEAM PROCESS

This involves a goal-planning cycle (Fig. 19.6) in which a patient is assessed, a problem identified, a recovery goal is set, an intervention provided and then the progress is assessed. This process can occur on several time scales, for example a short-term goal in a patient with mobility problems might be to enable transfers with one nurse, whereas a longer-term goal would be to promote independent walking.

A number of disciplines may carry out different assessments and identify a range of problems. Therefore, good coordination (through weekly multidisciplinary meetings) is essential to ensure that all members of staff have compatible goals and objectives and are providing a standard message to patients and carers. It is particularly important that nurses are involved in this process and that their daily interaction with the patient reflects the team goals. The team is also responsible for identifying failure to progress with rehabilitation and for reassessment of the patient to define

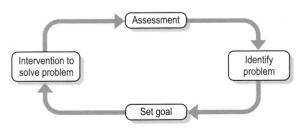

Figure 19.6   Goal-planning cycle.

Box 19.6   Practical markers of poorer prognosis

- Older age
- Pre-stroke dependency (Rankin scale > 2)
- Initially reduced consciousness level
- Severe hemiplegia (MRC scale < 3)
- Impaired mobility (e.g. no sitting balance)
- Urinary incontinence
- Visuo-spatial dysfunction

Note: No predictive systems are accurate for the individual patient. If in doubt, err on the optimistic side.

any potential barriers. These may be physical (e.g. pneumonia), psychological (e.g. depression), social (e.g. unsuitable housing) or cultural (e.g. the family's reaction to disability).

PROGNOSTICATION

It is evident that accurate prognostication is needed to ensure that goals are reasonable and achievable. Unfortunately, making an accurate prognosis in an individual patient can be very difficult and it is unwise to 'write off' anyone without a period of rehabilitation. Some simple practical (but not very accurate) markers of a poor prognosis are outlined in Box 19.6.

DISCHARGE PLANNING

Early on in the rehabilitation process the team should begin identifying a likely discharge date and identifying barriers to the patient returning home. A number of key issues to consider are:

- Previous functional level
- Severity of stroke
- Support available at home
- Wishes of the patient and family

Nearer the time of discharge (usually when the patient has regained some mobility) an occupational therapy home visit is often required to assess their function in their home and identify barriers to discharge. Social work input is often required at this stage to arrange services and allowances.

It is also important to use the appropriate voluntary sector services (such as clubs run by the Stroke Association or Chest, Heart and Stroke Scotland) which may be particularly useful for individuals with dysphasia. Post-discharge review can identify unexpected problems and pick up late complications such as the emotional impact of stroke on patients and carers. Recently, early supported discharge teams have been developed to help improve the transition from hospital to home.

WHAT CAN BE DONE TO PREVENT FURTHER VASCULAR EVENTS?

The management of stroke patients must address the risk of further vascular events. The risk of further stroke following a TIA or minor stroke is approximately 10% in the first year and 5% per year thereafter, the risk being highest in the first few days or weeks (Warlow et al 2001). Ischaemic heart disease and peripheral vascular disease are also common, with myocardial infarction being the commonest early cause of death after TIA or minor stroke. Strategies for preventing further vascular events can be outlined as follows.

TREAT THE UNDERLYING CAUSE IF POSSIBLE

A few stroke patients will have a specific pathology of thrombosis (e.g. polycythaemia, thrombocythaemia, thrombotic disorder), embolism (e.g. bacterial endocarditis) or of the vessel wall (e.g. giant cell arteritis, syphilis) requiring specific treatment of the underlying problem.

RISK FACTOR MANAGEMENT

The main vascular risk factors to be addressed are:

Blood pressure

There is good evidence that reduction of blood pressure is an effective primary and secondary prevention measure for stroke. Care should be taken to avoid over-aggressive blood pressure reduction early on (first 2 weeks) but subsequent target blood pressure is < 130/80 mmHg. The best evidence exists for a regimen incorporating an ACE inhibitor and thiazide combination (PROGRESS trial [PROGRESS Collaborative Group 2001]).

Internal carotid artery stenosis

For patients who have recently had a TIA or minor ischaemic stroke in the territory of a severely stenosed (greater than 70%) internal carotid artery, successful carotid endarterectomy almost abolishes the risk of further ipsilateral stroke (Warlow 2001). The benefits of surgery are greatest when performed as early as possible after the event when the risk of further stroke is highest. Surgery may be justified in patients with asymptomatic carotid stenosis but the risk–benefit ratio is less favourable. Therefore, patients require careful selection for this procedure. Routine carotid duplex scanning in patients with a posterior circulation stroke is inappropriate. Extracranial artery angioplasty and stenting show promise but require further investigation to clarify their place in routine clinical practice.

Atrial fibrillation

Non-rheumatic atrial fibrillation is a recognized risk factor for stroke and anticoagulation reduces the risk of further stroke (see 'Antithrombotic therapies' below). Cardioversion in atrial fibrillation may improve symptoms but is not proven to reduce stroke risk and elderly stroke patients often have underlying heart problems which render permanent cardioversion impossible.

Diabetes mellitus

Good diabetic control reduces the risk of microvascular complications and tight blood pressure control (< 130/80 mmHg) in type II diabetes mellitus reduces macrovascular complications including stroke (Gorelick et al 1999). It seems reasonable to optimize the diabetic control and blood pressure of any diabetic stroke patient.

Cholesterol

Lowering plasma cholesterol has been proven to reduce the risk of recurrent ischaemic stroke (Heart Protection Study [Heart Protection Study Collaborative Group 2004]) in all patient subgroups with a total cholesterol of > 3.5 mmol/L. Treatment with a high-dose statin (such as simvastatin 40 mg) should be used aiming for a target total cholesterol < 5.0 mmol/L (LDL < 3.5 mmol/L).

Lifestyle factors

Smoking should be stopped and alcohol should be taken only in moderation (up to one unit per day). Regular exercise should be encouraged and diet modified to reduce salt and fat intake and to increase fruit and vegetable consumption.

ANTITHROMBOTIC THERAPIES

Antithrombotic therapies have an established role in preventing recurrent stroke and other vascular events. They also have the additional benefit of preventing venous thromboembolism.

Antiplatelet therapy

Low-dose aspirin reduces the risk of serious vascular events (stroke, myocardial infarction, peripheral vascular disease) by about 25% in a wide range of patient groups. No aspirin dose has been shown to be more effective than 300 mg per day although a lower dose (75 mg) can probably be used without loss of efficacy. The combination of aspirin and modified-release dipyridamole (200 mg twice daily) may be more effective than aspirin alone and has been recommended as first-line therapy following stroke or TIA by NICE (NICE 2005). Clopidogrel (75 mg) is an alternative for patients who are aspirin intolerant. The combination of aspirin and clopidogrel has been evaluated post-stroke and TIA but was no more effective than clopidogrel alone, caused an excess of haemorrhagic complications and cannot be recommended routinely (Diener et al 2004).

Anticoagulant therapy

Adjusted dose warfarin (with an international normalized ratio between 2–3) is very effective in preventing stroke in patients with non-rheumatic atrial fibrillation but introduction is usually delayed until 2 weeks after stroke. However, it is often difficult in an elderly patient to judge accurately the balance of risks and benefits of such an approach. Aspirin is an appropriate alternative measure though less effective.

WHAT ADVICE SHOULD BE GIVEN TO THE PATIENT AND FAMILY?

Patients and carers often complain that they have not received appropriate information and advice following a stroke. Group meetings with patients and carers provide a useful forum for providing information and allowing discussion, and can prepare for the demands on carers and the roles expected of them. Advice should be provided in both written (e.g. Stroke Association booklets) and verbal form, covering the following areas:

- *What is a stroke?* Provide a simple explanation of stroke and the type of stroke the patient has experienced.
- *Why did it happen?* Explain the main risk factors and their management. It is often useful to dispel myths (e.g. that exercise or sexual activity will bring on a stroke).
- *Common aspects of the impact of stroke:* Explain the common sequelae of stroke (e.g. tiredness, depression, headache, loss of confidence).
- *General aspects of recovery:* It is useful to explain that recovery is usually more rapid early on but may continue slowly for many months (or even years).
- *Driving:* Driving is not allowed for 1 month after a stroke or TIA. The DVLA and insurer should be informed and progress reassessed. A formal driving assessment may be required, especially if there are cognitive deficits, in-attention and minor visual field defects. HGV and PCV licence holders will have their licences revoked for a year even after a single TIA and can reapply thereafter. The regulations relating to seizures and epilepsy also apply.
- *Sexual relationships:* There is rarely any reason not to resume sexual activity after a stroke.
- *Recurrence of stroke:* The risk of further stroke is higher than in the general population and averages 5–10% per year. We usually advise that non-recurrence is much more likely than recurrence.

CONCLUSIONS

We have tried to provide a framework for the assessment and management of stroke patients. As with most aspects of medicine there remain areas of ignorance where the best management is unknown; some of these are outlined in Box 19.7. Table 19.5 provides a summary of stroke classification together with some typical features of each section of the classification. Our description has involved some generalizations and individual patients may vary considerably from the 'typical' process, but we hope it provides a useful framework around which to plan patient management.

Acknowledgment

We are grateful to Dr Andrew Farrall, Consultant Neuroradiologist for providing the CT scans (Figs 19.2, 19.3 and 19.4).

Box 19.7   Areas of ignorance

- Control of blood pressure acutely after stroke – when and what to treat?
- Atrial fibrillation in acute stroke – how soon to anticoagulate?
- Does lowering blood glucose in acute stroke improve outcome?
- The optimal time window for administration of thrombolytic therapy in acute stroke
- The role of hypothermia in acute stroke
- The role of surgical evacuation following extensive total anterior circulation infarction with cerebral oedema
- Should lipid-lowering therapy be used in the elderly (> 75 years)?
- The role of balloon angioplasty and stenting in carotid and vertebral artery stenosis
- Optimal treatment of depression post stroke – choice of treatment and duration
- Optimal management of incontinence post stroke
- The optimal intensity and amount of physical and occupational therapy post stroke
- The relationship between stroke and cognitive impairment
- Prediction of stroke outcomes

Table 19.5 Summary of stroke classification

	Cerebral infarction				Primary intracerebral haemorrhage		
Classification	TACS	PACS	LACS	POCS	Lobar	Basal ganglia/ thalamus	Cerebellar/ brainstem
Typical presentation	HCD Hemiparesis Hemianopia	HCD Hemiparesis	Hemiparesis Hemisensory loss	Brainstem, cerebellar symptoms	HCD Hemiparesis	Hemiparesis Hemisensory loss	Brainstem, cerebellar symptoms
CT scan (look for...)	Large cortical infarct	Limited cortical infarct	Small subcortical infarct	Infarct in brainstem, cerebellum, occipital lobe	Haemorrhage in lobar white matter	Basal ganglia, thalamus haemorrhage	Brainstem, cerebellar haemorrhage
Cause (think of...)	Embolism from heart or carotids (atrial fibrillation)	Embolism from heart or carotids (atrial fibrillation)	Thrombosis (hypertension, diabetes)	Cardiac embolism, thrombosis	AVM Aneurysm	Vascular degeneration, AVM	Vascular degeneration, AVM
Problems (look for...)	Motor loss Sensory loss Dysphasia Neglect Hemianopia Dysphagia	Motor loss Dysphasia Neglect Dysphagia	Motor loss Sensory loss Ataxia	Ataxia Motor loss Cranial nerve palsy Dysphagia	Motor loss Dysphasia Neglect Dysphagia	Motor loss Sensory loss (dysphasia)	Ataxia Motor loss Cranial nerve palsy Dysphagia
Prognosis (at 1 year)							
Survival	60%	85%	90%	80%	50%?	?	?
Recurrence	5%	20%	10%	20%	5%	5%	5%
Independence	5%	60%	70%	70%	?	?	?
Mobility	40%	70%	80%	80%	?	?	?

HCD – higher cortical dysfunction

REFERENCES

*** Essential reading; ** recommended reading

Clarke J, Cranswick G, Dennis M S et al 2005 The FOOD Trial Collaboration. Effect of timing and method of enteral tube feeding for dysphagic stroke patients (FOOD): A multicentre randomised controlled trial. Lancet 365:764–772 **

Counsell C, Sandercock P 2003 Antiplatelet therapy for acute ischaemic stroke. Cochrane Database of Systematic Reviews, Issue 2. Art. No.: CD000029. DOI: 10.1002/14651858. CD000029 ***

Diener C-H, Bogousslavsky J, Brass L M et al for the MATCH investigators 2004 Aspirin and clopidogrel compared with clopidogrel alone after recent ischaemic stroke or transient ischaemic attack in high-risk patients (MATCH): randomised, double-blind, placebo-controlled trial. Lancet 364:331–337 **

Early Supported Discharge Trialists 2005 Services for reducing duration of hospital care for acute stroke patients. Cochrane Database of Systematic Reviews, Issue 2. Art. No.: CD000443. DOI: 10.1002/14651858. CD000443.pub2 **

Gorelick P B, Sacco R L, Smith D B et al 1999 Prevention of first stroke – a review of guidelines and a multidisciplinary consensus statement from the National Stroke Association. Journal of the American Medical Association 281:1112–1120 **

Gubitz G, Sandercock P, Counsell C et al 2004 Anticoagulants for acute ischaemic stroke. Cochrane Database of Systematic Reviews, Issue 2. Art. No.: CD000024. DOI: 10.1002/14651858. CD000024. pub2 ***

Heart Protection Study Collaborative Group 2004 Effects of cholesterol-lowering with simvastatin on stroke and other major vascular events in 20536 people with cerebrovascular disease or other high-risk conditions. Lancet 363:757–767 **

Langhorne P, Dennis M S, Kalra L et al 1999 Services for helping acute stroke patients avoid hospital admission. Cochrane Database of Systematic Reviews, Issue 3. Art. No.: CD00044. DOI: 10.1002/14651858. CD000444 **

Mendelow D A, Gregson B A, Fernandes H M et al for the STICH investigators 2005 Early surgery versus initial conservative treatment in patients with supratentorial intracerebral haematomas in the international surgical trial in intracerebral haemorrhage (STICH): a randomised trial. Lancet 365:387–397 **

National Institute of Neurological Disorders, Stroke rt-PA Stroke Study Group 1995 Tissue plasminogen activator for acute ischaemic stroke. New England Journal of Medicine 333:1581–1587 **

National Institute for Health and Clinical Excellence (NICE) 2005 Clopidogrel and modified-release dipyridamole in the prevention of occlusive vascular events. 2005. Online. Available: http://www.nice.org.uk **

Pound P, Sabin C, Ebrahim S 1999 Observing the process of care: a stroke unit, elderly care unit and general medical ward compared. Age and Ageing 28: 433–440 **

PROGRESS Collaborative Group 2001 Randomised trial of a perindopril-based blood pressure lowering regimen among 6105 patients with prior stroke. Lancet 358:1033–1041 **

Schrader J, Luders S, Kulschewski A et al 2003 The ACCESS Study: evaluation of acute candesartan cilexetil therapy in stroke survivors. Stroke 34: 1699–1703 **

Stroke Unit Trialists' Collaboration 2001 Organised inpatient (stroke unit) care for stroke. Cochrane Database of Systematic Reviews, Issue 3. Art. No.: CD000197. DOI: 10.1002/14651858. CD000197 ***

Wardlaw J M, del Zoppo G, Yamaguchi T 2003 Thrombolysis for acute ischaemic stroke. Cochrane Database of Systematic Reviews, Issue 3. Art. No.: CD000213. DOI: 10.1002/14651858. CD000213 ***

Warlow C P, Dennis M S, van Gijn J et al 2001 Stroke: a practical guide to management, 2nd edn. Blackwell Science, Oxford ***

Weir C J, Murray G D, Adams F G et al 1994 Poor accuracy of stroke scoring systems for differential clinical diagnosis of intracranial haemorrhage and infarction. Lancet 344:999–1002 **

RECOMMENDED READING

*** Essential reading

Clinical Effectiveness and Evaluation Unit 2004 National clinical guidelines for stroke, 2nd edn. Royal College of Physicians, London. Online. Available: http://www.rcplondon.ac.uk/pubs/books/stroke ***

Cochrane Library. Online. Available: http://www.cochrane.org/index.htm
The Cochrane Library is a useful source of information about stroke treatments.

Department of Health 2001 National Service Framework for Older People. Standard 5: Stroke. DoH, London, p 61–75 Online. Available: http://www.doh.gov.uk/nsf/olderpeople ***

Scottish Intercollegiate Guidelines Network (SIGN) 64
    Management of patients with stroke: rehabilitation,
    prevention and management of complications and
    discharge planning November 2002 (updated Jan
    2005). Online. Available: http://www.sign.ac.uk ***
Scottish Intercollegiate Guidelines Network (SIGN) 78
    Management of patients with stroke: Identification
    and management of dysphagia September 2004.
    Online. Available: http://www.sign.ac.uk ***
Warlow C P, Dennis M S, van Gijn J et al 2001 Stroke: a
    practical guide to management, 2nd edn. Blackwell
    Science, Oxford ***
A comprehensive text that provides an excellent general
reference.

Chapter 20

Clinical aspects of pressure sores

Mahendra Gonsalkorale

It is more rewarding and cost-effective to prevent pressure sores than to treat them. Pressure sores can cause misery and prolong hospital stay. They are costly, can lead to litigation and are largely preventable.

HISTORICAL ASPECTS

In 1815, William Heberden Junior recognized the influence of pressure on the causation of bed sores. He wrote: 'There is no one in the habit of attending the sick but must have reason to deplore the wretched condition of those who, being bed ridden through accident or infirmity, have contracted sores of a very painful and dangerous kind by long pressure, especially if the patient lies in the wet and filth of his own body which he is unable to restrain' (Heberden 1815). Sir James Paget in 1873 wrote: 'First of all look to the bed. Good bed-making is an indispensable thing in the prevention of bed sores. Several beds have been made especially for this purpose, of which the best is Dr Arnott's. It consists of a chest full of water on top of this is a waterproof sheet and over this an ordinary sheet on which the patient is laid. Here the patient is absolutely floating on the water. A patient might lie in this for years and never have a bed sore' (Paget 1873). Charcot's observations in 1868 that patients with spinal injuries develop pressure sores because of trophic disturbances (Charcot 1868) led unfortunately to a long period of nihilistic belief that little

could be done to prevent bed sores. In 1915, Pierre Marie and Gustav Roussy made a powerful plea for better management, their central theme being the alleviation of pressure and the prevention of infection.

Florence Nightingale is given credit for recognizing that good nursing care could prevent pressure sores. The medical profession has been slow to show an interest in this field, which largely remained the domain of nurses.

THE SIZE OF THE PROBLEM

The prevalence of pressure sores in hospitals varies from 5–15% (Agency for Health Care Policy and Research 1992, Allman et al 1986, O'Dea 1995). New pressure sores occur in 4–10% of patients admitted to a UK district general hospital, depending on the case mix (Clark & Watts 1994). The cost of preventing and treating pressure sores in a 600 bed large general hospital is between £600 000 and £3 million per year (Touche Ross & Co 1993). The financial cost to the NHS may be as high as £700 million per year (NICE press release, October 2003).

WHY ARE ELDERLY PATIENTS MORE PRONE TO DEVELOP PRESSURE SORES?

1. Age-related changes in the skin are a factor in the development of pressure sores, e.g. changes in collagen synthesis resulting in lower

mechanical strength of tissues, decrease in elastin content, loss of dermal vessels, thinning of the epidermis, flattening of the dermal-epidermal junction and increased skin permeability.

2. Ill old people are prone to vascular insufficiency, immobility, malnutrition, incontinence, hypoxia and sedative drug use.

WHAT IS A PRESSURE SORE?

A pressure sore is an ischaemic skin ulcer of variable depth caused by the application of excessive pressure or shear injury on skin and subcutaneous tissue. What determines whether the skin breaks down under these circumstances is the relationship between the health of the skin (susceptibility) and the degree and duration of pressure (the insult).

Apart from direct pressure which leads to capillary occlusion, shearing forces and direct frictional burns on the skin are important factors. Shear forces cause capillary wall damage, with thrombotic occlusion. Friction leads to direct trauma to the skin. Examples of friction sores are those caused on the heels by dragging patients upwards when they slide down on the mattress. The correct way to move such patients is to lift them up and place them higher up the bed. Dragging patients up also leads to shear forces being generated in the layers of tissue between the underlying bone and the skin.

Pressure sores most commonly develop over bony prominences, as very high occlusive pressures are reached when the skin gets sandwiched between the bone and the surface on which the patient lies. The commonest areas for pressure sore formation are the sacrum, ischial tuberosities, greater trochanters and heels. Patients lying on mattresses do not spread their weight evenly on the surface (unless it is a completely deformable surface like a water mattress), but do so mainly on many bony points, e.g. when lying supine, the main points are the heels, sacrum, scapulae, elbows and occiput.

The position in which a patient is nursed determines the sites at risk of developing pressure sores.

Supine position:	The sacrum, heels and occiput
Prone position:	The iliac crests, the knees and chest
Lateral position:	Greater trochanter, lateral malleoli, shoulders
Seated:	Ischial tuberosities

Other sites at risk are the lateral malleoli, elbows, pre-tibial area and ribs. Unusual sites should suggest pressure from external objects, e.g. inner surface of thigh from catheters, on temples from spectacle frames, mastoids from hearing aids.

CAN PRESSURE SORES BE PREVENTED?

The answer is almost always yes. How can this be achieved?

■ Increased awareness of the risk of pressure sores
■ Increased knowledge of causes and prevention of pressure sores among staff
■ Recognition and acceptance that all the members of the healthcare team (including the patient and the carer) have a role
■ Investment in preventive measures (proper mattresses, seating cushions, etc.)
■ A commitment by management to give manpower and financial support

In some very ill patients with multiple risk factors, it can be difficult or impossible to prevent pressure sores even with good preventive practices.

CAN THOSE AT RISK BE IDENTIFIED?

The most widely applied tools are pressure sore risk estimators such as the Norton, Douglas and Waterlow scales. These scales are similar in that points are awarded for a series of risk items concerning the patient and a total is calculated. They are not interval scales and a change from one point to another has no precise significance. The different items are weighted only in some scales. The total score provides some objective measure of risk. All these instruments have their limitations and are usually interpreted taking into account 'clinical judgment'. There is little evidence that these risk scales are better than clinical judgment and that their use produces better outcomes (Cullum et al 1995). In units that use a risk calculator as routine, the incidence of pressure sores is lower than in units that do not. This is probably because those units that do are more motivated and geared towards prevention. In addition to this, when a scale is used, the clinician is looking at known risk factors and dealing with them.

> **Practice point**
>
> A practical way of constructing the right environment to prevent pressure sores is to set up a team drawn from doctors, nurses, physiotherapists, occupational therapists, pharmacists, dieticians, and ideally a person responsible for purchase of equipment in the trust. The team must have management backing and set up local protocols and procedures for the prevention and treatment of pressure sores.

FACTORS THAT MAY CONTRIBUTE TO THE FORMATION OF PRESSURE SORES

EXTRINSIC FACTORS

- The nature of the support surface on which the patient is nursed, e.g. a mattress, or an overlay spread over the mattress
- Frequency of turning of the patient, which is often related to staffing levels
- How a patient is handled by staff (techniques of lifting and turning)
- Presence in the bed of urine, faeces, bed sheet folds, food crumbs and talcum powder

INTRINSIC FACTORS

1. Reduced blood supply
2. Nutritional state
3. Impaired mobility
4. Mental state and level of consciousness

5. Physical state, including loss of subcutaneous fat, generalized wasting
6. Age
7. Sensory impairment
8. Pain
9. Coexisting medical conditions such as diabetes mellitus, chronic lung disease and heart failure

> **Practice point**
>
> Any ill hospitalized elderly patient who is confined to bed should be regarded as being at risk of developing pressure sores.

> **Practice point**
>
> Prevention of pressure sores is a 24-hour job; regular turning (repositioning) and the use of specialized mattresses are of value while the patient is confined to bed. Once sitting out, attention must be paid to the pressure-relieving characteristics of the seat.

> **Practice point**
>
> Always show an interest in aspects of prevention when looking at patients with your team, e.g. show an interest in the support surface, look at the risk assessment done by the nurses, examine the areas of skin at risk. Your interest can have a positive effect on the whole team.

> **Practice point**
>
> The underlying damage to tissue may have occurred before the patient arrives in the ward. It may have occurred while the patient was lying on a hard trolley in the accident and emergency department or at home while lying on the floor. *Always record the state of the skin on arrival* and note any risk factors that may have operated before arrival. Never be judgmental about your nursing colleagues; a sore may have nothing to do with poor nursing.

MANAGEMENT PLAN TO PREVENT SORES

A plan of action must follow to prevent pressure sore formation. This must include:

1. Decision on the kind of support surface the patient needs in order to minimize the risk of developing a pressure sore. Water-filled gloves and doughnut-shaped rings should be avoided.

2. Identification and action on intrinsic factors that can be influenced, e.g. correct anaemia, add nutritional supplements, treat heart failure, COPD, etc.

3. Decision on how frequently the patient has to be turned. The 2-hourly turning or reposition-ing regimen that is widely used had its origins in Stoke Mandeville Hospital where they determined empirically that patients turned every 2 hours did not develop decubitus ulcers (Stewart 1997). (Decubitus ulcer is an alternative term for a pressure sore.) There are no studies to determine the optimum turning interval. It is probably impossible to arrive at a precise figure, as individual patients and their envi-ronments differ widely. The 2-hourly turn is a rough guide and each patient's needs should be individually determined.

4. A review process. Regular review includes re-examining risk factors and looking at areas of skin at risk for early warning signs, e.g. blanching erythema (an erythematous [red] area which becomes white [blanches] on application of digital pressure with the colour returning on release of pressure).

5. Application of agreed practices to prevent fric-tion and shear forces on the body. Lifting and handling guidelines are now in place in most trusts.

6. Ensuring that the patient's skin is protected from urine and faeces, food crumbs and folds in draw sheets. Attention to detail is important.

7. The use of positioning devices such as pillows or foam wedges to keep bony prominences away from each other, e.g. use of a pillow to separate knees in patients with adductor spasm.

8. Consider self-help devices such as monkey poles with slings or rope ladders which enable the patient to change the position of areas at risk.

9. The recognition that patients who need to sit out of bed should be provided with proper pres-sure relief seating cushions and should shift their position regularly. They should avoid long periods of uninterrupted sitting.

WHAT KINDS OF SUPPORT SURFACES ARE AVAILABLE AND HOW DO YOU DECIDE WHICH ONE TO USE?

Support surfaces include mattresses (patients nursed in beds) and seating cushions (patients nursed in chairs, including wheelchairs). The com-monest support surface for the recumbent patient is an ordinary mattress. Overlays are lightweight coverings placed directly on a mattress to make it more effective in spreading body weight over a larger area.

The standard hospital mattress is unsuitable for nursing moderate- to high-risk patients. There are many trials demonstrating the superiority of high specification foam mattresses over the standard hospital mattress (Cullum et al 2000). However, there is no accepted definition of what is a stan-dard hospital mattress and there is a wide varia-tion in them.

Two types of protective support surfaces are available.

1. Static surfaces   (Low-tech devices)
2. Dynamic surfaces (High-tech devices)

Static surfaces (also called constant low-pressure devices)

These deform and allow the patient gently to 'sink in', so that the weight is distributed over a larger surface area, thereby reducing the point pressure. The static surface could be the mattress itself or an overlay, which is laid on top of the mattress. They can be classified according to their construction, e.g. foam, foam and air, foam and gel, profiled foam (shaped to prevent patients from sliding), hammocks, air suspension, water suspension and air-particulate suspension/air-fluidized.

Practice point

Static mattresses have a finite useful life. With continued use, their efficiency deteriorates. With prolonged use, they often develop a depressed area (indentation) in the shape of the human body. If a patient of a different size and shape is then put on it, there may be areas of high pressure where the patient does not quite 'fit in'. Their purchase date must be written in indelible ink and they must be replaced according to guidelines. Most manufacturers provide information on mattress life but mattresses must be inspected regularly as their life depends on the types of patients who have been placed on them and how often they have been turned.

Water beds (a type of constant low-pressure device)

They are cumbersome, difficult for nursing patients and have been largely superseded by alternating pressure mattresses. They consist of a tank in which a plastic cushion filled with water is placed. The water is kept warm electrically. As it is difficult to nurse patients on this device and patients complain of feeling sea-sick, water beds are rarely used now.

Dynamic surfaces (alternating pressure devices)

These are mechanically driven, so the area of contact with the patient changes from time to time. This ensures that no part of the body is subject to high pressures (interface pressure) for too long. The most popular mattresses in use are the alternating pressure mattress systems. They can be either an overlay on a normal mattress (c.f. static overlays on normal mattresses) or mattresses in their own right. The earliest effective alternating system was the simple ripple system (Bliss et al 1967). A recent prospective study comparing seven mattress overlays again demonstrated that only the Large Cell Ripple bed mattress effectively prevented and healed sores in the elderly patients studied (Bliss 1995). There are now more sophisticated and reliable systems like the Nimbus or Pegasus. Their prices vary and little reliable evidence is available for their relative efficacy.

Interface pressure measurements are often quoted by manufacturers as a surrogate measure of clinical effectiveness, but there are no clinical studies to support this. More sophisticated methods involve continuous interface pressure measurement. This enables the proportion of time during a cycle where the interface pressure is below an accepted threshold to be determined (Rithalia & Gonsalkorale 1998).

OTHER COMPLEX SURFACES

Other complex surfaces include the low air loss bed (effective but costly), air fluidized beds, sand beds, automated assisted turning beds and net suspension beds. The low air loss bed is often used in intensive care units. It is effective but no comparative studies have been done between low air loss and alternating pressure mattresses.

There are very few randomized controlled trials to help us decide on the best support surface. The limitations of studies are described in the Cochrane Systematic Review by Cullum et al (2000). In general, for medium to high-risk patients, high specification constant low pressure mattresses are superior to the standard hospital mattress. The relative merits of alternating pressure devices are not very clear. Low air loss beds are effective in preventing and treating pressure sores but there are no trials to compare these very expensive beds with the far less costly alternating pressure systems. In the current state of knowledge, alternating pressure mattresses should generally be used for very high-risk patients. A good policy is to nurse medium- to high-risk patients initially on high specification constant pressure surfaces and be extremely vigilant about observing the skin at regular intervals and transfer on to an alternating pressure air mattress if there are early indications of possible skin breakdown. However, a policy of using an alternating pressure air mattress immediately for high-risk patients is acceptable.

A recent review by Rachael L. Fleurence from the Medtap Institute concluded as follows: 'Current information suggests that alternating pressure mattress overlays may be cost-effective for the prevention of pressure ulcers, whereas alternating pressure mattress replacements appear to be cost-effective for the treatment of superficial and severe pressure ulcers'.

Recently published NICE guidelines recommend the following.

Provision for all individuals vulnerable to pressure ulcers

All individuals assessed as being vulnerable to pressure ulcers should, as a minimum provision, be placed on a high-specification foam mattress with pressure-relieving properties.

Patients at elevated risk of developing pressure ulcers

Although there is no research evidence that high-tech pressure-relieving mattresses and overlays are more effective than high-specification (low-tech) foam mattresses and overlays, professional consensus recommends that consideration should be given to the use of alternating pressure or other high-tech pressure-relieving systems:

- As a first-line preventative strategy for people at elevated risk as identified by holistic assessment
- When the individual's previous history of pressure ulcer prevention and/or clinical condition indicates that he or she is best cared for on a high-tech device
- When a low-tech device has failed

CLASSIFICATION OF ESTABLISHED PRESSURE SORES

Stage 0   Skin hyperaemia only. Red area, which blanches on digital pressure showing that there is vasodilatation but no extravasation of blood. At this stage, it is really not a sore

Stage 1   Non-blanching erythema. This shows that there is capillary damage with extravasation of blood into the tissues

Stage 2   Partial thickness skin loss, involving epidermis and dermis

Stage 3   Full thickness skin loss with extension to subcutaneous tissues but not extending beyond deep fascia to the underlying bone, tendon or joint capsule

Stage 4   Full thickness skin loss, with extension to and beyond deep fascia involving bone, tendon or joint capsules

WOUND CARE MYTHOLOGY

- There is no evidence that rubbing the skin regularly to make it 'red' prevents pressure sores; indeed it could make it worse.
- There is no conclusive evidence that some idiosyncratic practices like applying honey, sugar, egg yolk, yoghurt, do any good. The use of sugar and honey is a very old practice dating back to the ancient Egyptians who packed honey combined with lard or resin into wounds sustained in battle. The low pH is unfavourable for bacterial growth. Sugar in high concentration has also been shown to inhibit bacterial growth. The high osmotic pressure draws in fluid. There are some studies suggesting that sugar and honey may have beneficial effects but a review of the published evidence in 1988 concluded that 'based upon available information, the use of sugar as the sole treatment of wounds cannot be recommended' (Keith & Knodel 1988).
- The old adage that 'it does not matter what you put on a sore so long as you don't put the patient on it' is only partly true, as some topical applications are harmful.
- There are 50 topical preparations used without any scientific basis (Parish 1997).

TREATMENT OF ESTABLISHED PRESSURE SORES

THREE MAIN PRINCIPLES

1. *Ensure relief of pressure.* This allows tissue perfusion, oxygenation and promotes healing. Support surfaces are important in prevention but are also of importance in managing the patient with an established sore.

2. *Treat predisposing factors.* Management of underlying medical conditions to provide the best conditions for wound healing by ensuring a good supply of oxygen, nutrients and vitamins is a common sense approach though there is no hard evidence that wound healing is influenced

by these measures. Attention to nutritional intake, correction of anaemia, dehydration, management of underlying medical problems such as diabetes mellitus, heart failure, obstructive airways disease may be required in individual patients. There is no evidence that routine zinc administration promotes pressure sore healing, unless the patient is zinc deficient. Vitamin C is essential for the synthesis of collagen. Vitamin C deficiency can impair healing but there is no evidence that large doses of vitamin C improve healing. The empirical administration of a daily multivitamin preparation sufficient to provide the normal daily requirement is advised in poorly nourished patients.

3. *Care of the wound.* This is essential before applying any dressing. Cleansing of the wound using cleansing agents (normal saline is probably the safest) and removal of dead tissue by wound debridement are essential, as dead tissue creates a physical barrier against tissue repair. Cleansing is followed by the application of a suitable dressing to provide the ideal moist environment for wound healing and to protect the wound from outside contamination. *Use of hydrogen peroxide and eusol for cleaning wounds is harmful as they are toxic and have an adverse effect on wound healing.*

TYPES OF DRESSINGS

Occlusive and semi-occlusive dressings

These create a moist micro-environment which promotes wound healing. Occlusive dressings are sometimes referred to as moisture-retaining dressings. Non-occlusive dressings are unsuitable but can be used as secondary dressings over the primary (next to the wound surface) occlusive dressing.

Types of occlusive dressings are:

- *Hydrocolloid dressings.* These are dressings manufactured from gel-forming agents combined with other materials, such as elastomers and adhesives. They are typically in the form of a flexible foam or film sheet, coated with a layer of hydrocolloid base and covered with a piece of release paper. They can be used for dry wounds and, by absorbing fluid, maintain a moist environment. The area in contact with the

wound always remains wet so that the dressing can be removed painlessly. The base is also provided as granules or paste which can be applied to the wound with the sheet to improve absorbency, e.g. Granuflex, Comfeel.

- *Hydrogel dressings.* These are dressings containing hydrophilic insoluble polymers which interact with aqueous solutions and retain significant volumes of water, e.g. Geliperm. Hydrogels tend to become dry earlier than hydrocolloids and may need more frequent changes. They are very soothing and easy to remove. Accurate placement and retention can also be a problem. Hydrogels also come in an amorphous form. When fluid is absorbed, the viscosity of the hydrogel is reduced and it flows to take up the shape of the wound, e.g. Scherisorb.

- *Semi-permeable film dressings.* Examples of these include Tegaderm and Opsite. These are said to be permeable to water and oxygen but impermeable to bacteria. They provide an effective barrier against contamination and maintain a moist environment. They are suitable for superficial pressure sores.

- *Low adherent dressings.* Examples such as silicone sodium and Mepitel appear to have no particular advantage.

- *Alginates.* Kaltostat and Sorbsan are extracted from seaweed and consist of sodium (soluble) and calcium (insoluble) salts. They are used in wounds with heavy exudation. They absorb the exudate and form a gel which maintains moisture. They are unsuitable for dry wounds.

- *Foam dressings.* These come as a product which is poured into a cavity wound where it expands to four times its original volume and forms into a sponge by releasing hydrogen (Silastic foam or Cavicare) and as a dressing (Lyofoam).

- *Odour absorbing dressings.* Some sores are malodorous and unpleasant for the patient, staff and visitors. Dressings incorporating activated charcoal, which acts as a filter, are useful in this situation, e.g. Kaltocarb and Actisorb.

There is no good evidence for the relative merits of various dressings. In general, dressings that provide a moist environment promote wound healing. There is no justification in using gauze directly on pressure sores, as it sheds fibres into the wound, does not maintain a moist environment and can be intensely painful when removed.

Systemic antibiotics are rarely necessary. The only indication is the presence of serious wound infection. Topical antibiotics should not be used. They only sensitize the skin and do not provide enough antimicrobial activity to overcome infection. Routine swabs for bacterial culture are unnecessary and wasteful. Almost all wounds are colonized with bacteria. A wound swab is only indicated where infection is suspected by the presence of clinical signs, or where infection control requires identification of methicillin-resistant *Staphylococcus aureus* (MRSA) contamination. Infection can be suspected by the presence of systemic signs such as pyrexia or local signs like cellulitis and induration around the sore (see Ch. 45). It may also be suspected when there is delayed healing, unusually friable granulation tissue or wound breakdown. Signs such as bad odour and discoloration can be misleading. Familiarity and experience could help in identifying infection. If a local tissue viability nurse specialist is available, she could be an extremely valuable resource. In general, in the absence of clear local signs around the ulcer or systemic signs of infection, systemic antibiotics should be withheld. Sending unnecessary wound swab specimens to the laboratory burdens an already over-stressed department and unnecessary use of antibiotics helps spread drug-resistant bacteria.

Use of enzymes

In theory, proteolytic enzymes are useful in removing necrotic tissue. The most widely used preparation is Varidase, which contains a mixture of streptokinase and streptodornase. Varidase is an expensive product and there is little evidence to support its routine use. There may be a place for its use in dry black eschars (or scabs), especially in the heels. Before it is applied however, the dead skin must be scored (cross-hatched) with a scalpel to allow penetration of the enzyme. Some inject Varidase under the dead skin – a practice which must be performed only by a skilled practitioner.

Management of pressure sores on the above principles should yield satisfying results. However, because of insufficient research in this area, many less well-established methods are in use. These include thermal therapy (heat lamps), electrical stimulation, electromagnetic stimulation, ultrasound and oxygen therapy. There is insufficient evidence to recommend these. The only other evidence-based intervention in pressure sore management is surgical treatment.

SURGICAL TREATMENT OF PRESSURE SORES

Wound debridement may be required to remove dead tissue in sores of grade 2 or more. More intensive surgical management, e.g. the use of skin flaps, excision of pressure sore followed at a later stage by closure, is sometimes necessary for large cavities to facilitate healing. This requires referral to a plastic surgeon.

The wound should be clean and free of infection. Surgical treatment consists of excision of the ulcer followed by closure at a later stage. Closure is by direct closure, use of cutaneous flaps or use of myocutaneous flaps.

REFERENCES

Agency for Health Care Policy and Research 1992 Pressure ulcers in adults: prediction and prevention. Clinical Practice Guidelines 3:1–63

Allman R M, Laprade C A, Noel L B 1986 Pressure sores among hospitalised patients. Annals of Internal Medicine 105:337–342

Bliss M R 1995 Preventing pressure sores in elderly patients – a comparison of seven mattress overlays. Age and Ageing 24:297–302

Bliss M R, McLaren R, Exton-Smith A N 1967 Preventing pressure sores in hospital: controlled trial of a large celled Ripple cell mattress. British Medical Journal 1:394–397

Charcot J M 1868 Sur quelques arthropathies qui paraissent dependere d'une lesion du cerveau ou la moelle epiniere. Archives de Physiologie Normale et Pathologique 1:161–178, 308–314

Clark M, Watts S 1994 The incidence of pressure sores within a National Health Service trust hospital during 1991. Journal of Advanced Nursing 20:33–36

Cullum N A, Deeks J J, Fletcher A W et al 1995 Preventing and treating pressure sores. Quality in Health Care 4:289–297

Cullum N, Deeks J, Sheldon T A et al 2000 Beds, mattresses and cushions for pressure sore prevention and treatment. Cochrane Database of Systematic Reviews, Issue 2. Art. No.: CD001735. DOI: 10.1002/14651858.CD001735

Heberden W 1815 Some account of a contrivance which was found of singular benefit in stopping the excoriation and ulceration consequent upon continued pressure in bed. Medical Transactions (published by College of Physicians, London), p 39–40

Keith J F, Knodel L C 1988 Sugar in wound healing. Drug Intelligence and Clinical Pharmacology 22: 409–411

O'Dea K 1995 The prevalence of pressure sores in four European countries. Journal of Wound Care 4:192–195

Paget J 1873 Clinical lecture on bed sores. Students Journal and Hospital Gazette 1:144–147

Parish L 1997 Medical management. In: Parish L C, Witkowski W C, Crissey J A (eds) The decubitus ulcer in clinical practice. Springer-Verlag, Berlin

Rithalia S V S, Gonsalkorale M 1998 Assessment of alternating air mattresses using a time based interface pressure threshold technique. Journal of Rehabilitation Research and Development 35:225–230

Stewart T P 1997 Support systems. In: Parish L C, Witkowski W C, Crissey J A (eds) The decubitus ulcer in clinical practice. Springer-Verlag, Berlin, p 148

Touche Ross & Co 1993 The cost of pressure sores. Department of Health Publications, London

RECOMMENDED READING

*** Essential reading; ** recommended reading*

Cullum N, Deeks J, Sheldon T A et al 2000 Beds, mattresses and cushions for preventing and treating pressure sores (Cochrane Review). The Cochrane Library 1. Update Software, Oxford ***
The reader is advised to read the most up-to-date and comprehensive review of the effectiveness of pressure sore prevention using beds, mattresses and cushions in the Cochrane database. The systematic review by Cullum and colleagues was last updated in May 1999.

Useful books on pressure sores

Dealey C 1997 Managing pressure sore prevention. Quay Books, Salisbury **

Lee B Y, Herz B 1997 Surgical management of cutaneous ulcers and pressure sores. Chapman & Hall, New York **

Parish W C, Witkowski J A, Crissey J T 1997 The decubitus ulcer in clinical practice. Springer-Verlag, Berlin **

Phillips J 1997 Pressure sores. Churchill Livingstone, London ***

Simpson A, Bowers K, Weir-Hughes D 1996 Pressure sore prevention. Whurr, London **

Webster J G (ed.) 1991 Prevention of pressure sores. Institute of Physics, London ***

SELF-ASSESSMENT QUESTIONS

Are the following statements true or false?

1. The most likely areas of the body to develop pressure sores in an elderly patient with pneumonia being nursed on his side are:
   a. The sacrum
   b. The ischial tuberosities
   c. The greater trochanter
   d. The lateral malleolus
   e. The occiput

2. In treating pressure sores:
   a. They should be kept open without dressings to encourage the formation of a scab to aid wound healing
   b. A clean sterile gauze dressing is useful as a wound dressing
   c. Topical antibiotics should not be used if a wound looks infected
   d. Occlusive dressings should be removed daily to inspect the wound
   e. High-dose vitamin C and zinc should be given to all patients with pressure sores

3. Are the following true or false?
   a. Low interface pressures quoted by manufacturers of alternating pressure air mattresses are a reliable way of selecting the most effective one
   b. Use of dynamic support surfaces eliminates the need for regular turning of patients
   c. The standard of the hospital mattress is suitable for medium- to high-risk patients provided patients are turned regularly
   d. Expensive equipment such as low air loss mattresses is essential in order to prevent pressure sores
   e. With good nursing and medical practice, most pressure sores can be prevented

Chapter **21**

Therapeutics

Teresa Donnelly and Stephen Jackson

INTRODUCTION

By 2031 those over 65 years will represent 30% of the total world population (Majeed & Aylin 2005). The proportion of those over 75 years is projected to double from 7% to 14% over the next 50 years. This older population has higher prevalence of chronic illness. Heart failure alone is predicted to increase by 53% by 2031 (Majeed & Aylin 2005). Advances in medical drug therapy have led to improved outcomes and quality of life in those living with chronic illness. Thus, the older patient is living longer with cardiovascular disease, dementia, osteoporosis, arthritis, Parkinson's disease and many other conditions. The increased medical needs are reflected in the increased drug use for this group. People over 60 years represent about 22% of the population yet receive over 54% of the medications prescribed. Those over 75 years represent 14% of the population yet receive 33% of medication prescribed. Up to 30% of them are on over three medications.

PHARMACOKINETICS

Pharmacokinetics is the description of how the body handles drugs after administration. It incorporates liberation, absorption, distribution, metabolism and excretion. There are a number of physiological changes associated with ageing that result in altered kinetics in the older patient. This is further altered in the presence of chronic illness and organ failure.

ABSORPTION

Following oral ingestion of a drug, there are a number of factors that determine its entry into the circulation. These include properties such as particle size, molecular weight, charge, solubility and pKa (the pH at which 50% exists in an unionized, lipid-soluble state). After liberation, some absorption takes place in the stomach depending on the pKa of the drug and the pH of the stomach. Reduction of parietal cell mass in the stomach with ageing increases the prevalence of gastric atrophy. This may be partly due to the prevalence of *Helicobacter pylori* infection which is estimated to be as high as 80% at 80 years. Bicarbonate secretion of the gastric cells after stimulation decreases with age, which further reduces the buffering capacity of the stomach. In theory, the altered pH could reduce the absorption of weak acidic drugs. In practice, lower levels of gastric acid have little impact. Gastric emptying is unaffected by ageing (Gainsborough et al 1993). For most drugs the large surface area of the small bowel makes this the main site of drug absorption.

BIOAVAILABILITY AND FIRST-PASS METABOLISM

Bioavailability is defined as availability of drug to the systemic circulation. In order to determine absolute bioavailability of a drug, a pharmacokinetic study must be undertaken to obtain a plasma drug concentration versus time plot for the drug after both intravenous (iv) and extravascular (e.g.

oral) administration. The absolute bioavailability is the dose-corrected area under the curve (AUC), extravascular divided by AUC intravenous. These areas are extrapolated to infinity (AUC [0–8]). According to this definition, a drug administered by the iv route is 100% bioavailable. In old age, studies using digoxin, paracetamol, lorazepam, bumetanide, theophylline and flumazanil have not shown significant differences in bioavailability with age.

Drugs that undergo substantial first-pass metabolism in the liver are avidly extracted from the blood. Drugs such as propranolol, verapamil and narcotics have a high extraction ratio. Such drugs are extremely dependent on hepatic blood flow. Liver volume declines by about 20–30% with ageing (Cope et al 1989). As a result, the bioavailability of highly extracted drugs, for example, propranolol, labetalol and verapamil are increased in the elderly patient.

DISTRIBUTION

The distribution of a drug throughout the body is dependent on its lipophilicity and the ability of the drug to bind to plasma proteins and tissue. Volume of distribution (V) is defined as the volume in which the amount of drug would need to be uniformly distributed to produce an observed blood concentration. V is important when considering the loading dose based on the desired steady-state blood level such as digoxin or amiodarone. Calculations of the loading dose are based on the desired steady-state blood level and V.

$$\begin{array}{c} \text{Loading dose} \\ \text{(mg/Kg)} \end{array} = \begin{array}{c} \text{desired blood} \\ \text{concentration} \\ \text{(mg/L)} \end{array} \times \begin{array}{c} \text{volume of} \\ \text{distribution} \\ \text{(L/Kg)} \end{array}$$

With ageing there is a decrease in lean body weight and body water and an increase in the proportion of body fat (Shock et al 1963). As a result, water-soluble drugs are distributed to a lesser extent in the elderly patient with decreased muscle mass and body water. These drugs will attain a higher initial plasma concentration after administration, e.g. ethanol and cimetidine.

Lipid-soluble drugs have a high volume of distribution due to their naturally high membrane permeability. The higher proportion of body fat associated with ageing increases the volume of distribution of fat-soluble drugs such as benzo-

diazepines, morphine, amiodarone, clomethiazole and amitriptyline.

The elimination half-life $\left(t\,\dfrac{1}{2}\,z\right)$ of a drug is the time it takes for the drug concentration in plasma to decrease by 50%. It is a function of the volume of distribution and clearance; the relationship can be represented as follows:

$$t\,\frac{1}{2}\,z = \frac{0.693\ V}{CL}$$

Where: CL = plasma clearance; 0.693 = natural logarithm of 2.

The elimination half-life tends to increase with increasing age. This may be due to an increase in the volume of distribution or a reduction in clearance (increasing the $t\,\dfrac{1}{2}\,z$). For water-soluble drugs the reduced V is more than offset by the reduced CL. For lipid-soluble drugs the rise in V and fall in CL have a multiplicative effect on the $t\,\dfrac{1}{2}\,z$.

PROTEIN BINDING

Many drugs bind to plasma proteins to varying degrees. Bound drugs are inactive. Unbound drug is free to mediate its effect. Most acidic drugs, such as warfarin and diazepam, bind to albumin (Hayes et al 1975). Basic drugs such as lidocaine (Cusack et al 1985) and tricyclic antidepressants bind to α1 acid-glycoprotein. There is little change in α1 acid-glycoprotein with age but it is an acute phase protein. Although healthy ageing is not associated with a significant fall in albumin per se (Greenblatt 1979), acute illness and chronic debilitating diseases decrease albumin and increase α1 acid-glycoprotein. A change in plasma protein tends to have its greatest effect on those drugs that are over 95% bound. A small reduction in albumin (from 99% to 98%) could double the pharmacologically active drug in the body (from 1% to 2%). The clinical relevance of these changes depends on the therapeutic index of the drug. The therapeutic index is a measure of the relationship between the concentrations of drug necessary to produce therapeutic and toxic effects. Heavily protein-bound drugs with a narrow therapeutic index are associated with clinically relevant changes in protein binding (Wallace & Verbeeck 1987).

CLEARANCE

Plasma clearance is defined as the volume of plasma that appears to be cleared of drug per unit time and is expressed as units of volume/time, e.g. mL/min. Hepatic and renal clearance are the predominant systems involved in drug clearance. Lipid-soluble drugs are metabolized in the liver, whereas water-soluble drugs tend to be excreted unchanged via the kidneys.

HEPATIC DRUG METABOLISM

Liver metabolism of drugs results in the formation of drug metabolites with enhanced hydrophilicity, facilitating excretion in the urine.

Phase 1 metabolism transforms parent molecules through the introduction of polar groups by oxidation, hydroxylation or hydrolysis. This is mediated largely through the cytochrome P450 system (CYP450) (Watkins 1992). The CYP450 enzymes are a large family of enzymes with greater than 50 subtypes active in man. In healthy populations there are 6-fold variations in the rates of the CYP450 metabolism observed. Antipyrine, a non-specific probe for the CYP system, is an example of a low-drug clearance. Wood et al reported an age-related decline of 19% in the clearance of antipyrine, suggesting a reduced CYP450 activity with age (Wood et al 1979). Studies looking at propranolol and theophylline have shown a decrease in clearance with ageing.

Induction of these enzymes decreases the bioavailability and inhibition increases the bioavailability of the parent drug. The effect of ageing on hepatic enzyme induction (e.g. by phenytoin, rifampicin) is not clear. Theophylline clearance was induced to a similar extent in old versus young smokers. This effect was not seen with antipyrine. Hepatic enzyme inhibition (e.g. by ciprofloxacin, macrolides) does not appear to be altered by the process of ageing.

Phase 2 reactions are synthetic and involve conjugation with glucuronic acid, sulphate, glycine or other groups. There is little evidence to show a significant reduction of the phase 2 pathways with age. Lorazepam and oxazepam, which are metabolized by glucuronidation, fail to show an age-related decline in clearance. A reduction in conjugation of paracetamol due to ageing has been reported. When corrected for liver volume there was little difference between the young and the fit elderly subjects, but clearance was significantly reduced in the 'frail' elderly people. This effect is thought to be as much related to a reduction in liver volume as to a reduction in the conjugation pathway.

RENAL CLEARANCE

Renal function in elderly subjects may not be accurately quantified by serum creatinine alone. Creatinine production is related to muscle mass. A fall in muscle mass and hence creatinine production occurs with age and disease. Clinically important reductions in renal function may be present despite a normal range serum creatinine. Renal clearance of drugs and creatinine relates closely to the glomerular filtration rate (GFR). This is best estimated using the Cockroft and Gault equation (Cockroft & Gault 1976):

$$GFR = \frac{\left(\dfrac{140 - age}{(years)}\right) \times \underset{(kg)}{weight} \times \underset{(men)}{1.23} \quad or \quad \underset{(women)}{1.04}}{Creatinine}$$

There is a decline in glomerular function with age due to a reduction in functioning nephrons. Estimation of GFR is appropriate where renal dysfunction is suspected. For drugs substantially excreted by the kidney, elderly patients need adjustment of dosage based on the renal function. In the case of drugs with a large therapeutic window, such as penicillin, little adjustment is needed. However, by contrast, those with a narrow therapeutic window need doses to be adjusted accordingly. For example, decline in renal function reduces digoxin clearance; therefore dose adjustment is required in the setting of a narrow therapeutic window.

PHARMACODYNAMICS

Pharmacodynamics is the study of the effects of drugs. The effect of ageing may result in increased or decreased response to equivalent serum drug concentrations in younger versus older individuals. These changes may result in either an increase in unwanted effects or an increase or decrease in wanted effects.

DECREASED DRUG SENSITIVITY

The response of the dorsal forearm vein to nor-adrenaline is reduced in old age. Similar reductions in sensitivity have been seen for the β_2, neuropeptide Y and the H2 receptor. Response of the acetylcholine receptor was equivocal. Impaired endothelium-dependent vasodilatation has been demonstrated in the ageing forearm, suggesting an age-related impairment of the nitric oxide system.

INCREASED DRUG SENSITIVITY

Warfarin sensitivity increases with age due to decreases in clotting factor synthesis.

Ageing is associated with increasing sensitivity to the adverse effects of non-steroidal anti-inflammatory drugs (NSAIDs). Reduced capacity to repair gastrointestinal mucosa, reduced prostaglandin levels and the high prevalence of *Helicobacter pylori* in the elderly population enhance the risk of gastrointestinal bleeding and perforation.

With advancing age, people are also more sensitive to the potential side-effects of benzodiazepines. The increased sensitivity is due to age-related alterations in the central benzodiazepine receptors in the brain causing increased sedation, unsteadiness and increased postural sway. These effects are independent of changes in drug kinetics (Greenblatt et al 1991).

Independent of reduced clearance, an increased brain sensivity to narcotics in the elderly patient has been demonstrated. Increased sensitivity to neuroleptics occurs in elderly patients with Lewy body dementia. Anticholinergic medication can exacerbate urinary retention or glaucoma in the elderly patient. Worsening cognitive function can also result from these drugs due to the cholinergic deficit seen in Alzheimer's disease.

A reduction in dopaminergic neuronal function that occurs particularly with Parkinson's disease alters the response to dopamine antagonists with ageing. This leads to an increased susceptibility to extrapyramidal symptoms (EPS). Antagonism of D2-receptors has been associated with antipsychotic-induced EPS. High-potency conventional antipsychotics have greater affinity for dopamine receptors and a greater tendency to cause EPS. Atypical antipsychotics have relatively lower affinity for D2-receptors and higher affinity for serotonin receptors and therefore cause minimal or no EPS.

HOMEOSTATIC MECHANISMS

Changes in autonomic function, reduced plasma volume, reduced vasomotor function and the presence of chronic disease all reduce the homeostatic reserve of the elderly patient.

Orthostatic intolerance increases with age. As well as reduced baroreceptor sensitivity, orthostatic intolerance may also be due to changes in vein capacitance with decreased baroreceptor activation (Lakatta 1980). This blunted orthostatic response is compounded by the addition of hypotensive or vasodilator drugs. In addition the increased postural sway seen with benzodiazepines in elderly people exacerbates the propensity to fall associated with ageing (Swift 1984).

Thermoregulation can be impaired in a subset of frail elderly patients. The normal response to hypothermia involves shivering, an increase in the metabolic rate, vasoconstriction and behavioural changes which serve to restore normal core body temperature. Drugs such as vasodilators, ethanol and neuroleptics can blunt this physiological response in susceptible frail elderly patients.

In the brain, cholinergic function tends to decrease with age.

OPTIMIZING PRESCRIBING FOR ELDERLY PATIENTS

The National Service Framework highlights the need for appropriate and rational prescribing for older people. Optimizing means ensuring that appropriate medications are prescribed for a given condition that are the most effective and that the safest dose is being used. There is little doubt that medication-related problems collectively form one of the geriatric giants. It has been said that *any symptom in an elderly patient should be considered a drug side-effect until proven otherwise* (Gurwitz et al 1995). Medication-related death is the fifth most common cause of death in the USA (Lazarou et al 1998). Hepler and Strand (1990) defined medication-related problems as 'an event or circumstance involving a patient's drug treat-

Box 21.1   Categories of medication–related problems

- Medical condition that requires new or additional drug therapy
- Patient taking unnecessary drug given present condition
- Wrong drug for the patient's medical condition
- Correct drug, dose too low
- Correct drug, dose too high
- Adverse drug reaction
- Drug interaction
- Patient not taking drugs correctly

ment that actually or potentially interferes with the achievement of an optimal outcome'. The eight categories of medication-related problems are outlined in Box 21.1.

POLYPHARMACY VERSUS APPROPRIATE PRESCRIBING

The term polypharmacy was originally used merely to refer to multiple drug use but has come to imply excessive prescribing or an inappropriately large number of drugs. A more meaningful concept is that of appropriate prescribing. This concept embraces both non-uses of drugs not indicated as well as the use of drugs where indications exist. The term polypharmacy therefore is probably best not used.

EVALUATING APPROPRIATE PRESCRIBING

There are much published data on methods of evaluating the appropriateness of prescribing. Beers et al developed a comprehensive set of criteria based on dosage, frequency and duration of therapy, which even with clinical data would be hard to relate to an evidence base (Beers et al 1991). We have developed prescribing indicators that measure purely descriptive markers such as the number of drugs, unnecessary or potentially harmful prescribing and evidence-based prescribing. This approach can be used in clinical practice to monitor and, if necessary, enhance the quality of prescribing (Batty et al 2003).

ADVERSE DRUG REACTIONS

Age-associated increases in the incidence of dose-related adverse reactions have been well described for certain groups of drugs, e.g. increased sedation and ataxia with benzodiazepines. These more commonly described adverse reactions are due to an accentuation of a drug's known pharmacological properties and are therefore predictable, often described as type A reactions. Idiosyncratic (type B) adverse reactions are unpredictable and often of unknown mechanism, e.g. rash or anaphylactic shock. Recent data indicate that half of the illness, disability and premature death caused by medication-related problems are preventable through vigilance at the prescribing and monitoring stage (although patient compliance was a factor in less than one-quarter of adverse incidents).

PRESCRIBING ADVICE

Much has been written regarding advice on appropriate prescribing in elderly patients. Some advice is general and some specific or particularly appropriate for elderly patients (Box 21.2). Here we summarize advice:

- *Establish a diagnosis.* It is highly desirable to have a diagnosis in order to define the appropriate therapeutic options. If this cannot be achieved, a therapeutic objective must be defined.

- *Review the patient's drug regimen regularly.* Patients with multiple chronic diseases and recurrent hospital admissions may see more than one prescriber. The patient's drugs must be clearly elicited at each visit, including over the counter preparations. While unnecessary drugs should be discontinued, patients should be offered drug prescriptions that will benefit them.

- *Consider adverse medication effects* as a potential cause of any presenting symptom, especially in those patients on sedative-hypnotics, antidepressants or anticholinergic medication. In the same way, always think of acute drug withdrawal as a potential cause of symptoms, e.g. delirium in benzodiazepine withdrawal.

- *Maximize drug compliance.* Strategies to improve compliance (such as patient education) should be instituted where appropriate. Use of dosette

Box 21.2 Prescription checklist

- What are the patient's views?
- What is the diagnosis?
- What is the aim of treatment?
- What are the treatment possibilities for the patient – pharmacological/non-pharmacological?
- How is your preferred drug (and its metabolites if relevant) cleared?
- Will other disease states affect your choice?
- Will physiological states affect your choice?
- Could one drug treat more than one problem?
- What is the best route and starting dose?
- How will your treatment be monitored?
- When will the dose be increased?
- What will the duration of treatment be?
- What are the potential treatment side-effects?
- What potential drug interactions are relevant?
- Would discontinuing another drug help?
- What information should you discuss with the patient?

boxes with careful labelling of drugs may be appropriate in individual cases. Family education may help. Involvement of the pharmacist and general practitioner may help to improve compliance with drug regimens.

- Where possible involve the patient in agreeing the therapeutic objectives. Consider a variety of strategies to meet the therapeutic objectives with particular regard to the patient's views and the full problem list. For example, choice of pharmacological versus non-pharmacological approaches, route of clearance of any drugs and metabolites (e.g. morphine is metabolized but an active metabolite, morphine-6-glucuronide, is cleared renally). Also consider whether there are drugs that could meet more than one therapeutic objective.

- Discuss the adverse effect profile with the patient.

CONCLUSION

Medications are probably the single most important healthcare technology in preventing injury, disability and death in the geriatric population.

With the increasing numbers of elderly patients and increase in medications available, optimizing drug prescribing is an essential part of geriatric medicine. Therapeutics in the elderly population is complex. The role of the geriatrician is the balancing of therapeutic goals against quality of life and minimizing the risk of adverse drug reactions.

Key points

- Drug utilization is significantly higher among the elderly population than among younger adults.
- Factors that result in the elderly patient being more at risk of drug-related adverse events include:
  - Reduction in total body water and a proportional increase in total body fat, increasing the volume of distribution and hence half-life
  - Impaired renal clearance of water-soluble drugs hence a prolonged half-life
  - Reduced liver volume resulting in reduced clearance of lipid-soluble drugs and hence a prolonged half-life
  - Reduced enzyme activity in the frail elderly patient may reduce clearance of lipid-soluble drugs further
  - Increased sensitivity to many drugs
  - Greater prevalence of disease processes leading to a larger number of concomitant drugs.
- Prescribing indicators are useful tools to monitor and enhance prescribing.
- The therapeutic goals are to maximize quality of life while minimizing adverse drug reactions.

REFERENCES

Batty G M, Grant R L, Agawal R et al 2003 Using prescribing indicators to measure the quality of prescribing to elderly medical in-patients. Age and Ageing 32:292–298

Beers M H, Puslander J G, Rollingehrer I et al 1991 Explicit criteria for determining inappropriate medication use in nursing home residents. Archives of Internal Medicine 151:1825–1832

Cockroft T W, Gault M W 1976 Prediction of creatinine clearance from serum creatinine. Nephron 16: 31–34

Cope E, Mutch E, Rawlins K W et al 1989 The effect of age upon liver volume and apparent liver blood flow in healthy man. Hepatology 9:297–301

Cusack B, O'Malley K, Lavern J et al 1985 Protein binding and disposition of lidocaine in the elderly. European Journal of Clinical Pharmacology 29: 323–329

Gainsborough N, Maskrey V L, Nelson M L 1993 The association of age with gastric emptying. Age and Ageing 22:37–40

Greenblatt D J 1979 Reduced serum albumin concentration in the elderly: a report from the Boston Collaborative Drug Surveillance Program. Journal of the American Geriatrics Society 27:20–22

Greenblatt D J, Harmatz D S, Shader R I 1991 Clinical pharmacokinetics of anxiolytics and hypnotics in the elderly. Clinical Pharmacokinetics 21:165–177

Gurwitz M, Monane M, Monane S 1995 Long-term care quality letter. Brown University, Providence, Rhode Island

Hayes M J, Langman M J S, Short A H 1975 Changes in drug metabolism with increasing age 1: Warfarin binding and plasma proteins. British Journal of Clinical Pharmacology 2:73–79

Hepler C D, Strand L M 1990 Opportunities and responsibilities in pharmaceutical care. American Journal of Hospital Pharmacy 47:533–543

Lakatta E G 1980 Age-related alterations in the cardiovascular response to adrenergic mediated stress. Federation Proceedings 39:3173–3177

Lazarou J, Pomeranz B H, Corey P N 1998 Incidence of adverse drug reactions in hospitalised patients: a meta-analysis of prospective studies. Journal of the American Medical Association 279:1200–1205

Majeed M, Aylin P 2005 The ageing population of the United Kingdom and cardiovascular disease. British Medical Journal 331:1362

Shock M W, Watkin D M, Yiengst M J 1963 Age differences in water content of the body as related to basal oxygen consumption in males. Gerontology Journal 18:1–8

Swift C G 1984 Postural instability as a measure of sedative drug response. British Journal of Clinical Pharmacology 18(Suppl):87S–90S

Wallace S M, Verbeeck R K 1987 Plasma protein binding of drugs in the elderly. Clinical Pharmacokinetics 12:41–72

Watkins B P 1992 Drug metabolism by the cytochrome P450 in the liver and small bowel. Gastroenterology Clinics of North America 21:511–526

Wood A J, Vestal R E, Wilkinson G R et al 1979 Effect of ageing and cigarette smoking on antipyrine and iodocyanine green elimination. Journal of Clinical Pharmacology and Therapeutics 26:16–20

RECOMMENDED READING

*** Essential reading; ** recommended reading; * interesting but not vital

Breckenridge A 2001 Optimal dose identification. Esteve Foundation Symposia, vol 9, 1st edn. Elsevier *

Chutka D S, Evans J M, Fleming K C 1995 Drug prescribing for elderly patients. Mayo Clinical Proceedings 70:685–693 ***

Jackson S H D, Mangoni A A, Batty G M 1999 Optimisation of drug prescribing. British Journal of Clinical Pharmacology 57:231–236 ***

Mangoni A A 2005 Cardiovascular drug therapy in the elderly patients; specific age related pharmacokinetic, pharmacodynamic and therapeutic considerations. Drugs and Aging 22:913–941 **

Simonson W, Feinberg J L 2005 Medication-related problems in the elderly: defining the issues and identifying solutions. Drugs and Aging 22: 559–569 ***

SELF-ASSESSMENT QUESTIONS

Are the following statements true or false?

1. Pharmacokinetics:
   a. Bioavailability describes the amount of drug which is absorbed following administration
   b. Renal clearance of a water-soluble drug is independent of the serum creatinine
   c. Decreases in plasma protein binding of drugs that are < 90% protein bound can still significantly increase volume of distribution
   d. Digoxin loading dose should be reduced

2. Drug treatment in elderly patients:
   a. Increased sensitivity to warfarin is due to altered plasma protein binding in the elderly patient
   b. Sensitivity to benzodiazepines is increased in older patients
   c. If amiodarone was discontinued following an adverse reaction, it would be cleared from the body over the following 6 months
   d. Sensitivity to the adverse reactions to β_2 agonists is increased in older patients

PART 3

Selected topics

SECTION 1

Central nervous system

Chapter 22

The management of Parkinson's disease

Jolyon Meara

WHAT IS PARKINSON'S DISEASE?

Parkinson's disease (PD) is a disease of elderly people with age-specific prevalence rates steeply increasing into extreme old age. In 2006, NICE published a full guideline document entitled Parkinson's Disease: Diagnosis and Management in Primary and Secondary Care (http://www.nice.org.uk/CG035).

In cross-sectional studies, two-thirds of subjects with PD will be aged over 70 years. PD results from dopamine deficiency in a part of the basal ganglia in the forebrain called the corpus striatum (caudate nucleus and putamen). This deficiency state arises from cell death in a large pigmented midbrain nucleus called the substantia nigra. The substantia nigra provides critical dopaminergic input to the basal ganglia via the nigrostriatal tract. With progression, PD can affect many parts of the brain and peripheral nervous system. Surviving neurons contain typical inclusions called Lewy bodies.

PD is primarily a disorder of voluntary motor control. There is a particular difficulty in the appropriate execution of automatic learnt motor plans.

HOW DO YOU DIAGNOSE PD?

The diagnosis of PD depends on bedside clinical skills. This may change as in vivo imaging of cerebral function based on SPECT scanning becomes more widely available and new investigative imaging agents are developed. Clinical diagnostic criteria for PD have been suggested (Hughes et al 1992).

The main clinical features of PD consist of:

- *Akinesia* (difficulty initiating voluntary movement, slowness of movement, difficulty with sequential complex movements, decreased amplitude of movement and rapid fatigability of repetitive movements)

- *Rigidity* (increased resistance of relaxed muscle to passive stretch)
- *Tremor* (rapid, involuntary rhythmic oscillation of a body part, typically occurring at rest when muscles are relaxed, with a frequency of 4–5 Hertz, tremor of the hand characteristically causing a pill-rolling tremor at rest)
- *Postural instability* in more advanced disease, resulting in falls

WHAT IS THE DIFFERENCE BETWEEN PARKINSONISM AND PD?

The presence of upper limb akinesia and rigidity, with or without tremor, indicates a diagnosis of parkinsonism. Parkinsonism can result from many causes, the commonest of which is PD. Overall, PD accounts for around 70% of cases of parkinsonism. However, with increasing age parkinsonism not due to PD (vascular, drug-induced, multiple system degeneration, parkinsonism in association with dementia) appears to become increasingly common. This impression needs to be established by careful clinical studies. The prevalence of parkinsonism increases even more steeply than PD with age, particularly if cases with akinesia and rigidity confined to the lower limbs associated with gait disturbance are also included.

HOW GOOD ARE WE AT DIAGNOSING PD?

Diagnostic accuracy decreases with increasing age of the patient. Clinicopatholological studies show that around 25% of patients under the care of experts thought to have PD at death will turn out to have other diagnoses at postmortem. In one large community study only 74% of people taking anti-parkinsonian medication had parkinsonism confirmed by examination. Only 53% of the subjects with parkinsonism met clinical diagnostic criteria for PD. Over half of the subjects had treatment initiated by their GP. Very few subjects had been seen by consultants with a specialist interest in PD. The diagnosis of both PD and parkinsonism can be very difficult in elderly people. A properly

conducted trial of anti-parkinsonian medication may be required to help resolve diagnostic difficulty.

WHAT CONDITIONS ARE COMMONLY MISDIAGNOSED AS PD?

- Essential tremor is commonly mistaken for PD, often leading to unnecessary treatment with expensive and toxic drugs and considerable anxiety for patient and family. Around 10–20% of cases misdiagnosed as PD will have this condition.
- Vascular parkinsonism (predominant involvement of the lower half of the body with leg and axial rigidity, gait apraxia and preservation of arm function).
- Drug-induced parkinsonism (DIP) can mimic PD and usually results from the use of neuroleptic (dopamine receptor blocking) drugs. Neuroleptic drugs used to treat major psychiatric illness commonly cause DIP. Elderly patients with delirium are also still regularly and often inappropriately prescribed these drugs. Newer atypical neuroleptic drugs much less commonly cause DIP. Drugs that can cause DIP are often prescribed for elderly people with dizzy spells (prochlorperazine and cinnarazine), and for those with gastrointestinal disturbances (metoclopramide).
- Parkinsonism in association with dementia, including dementia with Lewy bodies.

HOW DOES PD PRESENT IN OLDER PEOPLE?

Subtypes of disease in PD appear to exist, though further careful clinical studies are needed. Subjects with late-onset PD (arbitrarily defined as starting after 70 years of age) tend to have an akinetic-rigid presentation without tremor, respond less well to medication, progress more rapidly and develop dementia sooner than subjects with earlier-onset disease. The motor signs of PD can be overshadowed by other clinical features, including cognitive impairment, depression, anxiety, fatigue, muscle and joint pains, weight loss, autonomic failure, a general 'slowing down' and decreased functional ability with no apparent cause. Falls are not uncommon as a presenting feature of PD in elderly subjects in whom the diagnosis has been delayed. Dysarthria and dysphagia are distressing symptoms of PD that may be present at diagnosis or develop quite quickly in older people. The response to drug treatment is disappointing. Bladder and bowel symptoms due to autonomic failure, poor mobility and concurrent diseases are very common in older patients presenting with PD.

WHY IS THE DIAGNOSIS MISSED FOR SO LONG IN ELDERLY SUBJECTS WITH PD?

Elderly patients may have symptoms for longer before diagnosis than younger subjects, though this should be established through scientific study. Delay in diagnosis may occur because:

- Of the early non-specific presentation of PD
- Of concurrent diseases (dementia, stroke, arthritis, impaired mobility) which can make it difficult to detect the motor signs of PD
- The patient, family and doctor erroneously attribute many of the early signs of PD to the inevitable effects of ageing
- In some patients apparently presenting with advanced PD, the medical record indicates that the diagnosis had in fact been made earlier, but was not acted upon or communicated to the patient or family. This can occur if the diagnosis is made by chance after an acute admission to hospital or after consulting about an unrelated matter. In part, this may be to avoid causing unnecessary anxiety for the patient especially if the symptoms of PD (in the doctor's opinion) are mild and are not related to problems with which the patient presented

HOW SHOULD PD BE MANAGED AROUND THE TIME OF DIAGNOSIS?

As with most chronic and progressive diseases too little emphasis has been placed on how the diagnosis is communicated to the patient, spouse and family. How information-giving is handled can have long-lasting effects on how well individuals cope with this disease. A clear statement of the facts can be supported by the provision of explanatory leaflets, an early review by the doctor and the continuing input from the nurse specialist (if available). Details about voluntary bodies such as the Parkinson's Disease Society should also be given at this stage, or at the next review. Lying and standing blood pressure and pulse should be measured to detect postural hypotension. Co-morbidities should be assessed with particular emphasis on current medication. As PD is the only degenerative neurological disease for which effective treatment currently exists, the doctor may not appreciate the enormity of the problems faced by the patient and may be much more optimistic.

Comprehensive assessment of physical, cognitive and psychosocial function, as well as social-environmental factors should be undertaken. This will require the input from an interdisciplinary team and should ideally include the use of standardized assessment instruments to assess disease severity, cognition, mood, activities of daily living (ADL) and health-related quality of life. Early referral to physiotherapy, occupational therapy and speech and language therapy appears to be of benefit in delaying the onset of disability, though more studies are needed in this area. Objective measures of akinesia (simple motor tests and timed walking) can help with the overall assessment of response to treatment. Input from a social worker is important to assess social needs and to provide information about financial support, such as attendance allowance. Driving is often an important issue and fitness to drive should be discussed with the patient.

A key decision at this time is when and which drug therapy should be started. Patients should have life-long access to a specialist team and remain under specialist medical review.

WHEN SHOULD DRUG TREATMENT BE STARTED?

Since current drug treatment can improve the motor impairment in PD but does not delay the progression of the disease, treatment should be started when the disease is causing handicap and reducing quality of life. In many older patients, treatment will need to be started at or soon after diagnosis. If in the future treatments become available that can delay the progression of PD or favourably alter the clinical expression of later disease, then this strategy will no longer be appropriate.

WHAT DRUGS SHOULD BE USED TO START TREATMENT IN PD?

Levodopa is the mainstay of treatment for older patients with PD and is given in conjunction with a dopa decarboxylase inhibitor (Sinemet, Madopar). Levodopa should be started at a dose of 50 mg three times daily with food and then slowly titrated upwards by 50 mg every 4 days until a dose of 200 mg three times daily is achieved. Patients need to be reviewed after 6 weeks of treatment to establish the response to treatment and to either reduce or increase further the levodopa dose. Common side-effects from levodopa are nausea and vomiting, postural hypotension and drowsiness. At high dose and in any elderly patient with pre-existing cognitive impairment, levodopa can cause hallucinations, nightmares, delirium and psychosis. Nausea and vomiting can be controlled with domperidone 20 mg three times daily on starting levodopa. Domperidone can be withdrawn in nearly all patients after a few weeks of treatment.

The risk of levodopa-induced dyskinesias and motor fluctuations is strongly related to age at onset and therefore, in older patients, levodopa should not be withheld on this account. A recent retrospective case note study of dyskinesias reported that the incidence of dyskinesias after 5 years of treatment fell from around 40% in the 40–49 year age-at-onset group to around 16% in the 70–79 year-old group. The risk of disabling or troublesome dyskinesias was even less. The dose of levodopa should be the minimum necessary to control symptoms. As the disease progresses, the dose of levodopa usually needs to be increased, though older patients rarely tolerate doses of levodopa in excess of around 600 mg daily.

WHAT DRUGS CAN BE ADDED LATER TO IMPROVE DISEASE CONTROL?

After titrating the dose of levodopa to the maximally tolerated dose, other drugs can be used to try to improve worsening motor parkinsonism. These include COMT and MAO-B enzyme inhibition to improve the bioavailability of levodopa by preventing its peripheral (entacapone, tolcapone) or central (tolcapone, selegiline, rasagiline) breakdown. Selegiline and rasagiline also have intrinsic anti-parkinsonian actions and tolcapone may have central antidepressant effects. Tolcapone is available again in the UK, though patients on this drug require strict and regular monitoring of liver function. Dopamine agonist drugs can also be used, but are poorly tolerated in elderly patients with cognitive impairment, levodopa-induced hallucinosis or postural hypotension. Pergolide is best avoided as it may be rarely linked to the development of valvular heart lesions. Echocardiographic monitoring is now advised for patients on pergolide.

Wearing off in older patients (the loss of drug effect before the next dose is due) can be improved by the addition of entacapone/tolcapone, dopamine agonist drugs, or by the use of delayed-release or dispersible formulations of levodopa. Sudden 'off' periods that may take the form of motor freezing, panic attacks, painful crises, breathlessness or painful dystonia can respond dramatically to subcutaneous injections of apomorphine. Night-time problems of pain, restless legs and 'off' periods can be improved with the use of long-acting oral dopamine agonist drugs, such as cabergoline, or overnight subcutaneous infusion of apomorphine.

WHY IS THE RESPONSE TO TREATMENT OFTEN POOR IN OLDER PATIENTS WITH PD COMPARED TO YOUNGER SUBJECTS?

- The diagnosis may be wrong.
- Non-motor symptoms not responsive to dopaminergic drug therapy dominate the clinical picture.

- Multiple pathology in the cerebral cortex and basal ganglia, such as co-existing vascular disease, reduce the benefit of drug treatment.
- There may be poor tolerance of levodopa with failure to reach a maximally therapeutic dose.
- There may be under-treatment with anti-parkinsonian drugs.
- There may be poor compliance with complex and multiple drug regimens.
- Concurrent diseases are masking any drug benefit.

WHY DON'T PEOPLE REPORT FEELING BETTER ON DRUG TREATMENT DESPITE A REDUCTION IN AKINESIA, RIGIDITY AND TREMOR?

Many of the features of PD at presentation in older subjects that cause most of the handicap do not respond or may even be made worse by dopaminergic drugs. These include dysarthria, dysphagia, poor handwriting, impaired balance, falls, poor mobility, sudden freezing, dizziness on standing, and bladder and bowel symptoms. Generally, in older patients, over time, non-motor symptoms increasingly account for handicap and poor quality of life. Cognitive impairment due to PD or other pathology also limits the usefulness of drug treatment. Depression, anxiety and apathy are common in PD and are major determinants of quality of life for the patient, spouse and family. Depression and anxiety can respond well to specific drug and psychological interventions.

WHAT LONG-TERM STRATEGIES SHOULD BE USED IN PD?

Rehabilitation should form the central part of any strategy, with an emphasis on assessment, reassessment, goal setting and team working. A movement disorder clinic supported by a PD specialist nurse who can work in the community with patients and families is one effective model of care in PD. Education, information and health promotion are also key elements of long-term care.

HOW SHOULD ADVANCED PD BE MANAGED?

With disease progression, a situation can be reached where drug treatment no longer improves the major disabling features of PD (such as dementia, falls, immobility, dysarthria and dysphagia). At this stage, dopaminergic drugs may be doing more harm than good and can often be slowly reduced with good effect. Simple drug regimens should be used at this stage. Palliative care is an important aspect of the management in the final disease stages and requires good liaison with primary care teams and often the private nursing sector.

HOW CAN WE IMPROVE CARE THROUGH FURTHER RESEARCH IN THIS FIELD?

The clinical presentation and progression of PD in older people is poorly defined.

The impact of depression and cognitive impairment in PD needs further study in terms of prevalence, response to treatment and impact on health-related quality of life.

Elderly patients are poorly represented in industry-sponsored drug trials. The efficacy and tolerability of many drugs widely used to treat PD have never been established in older people. Methods of improving the care of people with PD in residential and nursing homes and after admission for medical and surgical emergencies need to be determined. There is little evidence for the effectiveness of rehabilitative strategies in PD, ranging from specific treatments used to improve motor impairments, through to the value of goal setting and multidisciplinary working. The impact of PD on families, spouses and carers is still poorly understood.

REFERENCES

Hughes A J, Daniel S E, Kilford L et al 1992 Accuracy of clinical diagnosis of idiopathic Parkinson's disease: a clinicopathological study of 100 cases. Journal of Neurology, Neurosurgery and Psychiatry 55: 181–184

RECOMMENDED READING

*** *Essential reading;* ** *recommended reading*

Bhatia K, Brooks D J, Burn D J et al 2001 Updated guidelines for the management of Parkinson's disease. Hospital Medicine 62(8):456–470 ***

Goetz C G, Poewe W, Rascol O et al 2005 Evidence-based medical review update: pharmacological and surgical treatments of Parkinson's disease: 2001 to 2004. Movement Disorders 20(5):523–539 ***

Hobson J P, Meara R J 2004 The risk and incidence of dementia in a cohort of elderly subjects with Parkinson's disease. Movement Disorders 18(9): 1043–1049 **

Hughes A J, Daniel S E, Kilford L et al 1992 Accuracy of clinical diagnosis of idiopathic Parkinson's disease: a clinicopathological study of 100 cases. Journal of Neurology, Neurosurgery and Psychiatry 55:181–184 **

Meara R J, Koller W C (eds) 2000 Parkinson's disease and parkinsonism in the elderly. Cambridge University Press, Cambridge ***

Quinn N 1995 Parkinsonism – recognition and differential diagnosis. British Medical Journal 310: 447–452 **

SELF-ASSESSMENT QUESTION

1. Which of the following are true or false?
   a. The commonest cause of hand tremor in older people is PD
   b. Cognitive impairment is usually mild and non-progressive in older subjects with PD
   c. PD progresses faster in older compared to younger subjects
   d. Drug-induced motor complications are less common in older subjects
   e. The sensation of breathlessness can be a distressing feature of 'off' periods in PD
   f. Disabling motor fluctuations and dyskinesias occur in around 40% of older patients with PD after 5 years of levodopa treatment

SECTION 1

Central nervous system

Chapter 23

Syncope and dizziness

Shona McIntosh and Joanna Lawson

SYNCOPE

'By Jove, what a rate my heart is galloping at! These confounded palpitations get worse instead of better ... Still he might only have fainted; it might only be a fit.

Sir Christopher knelt down, unfastened the cravat, unfastened the waistcoat, and laid his hand on the heart. It might be syncope; it might not – it could not be death. No! that thought must be kept far off.'

(George Eliot, 1858, *Scenes of Clerical Life*)

DEFINITION

Syncope is a loss of consciousness due to a temporary impairment of cerebral perfusion. (The word syncope is Greek in derivation and means abrupt interruption or pause.)

THE SCOPE OF THE PROBLEM

Older individuals are prone to syncope due to age-related changes in cardiovascular homeostatic mechanisms, co-morbid illness and (in particular) medications. The annual incidence of syncope in this age group is not known with certainty. Published figures may be underestimates as unwitnessed syncopal events are misreported as falls by elderly individuals with cognitive impairment (Shaw & Kenny 1997). A recurrence rate of 30% at 2 years has been reported (Lipsitz et al 1985).

Not surprisingly, the consequences of syncope are more serious for older patients than for their younger counterparts. The mortality rate is higher (although this probably reflects a higher prevalence of coexisting heart disease) and they suffer more major injuries (Kapoor 1996, Kapoor et al 1986). Falls in elderly subjects (with or without loss of consciousness) are associated with psychological morbidity and are frequently cited in nursing home applications (Linzer et al 1991, Tinetti & Speechley 1989). While a single syncopal event in a young patient with no evidence of cardiac disease may not require investigation, in older individuals the high morbidity coupled with the high recurrence rate mean that prompt assessment of all patients is warranted. A new chapter in the coronary heart disease National Service Framework includes care pathways for patients with syncope (DoH 2005).

CAUSES OF SYNCOPE

The mnemonic 'CORN' may assist in remembering some important causes of syncope:

- **C**ardiac:
  arrhythmia
  outflow obstruction   (e.g. aortic stenosis)
  circulatory failure   (e.g. pulmonary embolus)

- **O**rthostatic hypotension/post-prandial hypotension

- **R**eflex (neurally-mediated) syncope:
  vasovagal syncope   (also called neurocardiogenic, vasodepressor)
  carotid sinus syndrome
  situational syncope   (cough, micturition, defaecation, etc.)

- **N**eurological disease:
  vertebrobasilar   (other neurological
  transient ischaemic   symptoms/signs
  attack   usually present)
  subclavian steal   (uncommon)
  syndrome

Conditions which may mimic syncope but which do not reduce cerebral perfusion include:

- Epilepsy
- Metabolic disorders   (e.g. hypoglycaemia)
- Psychiatric disorders   (probably uncommon as a cause of syncope in elderly subjects – more research is needed)

WHY SYNCOPE OFTEN REMAINS UNEXPLAINED

Syncope is, by definition, intermittent and between attacks there may be no abnormal clinical findings. Thus, even in younger patients the cause of syncope may remain elusive. Indeed, studies in the 1980s reported that syncope remained unexplained in up to 40% of both young and elderly patients (Kapoor et al 1986).

In elderly patients an accurate history is frequently not available. Syncopal events may, therefore, be misreported as falls and may evade appropriate investigation. Even if the history is accurate, diagnostic difficulty may arise as a result of atypical disease presentation. For example, faints in elderly people may have many of the features of fits (including incontinence and slow recovery). The problem is often compounded by multiple pathology in this age group. Over one-third of older individuals have more than one cause of syncope (some will have both fits and faints). Nonetheless, using a systematic approach, a diagnosis can be achieved in the majority (McIntosh et al 1993).

INVESTIGATION OF SYNCOPE

We use the flow diagram in Figure 23.1 when investigating syncope. Mortality is increased in subjects with structural heart disease (Kapoor 1996). The guidelines indicate which patients should be admitted for investigation. The full syncope work-up may not be appropriate for frail older individuals in whom treatment may need to be based on limited data.

Notwithstanding the comments above, it is still important to obtain a detailed history. Ascertain whether the event was witnessed and contact the witness. (This will be of particular relevance if the patient has cognitive impairment.) Establish the circumstances of the event (e.g. the position of the patient and whether the episode occurred after medications, meals, micturition or exercise). Ask about any prodrome (e.g. dizziness, nausea or aura), any associated symptoms (e.g. nausea or palpitations), the subject's appearance during the attack (e.g. pallor or fitting) and their symptoms afterwards (e.g. confusion, incontinence, sweating or nausea). An enquiry about co-morbidity and medications will often be relevant in older subjects. It may, at this point, be possible to decide whether you are dealing with syncope or another cause of transient loss of consciousness such as epilepsy – transient myoclonic jerks can occur with syncope but begin *after* rather than *with* the loss of consciousness.

The examination should focus on the cardiovascular and neurological systems. It is important to assess gait and balance as changes in blood pressure insufficient to cause syncope may result in falls without loss of consciousness in older

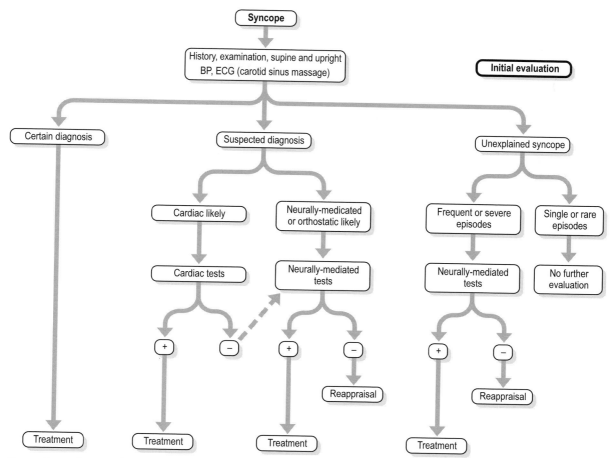

Figure 23.1 Syncope. (Modified from The European Society of Cardiology (ESC) 2004, reproduced with kind permission of Oxford University Press.)

patients. Blood pressure should be checked after 5 minutes of supine rest and at least once each minute for 3 minutes after standing (repeated morning readings may be necessary if orthostatic hypotension is strongly suspected). A 12-lead electrocardiogram (ECG) must be obtained in all patients. Carotid sinus massage should be considered in the initial assessment of older individuals. Recognized contraindications should be observed (Richardson et al 2000). Ideally, massage should be performed supine and upright with both ECG and beat-to-beat blood pressure monitoring (Parry et al 2000).

Following the initial evaluation it may be possible to make a definite diagnosis of orthostatic hypotension, carotid sinus syndrome, vasovagal syncope (if the history is typical and there is no

heart disease) or arrhythmia (if the ECG shows, e.g. a sinus bradycardia < 40 beats per minute, pauses > 3 seconds, Mobitz II second or third degree block or rapid paroxysmal ventricular or supraventricular tachycardia). The remaining patients are divided into those with a suspected diagnosis (either cardiac or neurally mediated) and those with unexplained syncope.

Features suggestive of cardiac syncope include the presence of structural heart disease, symptoms during exercise or when supine, symptoms associated with palpitations or an abnormal ECG. Tests for suspected cardiac syncope include echocardiography (which is rarely diagnostic but helps to risk-stratify patients) and prolonged ECG monitoring (a 24-hour ECG will only be helpful if symptoms are very frequent; an external or implantable loop recorder may be required). Electrophysiological studies are only undertaken if an arrhythmia is strongly suspected.

Features suggestive of neurally-mediated syncope include a long history, symptoms with prolonged standing or after exercise and symptoms associated with nausea or vomiting. Tests for suspected neurally-mediated syncope include carotid sinus massage (if not already performed) and head-up tilt testing with or without glyceryl trinitrate (Gieroba et al 2004). 24-hour blood pressure monitoring is useful to assess the need for medications and to detect post-prandial hypotension.

If symptoms remain unexplained following investigations, retake the history. The implantable loop recorder, which has a battery life of 18–24 months and which can be activated by the patient after the event, increasingly has a role here.

MANAGEMENT OF SYNCOPE

The management of the cardiac and neurological disorders which may cause syncope are discussed in the relevant chapters of this book.

Orthostatic hypotension

This is diagnosed when there is a 20 mmHg fall in systolic blood pressure or a fall in systolic blood pressure to less than 90 mmHg on standing. Patients should receive advice on avoiding sudden postural change, severe exertion, etc. Support hosiery is often recommended but poorly tolerated. Hypotensive medications should be reviewed (unfortunately, these patients often have a combination of orthostatic hypotension and supine hypertension – more research is needed in this area). Encouraging salt intake and raising the head of the bed may be appropriate in selected patients. If non-pharmacological methods fail, fludrocortisone may be considered if there are no contraindications. Midodrine (an unlicenced sympathetic vasoconstrictor) is occasionally given in centres specializing in this condition (Mathias & Kimber 1998).

Vasovagal syncope

The head-up tilt test is deemed diagnostic of vasovagal syncope if, in the absence of a cardiac cause for symptoms, the patient develops symptomatic hypotension with or without bradycardia. The pathogenesis of vasovagal syncope is not known. The mainstay of treatment is again explanation and advice on trigger events. Modification of hypotensive medications may be necessary. Isometric counterpressure manoeuvres (e.g. leg crossing and handgrip) may be helpful in selected patients (Krediet et al 2002). A number of therapeutic interventions have been used to treat recurrent vasovagal syncope but there have been few randomized controlled trials and even fewer looking specifically at older individuals. Cardiac pacing may be of benefit in a minority of patients who have a profound bradycardia or asystole during tilt-induced syncope (ESC 2004).

Carotid sinus syndrome

Abnormal responses to carotid sinus massage are cardioinhibitory (> 3 seconds asystole), vasodepressor (> 50 mmHg fall in systolic BP) or mixed. Carotid sinus syndrome is diagnosed if there is an abnormal response to carotid sinus massage and symptoms are reproduced or if there is an abnormal response and no other cause for symptoms (ESC 2004). Cardioinhibition is successfully treated with dual-chamber cardiac pacing, while the treatment of vasodepression remains unsatisfactory (McIntosh & Kenny 1994).

SYNCOPE AND DRIVING (see Ch. 10)

Remember to ask whether your patient drives a car! The DVLA guidelines divide patients without a cardiac or neurological cause for loss of consciousness into five categories. No driving restrictions are placed upon patients with a simple faint provided that the 3 Ps (provocation/prodrome/postural) apply on each occasion (DVLA).

DIZZINESS

'There can be few physicians so dedicated to their art that they do not experience a slight decline in spirits on learning that their patient's complaint is of giddiness.'

(Matthews 1975)

Table 23.1   Systems symptoms are arising from

	System	Symptom
a. Pre-syncope	Cardiovascular	This is the feeling of an impending faint often associated with pallor and relieved by sitting down. This suggests cerebral hypoperfusion due to hypotension, i.e. a cardiovascular cause
b. Vertigo	Peripheral or central vestibular	This is an illusion of movement (usually rotation – the word vertigo comes from the Latin *vere* meaning to turn). It suggests a lesion anywhere between the labyrinth of the inner ear (peripheral vestibular system) and the central vestibular system which includes the VIIIth nerve, vestibular nuclei and vestibulo-cerebellum. It occurs when there is an asymmetry in the input to the vestibular nuclei from the two sides
c. Disequilibrium	Gait disorder (Nutt & Marsden 1993)	This is a feeling of unsteadiness or veering when upright. This is the commonest type of dizziness seen

THE SCOPE OF THE PROBLEM

The prevalence of dizziness increases with age. In the USA it is the most common cause of primary care consultations for patients aged over 75 years (Sloane & Baloh 1989). Indeed, most dizzy patients are managed by their general practitioners. Older individuals are under-referred for a specialist opinion despite having more treatable disease and having had their symptoms for longer at diagnosis than their younger counterparts (Bird & Beynon 1998). Dizziness is associated with falls (with their attendant complications), syncope and a negative impact on quality of life and functional activity (Lawson et al 1999).

WHY IS IT SO DIFFICULT TO MAKE A DIAGNOSIS?

Faced with a dizzy patient, the problems are:

1. The patient has difficulty describing the symptom; many older patients have more than one type of dizzy symptom arising from different systems (usually a gait disorder and something else).
2. The list of differential diagnoses is depressingly long.
3. There is a misconception that there is no effective treatment anyway.

The solutions are:

1. Try to establish which system or systems the symptoms are arising from by the description of the dizzy sensation, associated symptoms and precipitating circumstances (Table 23.1).
2. Having identified the system that the symptoms are arising from, the potential causes should be easier to remember! Doctors often worry that they may be missing a central vestibular lesion but these are far less common than peripheral lesions and are invariably associated with other neurological signs.

Causes of dizziness are shown in Figure 23.2.

INVESTIGATION OF DIZZINESS

A thorough clinical evaluation will identify the cause (or causes) of dizziness in most elderly patients and will guide further investigation (Goebel 2001). The authors use the flow diagram in Figure 23.3 when investigating dizziness.

Notes on investigation

1. If the patient describes vertigo, ask about associated symptoms (tinnitus or deafness suggest a lesion in the ear; neurological symptoms a central cause). Ask about the duration of symptoms (benign paroxysmal positional vertigo lasts seconds, transient ischaemic attacks – minutes and Ménière's – hours). Ask about precipitating movements or circumstances in which the dizzy spells arise. Ask about the first ever episode of vertigo and the pattern of any subsequent

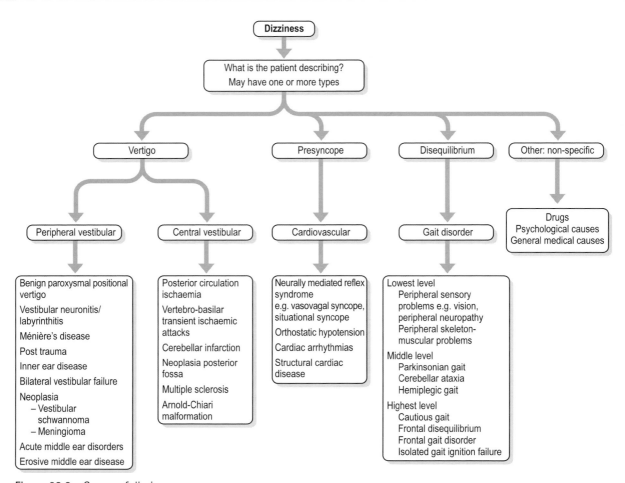

Figure 23.2   Causes of dizziness.

vertigo. Peripheral vestibular symptoms (e.g. due to vestibular neuronitis) usually resolve as a result of vestibular compensation. If this compensation process is inadequate, patients may experience ongoing symptoms associated with repeated quick head movements or in busy visual surroundings, such as supermarkets.

2. Include thorough examinations of the cardiovascular and neurological systems. Record visual acuity, assess gait and perform Romberg's test with both eyes open and eyes closed (this tests somatosensation and proprioception). Examine the eardrums. Look for sustained nystagmus. Down, upbeat or direction changing nystagmus is a central vestibular sign; horizontal nystagmus from a peripheral vestibular lesion is only seen immediately after an acute

lesion and is suppressed by optic fixation (Frenzel glasses block fixation and may be helpful). Assess saccades by asking the patient to look from your nose to a finger held up on each side without head movement. Abnormalities (such as the eyes not moving together or repeated under- or over-shooting of the target) are seen in central lesions. Smooth pursuit (the ability to track an object) is usually broken and, therefore, less helpful in older subjects. The vestibular ocular reflex (VOR) compensates for head movements by moving the eyes in the opposite direction to the head movement. This can be tested using dynamic head thrust, dynamic visual acuity and head shaking nystagmus (Halmagyi 2005). In the dynamic head thrust test, the examiner watches for catch-up saccades induced by a quick head movement

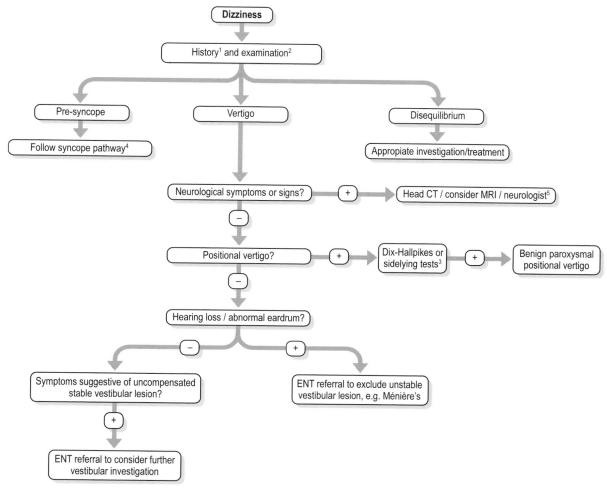

Figure 23.3 Investigating dizziness. ([1-5] See Notes on investigation in text.)

while the patient fixates on the examiner's nose – it is more difficult in older subjects due to restrictions in neck movement. Abnormalities suggest peripheral vestibular hypofunction. Dynamic visual acuity is a measure of visual acuity during horizontal head movement. A loss of acuity amounting to three or more lines on an eye chart when the head is in motion at a frequency of 2 Hz is suggestive of vestibular hypofunction. The head shaking nystagmus test involves oscillating the patient's head 20 times at 2 Hz while they are wearing Frenzel glasses. If this elicits nystagmus it suggests vestibular asymmetry between the two horizontal semicircular canals.

3. This is a test for benign paroxysmal positional vertigo and involves moving the patient from the sitting to the so-called head-hanging position while looking for characteristic symptoms and signs. The test is repeated on the right and left sides (Furman & Cass 1999) (Fig. 23.4). The sidelying test is a useful alternative in frailer patients (Fig. 23.5).

4. Head-up tilt is less likely to be positive with pre-syncope than with syncope (Fitzpatrick et al 1996). Carotid sinus massage should only be performed if the patient additionally has syncope, since dizziness is not an indication for pacing.

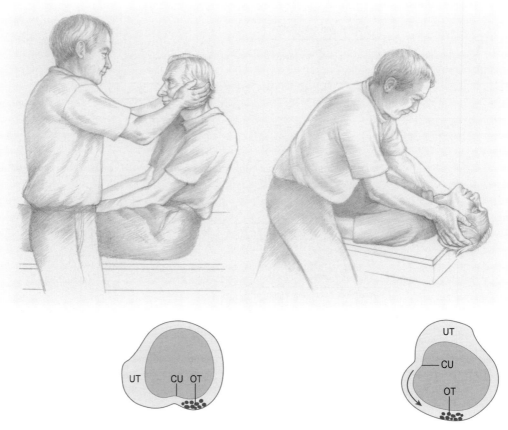

Figure 23.4 Test for benign paroxysmal positional vertigo that involves moving the patient from the sitting to the so-called head-hanging position, while looking for characteristic symptoms and signs. CU, cupula; OT, otoconia; UT, utricle.

5. Remember that cerebellar haemorrhage or infarct may not show up on computed tomography (CT); magnetic resonance imaging (MRI) is the investigation of choice for imaging the posterior fossa (Halmagyi 2005).

MANAGEMENT OF DIZZINESS

The management of presyncope is as for syncope. Gait disorders are covered elsewhere in this book (see Ch. 24). There are specific treatments for certain causes of vertigo such as Ménière's disease and benign paroxysmal positional vertigo (discussed below). In patients with an episode of peripheral vertigo due to, for example vestibular neuronitis, antiemetics and vestibular sedatives may be required in the short term to control symptoms. These should not be continued in the long term as they impair the compensation process. Vestibular rehabilitation is effective for vestibular hypofunction whether it is unilateral, for example after an episode of vestibular neuronitis or bilateral, for example post gentamicin (Shepard et al 1993). Central vestibular lesions often require a multidisciplinary team approach as the rehabilitation process is much slower than for peripheral lesions. Psychological problems may need to be addressed (Jacob & Cass 2003).

Benign paroxysmal positional vertigo (BPPV)

This may follow trauma or vestibular neuronitis but is often idiopathic. Patients with this condition experience transient severe vertigo or a sensation

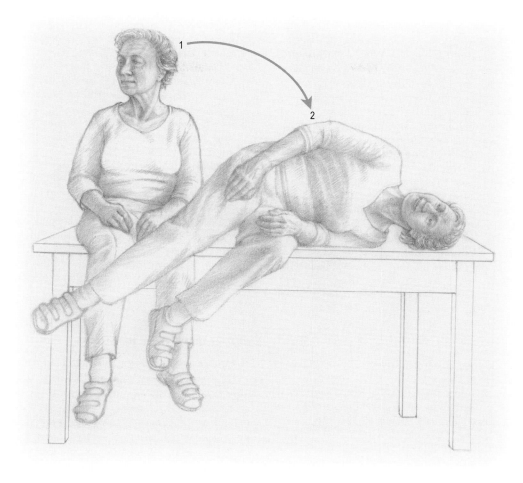

Figure 23.5 The sidelying test for benign paroxysmal positional vertigo.

of falling backwards with certain head movements (e.g. turning in bed and looking up – 'top shelf vertigo'). Debris in the posterior semicircular canal (usually) causes displacement of the cupula during these head movements. The condition can be successfully treated with canalith repositioning manoeuvres (e.g. Epley's) which disperse the debris (Epley 1992).

REFERENCES

*** *Essential reading;* ** *recommended reading;* * *interesting but not vital*

Bird J C, Beynon G J 1998 An analysis of referral patterns for dizziness in the primary care setting. British Journal of General Practice 48:1828–1832 *

Department of Health 2005 National Service Framework. Coronary heart disease, Ch. 8. DoH, London. Online. Available: http://www.dh.gov.uk ***

Driver and Vehicle Licensing Agency. Medical rules. Online. Available: http://www.dvla.gov.uk **

Epley J M 1992 The canalith repositioning procedure: for treatment of benign paroxysmal positional vertigo. Otolaryngology – Head and Neck Surgery 107:399–404 *

European Society of Cardiology (ESC) 2004 Taskforce on syncope. Guidelines on management (diagnosis and treatment) of syncope – update 2004. European Society of Cardiology. Europace 6:467–537. Online. Available: http://www.escardio.org ***

Fitzpatrick A P, Lee R J, Epstein L M et al 1996 Effect of patient characteristics on the yield of prolonged baseline head-up tilt testing and the additional yield of drug provocation. Heart 76:406–411 *

Furman J M, Cass S P 1999 Benign paroxysmal positional vertigo. New England Journal of Medicine 341:1590–1596 *

Gieroba Z J, Newton J L, Parry S W et al 2004 Unprovoked and glyceryl trinitrate-provoked head-up tilt table test is safe in older people: a review of 10 years' experience. Journal of the American Geriatrics Society 52:1913–1915 *

Goebel J 2001 Ten-minute examination of the dizzy patient. Seminars in Neurology 21:392–398 **

Halmagyi G M 2005 Diagnosis and management of vertigo. Clinical Medicine 5:159–165 **

Jacob R, Cass S 2003 Psychiatric consequences of vestibular dysfunction. In: Luxon L, Martini A, Furman J et al (eds) Textbook of audiological medicine. Martin Dunitz/Taylor & Francis, London, p 869–888 **

Kapoor W N 1996 Is syncope a risk factor for poor outcomes? Comparison of patients with and without syncope. American Journal of Medicine 100: 646–655 *

Kapoor W, Snustad D, Peterson J et al 1986 Syncope in the elderly. American Journal of Medicine 80: 419–428 *

Krediet P, van Dijk N, Linzer M et al 2002 Management of vasovagal syncope: controlling or aborting faints by leg crossing and muscle tensing. Circulation 106:1684–1689 *

Lawson J, Fitzgerald J, Birchall J et al 1999 Diagnosis of geriatric patients with severe dizziness. Journal of the American Geriatrics Society 47:12–17 **

Linzer M, Pontinen M, Gold D T et al 1991 Impairment of physical and psychosocial function in recurrent syncope. Journal of Clinical Epidemiology 44:1037–1043 *

Lipsitz L A, Wei J Y, Rowe J W 1985 Syncope in an elderly, institutionalised population: prevalence, incidence and associated risk. Quarterly Journal of Medicine 55:45–55 *

McIntosh S J, Kenny R A 1994 Carotid sinus syndrome in the elderly. Journal of the Royal Society of Medicine 87:798–800

McIntosh S, da Costa D, Kenny R A 1993 Benefits of an integrated approach to the investigation of dizziness, falls and syncope in elderly patients referred to a syncope clinic. Age and Ageing 22:53–58 *

Mathias C J, Kimber J R 1998 Treatment of postural hypotension. Journal of Neurology, Neurosurgery and Psychiatry 65:285–289

Matthews W B 1975 Practical neurology, 3rd edn. Blackwell Scientific, London *

Nutt J G, Marsden C D 1993 Human walking and higher-level gait disorders, particularly in the elderly. Neurology 43:268–279 **

Parry S W, Richardson D A, O'Shea D et al 2000 Diagnosis of carotid sinus hypersensitivity in older adults: carotid sinus massage in the upright position is essential. Heart 83:22–23 *

Richardson D A, Bexton R, Shaw F E et al 2000 Complications of carotid sinus massage – a prospective series of older patients. Age and Ageing 29:413–417 **

Shaw F E, Kenny R A 1997 The overlap between falls and syncope in the elderly. Postgraduate Medical Journal 73:635–639 **

Shepard N T, Telian S A, Smith-Wheelock M et al 1993 Vestibular and balance rehabilitation therapy. Annals of Otology, Rhinology and Laryngology 102:198–205 **

Sloane P D, Baloh R W 1989 Persistent dizziness in geriatric patients. Journal of the American Geriatrics Society 37:1031–1038 *

Tinetti M E, Speechley M 1989 Prevention of falls among the elderly. New England Journal of Medicine 320:1055–1059 *

RECOMMENDED READING

*** Recommended reading; * interesting but not vital*

Alexander N B 1996 Gait disorders in older adults. Journal of the American Geriatrics Society 44: 434–451 **

Baloh R W 1998 Vertigo. Lancet 352:1841–1846 *

Jansen R W M M, Lipsitz L A 1995 Postprandial hypotension: epidemiology, pathophysiology and clinical management. Annals of Internal Medicine 122:286–295 *

Kaufmann H, Wieling W (eds) 2004 Management of reflex syncope. Clinical Autonomic Research 14(Suppl 1) **

Kenny R A 1996 Syncope in the older patient. Chapman & Hall, London **

SELF-ASSESSMENT QUESTION

1. Are the following statements true or false?
   a. Vertebrobasilar ischaemia often causes isolated vertigo
   b. Benign paroxysmal positional vertigo is amenable to treatment
   c. Epilepsy is a common cause of syncope
   d. Patients with a simple faint should have no driving restrictions placed upon them

SECTION 1

Central nervous system

Chapter 24

Gait disorders

Jim George

INTRODUCTION

Assessment of gait (defined as the manner or style of walking) in the elderly patient should be an integral and essential part of the geriatrician's examination routine. Gait disorders contribute to common clinical presentations of elderly people, (e.g. immobility, falls and fractured neck of femur) and may result from pathologies, which are more common in old people (such as cerebrovascular disease, Parkinson's disease, dementia and osteo-arthritis). Gait and balance are inextricably linked and adequate gait and balance are both required for safe mobility. Impairment of mobility is common in old people with a prevalence of 9–42% in the community, 50–65% in nursing homes and 40–65% in hospital populations (Macknight & Rockwood 1995).

GAIT CHANGES WITH AGEING

Two major changes in the gait of healthy old people have been demonstrated (Whittle 2006):

1. Slowing of gait with reduction of stride length
2. Postural instability, with increased sway while standing still and deviation from a straight line when walking

In the past these gait changes with old age were probably exaggerated as it is difficult to rule out subclinical disease in very elderly subjects. A perfectly normal gait has been observed in 18% of a community-living sample aged between 88 years and 96 years (Bloem et al 1992). It has become apparent that so-called 'senile' gait disorder, which is characterized by caution and shorter strides and can occur in up to 24% of elderly people, is not due to age but to underlying neurological syndromes or stroke (see Table 24.1).

CLINICAL EXAMINATION OF GAIT

The gait may be the only abnormality present on clinical examination and it may lead you to the correct clinical diagnosis by encouraging you to look for the appropriate clinical association on the

Table 24.1 High-level gait disorders in the elderly (Nutt et al 1993)

Clinical classifications	Previous terms	Characteristics				Lesion
		Disequilibrium	Hesitancy	Wide base	Short steps and freezing	
1. Cautious	Elderly gait 'Senile gait'	–	–	+	+	Very non-specific Can be central nervous system or peripheral nervous system May be related to psychological factors – 'loss of confidence'
2. Disequilibrium	Tottering Gait apraxia Frontal ataxia	++	+/–	+/–	+/–	Midbrain Basal ganglia Frontal lobe
3. Isolated gait ignition disorder	Gait apraxia	–	++	–	–	Frontal lobe and basal ganglia
4. Frontal gait disorder	Marche à petit pas Magnetic gait apraxia Lower half parkinsonism	–	++	–	+	Frontal lobe

rest of the examination. Ask the patient to walk and observe for symmetry, size of the paces, posture, arm swing, distance between the feet, movement of the knees, pelvis and shoulders. This is an appropriate time to do a formal 'get up and go' test (see later).

If possible, ask the patient to walk as if on a tightrope (tandem gait) to test for a mild degree of ataxia. Ask the patient to stand with feet together and then close their eyes (Romberg's test). In a positive Romberg's test the subject is able to stand with eyes open but falls with eyes closed and it indicates a loss of joint position sense.

Finally, examine footwear for comfort and suitability, including the soles for abnormal wear, and examine any walking aids for length and condition (Mulley 1988).

To examine gait properly, the clinician needs adequate space, ideally at least 5 metres. Assessment of gait should involve the physiotherapist and occupational therapist. The day hospital may be a better environment rather than a busy medical out-patient department.

Gait disorders in elderly people may be classified into high-, middle- and low-level gait disorders (Box 24.1).

HIGH-LEVEL GAIT DISORDERS

Many of the gait disturbances found in elderly people, and in those with dementia, cannot be attributed to classical neurological disease or to normal ageing. Descriptions of such gait disorders include 'marche à petit pas', gait apraxia and 'senile' gait. Nutt et al (1993) describe a clinical classification of gait disorders. High-level gait disorders can be divided into four main types with differing aetiologies (Table 24.1). *Cautious gait* is described as a wide-based gait with a markedly shortened stride but maintenance of balance. *Disequilibrium syndrome* is associated with severe disturbance of balance. *Isolated gait ignition failure* is characterized by severe start/turn hesitation and freezing, but without other features of Parkinson's disease and with an otherwise normal

Box 24.1 Clinical classification of gait disorders (Nutt et al 1993)

High level
- Cautious gait
- Disequilibrium gait
- Isolated gait ignition disorder
- Frontal gait disorder

Middle level
- Spastic gait
- Hemiparetic gait
- Parkinsonian gait
- Choreiform gait
- Cerebellar ataxic gait

Low level
- Peripheral motor
  - arthritic
  - myopathic
  - neuropathic
- Peripheral sensory
  - sensory ataxia
  - visual ataxia

gait. *Frontal gait disorder* contains features of the other gait disorders in combination, including hesitation and freezing with poor balance and sometimes a wide base with a shortened stride.

Higher-level gait disorders and their possible causes are summarized in Table 24.1. The term 'senile gait disorder' is not recommended, as it is not descriptive and suggests that the cause is invariably idiopathic.

MIDDLE-LEVEL GAIT DISORDERS

At the middle level, the central nervous system selects the postural and locomotor responses but the execution is faulty. Middle-level gait disorders include hemiplegic gait with circumduction of the leg and hip adduction, and parkinsonian gait with small shuffling steps, hesitation, festination and absent arm swing.

Cerebellar ataxic gait is characterized by a wide base, increased sway and tendency to fall, particularly on turning.

LOW-LEVEL GAIT DISORDERS

Loss of proprioception leads to a sensory ataxic gait. Proximal myopathies may lead to a 'waddling' gait. 'Foot drop' leads to exaggerated hip flexion and lifting of the foot (high steppage gait) followed by 'foot slap'. Various arthropathies and foot disorders can cause abnormal gait due to difficulties with weight bearing, or due to a limited range of movement of the joints.

FUNCTIONAL ASSESSMENT OF GAIT

Geriatric assessment is not just about detecting disease, but also should encompass assessment of function as a basis for rehabilitation. Tinnetti (1986) explains that limiting the assessment of mobility problems to the standard physical examination and paraclinical tests is inadequate in elderly people. Gait disorders in older people often have multiple aetiologies. There is often a poor relationship between clinical signs and functional deficits. It is functional impairment which is more likely to predict falls (Tinetti et al 1994) and mobility problems. A good test of gait function should be relevant, sensible, sensitive and valid (Wade 1992). In this section we will limit discussion to tests which fulfil these criteria. Macknight & Rockwood (1995) give an excellent review of gait and mobility scales. Most of the tests described require no special equipment and are suitable as outcome measures in research or audit projects.

BALANCE AND MOBILITY SCALES

In 1986, Tinetti developed a performance orientated mobility assessment (POMA) intended for assessing older adults and, in particular, to identify those at risk of falls (Tinetti 1986). It is an objective and standardized assessment and the 'clinical equivalent of a gait and balance laboratory'. It includes simple tests of balance, including standing on one leg, as well as observation of gait. Each item is scored on an ordinal scale and summed to give a total of 24 or 40 (depending on the version used).

The functional ambulation classification is a gait measure originally developed in Boston but used in the UK, particularly for stroke patients. It is a simple 0–5 scale with 0 as non-ambulant and 5 as independently mobile. A more sophisticated scale which is more discriminative is the Rivermead Mobility Index (Wade 1992). This concentrates on activities that are considered likely to be undertaken by most people. These range from being able to turn over in bed at one extreme to a fast walk or run of 10 metres at the other extreme. A specific Elderly Mobility Scale (EMS) has been devised, which is particularly used by physiotherapists. This scale correlates well with the Barthel disability scale, but has poor predictive validity for discharge destination (Prosser & Canby 1997) (see Box 24.2).

TIMED WALK

The simple measurement of time taken to walk, for example, 10 metres at normal speed, using a walking aid if necessary, has been widely used in studies of frailty, falls, medical treatment and rehabilitation (Macknight & Rockwood 1995). This simple test correlates well with balance, limb power, fear of falling, stroke outcomes and general health.

'GET UP AND GO' TEST

The 'get up and go' test was originally developed in an English gait laboratory and refined in a Canadian geriatric day hospital (Macknight & Rockwood 1995). The test involves the subject rising from a chair, walking a distance of 3 metres, turning, walking back to the chair and sitting down again.

This simple test can be used at the bedside and demonstrates the subject's balance, gait, proximal muscle strength, speed and safety. A simple refinement is to time the test and the timed 'get up and go' is a good predictor of falls in old people living at home (Okumiya et al 1998). A time of 15 seconds or more identifies patients with a high risk of falling (Whitney et al 2005). This test is recommended for all patients reporting even a single fall to identify those who might benefit from a more in-depth interdisciplinary assessment (AGS/BGS on Falls Prevention 2001).

GAIT QUALITY

A criticism of the previous scales is that they do not attempt to measure gait quality. They tend to measure merely the ability to get from A to B. A poor quality gait may be unsafe, cause joint pain or may cause embarrassment to the elderly person. Physiotherapists will strive to help the patient achieve as normal a gait as possible, not just a purely functional gait. The Rivermead Visual Gait Assessment (RVGA) is a simple four point gait assessment scale which measures gait quality and is suitable for clinical use (Lord et al 1998).

LABORATORY–BASED GAIT ANALYSIS

There are many sophisticated ways of assessing gait using special walkways and video analysis to measure stride length and speed, including EMG analysis. These methods have limited clinical application (Wade 1992) However, the recent development of miniature, inexpensive accelerometer sensors, currently used mainly in research, have potential use in the clinical setting for a more objective assessment of gait and balance (Culhane et al 2005).

TREATMENT AND REHABILITATION OF GAIT DISORDERS IN THE ELDERLY

About one-quarter of gait disorders presenting in elderly patients may be treatable (Alexander 1996). This includes previously unrecognized Parkinson's disease, metabolic disturbances, intracranial tumours, normal pressure hydrocephalus, myelopathy due to compression of the spinal cord,

Box 24.3 Potentially treatable gait disorders in old age (Alexander 1996)

- Vitamin B12 deficiency
- Folate deficiency
- Hyperthyroidism, hypothyroidism
- Parkinson's disease
- Cervical myelopathy
- Normal pressure hydrocephalus
- Subdural haematoma
- Brain tumours
- Osteoarthritis
- Rheumatoid arthritis
- Stroke
- Peripheral neuropathy
- Proximal myopathy, particularly due to osteomalacia
- Drugs, e.g. major tranquilizers and hypnotics

inflammatory polyneuropathy, drug-related gait disorders and depression. Most of the information on treatment and rehabilitation of gait disorders in the elderly is from retrospective case studies. There are few controlled prospective studies and no randomized studies.

Positive outcomes with treatment, however, are reported with a large number of conditions (Box 24.3). Surgery for compressive cervical myelopathy and lumbar stenosis may improve gait in the individual patient. Similarly, shunting can improve the gait in normal pressure hydrocephalus, but this improvement may only be maintained in 5–20% of patients. Targeted exercise regimens aimed at strengthening leg muscles, improving joint flexibility and balance training have been shown to significantly improve gait and balance in frail elderly subjects (Hu & Woollacott 1996). Unfortunately, physiotherapy for high-level gait disorders in older people is often disappointing.

It is helpful to take a more pragmatic approach and advise on appropriate footwear and the use of suitable walking aids and environmental modification in order to prevent falls. Footwear should be non-slip with minimal heel lift. Use of a walking stick in the contralateral hand may help in relieving ipsilateral hip pain or, alternatively, using a walking stick in the ipsilateral hand may sometimes reduce the forces acting on the hip.

RESEARCH IN GAIT FOR THE SPECIALIST REGISTRAR

'Choose something common and you will find little is known about it.'

(H. Head)

The clinical assessment of gait is still very subjective, but sophisticated laboratory gait analysis, although objective, has not yet found a role in clinical practice. Further research is needed to refine our clinical assessment and to investigate further the community prevalence of gait disorders and their relationship to disease and the value of rehabilitation in improving outcomes, including falls and hospitalization. Rehabilitation techniques to improve the common high-level gait disorders are badly needed in older people.

CONCLUSION

The trainee should be able to:

1. Perform a clinical and functional assessment of gait
2. Recognize common abnormalities of gait and identify the probable cause, e.g. Parkinson's disease, frontal gait disorder
3. Be aware of physiotherapy techniques for treatment of gait disorders and how improvement can be measured

Assessment of gait, as with the overall assessment of older patients, should be functional as well as clinical and should provide the basis for successful rehabilitation.

Key points

1. Abnormal gait is not a feature of normal ageing and may be a predictor for falls.
2. About one-quarter of gait disturbances in elderly patients are treatable.
3. Gait can be assessed using simple clinical tests. Sophisticated gait analysis in the laboratory is mainly a research tool.
4. The 'get up and go test' is a simple clinical and functional test which is practical in old people.
5. More research is needed to identify the prevalence of gait problems in the community and to evaluate physiotherapy treatments.

REFERENCES

*** *Essential reading; ** recommended reading; * interesting but not vital*

Alexander N B 1996 Gait disorders in older adults. Journal of the American Geriatrics Society 44: 434–451 ***

American Geriatrics Society/British Geriatrics Society (AGS/BGS) on Falls Prevention 2001 Guidelines for the prevention of falls in older persons. Journal of the American Geriatrics Society 49:664–672 ***

Bloem B R, Haan J, Lagany A M et al 1992 An investigation of gait in elderly subjects over 88 years of age. Journal of Geriatric Psychiatry and Neurology 5:78–84 *

Culhane K M, O'Connor M, Lyons D et al 2005 Accelerometers in rehabilitation medicine for older adults. Age and Ageing 34:556–560 *

Hu M H, Woollacott 1996 Balance evaluation, training and rehabilitation of frail fallers. Reviews in Clinical Gerontology 6:85–99 *

Lord S E, Halligan P W, Wade D T 1998 Visual gait analysis: the development of a clinical assessment and scale. Clinical Rehabilitation 12:107–119 **

Macknight C, Rockwood K 1995 Assessing mobility in elderly people. A review of performance-based measures of balance, gait and mobility for bedside use. Reviews in Clinical Gerontology 5:464–486 ***

Mulley G P 1988 Everyday aids and applicances. Walking sticks. British Medical Journal 296:475–476 **

Nutt J G, Marsden C D, Thompson P D 1993 Human walking and higher level gait disorders particularly in the elderly. Neurology 43:268–279 ***

Okumiya K, Matsubayashi K, Nakamura T et al 1998 The timed 'up and go' test as a useful predictor of falls in community-dwelling older people. Journal of the American Geriatrics Society 46:928–929 *

Prosser L, Canby A 1997 Further validation of the Elderly Mobility Scale for measurement of mobility of hospitalised elderly people. Clinical Rehabilitation 11:338–343 *

Tinetti M E 1986 Performance-orientated assessment of mobility problems in elderly patients. Journal of the American Geriatrics Society 34:119–126 *

Tinetti M E, Baker D I, Mavay G et al 1994 A multifactorial intervention to reduce the risk of falling among elderly people living in the community. New England Journal of Medicine 331:821–827 **

Wade D T 1992 Measurement in neurological rehabilitation. Oxford University Press, Oxford *

Whitney J C, Lord S R, Close J T 2005 Streamlining assessment and intervention in a falls clinic using the timed up and go test and physiological profile assessments. Age and Ageing 34:567–571 *

Whittle M 2006 Gait analysis – an introduction, 4th edn. Butterworth Heinemann, Edinburgh ***

RECOMMMENDED READING

Bronstein A M, Brandt T, Woolacot M et al (eds) 2004 Clinical disorders of balance, posture and gait, 2nd edn. Arnold, London, especially Chs 4, 6, 21

Whittle M 2006 Gait analysis – an introduction, 4th edn. Butterworth Heinemann, Edinburgh

Acknowledgment

I wish to acknowledge the valuable contribution made by Dr Simon Lee to the earlier version of this chapter.

SELF–ASSESSMENT QUESTION

1. Are the following true or false?
   a. Parkinson's disease classically causes a high-level gait disorder
   b. Senile gait disorder is an accepted clinical entity
   c. Gait apraxia is associated with normal leg movement and power
   d. Foot drop causes a middle-level gait disorder
   e. Computerized gait analysis is superior to clinical assessment in detecting treatable gait disorders

SECTION 2

Cardiovascular system

Chapter 25

When to treat hypertension

Nigel S. Beckett

Elderly patients are often under-represented or excluded from clinical trials – even in conditions that predominately affect this age group (heart failure being a good example). Hypertension is common in elderly people, for which there is very good trial evidence of benefit from treatment. Many trials (such as those shown in Table 25.1) show that treating elderly patients who are hypertensive reduces the chance of them having a stroke. So do we simply have to make sure of a diagnosis of sustained hypertension, agree on a level of blood pressure as 'hypertensive' and then start treatment?

Elderly people, by whatever criteria we use, (age of retirement, over 70 years, etc.) are a heterogeneous group. There is good evidence from well-designed and well-conducted clinical trials for treating a fit elderly person up to the age of 80 years. However, many doctors may not treat a 74-year-old woman in a nursing home who has had two strokes and thus has limited mobility, is troubled with urinary incontinence and has marked cognitive impairment secondary to vascular dementia. This scenario may be thought to be at the extreme end of a spectrum, but where is the dividing line? What criteria should we use – the level of blood pressure, the overall risk to the patient, chronological age or even biological age? Is it simply fair to say 'when the benefits outweigh the risks'? What are the risks, what are the benefits? What evidence do we have to help with the question: 'when should we treat hypertension in older people?'

LEVEL OF BLOOD PRESSURE

Below the age of 75 years, there is a positive linear relationship between the relative risk of both stroke and coronary heart disease (CHD) and increasing diastolic blood pressure (over the range of about 76 to 105 mmHg). The relative risk of stroke between the highest (110 mmHg) and lowest (69 mmHg) is between 10 and 12 times, while the corresponding value for CHD is about 4 times. Lowering the casual diastolic blood pressure by only 7.5 mmHg is associated with a 46% decrease

Table 25.1 Level of blood pressure at entry and achieved blood pressure on active treatment in six major intervention trials in elderly subjects

	C+W[a]	EWPHE[b]	STOP-H[c]	MRC[d]	SHEP[e]	Syst-Eur[f]
SBP criteria for entry	> 170	160–239	180–230	160–209	160–219	160–219
DBP criteria for entry	> 105	90–119	90–120	< 115	< 90	< 95
BP at entry	196/99	182/101	195/102	185/91	170/77	174/85
BP obtained on active Rx	162/78	149/85	167/87	152/79	144/68	151/78

SBP = systolic blood pressure, DBP = diastolic blood pressure, Rx = treatment
[a]Coope & Warrender 1986; [b]Amery et al 1985, [c]Dahlof et al 1991; [d]MRC Working Party 1992; [e]Probstfield et al 1989, Cooperative Research Group 1991; [f]Staessen et al 1997

in the risk of stroke and a 29% decrease in the risk of CHD. If the relationships between risk and blood pressure are assumed to be linear, this equates in round figures to a reduction in risk of 6% for stroke and 4% for CHD for each 1 mmHg decrease in diastolic blood pressure. However, many of these data are based on studies of men, while the geriatrician sees more women than men. Although there would seem to be no reason to expect a different form of relationship between risk and casual diastolic blood pressure in women, the absolute values may vary. Indeed, studies of women have shown that they tolerate hypertension better then men and have lower coronary mortality rates with any level of hypertension (Kannel 1997, Pocock et al 2001).

Treatment decisions must not be based solely on diastolic pressure. Indeed, as a predicator of having a cardiovascular event, diastolic blood pressure is poor over the age of 50 years. Systolic pressure is a better predictor of morbidity and mortality. Because of arterial changes with age that lead to an age-related linear increase in systolic blood pressure, 65–75% of those over 65 years who have hypertension have isolated systolic hypertension (ISH). The pulse pressure (the difference between the systolic and diastolic pressure) may be an even better predictor. The higher the pulse pressure, i.e. the greater the difference between the systolic and diastolic readings, the greater the risk. However, irrespective of whether this is the case, we do not have drugs that specifically reduce the pulse pressure by effectively lowering systolic blood pressure without lowering diastolic pressure.

Large well-designed intervention trials and meta-analyses all show good evidence for benefit from treatment. Moreover, there is a strong consistency of results in the trials with percentage reductions in strokes ranging from 25–47%. The benefits for treatment have also been shown for ISH. The SHEP trial showed a 36% reduction in stroke events, a 27% reduction in cardiac events and a 32% reduction in all cardiovascular events. The absolute benefit was such that treating 33 patients for 5 years would prevent one event. In the Syst-Eur trial, active treatment reduced stroke events by 42% and the incidence of all cardiovascular complications by 31%. In absolute terms, treating 34 patients for 5 years would prevent one stroke and treating 19 patients for 5 years would prevent one major cardiovascular event.

When one considers the level of blood pressure (BP) at entry for the various trials, the evidence supports treatment for systolic BP equal to or above 160 mmHg and diastolic above 90 mmHg (Table 25.1). But, what should we do for pressures between 140 and 159 mmHg systolic? The current accepted definition of ISH is a systolic above 140 mmHg with a diastolic below 90 mmHg. However, to date, there is no randomized controlled trial evidence for making treatment decisions based on these levels alone. The guidelines on when to treat such individuals are based on an assessment of the level of their cardiovascular disease (CVD) risk. The risk tables recently published by the Joint British Societies (2005) only go up to the age of 69 years. Over the age of 60 years, anyone with a systolic blood pressure of 140 mmHg (even with a fairly low total cholesterol to high

Table 25.2	Results of six major trials with patients over 80 years of age				
C+W	EWPHE	MRC (Elderly)	STOP-H	SHEP	Syst–Eur
No patients over 80 years	No benefit (155 patients over 80 years)	No patients over 80 years	No benefit (269 patients over 80 years)	Reduction of non-fatal stroke events Fatal events not reduced	Reduction of non-fatal stroke events Fatal events not reduced

density lipoprotein ratio) has a CVD risk of over 20% in the next 10 years. Therefore treatment is warranted, even in non-diabetic, non-smoking men – this constitutes a very large group.

Most epidemiological data have been based on the brachial artery blood pressure, though logically it is the pressure at the point of potential arterial disease (e.g. the aortic root or carotid arteries) that is relevant. This may not be a practical problem unless there is a plausible reason to expect a disproportional central–peripheral pressure augmentation, or if a particular intervention is claimed preferentially to alter central pressure.

A confounding factor in future studies is likely to be the means of determining brachial blood pressure. The advent of automated blood pressure recording devices and ambulatory monitoring, with the phasing out of mercury sphygmomanometers for health and safety reasons, will require a number of assumptions about the equivalence of historical blood pressure data with values measured by newer techniques. For example, the Hypertension Optimal Treatment (HOT) trial (Hansson et al 1998) used automated oscillometric measurement of brachial blood pressure.

have been recruited into intervention trials to evaluate clearly the benefits/risks of treatment (Table 25.2). A meta-analysis of patients over 80 years recruited to intervention trials over the last 15 years did show a benefit in reduction in stroke, major cardiovascular events and incidence of cardiac failure (Gueyffier et al 1999). However, there was an increase in mortality of around 6%, suggesting that there may well be a trade-off between benefit and risk when treating the over-80s. The Hypertension in the Very Elderly Trial (HYVET) pilot (Bulpitt et al 2003) gave similar results to the meta-analysis. The authors concluded that treatment of 1000 patients for 1 year may reduce stroke events by 19 (9 non-fatal) but may be associated with 20 extra (non-stroke) deaths. The HYVET main trial is continuing and will hopefully clarify this conundrum.

How are we to assess biological age? To date, indices such as skin elasticity, arcus and baldness have been examined but there is no validated system that assesses the biological age of an individual. One potential tool is the assessment of arterial compliance, reinforcing the adage that a 'man is as old as his arteries'.

AGE

One of the biggest risks for CVD, whether or not it is related to hypertension, is increasing age. Does this mean we should treat patients of all ages? One might argue that as the absolute risk in elderly people makes them a high-risk group purely from their age, as a group they would all benefit. Certainly the risk tables allude to this. However, epidemiological data for the over 80s suggest that those with higher blood pressure live longer. To date, very few patients over 80 years

OVERALL RISK

Can we make some assessment based on co-morbidity and the overall risk, taking into account an individual's risk profile? By the fact of their age, older people are in a high-risk group – even before additional factors such as being a smoker, target organ damage, presence of diabetes mellitus, left ventricular hypertrophy and hypercholesterolaemia are considered. All these increase the risk in an individual and should encourage the doctor to start treatment to lower blood pressure.

Table 25.3 Comparison of prevalence of risk factors and cardiovascular diseases in the general population, hypertensive older patients and patients recruited to trials

	General population[a] (> 65 years) (%)	Hypertensive[a,b] older patients (65–89 years) (%)	Elderly trial patients since 1990 (%)
Smoker	13 (m), 15 (w)	11 (m), 11 (w)	7.3–18
Physically inactive	31 (m), 37 (w)	40 (m), 56 (w)	NR
Overweight (BMI > 25 kg/m²)	67 (m), 50 (w)	76 (m), 69 (w)	On average 55
Cholesterol > 6.5 mmol/L	24 (m), 42 (w)	23 (m), 48 (w)	On average 30
Angina	17 (m), 13.5 (w)	12.2 (m), 16 (w)	10–12
History of myocardial infarction	12.5 (m), 6 (w)	11.9 (m), 4.6 (w)	1–5
History of stroke	8.3 (m), 6.9 (w)	9.5 (m), 4.9 (w)	1.5–3.5
Diabetes mellitus	27 (m), 27.1 (w)	20.1 (m), 15.2 (w)	10.1–10.5

[a] = based on Health Survey for England 1998, [b] = definition of hypertension > 140/90 mmHg, m = men, w = women, NR = not recorded.

Older patients recruited to intervention trials tend to be relatively fit. They smoke less, have a lower prevalence of coronary disease and diabetes mellitus and are less likely to have had a stroke than hypertensive subjects in community surveys (see Table 25.3). Elderly people at home may be at greater risk, as they have a greater prevalence of risk factors and thus should gain more benefit from drug treatment. Conversely, the greater prevalence of co-morbidity might make them more susceptible to side-effects. In intervention trials in elderly hypertensive patients, the absolute benefit in reduction in stroke is proportional to the risk of a stroke event – despite the fact that the relative risk reduction is constant across the trials and reduces in old age. The greater the risk of a stroke in the placebo group, the greater the absolute benefit from active treatment. However, it is likely that at some stage the benefit is lost: co-morbidity may result in death before any benefit of treatment can occur. Where that line is crossed is uncertain. Even the Joint British Societies' (2005) guidelines on the prevention of cardiovascular disease in clinical practice state that, for people over 70 years, the treatment of hypertension and raised lipid concentrations is a matter for individual clinical management.

However, one has to use common sense when considering the risk to benefit ratio. Even if the benefits and risks are measured in the same units (e.g. events/1000 patient years), the events are unlikely to be of the same severity. In EWPHE for example, there were an additional four episodes of gout/1000 patient years of treatment but a reduction in non-fatal cerebrovascular events by 11/1000 patient years. We cannot simply divide the benefit by the risk in this case. There may also be potential benefits that are less easy to quantify. There is a suggestion from the Syst-Eur trial, and recently a meta-analysis, that the incidence of dementia may be reduced by antihypertensive treatment (Feigin et al 2005, Forette et al 2002).

WHEN TO TREAT

In conclusion, there is much evidence that we should treat fit elderly hypertensive subjects with systolic pressures over 160 mmHg (alone, or in combination with diastolic pressures over 90 mmHg), and that the benefits far outweigh the risks up to the age of 80 years. For individuals over 80 years, there is no strong evidence for starting treatment, though most doctors would treat systolic pressures over 200 mmHg or diastolic pressures above 110 mmHg.

Patients with severe orthostatic hypotension may not welcome antihypertensive treatment. In these cases, a rule of thumb is that the standing systolic blood pressure should be at least 140 mmHg. For those with mild ISH (systolic pressures between 140–159 mmHg), we need some evidence on which to base decisions. In the meantime, a sensible approach would be to address all the cardiovascular risk factors and consider drug therapy if life-style changes do not result in recordings consistently below 150 mmHg. As for the elderly patient with several co-morbidities, the clinician needs to make an informed sensible assessment of the risks and benefits in that individual. In the very frail elderly person more evidence is required on the benefits or otherwise of treatment before sound guidance can be given.

Key points

- Systolic blood pressure or pulse pressure is the best predictor of an event in the elderly.
- There are very clear benefits of treating fitter elderly patients up to the age of 80 years with sustained systolic blood pressures of 160 mmHg or more.
- An individualistic approach is required for those with sustained levels of 140–150 mmHg and for those with several co-morbidities.
- The benefits and risks of treating individuals aged 80 years or more remain unclear.

REFERENCES

Amery A, Birkenhager W, Brixko P et al 1985 Mortality and morbidity results from the European Working Party on High Blood Pressure in the Elderly trial. Lancet i:1349–1354

Bulpitt C J, Beckett N S, Cooke J et al 2003 Results of the pilot study for the Hypertension in the Very Elderly Trial. Journal of Hypertension 21:2409–2417

Coope J, Warrender T S 1986 Randomised trial of treatment of hypertension in elderly patients in primary care. British Medical Journal 293:1145–1151

Dahlof B, Lindholm L H, Hansson L et al 1991 Morbidity and mortality in the Swedish Trial in Old Patients with Hypertension (STOP-Hypertension). Lancet 338:1281–1285

Feigin V, Ratnasabapathy Y, Anderson C 2005 Does blood pressure lowering treatment prevent dementia or cognitive decline in patients with cardiovascular and cerebrovascular disease? Journal of the Neurological Sciences 229–230:151–155

Forette F, Seux M, Staessen J A et al 2002 The prevention of dementia with antihypertensive treatment: new evidence from the Systolic Hypertension in Europe (Syst-Eur) study. Archives of Internal Medicine 162:2046–2052

Gueyffier F, Bulpitt C, Boissel J P et al 1999 Antihypertensive drugs in very old people: a subgroup meta-analysis of randomised controlled trials. INDANA Group. Lancet 353:793–796

Hansson L, Zanchetti A, Carruthers S G et al 1998 Effects of intensive blood-pressure lowering and low-dose aspirin in patients with hypertension: principal results of the Hypertension Optimal Treatment (HOT) randomised trial. HOT Study Group. Lancet 351:1755–1762

Joint British Societies 2005 JBS 2: Joint British Societies' guidelines on the prevention of cardiovascular disease in clinical practice. Heart 91(Suppl V):v1–v52

Kannel W B 1997 Hazards, risks, and threats of heart disease from the early stages to symptomatic coronary heart disease and cardiac failure. Cardiovascular Drugs and Therapy 11(Suppl 1):199–212

MRC Working Party 1992 Medical Research Council trial of treatment of hypertension in older adults: principal results. British Medical Journal 304:405–412

Pocock S, McCormack V, Gueyffier F et al 2001 A score for predicting risk of death from cardiovascular disease in adults with raised blood pressure, based on individual patient data from randomised controlled trials. British Medical Journal 323:75–81

Probstfield J L, Applegate W B, Borhani N O et al 1989 The Systolic Hypertension in the Elderly Program (SHEP): an intervention trial on isolated systolic hypertension. SHEP Cooperative Research Group. Clinical and Experimental Hypertension. Part A, Theory and Practice 11:973–989

SHEP Cooperative Research Group 1991 Prevention of stroke by antihypertensive drug treatment in older persons with isolated systolic hypertension. Final results of the Systolic Hypertension in the Elderly Program (SHEP). Journal of the American Medical Association 265:3255–3264

Staessen J A, Fagard R, Thijs L et al 1997 Randomised double-blind comparison of placebo and active treatment for older patients with isolated systolic hypertension. The Systolic Hypertension in Europe (Syst-Eur) Trial Investigators. Lancet 350:757–764

RECOMMENDED READING

Bulpitt C, Rajkumar C, Beckett N 1999 Clinicians' manual on hypertension in the elderly. Science Press, London

Cochrane Collaboration. Online. Available: http://www.cochrane.org/index.htm

Ramsay L E, Williams B, Johnson G D et al 1999 Guidelines for management of hypertension: report of the third working party of the British Hypertension Society. Journal of Human Hypertension 13:569–592

Scottish Intercollegiate Guidelines no. 49. Hypertension in older people. Online. Available: http://www.sign.ac.uk

Acknowledgment

We wish to acknowledge the valuable contribution made by Professor Christopher Bulpitt to the earlier version of this chapter.

SELF-ASSESSMENT QUESTIONS

1. Are the following statements true or false?
   a. Cardiovascular risk is the same as coronary heart disease risk
   b. As men age, diastolic blood pressure increases in a linear fashion
   c. In the over-70s, casual systolic blood pressure is higher in men than women
   d. The effect of sodium restriction on blood pressure increases with increasing age
   e. Systolic blood pressure is a better predictor of events than diastolic pressure in elderly subjects

2. Are the following true or false? In the major intervention trials in elderly subjects with hypertension:
   a. Total mortality was usually significantly reduced
   b. Cardiac mortality was usually reduced
   c. Stroke events were usually reduced by at least 35%
   d. The relative reduction in stroke events increases with the increase in the stroke event rate in the placebo group
   e. The average reduction in systolic and diastolic blood pressures with treatment is similar

3. Are the following true or false in relation to the over-80s?
   a. High blood pressure is associated with longer survival in cross-sectional surveys
   b. There are data to suggest that treatment with antihypertensives might increase mortality
   c. The risk to benefit ratio from treatment of hypertension is well known
   d. By 2020 they will make up more than 10% of the general population of many European countries
   e. The prevalence of a casual recording of systolic blood pressure of greater than 159 mmHg is about 50% in women over 80

SECTION 2

Cardiovascular system

Chapter 26

Abdominal aortic aneurysm and peripheral vascular disease

David Berridge

'50% of octogenarians with abdominal aortic aneurysms will die from rupture of the aneurysm.'

(O'Donnell et al 1976)

INCIDENCE

Abdominal aortic aneurysms are a common cause of sudden death in old age. In an unselected population of men over the age of 60 years, about 1.5% will have an aneurysm of the abdominal aorta on ultrasound screening. In selected groups (those with a history of hypertension, coronary, cerebral or peripheral vascular disease), men over 60 years will have an incidence of 7–8%. Women have a much lower incidence: about 1–2% in similarly selected groups. Most (95%) abdominal aortic aneurysms are infrarenal in origin and hence can be considered for both endovascular and open repair. By contrast, those with a suprarenal aortic aneurysm will be unsuitable for any current endovascular device, with open surgery carrying a higher morbidity and mortality than infrarenal surgery. Devices are currently in development which may allow safer intervention in those elderly patients (> 75 years) with a suprarenal aneurysm. It may be wise to monitor with serial ultrasound scans at 6-monthly intervals those with asymptomatic aneurysms of less than 6 cm diameter.

It is important to detect aneurysms early, as they will be asymptomatic until the time of rupture in most individuals. A rapid ultrasound scan should be performed in the higher-risk groups mentioned above, in addition to those patients with any history of distal emboli (including 'blue toe syndrome'), sudden hypotension/collapse/back pain and even loin pain, as an aneurysm may masquerade as either a ureteric/renal calculus or a urinary tract infection.

EXAMINATION AND INVESTIGATION

Clinical exclusion of the presence of an abdominal aortic aneurysm is notoriously unreliable. While a 5–6 cm diameter abdominal aortic aneurysm should be readily palpable in a slim or medium build patient, it could easily be overlooked in even moderately obese patients. A high index of suspicion and a low threshold for performing ultrasound screening in high-risk groups, and in any cases of unexplained unproven abdominal or back pain, will allow an accurate aortic diameter to be recorded.

Although the UK Small Aneurysm Trial (1998) recommended surveillance for aneurysms < 5.5 cm in diameter, there was a survival advantage in the subgroup of 4.9–5.5 cm in diameter. *All patients with aneurysms less than 5.5 cm in diameter should undergo serial 6-monthly ultrasound scans* – providing they remain asymptomatic. Any development of symptoms, increase in diameter of > 0.5 cm in a 6-month period, or progressive increase up to and beyond 5 cm diameter should initiate detailed assessment and consideration of elective repair (although some authors continue to monitor aneurysms until they reach > 6 cm in diameter).

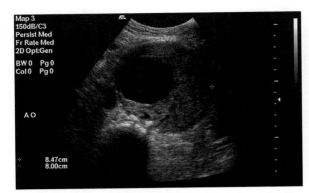

Figure 26.1 An aneurysm presenting at over 8 cm should be referred for urgent repair.

Asymptomatic aneurysms presenting at 8 or even 10 cm in diameter (Fig. 26.1) need urgent repair as rupture is almost inevitable. These patients should remain in hospital and be operated on in the next elective list.

IS IT WORTH DOING, DOCTOR?

Age itself should not be a bar to considering the merits of elective intervention for abdominal aortic aneurysms – it is biological age that matters, not chronological age!

This question may arise, particularly in very elderly subjects. It may be because the patients are anxious as to whether they will survive the procedure, or if they will be left with further morbidity on top of any existing limitations. All such discussions should include the patient's next of kin, and must take into account the patient's current medical status, including detailed investigation of pre-existing coronary, respiratory, diabetic, renal and neurological conditions. A realistic prognosis is needed from their elderly care specialist in addition to any other specialists involved with their care. The discussion for very large aneurysms (e.g. 8 cm in diameter) in the presence of multiple uncorrectable coexisting medical conditions should also include the consideration of emergency surgery in the case of rupture. If the patient and their partner/relative indicate that they would wish emergency surgery to be performed, then the risks for elective surgery, although high, will be much more favourable than emergency surgery and should therefore be reconsidered.

OPEN VERSUS ENDOVASCULAR REPAIR

The results of the randomized trials comparing open with endovascular stent graft repair (EVAR 1) and that between endovascular repair and best medical treatment have recently been published. In EVAR 1 (EVAR 2005a) there was a 3% reduction in aneurysm-related deaths in the endovascular group at up to 4 years follow-up (1082 patients randomized). However, there was no difference in all cause mortality, and endovascular repair was more expensive (£13 257 v £9946).

The lower mortality related to the procedure was offset by deaths due to rupture in the EVAR 1 group post procedure > 30 days, and also by increased coronary heart disease deaths in the endovascular group. At 4 years, 41% of the endovascular group had required reintervention compared to 9% in the open group. Long-term surveillance is deemed essential for the endovascular patient and not for the 'open' patient. Endovascular intervention proved feasible for about 50% of all patients considered.

Lower cardiorespiratory complications can be achieved with endovascular repair, which should be considered in those patients with marked cardiorespiratory compromise – though conversion to open repair is associated with high morbidity and mortality. Clearly, those patients who are severely compromised should not be subjected to a procedure designed to prevent future potential rupture, as the risk of intervention may equal or outweigh the likely risk of spontaneous rupture over that same period. EVAR 2 (2005b) showed clearly that at 4 years there was no difference in either overall all-cause mortality or aneurysm-related mortality between the two groups (4-year mortality 64%). Hence if a patient is considered unfit for open repair there is no justification for the use of an aortic stent graft in this group of patients.

Open repair, even in octogenarians, can be achieved with acceptable mortality even in the presence of co-morbidity (especially compared to results following emergency intervention for rupture).

ABDOMINAL AORTIC ANEURYSMS – SIZE DOES MATTER!

All patients with ruptures and symptomatic patients should be considered for urgent surgery. Current use of endovascular devices means that this type of intervention is unlikely to be able to be offered to most patients with ruptured or symptomatic abdominal aortic aneurysms, regardless of age. Rapid assessment of the patient, preferably by the consultant surgeon and consultant anaesthetist, should be both aggressive in terms of offering potentially life-saving major surgery, but also realistic in those patients who are already unconscious, those with negligible cardiac output or those with major life-limiting, co-morbid conditions (including metastatic neoplasia) with no realistic prospect of surviving surgery.

The risk of rupture depends on the size of the aneurysm. Small aneurysms can rupture, but this is relatively rare and is lower than the risk for elective surgery. Over 5.5 cm maximum transverse diameter, rupture can be expected in about 25% of patients within 5 years. Although the risk of rupture in the Small Aneurysm Study (UK Small Aneurysm Trial Participants 1998) (antero-posterior diameter) was only 1% per year for aneurysms < 5.5 cm diameter, 61% of those allo-cated to surveillance were actually repaired by the end of the study (6 years). This was due to either the development of symptoms, appreciable increase in size or patients' requests for operative repair.

RESULTS

Selection has a profound influence on operative results. 30-day mortality for elective aortic surgery in patients over 80 years can be as low as 3–8% (Harris et al 1986, O'Donnell et al 1976, Paty et al 1993). However, in a combined district and teaching hospital regional audit of elective surgery in the over-80s, mortality was found to be 24% compared to 71% in ruptured cases. Morbidity depends on the circumstances of the repair, varying from 29% in elective cases to 52% in those operated on as an emergency. In a series of 1131 patients (Berridge et al 1995), patients over 80 years of age accounted for only 6.4% of elective cases, but constituted 11.8% of emergency cases. All these emergency cases would have had a better chance of survival if they had had the opportunity of being assessed and offered elective surgery.

Key points: abdominal aortic aneurysms

- Abdominal aortic aneurysms are a common cause of death in old age.
- > 5.5 cm diameter should be considered for elective repair.
- Risk of rupture increases with diameter.
- Co-morbid factors need to be optimized.
- Endovascular repair can be considered.

PERIPHERAL VASCULAR DISEASE

INTERMITTENT CLAUDICATION

- Must be disabling
- Biological not chronological age
- Be realistic

Peripheral vascular disease may present in a number of different guises. Initially patients may complain of pain in the calf, thigh and/or buttock, which is brought on by walking and relieved rapidly by rest, i.e. vascular intermittent claudication. Similar pain with longer recovery times such as 10–15 minutes may suggest referred pain from the lumbosacral spine suggesting spinal claudication.

Risk factor management with the use of anti-platelet agents, statin therapy and the use of ACE inhibitors to control hypertension should be considered. Statins should be used in patients with peripheral vascular disease even if the cholesterol level is normal as there is now good evidence of reduced morbidity and mortality in patients on these agents. Diabetic control needs to be optimized, anaemia investigated and corrected and renal function assessed.

Claudication management needs to be medical in the first instance. Patients should be encouraged to stop smoking, keep walking, and to lose weight if they are obese. The claudication also needs to be disabling before intervention can be justified in terms of risk. Intervention needs to be considered in terms of biological age and not chronological age. Patients need to be realistic about their co-morbid factors as to their options for management. It is fruitless intervening, even with a small associated risk, if the patient's walking distance is actually limited by shortness of breath, angina or joint pains.

Once risk factors have been controlled, a period of conservative management of 3 months may reveal spontaneous improvement in 50% of patients. If this does not occur, a short trial of naftidrofuryl over 2–3 months may affect a modest increase in walking distance.

First-line intervention would usually be in the form of a duplex scan of peripheral arteries to determine if there is a lesion suitable for angioplasty and/or stent. There can then be informed discussion with the patient as to the relative merits of balloon angioplasty. If reconstruction is required, the degree of intervention will clearly influence whether reconstruction will be offered. For example, if a patient needs a femoro-distal bypass (below mid calf), then the risks are much greater than if a routine above-knee bypass or local groin procedure were required. Ankle–

brachial pressure index (ABPI) would usually be 0.5–0.8 in these patients (highest of maximum dorsalis pedis or posterior tibial pressure compared to brachial systolic pressure as measured by Doppler).

Ankle–brachial pressure index

This is performed using a hand-held Doppler to compare the systolic pressure at the brachial artery level with the highest ankle pressure in either the posterior tibial or dorsalis pedis (anterior tibial) arteries.

$$\frac{\text{Highest ankle pressure}}{\text{Highest brachial pressure}} \quad \text{Normal} = 1$$

CRITICAL ISCHAEMIA

Progression of peripheral vascular disease will see the development of rest pain. It is important to distinguish true ischaemic nocturnal rest pain from nocturnal cramps and other causes of intermittent nocturnal discomfort in the limbs.

Ischaemic nocturnal rest pain will occur in the toes and heal before any similar pains develop more proximally. They cause sleep disruption and are invariably progressive, though initially they may not necessarily occur every night. They occur because of four main factors:

- Reduction of cardiac output
- Loss of effect of gravity
- Vasodilatation of skin/subcutaneous tissue causing 'stealing' of blood from the deeper structures
- The weight of the bedclothes

Note: the diabetic patient with peripheral neuropathy may not develop rest pain, especially in the early stages, and this is at least in part why they have a tendency to present late with trophic and/or infective complications of peripheral arterial disease.

This latter point clearly has negligible impact when one's ankle/toe pressures are normal, however with severe peripheral arteriosclerotic disease, the ankle pressure may be inaudible. Hence the weight of the bedclothes under these circumstances may be sufficient to actually stop the local circulation subjected to the pressure. The disease process may then progress to develop trophic changes.

Management of these patients will then encompass endovascular angioplasty with or without stenting. If this is not possible, then reconstruction is necessary starting proximally initially and extending as necessary to include femoro-popliteal and femoro-crural grafting using saphenous vein grafts. The relative benefit of intervention compared to the risk of intervention needs to be carefully considered for each individual patient and their particular medical risk factors.

For the acute presentation, thrombolysis may be considered. Although the risks of major haemorrhage do increase with age, there are important contraindications and a recent meta-analysis showed no overall benefit compared to surgical intervention (Berridge et al 2001).

One must also consider the role of primary amputation. If the patient is already bedbound and unable to walk, there is little point in subjecting that patient to a long and potentially unsuccessful distal reconstruction if that is the only other option.

A primarily-healed amputation may offer a better overall outcome for that patient. Similarly, those patients presenting with extensive gangrene may have already progressed beyond the limits for limb salvage. Efforts therefore need to be made to maximize function with as distal an amputation site as possible to try to improve rehabilitation prospects. Ankle–brachial pressure index in this type of patient would be 0.3 or less. (Note: ankle Doppler signals may be inaudible in severe cases.)

Intervention for critical ischaemia

- No age limit
- Note functional restrictions
- Bedbound
- Wheelchair bound
- Extent of gangrene
- Note co-morbidites
- Remember primary amputation

REFERENCES

Berridge D C, Chamberlain J C, Guy A J et al 1995 Prospective audit of abdominal aortic aneurysm surgery in the northern region from 1988 to 1992. British Journal of Surgery 82:906–910

Berridge D C, Kessel D, Robertson I 2001 Surgery versus thrombolysis for acute limb ischaemia: initial management. Cochrane Review. The Cochrane Library 1, Oxford

EVAR Trial Participants 2005a Endovascular aneurysm repair versus open repair in patients with abdominal aortic aneurysm (EVAR trial 1): randomised controlled trial. Lancet 365(9478):2179–2186

EVAR Trial Participants 2005b Endovascular aneurysm repair and outcome in patients unfit for open repair of abdominal aortic aneurysm (EVAR trial 2): randomised controlled trial. Lancet 365(9478): 2187–2192

Harris K A, Ameli F M, Lally M et al 1986 Abdominal aortic aneurysm in patients more than 80 years old. Surgery, Gynecology and Obstetrics 162:536–538

O'Donnell T F, Darling R C, Linton R R 1976 Is 80 years too old for aneurysmectomy? Archives of Surgery 111(11):1250–1257

Paty P S K, Lloyd W E, Chang B B et al 1993 Aortic replacement for abdominal aortic aneurysm in elderly patients. American Journal of Surgery 166:191–193

UK Small Aneurysm Trial Participants 1998 Mortality results for randomised controlled trial of early elective surgery or ultrasonographic surveillance for small abdominal aortic aneurysms. Lancet 352:1649–1655

RECOMMENDED READING

Chetter I C, Spark J I, Scott D J A et al 1998 Prospective analysis of quality of life in patients following infrainguinal reconstruction for chronic critical ischaemia. British Journal of Surgery 85:951–955

Coghill T H, Landercasper J, Strutt P J et al 1987 Late results of peripheral vascular surgery in patients 80 years of age and older. Archives of Surgery 122:581–586

Gloviczki P 1995 Ruptured abdominal aortic aneurysms. In: Rutherford R B (ed.) Vascular surgery, 4th edn. WB Saunders, Philadelphia

Mitchell M B, Rutherford R B, Krupski W C 1995 Infrarenal aortic aneurysms. In: Rutherford R B (ed.) Vascular surgery, 4th edn. WB Saunders, Philadelphia

SELF-ASSESSMENT QUESTIONS

Are the following true or false?

1. Abdominal aortic aneurysms in the elderly may present as:
   a. Renal or ureteric colic
   b. Back pain
   c. Transient collapse in a normotensive patient
   d. Epigastric pain
   e. Chest pain

2. Abdominal aortic aneurysms in elderly patients:
   a. > 5.5 cm should be considered for elective repair
   b. Ruptured aneurysms should not be repaired in patients > 80 years of age
   c. Are more frequent in men with other features of atherosclerotic disease

   d. Clinical screening is reliable and cost-effective
   e. Cardiac status is a major determinant of outcome in both elective and emergency cases

3. Peripheral arterial disease:
   a. Patients with intermittent claudication will usually have a recovery time of up to 5–10 minutes
   b. Ankle pressure indices may be normal in patients with ischaemic rest pain
   c. Ankle–brachial pressure indices compare the lowest ankle pressure with the brachial systolic pressure
   d. Nocturnal rest pain is persistent, occurring in the calf and may be confused with night cramps
   e. Initial management should concentrate on identification and correction of risk factors

Cardiovascular system

Chapter **27**

The management of atrial fibrillation in the older patient

Anis Mamun

The improved survival of patients with congenital and acquired heart disease, the decreased prevalence of rheumatic heart disease and more importantly, an ageing population, have led to atrial fibrillation (AF) becoming predominantly a dysrhythmia of old age.

PREVALENCE AND PROBLEMS

SIZE OF THE PROBLEM

AF is the commonest *sustained* dysrhythmia (premature beats or extrasystoles are non-sustained) and its prevalence rises with age. About 0.5% of those aged 50–59 years have chronic AF; between 65–69 years the prevalence is about 4%, rising to 11.6% in subjects over 75 years. 5.6% of people aged ≥ 65 years living at home have chronic AF.

Thus, about 70% of those with AF are between 65 and 85 years. The absolute number of men and women with AF is about equal (Feinberg et al 1995). Other independent risk factors for an increased prevalence of AF are diabetes mellitus, hypertension, congestive heart failure and valve disease.

NATURE OF THE PROBLEM

AF is a marker for both increased morbidity and mortality (Onundarson et al 1987). The mortality rate in people with AF is twice those in sinus rhythm. Much of the increased morbidity and mortality is due to stroke and the negative haemodynamic consequences of AF. The annual stroke rate in subjects with AF is about 5%. It is more than twice this (12% per annum) for those with a recent history of stroke/transient ischaemic attack (TIA) and AF.

Individuals who have AF but no other cardiovascular risk factors have 'lone' atrial fibrillation. The likelihood of stroke in this group is not much different from age and sex matched controls: 0–0.5% per year in those under 60 years, 1.6% among 60–69-year olds, and 2.1% in

70–79-year olds. Most patients with AF have coexisting cardiovascular diseases, and lone AF is uncommon in elderly people.

TYPES OF ATRIAL FIBRILLATION

Acute (minutes to days) AF in old age is commonly due to a stressful event, such as a chest or urinary tract infection. In the younger age group, it is more commonly due to alcohol excess, drug abuse, rheumatic or congenital heart disease, or after surgery. Myocardial infarction, hypertension and thyroid disease are precipitants for AF in both age groups. About 50% of cases of new-onset AF spontaneously revert to sinus rhythm within 48 hours.

Paroxysmal (recurrent) AF on the other hand does not normally have a precipitating factor, and is usually seen in young and middle aged people (< 65 years) with no cardiovascular risk factors. It reverts to sinus rhythm spontaneously or with treatment. The natural history of paroxysmal AF is to proceed to chronic AF after a variable time.

When an episode of AF lasts for 7 days, spontaneous reversion is uncommon, and the condition is defined as persistent AF. Chronic or permanent AF (> 6 months duration) is the commonest type, particularly in those over 75 years. In the very old (≥ 85 years), most AF is chronic.

A UK community survey recorded a prevalence of 2.4% of AF in people aged 50 years or over, and nearly 80% of this was found in those over 70 (Lip et al 1997). About three-quarters had chronic AF, and the rest had paroxysmal AF.

CONSEQUENCES OF ATRIAL FIBRILLATION

SYMPTOMS

All three types may or may not be symptomatic. The most frequent symptoms experienced are breathlessness, palpitations, chest pain, dizzy spells and fatigue (Lip et al 1994). AF is commonly associated with heart failure or left ventricular dysfunction, particularly in older patients where both conditions are common (O'Connell & Gray 1996).

WHY TREAT ATRIAL FIBRILLATION?

There are three reasons:

- Symptom control
- Optimization of cardiac function
- Minimization of risk of thromboembolism

On average, AF reduces cardiac output by about 30%, but as much as 50% in people over 70 years or in those with impaired diastolic filling (i.e. people with left ventricular hypertrophy, mitral stenosis, and hypertrophic or restrictive cardiomyopathy) (Channer & Jones 1988). In addition, people with AF may have exercise-induced tachycardia, which may further diminish exercise tolerance. This is reversed when sinus rhythm is re-established.

MANAGEMENT

RHYTHM OR RATE CONTROL?

Rhythm control was previously thought to be preferable in AF. However, recent large trials have shown that there is no survival advantage or reduced rate of hospitalization with rhythm control over rate control strategy (AFFIRM Investigators 2002, van Gelder et al 2002). Besides, the incidence of adverse side-effects due to drugs may be lower in the latter. Despite this, in cases of new-onset AF and most cases of paroxysmal AF, rhythm control should be the aim, given the long-term effect of AF on the heart (anatomical and electrical remodeling of the atria) and symptomology. In chronic persistent AF one should still consider restoring sinus rhythm unless the patient is frail or has significant co-morbidity. Although duration of the dysrhythmia is important in the likelihood of reversibility, this is not an absolute criterion (Crozier et al 1987).

HOW DO WE ACHIEVE RHYTHM CONTROL?

DC cardioversion

The most effective and perhaps the safest method is transthoracic synchronized DC cardioversion. The success rate may be up to 90% (Dalzell et al 1990). In most cases cardioversion is achieved with 200 Joules or less. Pretreatment with an anti-arrhythmic (e.g. ibutilide or digoxin) improves the success rate and reduces the energy level required (Oral et al 1999). If the first attempt fails, a second attempt may be considered later.

A brief period of intravenous anaesthesia is required for this procedure, and this is usually well tolerated even in elderly people with cardio-respiratory compromise. Unfortunately, despite its efficacy and safety, it is thought that DC cardioversion is under-used in the UK (Lip et al 1994, 1997).

In general, patients with AF should be anti-coagulated. However, if the duration of dysrhythmia is less than 48 hours, cardioversion may be carried out with a small risk of thromboembolism (Stoddard et al 1995). Anticoagulation is needed for at least 3 weeks before, and 4 weeks after, a successful cardioversion (American College of Chest Physicians 1992). The first 3 weeks is needed to stabilize any intracardiac thrombus, and the next 4 weeks is to prevent any thrombus formation while the atrium is regaining its full contractile strength. Emergency cardioversion may override the need for full anticoagulation. Transoesophageal echocardiography (TOE) in expert hands may visualize left atrial thrombus, but this is not yet widely available.

Pharmacotherapy

Chemical cardioversion is common in those admitted as an emergency, and used more frequently than DC cardioversion (Lip et al 1994). It is less alarming to patients and easier to organize. Theoretically, many drugs from Class 1A (quinidine, disopyramide), 1C (flecainide, propafenone) or Class III (amiodarone, sotalol) may be used. Amiodarone (oral or parenteral) is the current favourite in the UK, particularly for older patients (flecainide should be avoided in patients with ischaemic heart disease and heart failure). Amiodarone is effective and has minimal negative inotropic effects. This is important, as many of these elderly patients also have heart failure or ventricular dysfunction. There is a success rate of > 60% for amiodarone, flecainide and propafenone (Strasberg 1991). However, when the duration of atrial fibrillation is > 10 days, the success rate drops to 40% or less (Borgeat et al 1986). In acute

situations, and when given parenterally, patients must be closely monitored because of potential pro-arrhythmic effects and possible aggravation of left ventricular dysfunction. In addition, amiodarone has many side-effects, which develop insidiously, and may not be reversible after withdrawal. This makes regular follow-up for any patients on amiodarone desirable.

Maintaining sinus rhythm

Following cardioversion – electrical or chemical – maintenance treatment with a drug is usually needed to maximize the chance of continuing in sinus rhythm. The most commonly used drug for this in Britain is probably amiodarone, while in North America it may be quinidine. There have been many trials of the effectiveness of drugs to maintain sinus rhythm. In general, all are more effective than placebo. The successful maintenance rate at 1 year is about 25% with a placebo and 50% with quinidine. Similar success rates are seen with disopyramide, procainamide, sotalol and amiodarone. Many of the trials which compared relative efficacy were unblinded, small and of short duration. There was a bias towards younger subjects, and the results may not apply to older people.

All anti-arrhythmic drugs are potentially harmful. They are known to have pro-arrhythmic effects, and retrospective analyses have suggested that such agents may increase mortality.

PAROXYSMAL AF

Class IA, IC and III drugs are effective in reducing the frequency of paroxysms. However, treatment is best individualized considering such factors as the frequency and severity of attacks, disruption in daily life and co-morbidity. Amiodarone is effective, but flecainide, propafenone and quinidine can be successful (Roy et al 2000, Singh et al 2005). Those having attacks of AF during times of stress may benefit more from a beta-blocker.

Paroxysmal AF has a similar type of risk for thromboembolism as persistent or permanent AF (Atrial Fibrillation Investigators 1994). However, as this group is relatively young, fit and may have lone AF, the decision for or against anticoagulation has to be carefully evaluated in each case.

RATE CONTROL IN ATRIAL FIBRILLATION

Rate control in AF is achieved through drugs that primarily act on the AV node to slow down conduction. They may be used singly or in combination. The commonest is digoxin, followed by calcium antagonists (diltiazem, verapamil) and beta-blockers. Since elderly subjects with established chronic AF often have ventricular dysfunction (± heart failure), digoxin is the drug of choice and is widely used (Lip et al 1997). It is well tolerated, cheap and a drug level can be measured if toxicity is suspected. However, the need for long-term rate control drugs in many elderly people who are otherwise restricted in their daily activities or have limited mobility is uncertain, as many maintain an acceptable ventricular rate for most of the time without intervention. In addition, with advancing age, nodal diseases are common, and ventricular response to AF is likely to decline in frail elderly subjects (> 75 years). However, fear of toxicity makes under-dosing common, and in otherwise active older people 125 microgram/day of digoxin may not be enough (Jeliffe & Brooker 1974).

The other two groups of drugs, although preferred, have restricted use because of their negative inotropic effect, frequent side-effects and poor tolerance. In younger people and those without heart failure, calcium antagonists or beta-blockers are favoured, as unlike digoxin these can control ventricular rate during exercise (exertional tachycardia).

Non-pharmacological approaches

When medical treatment is unsuccessful or not tolerated, an 'ablate and pace' strategy, i.e. catheter ablation of the His bundle and implantation of a pacemaker under local anaesthesia may be considered. The new discovery that some episodes of atrial fibrillation are initiated by rapid, repetitive firing of atrial myocytes in muscle sleeves located in the pulmonary veins has led to focal ablation and cure in selected cases of (paroxysmal) AF. This technique is evolving, and may be the first-line approach for paroxysmal AF with otherwise normal heart in the near future (Grubb & Furniss 2001).

The surgical option ('Corridor' and 'Maze' procedures) involves major operations and is not particularly suitable for elderly subjects (Cox et al 1991).

PREVENTION OF THROMBOEMBOLISM

The scientific evidence

Anticoagulation is beneficial in the young old (65–75 years old). In a pooled analysis of five major AF trials, warfarin reduced the risk of thromboembolic stroke by 68% (or 31 events per 1000 patients treated), and annual mortality by 33% (Atrial Fibrillation Investigators 1994). There was a 25% risk reduction with aspirin (Aronow et al 1999, Stroke Prevention in Atrial Fibrillation Investigators 1994).

In general, the risk of serious haemorrhage is low (1% per annum both in the warfarin and aspirin group). The average age of patients in these trials was 69 years, and the results may not necessarily apply to the over-75s. However, in those over 75 years the risk of thromboembolism is higher and so the benefit may be greater. This uncertainty needs to be resolved by a large controlled trial with adequate power to ascertain if benefits and low risks also occur in elderly subjects.

In younger patients (< 65 years) with lone AF, the annual risk of stroke is no different from the general population (0.5%), and so warfarin may not be indicated. Our suggested practice for anticoagulation in AF is shown in Table 27.1.

Table 27.1 Anticoagulation recommendations (Sager 1997)		
Age	Risk factors	Recommendations
< 65 years old	None Yes	Aspirin or no Rx Warfarin
65–75 years old	None Yes	Aspirin or warfarin Warfarin
> 75 years old	Yes or No	Warfarin

Risk factors: stroke or TIA, left ventricular dysfunction, congestive heart failure, valvular heart disease, hypertension and diabetes mellitus.

Problems with widespread use of warfarin

Anticoagulation in AF is under-used in primary and secondary care (Lip et al 1997). There are three main reasons for this. First, there are still reservations about a favourable risk–benefit profile for anticoagulation in those over 75 years. Second, a physician's attitude to anticoagulation in the frail elderly patient may be guarded for other reasons, including cognitive deficits, problems with effective communication and difficult social circumstances (McCrory et al 1995, Monette et al 1997). Third, we need a big organizational change to introduce optimal anticoagulation for all eligible elderly subjects. Recent data suggest that doctors' experiences of bleeding events associated with warfarin use may reduce subsequent warfarin prescribing, but the reverse may not be the case (i.e. adverse events associated with underuse of warfarin may not increase the prescribing habit) (Choudhury et al 2006).

THERAPEUTIC OPTIONS

Elderly patients often present to emergency departments with fast acute or acute-on-chronic AF due to an underlying cause, usually a chest or urinary tract infection. Most improve with treatment of the precipitating cause. However, if there is important haemodynamic compromise (systolic blood pressure < 90 mmHg, or ventricular rate > 200/min) or chest pain, cardioversion (preferably electrical) should be considered. All patients with AF should have their thyroid function (only a small minority of these are due to thyroid dysfuntion) and electrolytes checked (Bath et al 1993). The scope for rhythm control should be reviewed in each case, but may not be possible or appropriate in many older people. However, if sinus rhythm is established following intervention, many will require maintenance therapy, and these people should be followed up regularly.

The most important preventative treatment in AF is anticoagulation, and for some this may be the only treatment required. A target international normalized ratio (INR) of 2.5 with a range of 2–3 is safe and effective (Stroke Prevention in Atrial Fibrillation Investigators 1996). A lower fixed INR of 1.5 in combination with aspirin is ineffective and should not be considered. In patients over 75 years, close surveillance of anticoagulation is needed because of possible increased risk of bleeding. Patients who cannot be prescribed warfarin should be given aspirin 300 mg a day (Royal College of Physicians of Edinburgh 1998).

There is no randomized controlled trial data about the optimum timing for starting anticoagulation after a stroke. However, for secondary prophylaxis, it is wise to avoid anticoagulation for up to 14 days or until the neurological deficits have stabilized after a large embolic stroke, because of the risk of haemorrhagic transformation. For small embolic cerebral infarcts confirmed by imaging, anticoagulation may be restarted after 48 hours.

Common contraindications for warfarin therapy are frequent falls, dementia, immobility, poor health-related quality of life, alcoholism, haemorrhagic infarction and other bleeding problems.

CONCLUSION

Our understanding of the management of AF both in terms of rhythm and rate control and use of anticoagulation are evolving. Although we have much more information than we had a decade ago, we are still unsure about the answers to many questions, particularly those involving older people.

Key points

- AF is the commonest sustained dysrhythmia whose prevalence rises with age.
- It is a marker of increased morbidity and mortality.
- Rhythm control is no longer considered preferable over rate control.
- Anticoagulation with warfarin needs to be considered unless contraindicated or in cases of lone atrial fibrillation ≤ 65 (although this is now being questioned).

REFERENCES

AFFIRM Investigators 2002 A comparison of rate control and rhythm control in patients with atrial fibrillation. New England Journal of Medicine 347: 1825–1833

American College of Chest Physicians 1992 Third American College of Chest Physicians Conference on Antithrombotic Therapy. Chest 102:3035–3055

Aronow W S, Ahn C, Kronzon I et al 1999 Incidence of new thromboembolic stroke in persons 62 years and older with chronic atrial fibrillation treated with warfarin versus aspirin. Journal of the American Geriatrics Society 47:366–368

Atrial Fibrillation Investigators 1994 Risk factors for stroke and efficacy of antithrombotic therapy in atrial fibrillation: analysis of pooled data from five randomized trials. Archives of Internal Medicine 154:1449–1457

Bath P M W, Prasad A, Brown M M et al 1993 Survey of use of anticoagulation in patients with atrial fibrillation. British Medical Journal 307:1045

Borgeat A, Goy J J, Maendly R et al 1986 Flecainide versus quinidine for conversion of atrial fibrillation to sinus rhythm. American Journal of Cardiology 58:496–498

Channer K S, Jones J V 1988 Atrial systole: its role in normal and diseased hearts. Clinical Science 75:1–4

Choudhury N K, Anderson G M, Laupacis A et al 2006 Impact of adverse events on prescribing warfarin in patients with atrial fibrillation: matched pair analysis. British Medical Journal 332:141–143

Cox J L, Schuessler R B, D'agostino H J J et al 1991 The surgical treatment of atrial fibrillation, III: development of a definitive surgical procedure. Journal of Thoracic and Cardiovascular Surgery 101:569–583

Crozier I G, Ikram H, Kenealy M et al 1987 Flecainide acetate for conversion of acute supraventricular tachycardia to sinus rhythm. American Journal of Cardiology 59:607–609

Dalzell G W, Anderson J, Adgey A A 1990 Factors determining success and energy requirements for cardioversion of atrial fibrillation. Quarterly Journal of Medicine 76:903–913

Feinberg W M, Blackshear J L, Laupacis A et al 1995 Prevalence, age distribution, and gender of patients with atrial fibrillation – analysis and implications. Archives of Internal Medicine 155:469–473

Grubb N R, Furniss S 2001 Radiofrequency ablation for atrial fibrillation. British Medical Journal 322: 777–780

Jeliffe R W, Brooker G 1974 A nomogram for digoxin therapy. American Journal of Medicine 57:63–68

Lip G Y H, Tean K N, Dunn F G 1994 Treatment of atrial fibrillation in a district general hospital. British Heart Journal 71:92–95

Lip G Y H, Golding D J, Nazir M 1997 A survey of atrial fibrillation in general practice: the west Birmingham atrial fibrillation project. British Journal of General Practice 47:285–289

McCrory D C, Matchar D B, Samsa G et al 1995 Physician attitudes about anticoagulation for nonvalvular atrial fibrillation in the elderly. Archives of Internal Medicine 155:277–281

Monette J, Gurwitz J H, Rochon P A 1997 Physician attitudes concerning warfarin for stroke prevention in atrial fibrillation: results of a survey of long-term care practitioners. Journal of the American Geriatrics Society 45:1060–1065

O'Connell J E, Gray C S 1996 Atrial fibrillation and stroke prevention in the community. Age and Ageing 25:307–309

Onundarson P T, Thorgeirsson G, Jonmundsson E et al 1987 Chronic atrial fibrillation: Epidemiologic features and 14 years follow up: A case control study. European Heart Journal 8:521

Oral H, Souza J, Michaud G F et al 1999 Facilitating transthoracic cardioversion of atrial fibrillation with ibutilide pretreatment. New England Journal of Medicine 340:1849–1854

Roy D, Talajic M, Dorian P et al 2000 Amiodarone to prevent recurrent atrial fibrillation. New England Journal of Medicine 342:913–920

Royal College of Physicians of Edinburgh Consensus Conference on Medical Management of Stroke 1998 Consensus statement. Age and Ageing 27:665–666

Sager P T 1997 Atrial fibrillation: antiarrhythmic therapy versus rate control with antithrombotic therapy. American Journal of Cardiology 80(8A):74G–81G

Singh B N, Singh S N, Reda D J et al 2005 Amiodarone versus sotalol for atrial fibrillation. New England Journal of Medicine 352:1861–1872

Stoddard M F, Dawkins P R, Prince C R 1995 Left atrial appendage thrombus is not uncommon in patients with acute atrial fibrillation and a recent embolic event: a transoesophageal ecocardiographic study. Journal of the American College of Cardiology 25:452–459

Strasberg B 1991 Intravenous amiodarone for conversion of atrial fibrillation to sinus rhythm. American Journal of Cardiology 67:325

Stroke Prevention in Atrial Fibrillation Investigators 1994 Warfarin versus aspirin for prevention of thromboembolism in atrial fibrillation: Stroke Prevention in Atrial Fibrillation II (SPAF II) Study. Lancet 343:687–691

Stroke Prevention in Atrial Fibrillation Investigators 1996 Adjusted-dose warfarin versus low-intensity, fixed dose warfarin plus aspirin for high-risk patients with atrial fibrillation: Stroke Prevention in Atrial Fibrillation III (SPAF III) randomized clinical trial. Lancet 348:633–638

van Gelder I C, Hagens V E, Bosker H A et al 2002 A comparison of rate control and rhythm control in patients with recurrent persistent atrial fibrillation. New England Journal of Medicine 347: 1834–1840

Acknowledgments

We wish to acknowledge the valuable contribution made by Dr Jeffrey Ball and Professor Michael Lye.

SELF-ASSESSMENT QUESTIONS

1. Are the following true or false?
   a. AF is the commonest sustained dysrhythmia
   b. About a quarter of people with AF are ≥ 75 years of age
   c. Based on a 1991 census, a figure of 160 000–644 000 subjects over 65 years of age are estimated to have AF in the UK
   d. The risk of stroke in rheumatic AF is 10-fold higher than in controls
   e. The likelihood of stroke in lone AF is low; it therefore may be treated with aspirin instead of warfarin

2. Are the following true or false?
   a. The natural history of paroxysmal AF is to proceed to chronic AF after a variable time
   b. AF reduces cardiac output by 15%
   c. In elderly people with AF, rate control is preferable to rhythm control
   d. As a rule, full anticoagulation is advised for elective DC cardioversion as a stroke rate of up to 7% occurs without it
   e. Drugs from Class 1A, 1B, 1C and Class III may be used for chemical cardioversion

3. Are the following true or false?
   a. Recent trials have shown huge benefits of anticoagulation in people with AF
   b. In the over-75s, anticoagulation is less effective than in younger subjects in preventing thromboembolic stroke
   c. The risk of intracranial haemorrhage in the over-75s may be as high as 2.8% compared to < 1% in those under 75 years
   d. The average age of subjects participating in the five major atrial fibrillation trials (pooled data) was 69 years, and only 15% were over 75 years
   e. The over-75s, who are more likely to have a thromboembolic stroke, are more commonly anticoagulated than their younger counterparts

4. Is it true or false that the following are primary prevention trials?
   a. Placebo controlled, randomized trial of warfarin and aspirin for prevention of thromboembolic complications in chronic AF: the Copenhagen atrial fibrillation (AFASAK) study
   b. Boston Area Anticoagulation Trial for Atrial Fibrillation (BAATAF). The effect of low-dose warfarin on the risk of stroke in patients with non-rheumatic AF
   c. Stroke Prevention in Atrial Fibrillation (SPAF-I) study
   d. European Atrial Fibrillation Trial (EAFT) in people with non-rheumatic AF
   e. Canadian Atrial Fibrillation Anticoagulation (CAFA) study

SECTION 3

Respiratory system

Chapter 28

Asthma and chronic obstructive pulmonary disease

Gurcharan S. Rai

Up to 60% of older people living at home will have one or more respiratory symptoms, either intermittently or chronically (Dow et al 1991). Respiratory symptoms such as wheeze, breathlessness and cough (with or without phlegm) do not specify a diagnosis in their own right. Some patients will have multiple causes of these symptoms – this is more likely in heavy tobacco smokers, as the risk factors for chronic obstructive pulmonary disease (COPD) and ischaemic heart disease are shared.

Other information obtained from further questioning, examination (particularly of the respiratory and cardiac systems) and investigations will be necessary before one or more diagnoses can be made. Several appointments will usually be necessary so that the appropriate information (including results of investigations) is finally obtained for interpretation.

What additional information should you seek on history taking, examination and investigation to decide whether a patient may or may not have asthma or COPD (see Fig. 28.1)?

From the history, find out whether the wheeze is due to prolongation of expiration rather than retained secretions in the throat or stridor (possibly caused by upper airway obstruction). Are the symptoms intermittent and variable (asthma) or chronic and slowly progressive (COPD)? What triggers the symptoms? Patients with asthma are more likely to report symptoms being brought on by cold air, smoke, allergens or chemical irritants.

Always take a full drug history. Airway obstruction from asthma or COPD can be triggered by certain drugs such as beta-blockers (topical or oral) and, less frequently, aspirin or NSAIDs. What is the smoking history? How many pack years (1 pack year = 20 cigarettes per day per year)? This is important but, even in very heavy tobacco smokers, asthma can still be present so do not assume that all smokers have COPD. COPD is a gradually progressive disease and by the time a diagnosis is made, it has usually been present and associated with gradually deteriorating lung function over many years. See if the history of the symptoms supports this pattern of illness (see Table 28.1).

There may be a history of allergies but, for reasons poorly understood, asthma in older people is not as strongly associated with eczema or hay

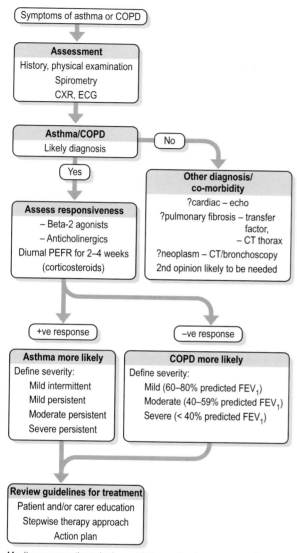

Symptoms of asthma or COPD

Assessment
History, physical examination
Spirometry
CXR, ECG

Asthma/COPD
Likely diagnosis — No

Yes

Other diagnosis/co-morbidity
?cardiac – echo
?pulmonary fibrosis – transfer factor,
– CT thorax
?neoplasm – CT/bronchoscopy
2nd opinion likely to be needed

Assess responsiveness
– Beta-2 agonists
– Anticholinergics
Diurnal PEFR for 2–4 weeks
(corticosteroids)

+ve response

–ve response

Asthma more likely
Define severity:
Mild intermittent
Mild persistent
Moderate persistent
Severe persistent

COPD more likely
Define severity:
Mild (60–80% predicted FEV_1)
Moderate (40–59% predicted FEV_1)
Severe (< 40% predicted FEV_1)

Review guidelines for treatment
Patient and/or carer education
Stepwise therapy approach
Action plan

Monitor progress through planned follow-up in primary or secondary care.

COPD – Chronic obstructive pulmonary disease
PEFR – Peak expiratory flow rate
FEV_1 – Forced expiratory volume in 1 second
CT – Computerized tomography

Figure 28.1 Diagnosing asthma and COPD.

Table 28.1 Differentiating asthma and COPD from the history

	Clinical features	
	COPD	Asthma
Chronic productive cough	Common	Uncommon
Breathlessness	Persistent and progressive	Variable
Night time breathlessness and/or wheezing	Uncommon	Common
Diurnal variation	Uncommon	Common

EXAMINATION

Look not only for the typical signs of severe chronic airflow obstruction (pursed lip breathing, barrel chest) but also for the other signs that may indicate another disease (or co-morbidity) such as ischaemic heart disease with atrial fibrillation and congestive cardiac failure. There may be no abnormal physical signs in patients with asthma/COPD as the signs generally become present when the disease is more advanced. The degree of airway obstruction cannot always be predicted from signs or symptoms.

INVESTIGATIONS

The most important investigations are spirometry and home recording of peak expiratory flow rate (PEFR). If it remains unclear whether the symptoms are caused by cardiac or respiratory disease, chest X-ray, ECG and, occasionally, echocardiography are indicated. Most people aged 65 years and over are able to perform lung function to the required standard laid down in national and international guidelines. It is important that patients are carefully instructed and lung function results are interpreted appropriately. As most geriatricians do not have expertise in lung function testing, referral of the patient to the lung function laboratory is usually a sensible option for the patient, particularly where the cause of shortness of breath is not clear.

fever as in younger people with asthma. Are there any other respiratory or non-respiratory symptoms such as haemoptysis or rapid weight loss – is there dual pathology, with lung cancer complicating a pre-existing condition, such as COPD or asthma?

Spirometry will identify whether the patient has airflow obstruction (forced expiratory volume in 1 second (FEV_1) < 80% predicted value for age, sex and height and FEV_1/vital capacity < 70%). In young adults, asthma is not normally associated with airflow obstruction but in older adults airflow obstruction is frequently present. In the presence of airflow obstruction, spirometry should be repeated following inhaled beta-2 agonists and anticholinergics administered via a volume-spacer device or nebulizer or after a 2-week trial of steroids (prednisolone 30 mg/day). A clinically significant response is defined as at least a 15% increase in the pre-bronchodilator FEV_1, providing that the size of the increase is at least 200 mL; if the increase is equal to or greater than 400 mL this is even more significant and helps identify asthma. The size of a significant bronchodilator response does not discriminate between asthma and COPD unless the post-bronchodilator FEV_1 returns to near-normal, reflecting full reversibility – which is almost certainly due to asthma.

Following a bronchodilator or corticosteroid trial, the patient can be provided with a peak flow meter to record the highest of three blows in the morning and evening for 2 to 4 weeks in order to look for 20% or more variation between morning and evening values. If the patient is agreeable, four measurement points within the day make the test more likely to pick up important variation than measurements made only twice daily. PEFR variation is calculated for each 24-hour period as the highest–lowest value divided by the highest. The presence of 20% or more variation in PEFR suggests asthma but if PEFR is low then spontaneous variability of the measurement may exceed this. Patients should be treated with regular inhaled antiinflammatory drugs and intermittent bronchodilators. They should be reviewed regularly as treatment is stepped down or stepped up (as recommended in the British Thoracic Society guidelines [BTS 1997a, NICE 2004]).

COPD is diagnosed when the patient has chronic and progressive airflow obstruction with one or more symptoms of exertional dyspnoea, chronic cough, regular sputum production, frequent winter 'bronchitis' and wheeze. Home records of PEFR will tend not to show 20% or more variability. A corticosteroid trial (prednisolone 30 mg/day for 2–4 weeks) or a high-dose inhaled corticosteroid trial (beclometasone or equivalent 2 mg/day through a volume-spacer device) are recommended for patients with severe COPD (FEV_1 < 30% of the predicted value.) A further assessment that is also important for patients with more severe disease is estimation of arterial gases: if oximetry is less than or equal to 92%, patients may require home oxygen for prolonged periods. Oximetry cannot be relied upon if the patient is deteriorating clinically or when complications have developed.

Key points to remember

- There is no single diagnostic test for COPD.
- For the diagnosis of COPD, history, physical examination and confirmation of airflow obstruction (spirometry) are necessary.
- The diagnosis of asthma is supported by 20% or greater diurnal variation or day-to-day variability in peak flow measurements, response to bronchodilator or response to oral steroid (prednisolone 30 mg daily for 2 weeks) with return of FEV1 and FEV1/FVC ratio to normal.

TREATMENT

For both asthma and COPD, the British Thoracic Society guidelines (BTS 1997a,b, NICE 2004, SIGN & BTS 2004) are available and provide clear and concise information on treatment of both diseases.

In asthma, inhaled corticosteroids (and leukotriene antagonists) reduce airway inflammation as the mainstay preventative approach. Short-acting inhaled bronchodilators are used for relief of symptoms and longer-acting bronchodilators (such as salmeterol) are prescribed when sufficient control has not been obtained with preventative and relief therapy. There is much less need to use oral bronchodilators in airways disease in older people because of the availability of longer-acting inhaled bronchodilators. Oral bronchodilators (such as theophyllines) can be associated with serious side-effects (such as cardiac dysrthymias and seizures) when plasma levels become raised because of over-dosage or impaired metabolism (due to intercurrent illness, such as respiratory tract infection or cardiac failure).

Relief and/or long-acting bronchodilators are the mainstay of treatment in COPD. Smoking cessation is one of the most important components of management and advice should be combined with use of nicotine replacement therapy. New guidelines recommend adding inhaled corticosteroids to the long-acting bronchodilators. This reduces exacerbations in patients with an FEV_1 $\leq 50\%$ predicted and in those who have had > 2 exacerbations in the past year.

Benefits of pulmonary rehabilitation (see Ch. 30) are clear and should be offered to all patients with moderate/severe COPD. Patient and/or carer education is important for both diseases. Many patients will benefit from a simple management plan drawn up in conjunction with their general practitioner or hospital physician. Agreement about clinical indicators that define when to use antibiotics or prednisolone, when to seek medical help and when to call for an ambulance are examples of the topics covered in such a plan.

INHALER DEVICES

Because of the higher prevalence of clinical problems in old age that may limit the competent use of drug delivery devices, selecting the correct device for patients needs to be done with great care. There are many different inhaler devices and time is required when the patient (and preferably the respiratory nurse in primary or secondary care in conjunction with the patient and/or carer) can try the different devices and find the most suitable one. Metered dose inhalers together with an Aerochamber are recommended. Rinsing of the chamber and gargling afterwards reduces steroid deposition in the oropharynx and therefore oropharyngeal candidiasis. In very frail breathless patients, inspiration may be at too low a flow rate to adequately activate drug release and allow sufficient lung drug deposition. The proportion of patients with asthma or COPD in whom a nebulizer is required is small.

There are several groups of older patients in whom management of asthma/COPD may be less than adequate. One such group is people with cognitive impairment, who may not be able to carry out satisfactory lung function tests, may be unable to coordinate correct inhaler technique and might be unable to pick up signs of worsening disease requiring medical help. These patients and their carers need a lot of attention. Their inhaler devices should be simple to use, such as the metered dose inhaler attached to a volume spacer. The carer can administer the drugs with the patient being encouraged to tidal breathe (take normal breaths). An anaesthetic mask over the mouth can be attached if the patient will not keep their mouth closed around the mouthpiece.

Another group of vulnerable patients is those who are generally weak and unwell from severe disease (with or without co-morbidity) and who do not have the strength to carry out repeated lung function tests or generate sufficient inspiratory flow to allow deposition of drugs in the airways. This situation is particularly common in acutely unwell older people admitted into hospital. Attempts at diagnosis are better delayed until recovery has taken place. Nebulizers may be needed during the acute period.

Sometimes patients do not seem to recover for long enough between attacks. Here referral to a chest physician may be helpful.

Follow-up to reassess the effectiveness of treatment and how the patient is coping with the inhaler devices prescribed is essential. As geriatricians, unless there is a specific respiratory interest, this is best done in primary care by the asthma/COPD nurse and GP, who would be able to offer pneumococcal vaccination and annual influenza vaccination as well as osteoporosis prophylaxis to patients on long-term corticostroids or who are requiring frequent courses of oral corticosteroids.

As with other aspects of respiratory disease, most research has concentrated on young and middle-aged adults. In relation to asthma, there is little or no information on the importance of allergy and the relationship with other atopic disorders, such as eczema.

REFERENCES

British Thoracic Society (BTS) 1997a Guidelines for the management of chronic obstructive pulmonary disease. Thorax 52 (Suppl 5):S1–S28
British Thoracic Society (BTS) 1997b National asthma campaign, Royal College of Physicians. Thorax 52 (Suppl 1):S1–S2

Dow L, Coggon D, Osmond C et al 1991 A population survey of respiratory symptoms in the elderly. European Respiratory Journal 4:267–272

National Institute for Clinical Excellence (NICE) 2004 Chronic obstructive airways disease, clinical guideline 2. NICE, London. Also published in Thorax 59:2

Scottish Intercollegiate Guidelines Network (SIGN), British Thoracic Society (BTS) 2004 British guideline on management of asthma. Royal College of Physicians, Edinburgh, British Thoracic Society, London

Acknowledgment

I wish to acknowledge that the earlier chapter, on which this chapter is based, was written by Dr Lindsey Dow. I am grateful to Dr Dow for her valuable contribution.

SELF-ASSESSMENT QUESTION

A 72-year-old ex-smoker of 40 pack years (smoking 20 cigarettes a day for 40 years) attends out-patients with a history of progressive breathlessness and wheeze over 2 years. Are the following true or false?

1. The factors that support use of inhaled corticosteroids in combination with inhaled bronchodilators are:
   a. Post-bronchodilator FEV_1 change of 10% increase over the pre-bronchodilator FEV_1
   b. Family history of asthma
   c. Twenty per cent or greater variation of with-day peak expiratory flow (PEF) on one or more days out of a 2-week PEF record
   d. Early morning haemoptysis
   e. A change in FEV1 from 1.9 L to 2.4 L following a trial of prednisolone 40 mg daily for 2 weeks

SECTION 3

Respiratory system

Chapter 29

Tuberculosis

Charlie Teale

INTRODUCTION

Tuberculosis causes some 3 million deaths per year worldwide – a quarter of all preventable deaths (Maher et al 1997). Although more common in the developing world, recent increases in incidence in some developed countries (Reider 1992) make it an important threat to health. In the UK around 30% of notifications for tuberculosis are in subjects over 65 (Teale et al 1993). In this chapter I shall review the condition with particular reference to differences between older and younger subjects.

EPIDEMIOLOGY

In the UK the incidence of tuberculosis per 100 000 fell from over 200 to 10 in the 20th century. This was mainly because of improvements in public health, poverty and nutrition, with a lesser effect of more recent screening programmes and effective chemotherapy (Seaton et al 2000). This fall was accompanied by a doubling in the proportion

of notifications in older subjects from 14% to 29% between 1953 and 1979 (Powell & Farer 1980). A recent survey in Scotland (Driffield et al 1996) reported the incidence of tuberculosis to be three to five times higher in subjects aged 65 years and over compared to those aged 15 to 44 years; the absolute number of notifications in subjects aged 65 years and over may be increasing, perhaps due to increases in the numbers of the very old in the population. Increases in the proportion of tuberculosis diagnosed in older people have been reported outside the UK (Chan-Yeung et al 2002). Notification rates for tuberculosis increase with age regardless of race, gender or ethnic group (Centers for Disease Control 1990). There have been outbreaks of tuberculosis in nursing homes but a study from the UK suggest residents are not generally at increased risk (Nisar et al 1993).

PATHOGENESIS

In the early 1900s, 80% of the population was infected by the age of 30 years (Rich 1951). Most cases now occurring in older subjects reflect reactivation of old 'healed disease' (Stead & Dutt 1991). This occurs because of impaired immunity, related to such factors as disease, poor nutrition, poverty and ageing (Teale & Pearson 1996). A reduction in the incidence of tuberculosis in older subjects is unlikely for some decades, when there will be a new cohort of elderly people with a lower prevalence of previous infection.

CLINICAL FEATURES

Several recent studies have examined the presentation and clinical features of tuberculosis in old and younger adults (Katz et al 1987, Korzeniewska-Kosela et al 1994, Teale et al 1993, Umeki 1989, van der Brande et al 1991) although none have reported specifically on the very old (e.g. 80 years and over). The commonest presenting features of tuberculosis in both younger and older adults are cough, anorexia and lethargy while weight loss, fever, sweats and haemoptysis are all well recognized. The frequency of symptoms is broadly similar in both groups. In both elderly and younger subjects 80–90% of notifications with tuberculosis are for pulmonary disease. Non-pulmonary disease is rare in the UK but may affect particularly the skeleton, the urogenital system and the meninges (Teale & Pearson 1996).

INVESTIGATIONS

The most important investigations in diagnosing tuberculosis are sputum microscopy and culture plus chest radiography. Upper-zone involvement on chest radiograph is reported in about 70% of young and older subjects but mid- and lower-zone involvement is more common in old people, seen in around 20% of cases in European and American studies (Korzeniewska-Kosela et al 1994, Teale et al 1993); interestingly, these ratios were reversed in an African study (Morris 1989). Miliary changes are seen in about 5% of older cases but are very rare in the young (Korzeniewska-Kosela et al 1994, Teale et al 1993); miliary tuberculosis is caused by blood-borne spread of many tubercules to the lung and other organs and may appear as

small 'millet-size' nodules on the chest radiograph. Skin testing can be of value but a grade 3–4 Heaf reaction is seen in around a third of older subjects due to previous infection and may not help diagnosing new disease (Capewell & Leitch 1986). In addition, false negative results may be obtained in several circumstances such as miliary disease, immunosuppressant drugs and diseases such as lymphoma (Teale & Pearson 1996). A raised sedimentation rate is common in younger and older subjects with tuberculosis (van der Brande et al 1991) but anaemia and a reduced white count are more frequently seen in older subjects (Umeki 1989, van der Brande et al 1991).

MANAGEMENT

Management is similar in older and younger subjects and requires curative chemotherapy and prevention of infection. Specialist referral is recommended because of the relative infrequency with which most geriatricians will manage such patients and the high mortality and incidence of side-effects in older subjects. Standard therapy for fully sensitive organisms consists of 2 months of rifampicin, isoniazid and pyrazinamide and a further 4 months of just rifampicin and isoniazid (ethambutol may be added in the initial 2 months but is usually avoided in older subjects because of its ocular toxicity, while pyridoxine is generally given to protect against isoniazid-induced neuropathy [Ormerod 1990]). Drug resistance is rare in old people, seen in only 2% of a survey in the UK (Teale et al 1993). Relapse usually reflects poor compliance and may be helped in some regimes using once-daily combination preparations such as Rifater and Rifinah. Side-effects are more common in older subjects; they necessitated stopping drugs on 18% of patients in one series compared with only 7% of younger subjects (Teale et al 1993).

OUTCOME

Advanced age is an adverse risk factor for outcome. In one survey, 21% of tuberculosis in subjects 65 years and older was diagnosed post mortem compared to only 1% under 65 years (Teale et al

1993). Even after diagnosis and starting treatment, there is a high mortality (16%) from tuberculosis in subjects aged 65 years and older compared with 3% under 65 years (Humphries et al 1984). It is not known whether mortality has improved over the past 20 years.

SUMMARY

Tuberculosis is an important cause of preventable death which may often enter the differential diagnosis of ill older people. There are broad similarities between tuberculosis in older and young subjects, though important differences exist. About 30% of cases diagnosed in the UK are diagnosed in subjects over 65 years and are usually due to reactivation of old 'healed' disease. Tuberculosis usually presents with cough, anorexia and lethargy plus upper-zone changes on chest radiograph. Lower-zone and miliary disease are more frequent in older subjects. Treatment is similar in older and younger subjects but side-effects are more common in the old. Death is much more frequent in older subjects, with around 20% of cases diagnosed post mortem and up to 20% dying despite treatment. A high index of suspicion is required to reduce the mortality from this potentially curable condition.

Key points

- *Epidemiology:* 30% of notifications for TB in the UK are aged 65 years and over.
- *Pathogenesis:* usually reactivation.
- *Presentation:* typically cough/anorexia/weight loss with upper-zone shadowing on chest radiograph.
- *Management:* the same as in young people – it is best to refer to the specialist.
- *Outcome:* one in six may die despite treatment.

REFERENCES

*** *Essential reading; ** recommended reading; * interesting but not vital*

Capewell S, Leitch A G 1986 Tuberculin reactivity in a chest clinic: the effects of age and prior BCG vac- cination. British Journal of Diseases of the Chest 80:37–41 **

Centers for Disease Control 1990 Screening for tuber- culosis and tuberculosis infection in the United States. Recommendations of the Advisory Com- mittee for Elimination of Tuberculosis; MMWR 39 (RR-8),1 *

Chan-Yeung M, Noertjojo J, Tan J et al 2002 Tuberculosis in the elderly in Hong Kong. International Journal of Tuberculosis and Lung Disease 6:771–779

Driffield J S, Adams W H, Anderson M et al 1996 Increasing incidence of tuberculosis in young and elderly in Scotland. Thorax 51:140–142 ***

Humphries M J, Byfield S B, Darbyshire J H et al 1984 Deaths occurring in newly notified patients with pulmonary tuberculosis in England and Wales. British Journal of Diseases of the Chest 78: 149–158 ***

Katz P R, Reichman W, Dube D et al 1987 Clinical features of pulmonary tuberculosis in young and old veterans. Journal of the American Geriatrics Society 35:512–515 **

Korzeniewska-Kosela M, Krysl J, Muller N et al 1994 Tuberculosis in young adults and the elderly. Chest 106:28–32 **

Maher D, Chaulet P, Spinachi S et al 1997 Treatment of tuberculosis: guidelines for national programmes, 2nd edn. WHO, Geneva, p 13 *

Morris C D W 1989 The radiography, haematology and bronchoscopy of pulmonary tuberculosis in the aged. Quarterly Journal of Medicine New Series 71:259–265 **

Nisar M, William C S D, Ashby D et al 1993 Tuberculin testing in residential homes for the elderly. Thorax 48:1257–1260 **

Ormerod L P 1990 Chemotherapy and management of tuberculosis in the United Kingdom: recom- mendation of the joint tuberculosis committee of the British Thoracic Society. Thorax 45:403–408 **

Powell K E, Farer L S 1980 The rising age of the tuber- culosis patient. Journal of Infectious Diseases 142: 946–948 **

Reider H L 1992 Misbehaviour of a dying epidemic: a call for less speculation and better surveillance (Edi- torial). Tuberculosis and Lung Disease 73:181–182 *

Rich A R 1951 The pathogenesis of tuberculosis. Charles C Thomas, Springfield, IL **

Seaton A D, Haslett C, Seaton D et al 2000 Crofton and Douglas's respiratory diseases, 5th edn. Blackwell Scientific, Oxford, p 476–564 **

Stead W W, Dutt A K 1991 Tuberculosis in elderly persons. Annual Review of Medicine 42:267–273 **

Teale C, Pearson S B 1996 Tuberculosis and other myco- bacterial diseases in elderly patients. In: Connolly

M J (ed.) Respiratory disease in the elderly patient. Chapman and Hall, London, p 126 **

Teale C, Goldman J M, Pearson S B 1993 The association of age with the presentation and outcome of tuberculosis: a five year survey. Age and Ageing 22:289–293 ***

Umeki S 1989 Comparison of young and elderly patients with pulmonary tuberculosis. Respiration 55:75–79 **

van der Brande P, Vijgen J, Demedts M 1991 Clinical spectrum of pulmonary tuberculosis in older patients: comparison with younger patients. Journal of Gerontology 46:M204–209 **

SELF–ASSESSMENT QUESTION

1. Are the following true or false?
   a. Notifications for tuberculosis in old age in the UK are falling
   b. Apical shadowing on chest radiographs is typical of tuberculosis in older subjects
   c. Tuberculosis is usually associated with a blood leucocytosis in older subjects
   d. Death from tuberculosis is rare once an older patient is started on treatment
   e. In the UK, nursing home residents should usually be considered to be at increased risk of tuberculosis
   f. A strong positive Heaf test (grade 3–4) is highly suspicious of active tuberculosis

SECTION 3

Respiratory system

Chapter 30

Respiratory rehabilitation

Martin J. Connolly

INTRODUCTION

Respiratory disease ranks second only to musculoskeletal disease (and above stroke) as a cause of overall disability in elderly people (Hunt 1976). Over 15 years ago, Cockcroft defined respiratory rehabilitation as 'returning patients with respiratory disability to as normal a life as possible, aiming for them to achieve independent function in all their life activities' (Cockcroft 1988). With the removal of the word 'respiratory' from this definition, geriatricians would recognize Cockcroft's phraseology as an excellent definition of rehabilitation in general. Given this, and the numerical importance of respiratory disease as a cause of disability, it is surprising that respiratory rehabilitation has not hitherto occupied the thoughts and practices of most geriatricians. The possible reasons for this have been reviewed (Connolly 1996). Hospital-based pulmonary rehabilitation programmes in the UK tend to exclude elderly patients with COPD, despite the age-related demographics of this condition (Yohannes & Connolly

2004). Atypical presentation and difficulties in detection of respiratory disease and disability are discussed elsewhere in this volume (see Ch. 28).

The main aim of this chapter is to review the evidence (or frequently lack of it) for the value of respiratory rehabilitation in elderly patients. I will extrapolate data on studies of younger patients (often a dangerous thing to do). I will also point out where evidence is lacking, and this may help direct the trainee to areas of further potentially fruitful research.

COMPONENTS OF RESPIRATORY REHABILITATION

Respiratory rehabilitation requires an interdisciplinary approach comprising: best medical therapy; smoking cessation (with help and support); patient and family education; exercise training and respiratory muscle training; nutritional assessment and possibly support; psychological assessment and often intervention; and assessment for long-term oxygen therapy (LTOT). To be most effective, respiratory rehabilitation should be started as soon as possible and preferably before the patient becomes so disabled as to be housebound.

SMOKING CESSATION

Most elderly patients requiring respiratory rehabilitation will have smoking-related chronic obstructive pulmonary disease (COPD) and many will still be smoking at the time of initial assessment. The value and feasibility of smoking cessation in old age have been reviewed recently (Connolly 2000). It is one of only two measures (the other being LTOT for some patients) that prolong life in COPD. It is of value even in very elderly people. Patients who are unable or unwilling to stop smoking should not, however, be denied access to respiratory rehabilitation programmes. There is evidence for the value of nicotine replacement therapy in smoking cessation support in old age. Nicotine replacement can increase quit rate in the motivated smoker up to 20% at 1 year (Connolly 2000). Smoking cessation is only part of the range of measures in a respiratory rehabilitation programme and should probably be addressed only after a trusting relationship has developed between the interdisciplinary team and the patient. Unfortunately, there is evidence that offers of smoking cessation by health personnel to patients both within and outwith the hospital context have an age-related bias (Buckland & Connolly 2005).

EXERCISE TOLERANCE TESTING

Exercise tolerance testing is a mainstay of assessment in pulmonary rehabilitation. It helps provide a baseline for the patient and the interdisciplinary team and, when repeated occasionally throughout the rehabilitation programme, its gradual improvement may provide continued motivation for the patient. Some elderly patients have been put off by technology such as treadmills and bicycle ergometers, and thus exercise assessment should be as simple as possible. The 6-minute walk test has been validated in elderly patients with COPD (Roomi et al 1996). Other tests such as the 2-minute walk test, the 12-minute walk test, and the shuttle walk test (a progressive, externally paced exercise test requiring the subject to walk/run back and forth between two fixed points) may be equally valuable.

EXERCISE TRAINING

This is an essential component of all respiratory rehabilitation programmes. It should be done in out-patient units and comprises aerobic conditioning (both upper and lower body) together with inspiratory and expiratory resistance training (respiratory muscle training). In younger patients, training improves not only exercise capacity but also quality of life (Lacasse et al 2003, Ries et al 1997). Pulmonary rehabilitation also reduces breathlessness (Ries et al 1997) and is cost-effective compared to usual care (Griffiths et al 2001). The data on rates of hospitalization and time spent in hospital are equivocal.

The duration of benefit is also a matter of debate, with some studies suggesting that the improvements (at least in exercise tolerance) may last for up to 12 months in the absence of any maintenance programme, and other data suggesting the converse (Swerts et al 1990, Vale et al 1993). There is very little evidence concerning the benefits of attendance at further 'top-up' pulmonary rehabilitation programmes.

In practice, a 6–8 week programme should comprise a physiotherapy-directed assessment session followed by individualized programmes of daily aerobic exercise (or small amounts of exercise 3 or 4 times daily). As many muscle groups as possible should be involved in the exercises which might include walking, step aerobics (bottom step of the staircase), *light* weightlifting for upper body exercise, alternate standing and sitting, 'punching the air', etc. There should be a supervised group session at least once weekly to check on techniques and progress and to facilitate the positive support of a group environment. Exercise to music may help add variety and maintain motivation. Home-based programmes may be particularly appropriate for elderly people (Wijkstra et al 1996).

Areas for further research here include: duration of benefits of pulmonary rehabilitation in old age, the effect on activities of daily living, and whether such programmes affect the frequency of falls.

PSYCHOLOGICAL ASSESSMENT

Clinical psychology input is important in treating patients disabled with respiratory disease. In practice, however, such input is not always readily available. This is unfortunate as the prevalence of depression in elderly patients with COPD is over 40% (Yohannes et al 2000a), and the prevalence of sub-threshold depression which significantly affects quality of life is commoner still (Yohannes et al 2003). Clinical anxiety is also common but seems to be strongly associated with depression, with anxiety being uncommon in those who do not have depressive symptomatology.

Unfortunately, most older patients will not volunteer depressive symptoms and the detection rate in the absence of screening questionnaires is poor. This is a well-recognized phenomenon in depression associated with chronic illness in old age (Jackson & Baldwin 1993). The BASDEC questionnaire has proved useful in detection of depressive symptomatology (Yohannes et al 2000a) and is highly sensitive and specific in this subject group.

However, treatment of depressive problems in elderly COPD patients is often difficult. Frequently a patient is reluctant to accept the diagnosis and even more reluctant to take antidepressant medication (Yohannes et al 2002). This is also seen in depression associated with many other chronic diseases in old age and merits further research.

Depression is not only a predictor of poor quality of life but also appears to predict mortality in elderly patients with severe COPD (Yohannes et al 2005). Whether the treatment of depression in this patient group will reduce mortality from COPD is unknown and worthy of further research, though the ethical dilemmas involved in this might be considerable.

ASSESSMENT OF DISABILITY

It is not possible to assess a patient's level of function from clinical examination and simple investigations such as spirometry or even exercise tolerance testing. Until recently there had been little validation of scales of activities of daily living (ADL) in people with chronic lung disease. The Barthel Index underestimates disability in this subject group but the Nottingham Extended ADL Scale is a good discriminator between normal elderly people and those disabled by COPD (Yohannes et al 1997). However, the Nottingham scale is not responsive to improvement resulting from treatment. Two new scales, the Manchester Respiratory Activities of Daily Living Scale (MRADL) and London Chest ADL Scale (Garrod et al 2000, 2002, Yohannes et al 2000b), are both sensitive and specific for COPD in old age and also responsive to treatment in pulmonary rehabilitation. Activities of daily living are a more powerful predictor of mortality in COPD than spirometry (which has previously been regarded as the best mortality predictor [British Thoracic Society 1997, Yohannes et al 2005]). The use of a validated ADL scale is essential in the assessment of elderly patients with COPD whether or not they are participating in a respiratory rehabilitation programme. With such an assessment, we can determine the impact of the illness on the patient's life; this may help in the design and tailoring of rehabilitation to each patient and in the planning of an individual care package.

COMMUNITY SUPPORT

Elderly patients disabled by COPD seem to receive less statutory community support than patients of the same age equally disabled by other conditions (Yohannes et al 1998). This is despite evidence that such provision helps increase social interaction and self-esteem. Community support also reduces hospitalization (Bergner et al 1998, Cummings et al 1990, Haggerty et al 1991, Miles-Tapping 1994). The respiratory rehabilitation team should assess the needs for home care and for the provision of 'meals on wheels'. The value of occupational therapy assessment is unproven, though recommended in national guidelines (National Collaborating Centre for Chronic Conditions 2004). The value of occupational therapy in the assessment of patients with COPD is an area worthy of further study.

Where patients are provided with nebulizers or LTOT, there should be home-based assessment of patients and carers and abilities to use such devices, together with provision for regular servicing and an emergency telephone number for use in the case of breakdown of nebulizers or concentrators.

PATIENT SUPPORT, SELF-MANAGEMENT AND EDUCATION

In contrast to self-management plans in asthma there is little evidence of the value of self-management in COPD. We need more research in this area as well as on the effectiveness (and indeed the content) of educational packages for such patients. Many (though not all) patients find contact with patient support groups helpful.

PALLIATIVE CARE

Many patients will not wish to participate in respiratory rehabilitation or will be too ill, frail or cognitively impaired to do so. Simple advice to patients to lie propped up on their side (high-sided lying) often improves breathlessness at night in patients with severe COPD. These patients can be helped symptomatically by the use of high walking frames which reduce breathlessness (Grant & Capel 1972, Roomi et al 1998). Self-propelled wheelchairs are seldom useful because of the high levels of aerobic work needed to propel them, but outdoor battery-operated chairs or pushchairs may reduce social isolation and increase independence. Chair lifts for patients unable to climb stairs may be helpful. Provision of emergency alarm systems may help reduce anxiety, particularly in patients prone to severe attacks of breathlessness.

Following hospitalization for acute exacerbation, those patients surviving to discharge have a 1-year mortality usually in excess of 30% (Yohannes et al 2005). This is higher than that for many cancers and yet, in common with other non-neoplastic conditions with high mortality (most notably congestive cardiac failure), the provision of expert end-of-life care for such patients is patchy at best. Further evaluation and an expansion of the service in this area is urgently needed.

REFERENCES

Bergner M, Hudson L D, Conard D A et al 1988 Cost and efficacy of home care for patients with chronic lung disease. Medical Care 26:566–579

British Thoracic Society 1997 BTS guidelines for the management of chronic obstructive pulmonary disease. Thorax 52(Suppl 5):S1–S28

Buckland A, Connolly M J 2005 Age-related differences in smoking cessation advice and support given to patients hospitalised with smoking-related illness. Age and Ageing 34:639–642

Cockcroft A 1988 Pulmonary rehabilitation. British Journal of Diseases of the Chest 82:220–225

Connolly M J 1996 Obstructive airways disease: a hidden disability in the aged. Age and Ageing 25:265–267

Connolly M J 2000 Smoking cessation in old age: closing the stable door? Age and Ageing 29:193–195

Cummings J E, Hughes S L, Weaver F M et al 1990 Cost-effectiveness of Veterans Administration Hospital-based home care: a randomised clinical trial. Archives of Internal Medicine 150:1274–1280

Garrod R, Bestall J C, Paul E A et al 2000 Development and validation of a standardized measure of activity of daily living in patients with severe COPD: the London Chest Activity of Daily Living scale (LCADL). Respiratory Medicine 94:589–596

Garrod R, Paul E A, Wedzicha J A 2002 An evaluation of the reliability and sensitivity of the London Chest Activity of Daily Living Scale (LCADL). Respiratory Medicine 96:725–730

Grant B J B, Capel L H 1972 Walking aids for pulmonary emphysema. Lancet ii:1125–1127

Griffiths T L, Phillips C J, Davies S 2001 Cost effectiveness of an outpatient multidisciplinary pulmonary rehabilitation programme. Thorax 56:779–784

Haggerty M C, Stockdale-Wolley R, Nair S 1991 Respicare: an innovative home care program for the patient with chronic obstructive pulmonary disease. Chest 100:607–612

Hunt A 1976 The elderly at home: a study of people aged sixty-five and over living in the community in England 1976. OPCS/HMSO, London

Jackson R, Baldwin B 1993 Detecting depression in elderly medically ill patients: the use of the Geriatric Depression Scale compared with medical and nursing observation. Age and Ageing 22:349–353

Lacasse Y, Brosseau L, Milne S et al 2003 Pulmonary rehabilitation for chronic obstructive pulmonary disease. Cochrane Database of Systematic Reviews, Issue 3. Art. No.: CD003793. DOI: 10.1002/14651858. CD003793

Miles-Tapping C 1994 Home care for chronic obstructive pulmonary disease: impact of the Iqualit programme. Archives of Medical Research 55:163–175

National Collaborating Centre for Chronic Conditions 2004 Chronic obstructive pulmonary disease. National clinical guideline on management of chronic obstructive pulmonary disease in adults in primary and secondary care. Thorax 59(Suppl 1):1–232

Ries A L, Carlin B W, Carrieri-Kohlman V et al 1997 Pulmonary rehabilitation: joint ACCP/AACVPR evidence-based guidelines. Chest 112:1363–1396

Roomi J, Johnson M M, Waters K et al 1996 Respiratory rehabilitation, exercise capacity and quality of life in chronic airways disease in old age. Age and Ageing 25:12–16

Roomi J, Yohannes A M, Connolly M J 1998 The effect of walking aids on exercise capacity and oxygenation in elderly patients with chronic obstructive pulmonary disease. Age and Ageing 27:703–706

Swerts P M, Kretzers L M, Terpstra-Windevean E et al 1990 Exercise reconditioning in the rehabilitation of patients with chronic obstructive pulmonary disease: a short and long-term analysis. Archives of Physical Medicine and Rehabilitation 71: 570–573

Vale F, Reardon J Z, Zuwallack R L 1993 Long-term benefits of out-patient pulmonary rehabilitation on exercise endurance and quality of life. Chest 103: 42–45

Wijkstra P J, van der Mark T W, Kraan J et al 1996 Long-term effects of home rehabilitation on physical performance in chronic obstructive pulmonary disease. American Journal of Respiratory and Critical Care Medicine 153:1234–1241

Yohannes A M, Connolly M J 2004 Pulmonary rehabilitation programmes in the UK: a national representative survey. Clinical Rehabilitation 18:444–449

Yohannes A M, Roomi J, Waters K et al 1997 A comparison of the Barthel Index and Nottingham extended activities of daily living scale in the assessment of disability in chronic airflow limitation in old age. Age and Ageing 27:369–374

Yohannes A M, Roomi J, Connolly M J 1998 Elderly people at home disabled by chronic obstructive pulmonary disease. Age and Ageing 27:523–525

Yohannes A M, Baldwin R C, Connolly M J 2000a Depression and anxiety in elderly outpatients with chronic obstructive pulmonary disease: prevalence, and validation of the BASDEC screening questionnaire. International Journal of Geriatric Psychiatry 15:1090–1096

Yohannes A M, Roomi J, Winn S et al 2000b The Manchester Respiratory Activities of Daily Living Questionnaire: development, reliability and responsiveness. Journal of the American Geriatrics Society 48:1496–1500

Yohannes A M, Connolly M J, Baldwin R C 2002 A feasibility study of antidepressant drug therapy in depressed elderly patients with chronic obstructive pulmonary disease. International Journal of Geriatric Psychiatry 16:451–454

Yohannes A M, Baldwin R C, Connolly M J 2003 Prevalence of sub-threshold depression in elderly patients with chronic obstructive pulmonary disease. International Journal of Geriatric Psychiatry 18:412–416

Yohannes A M, Baldwin R C, Connolly M J 2005 Predictors of 1-year mortality in patients discharged from hospital following acute exacerbation of chronic obstructive pulmonary disease. Age and Ageing 34:491–496

RECOMMENDED READING

Chauhan A J, Leahy B C 1996 Pulmonary rehabilitation in the elderly patient. In: Connolly M J (ed.) Respiratory disease in the elderly patient. Chapman and Hall, London, p 261–295

Connolly M J 1993 Respiratory rehabilitation in the elderly patient. Clinical Gerontology 3:381–394

Patient self-help
The UK national self-help group for COPD patients is known as Breathe Easy. There are over 100 Breathe Easy groups throughout the United Kingdom that provide support for both patients and their carers. Information can be accessed from the British Lung Foundation website: http://www.britishlungfoundation.com

SELF-ASSESSMENT QUESTIONS

Are the following statements true or false?

1. Stroke is a commoner cause of disability in old age than respiratory disease

2. The 1-year smoking quit rate for motivated elderly people given nicotine replacement therapy may be up by:
   a. 5%
   b. 20%
   c. 30%

3. The prevalence of depressive symptoms in elderly patients disabled by COPD is about 20%

4. Self-propelled wheelchairs may improve independence of elderly patients disabled by COPD

5. Patients discharged from hospital following acute exacerbations of COPD have an approximate 1-year mortality of:
   a. 7%
   b. 15–20%
   c. Over 30%

6. Exercise tolerance testing is the best method of assessing level of disability in elderly patients with COPD

SECTION 4

Gastrointestinal system

Chapter 31

Oral health

Angus Walls

STEREOTYPES AND CHANGES

The traditional image of the older person is of someone with few or no natural teeth who relies on dentures for adequate oral function. While this was true, the situation is changing rapidly. The reasons for this are complex but there are two fundamental alterations:

- People are no longer content with extraction as a generic solution for dental problems
- By means of dental care, dentists have increasing capability of saving teeth that once would have been regarded as beyond rescue

This alteration in the oral health status of the population will continue over the next 30 to 40 years (Fig. 31.1) (Kelly et al 2000). The reason for the protracted timescale for change is that tooth extraction and edentulism (having no natural teeth) are irreversible. Humankind only has two 'sets' of natural teeth. Once the adult teeth are removed people have to rely increasingly on artificial substitutes.

Fortunately, not only are fewer people being rendered edentulous but fewer teeth are also being removed in those who have teeth. The result is that the oral health of the next generations of older people will be markedly different. There will be more people with natural teeth and those who have teeth will tend to have more of them than today's age-matched cohorts currently.

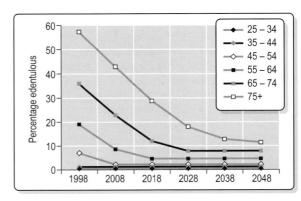

Figure 31.1 Projected changes in the rates of edentulism in the UK over the next 40 years (Kelly et al 1998).

This change will necessitate changes in oral healthcare pathways for older patients, particularly those who rely on others for personal care and hygiene. It also means that the patterns of oral disease seen in older people will change. Currently, most problems relate to oral mucosal disease. However, with increasing numbers of people having teeth, there will be an increase in older people having problems with their natural teeth: tooth decay leading ultimately to abscess formation (with the associated symptoms of pain) and gum disease leading to loosening of the teeth.

THE EDENTULOUS

Edentulism is the state of having no natural teeth. There is some social inequality in rates of edentulism in all age groups with greater proportions of people from less advantaged social backgrounds having no natural teeth. Edentulous people mainly rely on dentures for oral function and appearance. There are small numbers of people who do not use dentures as a matter of choice. They rely on gumming their food and require a soft diet to allow them to maintain nutrition. Dentures are often regarded erroneously as a replacement for teeth. They are not; rather they are poor substitutes for natural dentition. Essentially they are two large pieces of plastic which rest against the oral mucosal lining. They are held in place by three variables:

- *Gravity.* This acts in favour of a lower denture and serves to displace an upper denture.
- *Adhesion and cohesion.* When dentures are relatively new, the shape of the fitting surface of the denture should correspond quite closely to the shape of the gum. The procedures that a dentist uses to make dentures are designed to maximize the quality of this relationship. When the dentures fit well, there is a thin and even film of saliva between the denture surface and the gum. The saliva adheres to both surfaces and has intrinsic cohesive strength which results in stabilization of the denture. This can be likened to two plates of glass being glued together by a thin film of water. When the film is thin it is very difficult to pull the glass plates apart, they need to be separated by sliding. As

the thickness of the water film increases, the attachment between the surfaces is reduced exponentially.

- *Juggling.* Dentures only fit well for a relatively short period as the shape of the supporting bone changes with time. The bone progressively resorbs, resulting in a loss in both height and width of the supporting ridge. The rate of change varies from individual to individual, but after about 4–5 years of use the closeness of adaptation of a denture base to the gum will reduce to such an extent that it is no longer held in place by the salivary film. Furthermore the retentive forces that are generated by the salivary film are relatively low. The dentures are stabilized in the mouth by their owner with carefully controlled neuromuscular activity pushing the denture back in to place. As an example: when someone wearing dentures wants to bite something with their front teeth, they curl the back of the tongue up to press the back of the upper denture against the palate and the sides of the tongue down to stabilize the back of the lower denture and allow pressure to be applied by the teeth at the front of the mouth.

The reported average age of dentures in an older population is 10–15 years. Thus most denture users are relying on their oral juggling skills for denture stability and retention. This is a complex learned neuromuscular skill that must be practised regularly for the skill to be maintained. If someone leaves their dentures out for any length of time, for example during chemotherapy when the mouth is sore, then this skill will be lost and dentures that previously appeared to function well will suddenly become loose. Equally, patients after a stroke who have some loss of control of the tongue often experience problems trying to stabilize their dentures.

Dentures should be worn when the person using them is awake (if they wish) but should not be worn during sleep.

THE DENTATE

Nowadays, between 30 and 40% of people aged 75 years and over will have some natural teeth, with a greater proportion of people being from more affluent social backgrounds. Of these, about 30% will also have a complete denture in one jaw, usually the upper, and a further 40–50% will use a partial denture to facilitate oral function and appearance. The partially dentate who use dentures as well, and particularly those who have a compete denture in one jaw, are at risk both from disease associated with teeth and those problems that are attributable to denture wear (Baum et al 1992, Steele et al 1998).

ORAL DISEASE AND ITS MANAGEMENT

The pattern of oral diseases seen will depend on whether or not a person has some natural teeth and whether or not they use dentures.

SALIVA

Historically, salivary flow was thought to reduce with increasing age. However, recent studies have demonstrated that in healthy, non-medicated older people there are few changes in flow rate from the major salivary glands. Alterations are seen, however, in salivary composition with some variation in the mineral balance of saliva along with alterations in mucins. The clinical significance of these changes is unclear. However, the alterations in ionic content may be related to variations in taste perception found in older subjects.

There are alterations in minor salivary gland output with age (the minor glands lie immediately beneath the oral mucosa and empty directly onto the mucosal surface). These glands have a highly mucous secretion as well as being responsible for much of the secretory IgA and IgG in the mouth. Again, the clinical significance of these changes is unclear; however there will be reduced mucosal immunity as a consequence of this change (Baum et al 1992, Ship 2002).

Pathological change in gland function

The most common cause of dry mouth (xerostomia) in older people is as a side-effect of drugs. The secretory control of saliva is complex, but involves α and β adrenergic receptors, muscarinic cholinergic receptors as well as intracellular calcium channel signalling. Xerostomia is also influenced by hydration.

> Any drugs that impact on these receptors have the potential to reduce salivary output. Unfortunately these drugs are commonly given in combination and their effects are synergistic in relation to salivary output (Narhi et al 1992).

Other causes of xerostomia are Sjögren's syndrome and either surgical removal of gland tissue or destruction of the gland as a secondary effect of radiotherapy for head and neck malignancy.

Dry mouth is a cause of morbidity for sufferers and can result in difficulties in speech, chewing and swallowing and derangement of taste (Chambers 2004).

There are a number of potential strategies to stimulate salivary flow or to replace the fluid, should this be required.

Mechanical/taste
Chewing food and having a pleasant taste in the mouth both stimulate salivary output. One potentially simple adjunct for patients with dry mouth is to encourage them to use chewing gum regularly. Gums that are sugar free are preferred (see below) (Bots et al 2005).

Chemical
It is possible to use drugs that will simulate salivary flow, for example the cholinergic agonist pilocarpine. The utility of such drugs is limited by their side-effects of increased cholinergic tone (including sweating, increased frequency of micturition, hair loss and tachycardia). Pilocarpine is licensed for use in the UK for patients with radiation-induced salivary gland damage. Cimeviline also stimulates salivary flow and has fewer side-effects than pilocarpine.

Substitution
Commercial salivary substitutes may be of benefit for people with a dry mouth. However, care is required to ensure that the artificial saliva does not cause problems. Some artificial salivas have a pH which is lower than that which can cause the tooth surface to dissolve so should not be used

in people with natural teeth (the liquid should have a pH above 5.9). Palliation of symptoms with water is often used by patients.

ORAL MUCOSAL DISEASE

There are a wide number of diseases of the oral mucosa, many of which are oral manifestations of common dermatological problems. The scope of this chapter is too wide to cover all of these in detail. Remember that *if a patient has a dermatological problem and is also complaining of discomfort or ulceration in their mouth, then the two may be linked.* One classical example would be lichen planus, and particularly lichenoid drug reactions, which often manifest in the mouth. Indeed oral signs of lichen planus often precede cutaneous manifestations. The diagnosis and management of specific conditions should be undertaken by an individual with training and expertise in oral medicine.

Oral ulceration

Mouth ulcers are a common complaint and are a source of considerable morbidity. Again, there are many causes of ulcers, from simple trauma through nutritional deficiencies to oral mucosal disease and malignancy. Most individual oral ulcers will heal over 7 to 10 days; *any ulcer that persists for longer than this must be investigated to determine its aetiology.* Obviously, a traumatic ulcer will not heal unless the source of the trauma is removed, so an over-extended denture base rubbing on the gum should be adjusted to correct the extension before a related ulcer will resolve. Equally, ulcers associated with iron or B complex vitamin deficiency will heal as individual units but will recur unless the underlying pathology is corrected. Oral ulceration is also the most frequent presentation of oral squamous cell carcinoma: any persistent ulcer that does not resolve after simple treatment to remove sources of trauma must be regarded with suspicion until it is proven that the lesion is benign (Ship et al 2000).

A patient with a persistent ulcer should be referred to the local head and neck oncology unit as a matter of urgency. This service is often provided by a combination of oral and maxillofacial, ear, nose and throat, and plastic surgeons. In the best units they work in large interdisciplinary teams alongside clinical oncologists and rehabilitation teams (including restorative dentists) to achieve the best outcome for each individual patient. Treatment, particularly for late presentation disease, is often a combination of radiotherapy and surgical removal of tissue and the associated regional lymphatic drainage. Such care has high morbidity.

Oral cancer

Oral malignancies are predominantly squamous cell carcinomas. Mesothelial tumours do occur as do malignancies in specialized oral tissues such as salivary gland tissue. However, they are rare. Oral malignancy is unfortunately characterized by late presentation and has a poor prognosis. As with most malignancies, the chances of successful treatment are improved with early diagnosis and management.

The risk factors for oral malignancy are iron deficiency, high levels of habitual alcohol intake (particularly spirits rather than beer and wine) and tobacco use. There is little difference between most forms of tobacco when smoked, although reverse smoking (where the burning end of the cigarette is held inside the mouth) is associated with particularly high risk. Another group of tobacco products that are dangerous are those that are chewed or held against the cheek for long periods of time, e.g. chewing tobaccos, tobacco or snuff pouches designed to be held in the mouth and a variety of quids (commonly used in the Indian subcontinent). This include both Betel and Areca nut quid. These quids are thought to be particularly harmful as they contain a mixture of both tobacco and slaked lime, in addition to nut product (Scully et al 1994, Warnakulasuriya 2004).

Oral mucosal infections

The most common oral mucosal infection, particularly in elderly subjects, is oral candida. The manifestation will vary (depending on the severity of the condition) from a debilitating acute infection with generalized erythema of the oral mucosa (including the surface of the tongue) and white plaques, that can be easily scraped off the surface of the mucosa, to chronic oral disease (most commonly associated with complete dentures). The characteristic appearance here is of reddening and soreness of the gum which underlies the denture, sometimes with a granulomatous appearance that has been likened to a raspberry. Oral candidiasis is often also associated with inflammatory disease at the angles of the mouth (angular cheilitis).

In the acute form, oral candidiasis is usually a manifestation of a more general debilitating illness or immunosuppression. It may or may not be associated with denture use and usually responds well to topical antifungal treatment with nystatin or amphotericin B lozenges/pastilles or miconazole oral gel. Any underlying debilitating condition must be addressed. In its most severe form, systemic antifungal treatment with ketoconazole may be appropriate – particularly if the candidal infection is spreading down the oesophagus.

Chronic oral disease, particularly associated with old and ill-fitting dentures and in people who habitually wear their dentures continually (rather than leaving them out at night) is relatively common. Successful management is underpinned by three principles: treating the infected mucosa, removing the source of infection, and allowing the mucosa to recover from supporting dentures.

The mucosal infection itself is best treated with topical antifungal agents, e.g. miconazole oral gel, which can be applied to the surface of the denture and is then held in place against the mucosa by the denture itself.

The *Candida* species responsible for the infection can invade the mucosae and may colonize a porous denture surface. The surface of the plastic from which dentures are made degrades with time in the mouth, becoming increasingly porous, particularly the relatively rough plastic surface that is in contact with the oral mucosae. This surface will become colonized and any effort to manage candidiasis will be unsuccessful unless the dentures are also disinfected. The most effective way of doing this is to store the dentures out of the mouth overnight in cold dilute sodium hypochloride (the easiest product to use is Milton which is used for sterilization of babies' bottles and nappies).

The dentures must be left out of the mouth while the person is asleep; this allows for disinfec-

tion of the denture and permits mucosal recovery from the trauma of denture wear.

Once the condition has been treated, it is often advisable to make new dentures for the person to remove the porous denture surface from the mouth. If this is not done there is an increased risk of reinfection of the denture surface.

Angular cheilitis

Angular cheilitis may also respond to the use of topical antifungal agents. These lesions are commonly infected with staphylococci and a topical antimicrobial may also be of benefit. The most effective agent is chloramphenicol ointment.

One of the factors that can influence the development of angular cheilitis is a reduction in support for the lips as a consequence of skeletal changes resulting in loss of support for old dentures. The provision of new dentures is essential for satisfactory outcome as support for the lips and cheeks will help eliminate skin folds at the corner of the mouth (Scully et al 1994).

DISEASE OF THE TEETH AND SUPPORTING TISSUES

Tooth decay

The teeth in an older person are at greater risk of developing decay than in a younger individual. This increased risk is present because of the loss of bone support with increasing age as a consequence of gum disease. This in turn results in the exposure of the root of a tooth into the mouth as we become long in the tooth. The root of a tooth is made up of dentine which is less well mineralized than the enamel and as a consequence is more susceptible to decay. Caries of the roots of teeth along with decay which occurs at the edges of existing restorations on teeth are the principle manifestations of tooth decay in older people.

An individual's susceptibility to decay will depend on their diet, personal oral healthcare (both of these variables are under the control of the medical team in both acute and long-stay residential care settings) and any alterations to the host's protective mechanisms, particularly variation in salivary flow.

Diet

Sugars are an important component of all diets and yet they are also responsible for the source of acids that are primarily responsible for the development of tooth decay. One particular area of concern is the high level of untreated dental caries in institutionalized older people. This is the result of a combination of poor access to dental care, compromised provision of personal oral hygiene and a cariogenic diet, with a high frequency of sugar intake. Three variables that determine the impact of dietary sugars on the teeth are: frequency of intake, type of sugar and sugars in medicine.

Frequency of intake

Acids are produced by mature plaque on the surface of teeth every time fermentable sugars are taken into the mouth. With low frequency of intake of sugars, the natural defence and repair mechanisms in saliva are effective, providing these mechanisms are intact. However, when frequencies of intake are high the demineralization phase dominates, tipping the balance away from repair towards decay.

There is no evidence on what frequency of sugar intake is safe in preventing caries in older adults. This problem is confounded by most of the preventive advice which is designed to prevent decay of tooth enamel rather than dentine. Dentists would normally recommend no more than four or five intakes of sugar-containing foods/drinks per day. (This includes sugar used to sweeten tea and coffee.)

All sugars that are consumed during a meal equate to one episode of sugar intake for this purpose, so three or four intakes of sugar-containing food (e.g. a sweetened drink, baked beans and a desert) would only count as one episode of intake when assessing decay risk.

One specific problem in elderly infirm individuals is the use of high-energy liquid or syrup supplements to try to maintain an adequate calorific intake. These are often sipped over long periods of time by their users resulting in prolonged exposure of the teeth to plaque acid. The syrupy nature of these preparations is of particular relevance because their rate of oral clearance will be low, particularly in individuals with impaired salivary flow.

The type of sugar

Refined carbohydrates are the most cariogenic sugars, particularly sucrose but also glucose. Natural sugars (like fructose and lactose) can also be metabolized by plaque bacteria to produce acids but are more difficult for the bacteria to metabolize and hence are less acidogenic. Natural sugars are often also consumed in a form that helps to resist decay. For example, sweetened yoghurt contains sugars and has an intrinsically low pH; however it is also a supersaturated solution of calcium, which helps to limit its potential effects on the tooth surface.

Refined sugars are widely used in the food industry both as sweetening agents and as preservatives (hidden sugars). Many savoury foods contain much added sugar (prime examples would be tomato ketchup and many canned vegetables, but there are many others).

Sugars in medicines

Sugars are used in medicines, as preservatives in syrups and mixtures and to mask the bitter flavour of drugs. Drugs delivered to adults are commonly taken in tablet or capsule form, but there is increasing use of liquid preparations in older adults and also of drugs which have prolonged oral clearance (tablets that are sucked or chewed, for example, rather than swallowed). Sugar-free versions of many of these medications are available, but they must be specifically prescribed and are often more expensive than their sugar-containing alternatives (Baqir & Maguire 2000).

Caries prevention

There are three strategies that can assist with preventing caries: reducing frequency, sugar replacement and salivary stimulation.

Reducing frequency

With intakes at four to five times daily, the normal remineralizing capacity of the mouth should be able to cope with resulting acid challenge, providing there are normal levels of salivary flow.

Sugar replacement

Wherever possible the replacement of added sugars with artificial sweeteners will allow between-meals consumption of sweetened foods that do not cause decay. Foods designed for people with diabetes mellitus would be one example, as would those marked with the tooth-friendly symbol.

Artificial sweeteners come in 2 forms:

■ Intense sweeteners (e.g. saccharin and acesulfam K) which are commonly used to sweeten drinks
■ Bulk sweeteners (e.g. isomalt, sorbitol, xylitol) which are used in prepared foods to replace the bulking effect of sugars. One complication of their use is that they are not absorbed across the gut wall and hence remain in the large bowel, where they are osmotically active, reducing the capacity for water uptake from the stool. If taken in large quantities, this can result in osmotic diarrhoea

Salivary stimulation

Chewing has the effect of stimulating salivary output. The fall in pH associated with sugar intake is dramatically modified if it is followed by a period of chewing gum to stimulate salivary flow (Dodds et al 1991) (Fig. 31.2). Sugar-free gum is recommended.

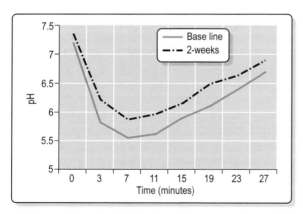

Figure 31.2   The response to a sugar challenge in people before and after chewing gum regularly for 2 weeks. The reduction in pH (the Stephan curve) is less and of shorter duration after chewing gum regularly due to the increased rate of salivary flow. (From Dodds M W J, Hsieh S C, Johnson D A 1991 The effect of increased mastication by daily gum-chewing on salivary gland output and dental plaque acidogenicity. Journal of Dental Research 70(12): 1474; reproduced with kind permission of the Journal of Dental Research.)

ORAL HEALTH–RELATED QUALITY OF LIFE

Quality of life (QoL) is an important part of an individual's well-being. Oral health affects quality of life of all age groups in relation to comfort, appearance and function. On a population basis the overall impact of oral health on personal QoL is similar to the impact from cardiovascular disease. This may seem surprising, but if someone cannot/will not eat because it hurts, or hates the appearance of their teeth, these daily experiences produce an adverse overall impact (Locker 1992).

Paradoxically, older people are relatively poor at accessing oral healthcare, with reduced frequency of attendance even among those who have some teeth and very low rates of attendance among the edentate. Stoicism can be part of some older people's attitude towards oral healthcare, exemplified by these quotations from a sample of older Canadians (MacEntee et al 1997):

> 'I don't think I need to go to a dentist because my mouth is free of pain and I'm chewing fairly well.'

> 'If your general health is good, you've got enough on the ball to look after your teeth. If your general health isn't good, maybe you haven't got the energy to get out to the dentist.'

RELATIONSHIP BETWEEN ORAL AND GENERAL HEALTH

There are three mechanisms through which the state of the mouth can have an effect on general health: nutrition, the mouth as a source of chronic inflammation and the mouth as a source of bacteria.

Nutrition

The dietary needs of an older person are different to those of a younger individual. There is a reduced need for calories as older people tend to be less physically active and also have less metabolically active tissue (e.g. muscle) in their body. The diet therefore needs to be less calorific but needs to maintain the levels of micronutrients required for healthy tissue function. It needs to be nutrient dense, with a diet that is high in

Table 31.1	Data from two large cross-sectional epidemiological studies of ageing and nutrition					
	Intact		Compromised		Edentulous	
	UK	*US*	*UK*	*US*	*UK*	*US*
Protein (63 g/day)	72.3	80	66.6	74	60.1	68
NSP (non-starch polysaccharide) (25 g/day)	16.2	21	12.9	19	11.0	16
Calcium (800 mg/day)	883	773	812	677	722	689
Niacin (15 mg/day)	33.8	32	31.0	28	27.0	34
Vitamin C (60 mg/day)	82	156	73	146	60	127

This table shows data from two large cross-sectional epidemiological studies of ageing and nutrition. The data are divided into three groups, people with an 'intact' dentition (defined as having 21 or more natural teeth), a compromised dentition (defined as having some natural teeth, but fewer than 21) and no natural teeth (edentulous). For both population samples in the US and UK, people with more teeth consume more of all of these dietary components and there is a progressive reduction from the intact through the compromised to the edentulous group. The intakes from NSP and some of the calcium intakes fall below the recommended daily intake levels which are given in parentheses in the first column (Krall et al 1998, Sheiham et al 2001).

micronutrients, particularly, compared with its calorie/protein content so that individuals can maintain micronutrient intakes at 'normal' levels while consuming less protein and carbohydrate.

Oral function is essential for chewing and swallowing foods and for our enjoyment of eating (Walls & Steele 2004). People who have a limited number of teeth or no natural teeth consume a diet that is characterized by a reduction in fibre (non-starch polysaccharide) and increase in consumption of sugars and potentially fats. This diet has a reduced intake of fruits and vegetables, and tends to have relatively low nutrient density (Table 31.1) (Krall et al 1998, Sheiham et al 2001). This dietary pattern affects haematological measures of micronutrient status, with levels of vitamin C being of particular concern in edentulous residents of care homes (Table 31.1). The median value for plasma ascorbate in this group in the UK National Diet and Nutrition Survey was only just above the reference level for scurvy (11.4 µmol l^{-1} compared with a reference value of 11 µmol l^{-1}) (Sheiham et al 2001).

Not surprisingly, there are many reasons for this dietary pattern including social and attitudinal factors. All the same, oral health status does play a part and improving oral health status provides an opportunity to deliver a targeted dietary intervention which improves fruit and vegetable intakes by 200 g per day (this is an improvement

of just under 50% of the recommended daily intake) (Bradbury et al 2006).

In addition to the influence of oral health status, there are other changes in the mouth that alter an individual's enjoyment of foods. There are reductions in taste perception for bitter, sweet, sour and salty but not for the fifth taste modality unami (the taste of 'savoury' as opposed to bitter, salt, sour and sweet. It is sometimes likened to the taste of tofu or to the taste-enhancer monosodium glutamate) and reduced ability to smell. Taste and smell are central to our enjoyment of foods and there has been some success in improving food consumption by adding taste stimulants (such as monosodium glutamate) to food for older people.

Salivary flow and function are also important in relation to a person's ability to consume foods. Saliva has a number of important roles in the mouth including lubricating the process of chewing, acting as a glue to bind the food bolus together and to lubricate swallowing. In people with a limited number of teeth or those with dentures, there is a tendency to chew foods less well leaving coarse particles in the bolus. Good salivary function is then required both to stick the bolus together and to lubricate its passage down the oesophagus. People who report impaired salivary function also report an increased number of problems with chewing and swallowing foods.

Chronic inflammation

Inflammation is important in a number of chronic disease processes including diabetes mellitus and cardiovascular disease. Oral inflammatory diseases are very common. Among the dentate, gum disease is almost universally prevalent, and in those who wear dentures, chronic irritation of the mucosae through trauma or infection is common. The extent and severity of this chronic inflammation is often unclear. Gum disease does not cause a painful response, nor does chronic, low-grade denture-induced stomatitis. However, the area of inflamed tissue has been estimated at 100 mm^2 per tooth for dentate subjects with established chronic adult periodontal disease. The average dentate older adult will have 12 standing teeth, giving an inflamed mucosal surface of 1200 mm^2.

Cardiovascular disease

Much of the evidence links oral inflammatory conditions to increased risk of both myocardial infarction and stroke. The mechanisms for this linkage are unclear at present. It may be that such subjects are simply part of a hyperinflammatory phenotype and as such all inflammatory processes are exaggerated. Equally, the inflammation associated with established periodontal disease will result in elevated levels of circulating markers such as C reactive protein. Such markers may be associated with increased atheroma formation. There have been some links drawn between at least one common periodontal pathogen (*Porphyromonas gingivalis*) and the severity of atheroma formation. There may be co-reaction between circulating leukocytes and high levels of advanced glycation end products, to which a poor diet may contribute (Meurman et al 2004).

Diabetes mellitus

There is a bi-directional relationship between periodontal (gum) disease and diabetes (Genco et al 2005). Periodontal disease occurs more frequently and progresses at a greater rate in subjects with diabetes, particularly if their glycaemic control is poor. This relationship may occur as a consequence of alterations in both the immune response and in leukocyte function. This pattern of aggravation of disease extends to sub-clinical

levels of impaired glucose tolerance as well as to subjects with established disease of either type. Recent evidence has also suggested a link between the glycaemic control in subjects with type 2 diabetes (where inflammation is thought to play a role in the pathogenesis of the disease process). A recent meta-analysis demonstrated a consistent (but non-significant) reduction in HbA1c levels from a number of relatively small studies. Larger clinical trials are in progress (Janket et al 2005).

The mouth as a source of bacteria

The mouth is a source of bacteria implicated in the development of pneumonia in debilitated subjects. This includes people who are having prolonged periods of anaesthesia, those in the acute phase of a stroke (particularly those with dysphagia) and debilitated subjects in long-term care. Oral hygiene is important when trying to eliminate the risk of nosocomial infection of this sort (Shay et al 2005). One recent paper has shown that the use of a chlorhexidine gel as part of a regular oral hygiene programme significantly reduced the risk of oral carriage of aerobic Gram-negative bacteria and resulted in a reduction in the prevalence of pneumonia in the sample (of 203 subjects divided into two groups, seven controls developed pneumonia compared with one on active treatment) (Gosney et al 2006). There was no difference in mortality between the groups but the sample size was too small to be able to show this. There are studies that suggest strategies for managing oral healthcare in at-risk groups. However, this remains an area where optimal care is not often delivered.

ORAL HEALTHCARE NEEDS OF OLDER PEOPLE

The oral healthcare needs of older people will depend on their dental status.

EDENTULOUS

One of the most important tasks for people with dentures is to mark their prostheses with their name so that they are not lost or confused with another patient's dentures during cleaning. The easiest way to mark dentures is by writing the patient's name or hospital number on the pink plastic gum work of a denture towards the back of the mouth using an indelible marker pen (a laundry marker is ideal). Dentures need to be cleaned regularly. This will not harm dentures unless the solutions in which they are soaked are hot. Routine cleaning is best achieved simply by using a brush, soap and water. A proprietary denture brush is useful as the bristle head is large enough to clean the denture surfaces efficiently while still being of an appropriate size to clean both the upper and the lower surfaces of the denture. Toothpaste can be used but is relatively abrasive to the acrylic material from which dentures are made if used often over a long time period.

Proprietary cleaning agents can also be used. These usually come as a dispersible tablet that effervesces when placed in water. Gross debris should be removed from the acrylic surface before the denture is placed in the solution. Once again, the solution should be cool.

Some hard accretions of calculus can also form on the surface of the plastic, usually adjacent to the opening of the salivary glands (on the middle of the inside of a lower denture and the sides of an upper denture). These can only be removed with an acidic cleanser (e.g. DenClen) or by placing the denture into an ultrasonic cleaning bath.

Dentures should be cleaned at least once a day, ideally last thing at night. The denture is then placed in water for overnight storage. *Dentures should NOT be worn overnight.*

One of the common complaints from patients who have been ill is that their dentures are loose. This is often (falsely) attributed to weight loss through illness, particularly during chemotherapy. The shape of the mouth remains remarkably constant in people during illness (with the exception of some patients on renal dialysis when there can be some cyclical changes to the mucosae depending on the state of hydration of the individual). It is usually associated with leaving the prosthesis out during a period of acute illness or while the oral mucosae are sore during chemotherapy. The dentures are most likely to be old and will be poorly adapted to the supporting oral mucosa. During the time when the denture is not being worn, some of the learned skill for stabilizing the denture will be lost. The patient has simply forgotten how to juggle the denture and, consequently, its poor stability from lack of contact with the oral mucosa becomes obvious and it is perceived to be loose. The only solution for this is to renew the surface of the denture that contacts the gum with a material that will make the denture much more stable and help the patient to relearn their juggling skills. A dentist will do this for you with a proprietary soft lining kit. The procedure is simple and does not take long. However, these are temporary solutions, do not last long, and the permanent answer is to have new dentures made which fit better.

THE DENTATE

People with teeth have different needs in terms of their personal healthcare. Many will also have either partial dentures or a full denture in one jaw opposed by a partial denture in the other. These dentures need to be maintained using the procedures outlined above with one cautionary note: *if a denture has a metal base (rather than plastic) then it should not be placed in a soaking solution, particularly in Milton, as this will corrode the metal.*

In most oral disease, the mainstay of protection and prevention is the use of effective personal oral healthcare. The patient may be able to undertake this for themselves; carers may be required to provide assistance for the more debilitated subject. There are barriers to the achievement of adequate oral healthcare for dependent older people that need to be surmounted before an optimum standard of care can be delivered (Eadie & Schou 1992).

Theoretically, there is a wide range of devices that could be used for this purpose but the practicality of using some of them is limited – particularly in people with reduced dexterity or where care is being provided by a carer. For example the use of dental floss requires considerable dexterity and is difficult to use on someone else without both training and good lighting and relative positioning of the patient and the carer. This latter is a problem when working in hospital wards or in out-patient clinics, where patients are usually in a bed or chair which are not designed to facilitate oral healthcare.

Conversely, the use of sponge pads and mouth-wash (which is a common practice in the UK) can be of limited value in terms of cleaning plaque from the surfaces of teeth efficiently and thoroughly.

The mainstay of any oral hygiene regimen is a toothbrush. There is some evidence that a mechanical brush is best, particularly if a caregiver is delivering the oral hygiene (Hellstadius et al 1993, Robinson et al 2005). This should be used in conjunction with a toothpaste, and there are pastes that contain a higher concentration of fluoride which will be of benefit in helping to prevent decay in older people (e.g. Duraphat® paste from Colgate which contains 2800 ppm fluoride compared with about 1000 ppm for a standard paste; this is also available as a prescription item in the UK).

The oral hygiene needs of people alter with age. The architecture of the mouth changes with exposure of root surfaces and irregularities on the surface of the tooth. Consequently, both patients and caregivers need to be aware of these changes and apply oral health interventions appropriately. There is currently very little emphasis on the delivery of oral hygiene in the training programmes for nurses and nursing assistants. Any carer who is involved in providing oral healthcare should receive some training on the best approach to achieve optimal outcomes. Simple advice (e.g. it is easier to brush someone's teeth when standing behind and above them, using gloves to protect your hands) and teaching how to identify oral deposits with dyes are vital to the acceptance of this task by caregivers. There is an aversion on the part of many people to *invade* the personal space that is someone else's mouth. This can be overcome with training and motivation.

Discomfort beneath a denture is often associated with it rubbing against the oral mucosa. When hard acrylic does irritate the oral mucosa the result is often a traumatic ulcer associated with the border of the denture. On occasion, the irritation is more chronic and results in granuloma formation at the border of the denture. Professional dental advice should be sought to attempt to adjust the prosthesis to make it more comfortable.

Denture trauma can be a particular problem in patients with reduced salivary flow where the lubricating effects of the salivary film are missing.

It is possible to make dentures for patients with xerostomia that contain a reservoir for artificial saliva. This can then be expressed into the mouth on demand by the patient. Again professional advice and intervention are required. People who are edentulous with severe xerostomia may benefit from having an oral reconstruction based on osseointegrated dental implants. Implants are essentially artificial tooth roots in the form of titanium bolts screwed onto the bone of the jaw. These can then be used to support a fixed replacement for the teeth that does not contact the gum at all and hence does not cause the problems of irritation associated with a plastic prosthesis.

Pain from teeth can be spontaneous or it can be triggered by stimuli such as temperature, sweet tastes and pressure. The nature of the pain usually gives some indication of its origin.

Transient discomfort (a sharp pain that lasts for seconds after application of the stimulus) with temperature change or biting will often be associated with sensitivity from the dentine of the tooth, either through exposure of the dentine into the mouth or when the tooth bends under biting forces. Dentists may ease this discomfort with the use of desensitizing pastes/solutions.

Discomfort associated with temperature, taste or biting that lingers for a significant time after the stimulus (particularly that which is a dull ache rather than a sharp stabbing pain) is associated with advanced tooth decay and requires prompt professional intervention. This is particularly important if the discomfort wakes somebody from their sleep, when it is usually associated with dental abscess formation: again, prompt attention is essential. If it is not possible for a patient to be seen by a dentist, a dental abscess will respond to antibiotics in the short term to alleviate pain. However, it will always recur unless the underlying cause of the infection is addressed by a dental professional. Broad-spectrum antimicrobials (for example amoxicillin) are usually effective in managing an acute infection of dental origin, although anaerobic organisms are often involved in such lesions and metronidazole may also be of benefit. Conventional oral delivery is all that is required unless there is a problem with drug compliance or there is an acute swelling associated with the infection.

Key points

- Older people are retaining natural teeth and need different patterns of oral healthcare as a consequence.
- Teeth are a potential source of pain and acute infection which can be difficult to identify.
- Poor oral health and oral cleanliness have been linked to increased risk of pneumonia in vulnerable population groups.
- Caregivers need to be trained in the provision of oral hygiene to others.
- Oral health status is one of the variables that influences food choice, with people who have no teeth choosing a less healthy diet.
- Drugs can have a significant effect on salivary flow and associated quality of life.

REFERENCES

*** Essential reading; ** recommended reading; * interesting but not vital

Baqir W, Maguire A 2000 Consumption of prescribed and over-the-counter medicines with prolonged oral clearance used by the elderly in the Northern Region of England, with special regard to generic prescribing, dose form and sugars content. Public Health 114:367–373 **

Baum B J, Ship J A, Wu A 1992 Salivary gland function and aging: a model for studying the interaction of aging and systemic disease. Critical Reviews in Oral Biology and Medicine 4:53–64 ***

Bots C P, Brand H S, Veerman E C et al 2005 Chewing gum and a saliva substitute alleviate thirst and xerostomia in patients on haemodialysis. Nephrology, Dialysis, Transplantation 20:578–584 *

Bradbury J, Thomason J M, Jepson N J et al 2006 Nutrition counseling increases fruit and vegetable intake in the edentulous. Journal of Dental Research 85:463–468 **

Chambers M S 2004 Sjögren's syndrome. ORL Head and Neck Nursing 22:22–30; quiz 32–33 **

Dodds M W, Hsieh S C, Johnson D A 1991 The effect of increased mastication by daily gum-chewing on salivary gland output and dental plaque acidogenicity. Journal of Dental Research 70:1474–1478 *

Eadie D R, Schou L 1992 An exploratory study of barriers to promoting oral hygiene through carers of elderly people. Community Dental Health 9:343–348 *

Genco R J, Grossi S G, Ho A et al 2005 A proposed model linking inflammation to obesity, diabetes, and periodontal infections. Journal of Periodontology 76:2075–2084 *

Gosney M, Martin M V, Wright A E 2006 The role of selective decontamination of the digestive tract in acute stroke. Age and Ageing 35:42–47 **

Hellstadius K, Asman B, Gustafsson A 1993 Improved maintenance of plaque control by electrical toothbrushing in periodontitis patients with low compliance. Journal of Clinical Periodontology 20: 235–237 *

Janket S J, Wightman A, Baird A E et al 2005 Does periodontal treatment improve glycemic control in diabetic patients? A meta-analysis of intervention studies. Journal of Dental Research 84:1154–1159 **

Kelly M, Steele J G, Nuttal N et al 2000 Adult dental health survey, oral health in the United Kingdom 1998. The Stationery Office, London *

Krall E, Hayes C, Garcia R 1998 How dentition status and masticatory function affect nutrient intake. Journal of the American Dental Association 129: 1261–1269 *

Locker D 1992 The burden of oral disorders in a population of older adults. Community Dental Health 9:109–124 **

MacEntee M I, Hole R, Stolar E 1997 The significance of the mouth in old age. Social Science and Medicine 45:1449–1458 **

Meurman J H, Sanz M, Janket S J 2004 Oral health, atherosclerosis, and cardiovascular disease. Critical Reviews in Oral Biology and Medicine 15: 403–413 ***

Narhi T O, Meerman J H, Anaimo A et al 1992 Association between salivary flow rate and the use of systemic medication among 76–81 and 86 year old inhabitants of Helsinki, Finland. Journal of Dental Research 71:1875–1880 **

Robinson P G, Deacon S A, Deery C et al 2005 Manual versus powered toothbrushing for oral health. Cochrane Database of Systematic Reviews 2. Art. No.: CD002281. DOI: 10.1002/14651858.CD002281. pub2 *

Scully C, el-Kabir M, Samaranayake L P 1994 Candida and oral candidosis: a review. Critical Reviews in Oral Biology and Medicine 5:125–157 **

Shay K, Scannapieco F A, Terpenning M S et al 2005 Nosocomial pneumonia and oral health. Special Care in Dentistry 25:179–187 **

Sheiham A, Steele J G, Marcenes W et al 2001 The relationship among dental status, nutrient intake, and nutritional status in older people. Journal of Dental Research 80:408–413 **

Ship J A 2002 Diagnosing, managing, and preventing salivary gland disorders. Oral Diseases 8:77–89 ***

Ship J A, Chavez E M, Doerr P A et al 2000 Recurrent aphthous stomatitis. Quintessence International 31:95–112 **

Steele J G, Sheiham A, Marcenes W et al 1998 National diet and nutrition survey: people aged 65 years or over, vol 2: report of the oral health survey. Stationery Office, London *

Walls A W, Steele J G 2004 The relationship between oral health and nutrition in older people. Mechanisms of Ageing and Development 125:853–857 ***

Warnakulasuriya S 2004 Smokeless tobacco and oral cancer. Oral Diseases 10:1–4 **

SELF-ASSESSMENT QUESTIONS

Are the following statements true or false?

1. Oral mucosal inflammatory disease:
   a. Is associated with increased risk of atherosclerosis leading to MI and stroke
   b. Can influence glycaemic control in patients with type 2 diabetes
   c. Results in pain on ingestion of hot or sweet foods
   d. Results in alterations in food choice
   e. Is universally prevalent in dentate people

2. Oral function in older people:
   a. Is affected by the number and distribution of teeth in their mouths
   b. Is affected by polypharmacy
   c. Influences food choice in a 'harmful' way
   d. Affects speech
   e. Has a significant effect on quality of life

SECTION 4

Gastrointestinal system

Chapter 32

Faecal incontinence and constipation

James A. Barrett

ANORECTAL CONTINENCE MECHANISMS

The following all contribute to the maintenance of anal continence:

- Internal anal sphincter activity produces anal resting tone
- External anal sphincter activity produces voluntary anal squeeze and reflex anal contraction when the rectum is initially distended
- Anorectal angle
- Anal sensation including sampling reflex
- Slit shape of anal canal
- Vascular and mucosal components

DEFECATION

- Defecation requires relaxation of the anal sphincters (recto-anal inhibitory reflex)
- It varies with stool consistency
- It often follows a gastrocolic reflex (whole gut mass movement following eating and/or exercise)
- Normal frequency varies between twice per week to three times per day

Constipation and faecal incontinence are common in older people, especially in those who are frail or disabled. There are a number of age-related changes that increase the risk of faecal incontinence in old age (background factors) with other specific factors that lead to loss of continence.

BACKGROUND FACTORS

External anal sphincter weakness

Anal squeeze pressures fall with age and probably also with immobility but this does not necessarily need to lead to loss of bowel control.

Pudendal neuropathy may occur as a result of an old childbirth stretch injury (especially if forceps were used) or chronic straining at stool.

Loss of anal sensation

Anal sensation is impaired in many asymptomatic older people and in incontinent patients but does not necessarily result in faecal incontinence, even when totally absent.

Immobility

Immobility may contribute to faecal incontinence because of either of the following:

■ Physical factors, i.e. loss of gastrocolic reflex
■ Dependency upon others, especially if there is urgency of defecation

SPECIFIC FACTORS

Faecal loading

■ *Faecal loading, especially with soft faeces is the most common cause of faecal incontinence in elderly subjects*
■ Faecal soiling in faecally-loaded patients is more common when soft stool is present and leakage usually occurs before a call to stool is experienced
■ It is usually associated with loss of anorectal angle

How do you define constipation?

Common answers

■ Infrequent bowel movements
■ Straining to pass stool
■ Hard stools

The faecally-loaded elderly incontinent patient, however, may leak up to 10 times per day, does not have to strain and usually has *very soft* stools.

What does the term faecal impaction mean?

Possible answer

■ Rectum and colon full of *hard* faeces

However, less than 10% of faecally-loaded patients have a rectum loaded with hard stool.

Constipation can be the presenting symptom of colonic disease and may require investigation.

> ### Correction to an old wives' tale
>
> *Spurious diarrhoea* around a large mass of hard faeces in the rectum is not common in frail elderly patients. *Overflow incontinence* is due to massive amounts of soft faeces in the rectum leaking out.

'Idiopathic constipation' can be classified as either slow transit or normal transit constipation.

Slow transit (usually due to reduced colonic propulsion) predominates in frail elderly subjects. Whole gut transit times often exceed 14 days (normal < 5 days). Some of these patients develop a megarectum. Abdominal radiographs will often demonstrate extensive faecal loading throughout the colon (a typical 'ground-glass' appearance).

Normal transit patients tend to experience major problems with the process of defecation, e.g. inappropriate sphincter contraction on attempted defecation or obstructed defecation due to rectocele or intussusception. Defecating proctography may help in diagnosis.

Loss of rectal awareness of the call to stool may also contribute towards the development of constipation.

Internal sphincter weakness with low anal resting tone

Anal resting tone does not change with ageing.

Low resting pressures are found in incontinent patients of all ages. One possible cause of this is physical disruption of the sphincter. This can be demonstrated in special centres by the use of anal ultrasound.

In some incontinent patients, the anus gapes open. It cannot therefore delay the passage of liquids but it can still delay the passage of solid material. Continence may be restored therefore by changing stool consistency.

Diarrhoea

Acute and/or chronic diarrhoea may lead to faecal incontinence.

Clostridium difficile is now a major problem among hospital in-patients. The profuse diarrhoea and malaise tend to overwhelm continence mechanisms. Prevention measures should include adoption of strict antibiotic policies and hand washing by all staff before and after contact with patients.

Loss of cognitive awareness

Unconsciousness

The most basic requirement for control of bowel evacuation is for a person to be awake. Loss of this will inevitably lead to faecal leakage as voluntary control is not possible.

Dementia

Some patients with advanced dementia are incontinent of faeces, usually due to severe mental confusion and loss of awareness of the call to stool.

Behavioural

Patients with severe behavioural problems may defecate in inappropriate places, e.g. in the lounge of a residential home. This may also be associated with faecal smearing and/or coprophagia. This is presumably due to severe frontal lobe damage or degeneration and can prove very difficult to manage.

HISTORY AND PHYSICAL EXAMINATION

The *history* should include enquiry into:

- Bowel habit past and present including awareness of call to stool, defecation, stool consistency and episodes of leakage
- Diet – ask specifically about fibre content
- Laxative use
- Mobility

Physical examination should include:

- Abdominal examination for presence of palpable faecal mass(es)
- Anorectal examination, looking for evidence of perineal descent, gaping anus, rectal prolapse, perianal scarring and/or soiling
- Digital examination to assess anal resting tone and squeeze and to determine whether there are any abnormal rectal lesions or faecal loading

of the rectum. If the rectum is loaded, then determine the stool consistency
- Cognitive assessment

Bowel investigations will occasionally be indicated to exclude bowel pathology. If requesting investigations such as barium enema in patients with faecal incontinence, remember that they are likely to experience profuse diarrhoea and incontinence during the bowel clearance in preparation for the test and there is a high chance that they will not retain the barium. You may put them through the test without obtaining any useful clinical information. CT colonography is now becoming the preferred investigation.

> In a survey 100 patients who had had a barium enema were asked: 'Would you like another one?' 100% replied 'no way!'

HOW TO HELP SOMEONE WITH BOWEL PROBLEMS

The management plan that is proposed below for faecal incontinence and constipation is goal-orientated. (The aim should also be to educate mentally competent patients about how their bowels work, how to regain control and how to respond to changes in their bowel habit as the problems are often ongoing.)

The two main aims in bowel management in old age are:

1. To produce stools of the ideal consistency which are neither too hard nor too soft
2. For bowel emptying to occur at a predictable time

The first aim is usually the initial target for patients seen in a community setting whereas the second aim is usually the initial target for patients in hospital or care home settings.

The ideal stool has been christened the 'Goldilocks stool' because it is neither too hard nor too soft but 'just right'. Most old people with faecal incontinence, however, produce stools that resemble Goldilock's porridge, i.e. soft and gooey. This would not be 'just right' as this is precisely the type of stool that leaks easily and is very messy to clean up.

PRODUCTION OF STOOLS OF IDEAL CONSISTENCY

The following is a guide to producing stools of the ideal consistency that are neither too hard nor too soft.

If stools are too hard, the aim should be to soften them to produce a firm stool that is easy to pass when defecation is attempted.

Increase the dietary fibre intake? 'Healthy eating' is widely promoted and appears to be desirable for otherwise healthy people to reduce their risk of diverticular disease and other colorectal abnormalities including constipation.

Fibre is effective at softening stool, increasing its bulk and stimulating defecation. This, however, is not usually desirable as a treatment for frail elderly subjects with constipation or anyone with faecal incontinence, as the high-fibre intake adds to the existing colonic faecal loading and increases the risk of faecal incontinence. Fibre also causes flatulence.

An alternative is to soften hard stool with an osmotic laxative, e.g. lactulose. Lactulose exerts its osmotic effect only in the small bowel. It increases faecal weight, volume and water content as well as bowel movements and usually acts within 2 days. Alternatives include docusate, which is a faecal softener but a poor laxative. Movicol or magnesium sulphate are potent osmotic laxatives which are reserved for some resistant cases of constipation.

Diarrhoea is often associated with faecal incontinence. While the cause is sought, use of anti-diarrhoeal agents (constipating drugs) can considerably improve patients' symptoms. The most popular drug in this class is loperamide, which is effective in altering stool consistency from soft to firm (and if too much is used, to hard). It may prevent faecal incontinence by mechanisms other than by just changing stool consistency – loperamide has been shown to influence internal sphincter function. Other agents in this class include codeine phosphate.

The main challenge when using loperamide to alter the stool consistency for patients with soft stools is to get the dose right, as too much induces severe constipation. The following starting doses are suggested:

- Soft stool: 0.5 mg/day of the syrup preparation titrated slowly up or down depending on result
- Liquid stool: 2–4 mg/day but may require much higher doses initially until stool becomes firmer

Maintenance doses of loperamide tend to fluctuate, depending upon stool consistency in individual patients. Some patients require very little, i.e. 0.5 mg once per week, whereas others require large doses. A patient education programme leading to the patient modifying their own dose of loperamide to achieve the goal of the ideal stool consistency appears to be the most effective regimen to follow.

This is achieved in normal circumstances by defecating in an appropriate place by consciously responding to the call to stool.

The method used to assist patients who are experiencing problems either opening their bowels or controlling when their bowels open depends on a number of factors. These include the presence of faecal incontinence, discomfort due to a loaded colon and/or rectum, which the patient cannot empty, and the patient's mental state.

In the presence of faecal incontinence, the initial aim of treatment should be to empty the rectum and colon within a few days to prevent faecal soiling. The preferred treatment is to empty the rectum by administering an enema or suppository each day until the faecal mass is cleared.

A quote from a caring daughter soon after her mother's death:

'In the later stages of her dementia, Mum didn't have a clue where she was or what she was doing. I thought that the district nurses were marvellous giving her the suppositories every Monday and Thursday. We knew when her bowels were going to work and it helped us to be able to keep her at home right up to the end. We had very few accidents once they started giving the suppositories.'

When suppositories are used to stimulate defecation, glycerine suppositories are usually used. More potent stimulation of defecation may be obtained by use of bisacodyl. It is now recognized that suppositories are best inserted blunt end first as they are easier to insert and better retained than the traditional sharp end first method.

Microenemas are now the preferred type of enema, principally because they are effective and easy to administer and are free of the adverse effects associated with phosphate enemas.

Occasionally, suppositories or enemas are ineffective at inducing defecation in either the acute or chronic situation, and manual removal of faeces may be required – especially if the stool is very hard. For patients with an atonic rectum, this is often the only treatment available. This problem is particularly prevalent among patients with severe spinal cord lesions, e.g. multiple sclerosis, traumatic cord lesions, in whom the parasympathetic supply to the rectum is deficient.

In patients who are faecally loaded with soft or formed stool but who are not incontinent or in discomfort, the preferred treatment is a stimulant laxative given orally. The most commonly used are senna (Senokot), sodium picosulphate and bisacodyl. These act directly on the myenteric plexus. They should be given at night as they take 10–14 hours to reach the colon, where they exert their effect (ideally during the day time). Long-term use of stimulant laxatives should be avoided, if possible, especially in younger patients as this may cause myenteric plexus degeneration.

Occasionally, a combined osmotic and stimulant laxative, e.g. codanthramer, is required when softening stool has not induced defecation or in patients with drug-induced constipation, e.g. secondary to opiates.

MAINTAINING A REGULAR PATTERN OF BOWEL EMPTYING

In about 50% of elderly patients who are constipated during hospitalization for an acute illness, the problem resolves with the treatment of their underlying illness. Other patients, however, have a continuing tendency to constipation. Their whole gut transit time is not necessarily reduced by the clearance of the faecal loading. Laxatives are the main treatment for these patients but some require regular emptying of their bowel from below using either enemas or suppositories.

TREATMENT OF THE FAECALLY INCONTINENT DEMENTED PATIENT

Incontinence in these patients is usually secondary to faecal loading, which should be cleared as above. A regimen of planned defecation should be implemented by the use of an enema one to three times per week if there is a continuing tendency to faecal incontinence or constipation. A constipating drug may be needed to prevent leakage between enemas. Poor compliance with treatment tends to limit success, especially in patients with severe behavioural problems. Strategies that may help these patients include the administration once weekly of a potent stimulant laxative, e.g. sodium picosulphate (initial dose 5 mg).

TREATMENT OF ANORECTAL INCONTINENCE, I.E. WEAK ANAL SPHINCTERS

The principles of treatment are similar to those described above. Maintaining a firm stool will help in most cases. Moderate success (about 60%) has been reported with surgical repairs in young and middle-aged incontinent patients, but its use cannot be recommended for elderly subjects as the problems tends to be multifactorial.

OUTCOME OF TREATMENT FOR FAECAL INCONTINENCE

In most cases, the simple measures described above are effective. The outcome of treatment is, however, influenced by the presence of other problems, e.g. dementia, especially when behavioural problems are present. The main anorectal factor that influences outcome is rectal prolapse; ideal stool for a prolapse patient is soft rather than firm.

'I have been able to go on coach trips to Scotland again since I started taking the loperamide. I thought I would never be able to travel again. It's wonderful to have my life back again after the miserable time I've had with my bowels. I never thought the answer would be so easy. I just give myself an extra dose before I leave home and I can be confident I won't embarrass myself on the bus.'

RECOMMENDED READING

*** Essential reading; ** recommended reading; * interesting but not vital

Barrett J A 1993 Faecal incontinence and related disorders in the older adult. Edward Arnold, Sevenoaks *

Barrett J A 1996 Disorders of the lower gastrointestinal tract. Reviews in Clinical Gerontology 6:129–146 *

Barrett J A, Chew D 1991 Disorders of the lower gastro-intestinal tract. Reviews in Clinical Gerontology 1:119–134 *

National Institute for Health and Clinical Excellence (NICE) 2007 Guideline on faecal incontinence. (In press) ***

Potter J, Norton C, Cottenden A 2002 Bowel care in frail older people – research and practice. Royal College of Physicians Clinical Effectiveness and Evaluation Unit, London ***

Tobin G W, Brocklehurst J C 1986 Faecal incontinence in residential homes for the elderly: prevalence, aetiology and management. Age and Ageing 15: 41–46 **

SELF-ASSESSMENT QUESTIONS

Are the following statements true or false?

1. Faecal incontinence in elderly people is more likely to occur in men than women

2. The most common cause of faecal incontinence in elderly people is faecal loading with soft faeces

3. A barium enema should be performed in the investigation of all older people with faecal incontinence

4. Rectal examination rarely provides useful information in the incontinent patient

SECTION 5

Genitourinary

Chapter 33

Prostate diseases

Ian Eardley and Mary Garthwaite

INTRODUCTION

Three main disease processes can affect the prostate:

- Prostatitis (infection of the prostate)
- Benign prostatic hypertrophy
- Prostatic carcinoma

Of these, prostatitis is most commonly seen in young men, while benign prostatic hyperplasia (BPH) and prostatic carcinoma are almost exclusively seen in elderly men. Urologists will manage most of these men, but an understanding of these conditions will be valuable to the geriatric physician in order to guide appropriate investigation, treatment and referral.

BENIGN PROSTATIC HYPERPLASIA

INTRODUCTION AND EPIDEMIOLOGY

Terminology is unfortunately confusing when discussing the benign prostate. Benign prostatic hyperplasia is a histological term, though it is often used as a clinical diagnosis. The incidence of BPH increases with age with more than 60% of men over the age of 60 years having histological evidence of BPH. About 50% of these men will have symptoms as a result, and these symptoms are referred to as lower urinary tract symptoms (LUTS). In some of these men, there will also be bladder outflow obstruction (BOO) as a direct consequence of the enlarged prostate. Bladder outflow obstruction is a urodynamic diagnosis (see Ch. 13).

While some men will have BPH, LUTS and BOO, not all men with BPH have symptoms, and not all are obstructed. Furthermore, LUTS can arise as a result of other conditions (e.g. detrusor overactivity, neurogenic bladder) and BOO can also be caused by other diseases (e.g. urethral stricture, prostatic carcinoma) (Fig. 33.1).

PATHOGENESIS AND COMPLICATIONS OF BPH

An insight into the symptoms (Box 33.1) and complications (Box 33.2) of BPH can be gained by reviewing the pathophysiological consequences of

Box 33.1 Symptoms of BPH (lower urinary tract symptoms)

Symptoms due to increased prostatic resistance (voiding symptoms)	Symptoms due to detrusor hypertrophy and detrusor overactivity (storage symptoms)
Hesitancy	Frequency
Poor stream	Nocturia
Terminal dribbling	Urgency
	Urge incontinence

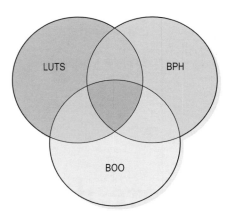

Figure 33.1 The relationship between benign prostatic hyperplasia (BPH), lower urinary tract symptoms (LUTS) and bladder outflow obstruction (BOO).

benign enlargement of the prostate. BPH restricts the flow of urine from the bladder, leading to hesitancy of micturition and a reduced urinary stream. The bladder must work harder to overcome the increased resistance of the prostate. It hypertrophies and may develop secondary detrusor overactivity, with frequency of micturition, nocturia, urgency and occasionally urge incontinence. Later in the disease, the bladder is unable fully to overcome the increased resistance, and it fails to empty. There is an increased risk of urinary tract infections and bladder calculus formation. In some cases the bladder hypertrophy, together with the residual urine, results in very high pressures within the bladder. This high pressure is transmitted to the kidneys and can lead to hydronephrosis and renal failure. In others, the smooth muscle of the bladder is gradually replaced by fibrous tissue resulting in a large floppy bladder with overflow incontinence.

One of the commonest complications of BPH is acute urinary retention (AUR). The exact pathogenesis of AUR is unknown but there is an increased risk in older men, in those with large prostates, in those with more severe symptoms and in those with the lowest urinary flow rates. Haematuria may also complicate BPH, due to the hypervascularity of the prostate, which is commonly associated with the BPH process.

COMMON CLINICAL PROBLEMS

Lower urinary tract symptoms

Assessment
Lower urinary tract symptoms (Box 33.1) are not solely a feature of BPH, and indeed are not only confined to men! A number of other conditions can give rise to LUTS (Box 33.3) and the first objective of the clinical assessment must be to distinguish between the different causes. A second objective is the identification of complications with the third being to ascertain the degree to which

Box 33.2 Complications of BPH

- Acute painful urinary retention
- Chronic painless urinary retention
- Overflow incontinence
- Urinary tract infection
- Bladder calculus
- Hydronephrosis
- Renal failure
- Haematuria

Box 33.3 Causes of lower urinary tract symptoms (LUTS)

- Benign prostatic hyperplasia
- Prostatic carcinoma
- Detrusor overactivity
- Urethral stricture
- Neurogenic bladder
- Hypocontractile bladder
- Nocturnal polyuria

Table 33.1   Important findings on clinical examination

Neurological disease	→	possible cause of LUTS
Anaemia	→	possible result of uraemia
Palpable bladder	→	complication of BPH
Phimosis	→	possible cause of LUTS
Meatal stenosis	→	possible cause of LUTS
Hard irregular prostate	→	possible carcinoma of prostate

symptoms affect the quality of life of the patient. These latter two features – namely the presence or absence of complications and the degree to which the condition affects quality of life – will usually direct treatment, as will the presence of any co-morbid conditions. The symptoms that typically arise from BPH are outlined in Box 33.1 and some of the more important features that may be seen on clinical examination are listed in Table 33.1. Baseline investigations include a mid-stream urine (MSU), serum electrolytes, an ultrasound scan of the urinary tract and a urinary flow rate (Table 33.2). Other occasional tests include the prostate-specific antigen (PSA), transrectal ultrasonography, urine cytology, cystoscopy and urodynamic studies (Table 33.3).

Treatment

Treatment options in elderly patients include surgery (transurethral prostatectomy, TURP), medication (α-adrenoceptor blocking agents, 5α-reductase inhibitors or a combination of the two), catheterization or 'watchful waiting'.

Table 33.2   Baseline investigations in LUTS

Test	Purpose	Notes
Mid-stream urine	Identification of haematuria, pyuria or infection	–
Serum electrolytes	Identification of uraemia	–
Ultrasound of urinary tract	Identification of hydronephrosis, poor bladder emptying or calculi	Post-void residuals greater than 100 mL are significant. If greater than 300 mL, the upper tracts are at risk
Urinary flow rate	Identification of reduced flow	Need a voided volume greater than 125 mL. Peak flow rates less than 12 mL/second are significant

Table 33.3   Occasional investigations in LUTS

Test	Indication	Purpose
PSA	Irregular prostate on rectal examination. Case finding for prostate cancer (controversial)	Identification of prostate cancer
Transrectal ultrasound	Raised PSA or hard irregular prostate	Identification of prostate cancer
Urine cytology	Haematuria or pyuria	Identification of bladder cancer
Cystoscopy	Haematuria	Identification of bladder cancer
Urodynamics	Neurological disease. Prior to prostate surgery. Previous prostate surgery. Equivocal urinary symptoms	Confirm urodynamic diagnosis

■ *Transurethral prostatectomy (TURP).* Given appropriate patient selection, around 80–90% of men will achieve a successful result. Complications include retrograde ejaculation (~ 80%), impotence (~ 10%), urethral stricture (~ 4%), incontinence (~ 1%) and the requirement for repeat surgery (~ 10% over 5 years). There is about a 1% mortality rate.

■ *Alpha-adrenoceptor blocking agents.* These drugs probably act by relaxing smooth muscle within the prostate, thereby reducing the resistance to flow. About 60–70% of men respond to treatment, although the magnitude of improvement is less than that seen following TURP. They are rapidly effective but side-effects include postural hypotension (5%) and flu-like symptoms (5%).

■ *5α-reductase inhibitors.* These drugs inhibit the conversion of testosterone to dihydrotestosterone leading to shrinkage of the prostate by about 30%. About 50% of men have modest improvements in symptoms and flow rate. Men with larger prostates respond best, and there appears to be a long-term reduction in the risk of urinary retention. They take about 6 months to be effective and side-effects include impotence (5%).

■ *Combination therapy.* A recently published long-term, double-blind trial of 3047 men (the Medical Therapy of Prostatic Symptoms or MTOPS Trial, McConnell et al 2003) compared the effects of placebo, an alpha-blocker (doxazosin), a 5α-reductase inhibitor (finasteride) and combination therapy on the clinical progression of BPH. The mean follow-up time was 4.5 years. The authors concluded that combination therapy with doxazosin and finasteride was safe and reduced the risk of overall clinical progression of BPH significantly more than treatment with either drug alone. Both combination therapy and treatment with finasteride alone led to a reduction in the long-term risk of acute urinary retention and the need for invasive therapy. In the light of this trial, the place of combination therapy in the treatment of men with BPH has been reappraised and a number of clinical guidelines have been produced to take account of this.

■ *Catheterization.* This is only indicated when other treatments are not possible.

■ *Watchful waiting.* Natural history studies suggest that at least 50% of men do not deteriorate over a 5-year period if treated conservatively. If the man has modest symptoms and no complications, he may wish to avoid surgical or drug treatment. He will have a ~ 5–10% risk of urinary retention over a 5-year period (depending upon his age and prostatic size).

The treatment of an individual with LUTS secondary to BPH is influenced by:

■ *The presence (or otherwise) of complications.* If complications are present, then surgical treatment is usually necessary.

■ *Co-morbid conditions.* These may preclude surgery or anaesthesia. Occasionally, the presence of cardiovascular disease may also prevent the use of α-adrenoceptor blocking agents.

■ *Patient choice.* Surgery provides the greatest subjective and objective improvement compared with other treatments. However, it has more complications. In many cases, the degree to which the patient is bothered by his symptoms will determine the treatment that he is willing to undergo.

In all cases, thorough counselling of the patient is vital so that the treatment can be tailored to the individual.

Painful (acute) urinary retention

Assessment

Painful urinary retention in men can be due to BPH or it may arise as a complication of another condition or therapy (Box 33.4). If present, these

---

Box 33.4   Precipitating (transient) causes of acute urinary retention (AUR)

■ Constipation
■ Urinary tract infection
■ Surgery
■ Excessive alcohol intake
■ Use of anticholinergic drugs (e.g. tricyclic antidepressants)
■ Neurological disease (e.g. multiple sclerosis)
■ Bladder calculi

causes must be identified, and any other complications of BPH should also be identified. Following catheterization, investigation includes a midstream urine, serum electrolytes and an abdominal X-ray (to identify urinary calculi).

Treatment

Urethral catheterization with a 12 or 14 Fr Foley catheter is appropriate. The amount of urine drained from the bladder should be recorded. Any precipitating cause for the urinary retention that can be treated should be treated before a trial without catheter (TWOC). In men who have developed urinary retention following some other surgery, a period of 4–6 weeks is usually necessary before the TWOC is performed. If there are no obvious precipitating causes for the retention, a TWOC is only indicated if there is less than 800 mL in the bladder at the time of catheterization *and* if there are no pre-existing LUTS. Under these circumstances, there is a reasonable (30–50%) chance that the patient will be able to void without any further treatment. There is emerging evidence that alpha-blockers may help to improve the ability of a man to void under these circumstances, although the long-term outcome of alpha-blockers in men with acute urinary retention is as yet unclear.

When the cause of the retention is BPH, and when there is a large residual volume at catheterization (i.e. = 800 mL), or when the patient has failed a TWOC, then the only therapeutic options are TURP or catheterization (either permanent or intermittent). In most cases, unless the patient is unfit for surgery, TURP is the best option.

Painless (chronic) urinary retention with renal failure

Assessment

There are often only mild LUTS, although there is often a history of nocturnal incontinence. On examination the bladder is distended and painless. The renal function may be considerably impaired, and ultrasound scanning confirms bilateral hydronephrosis. Occasionally, such cases can present with gross peripheral oedema or with hypertension.

Treatment

Catheterization will relieve the retention, but caution is needed in the following cases:

- *Sepsis*. Patients with chronic retention of urine often have infected urine, and catheterization may precipitate a septic episode. Parenteral antibiotics (gentamicin 8–120 mg as a single dose) are needed before catheterization.

- *Haematuria*. Decompression of a grossly distended bladder can lead to haematuria, which may be severe. The haematuria usually settles within 24 to 48 hours and no extra precautions or treatment are needed.

- *Post-obstructive diuresis*. In men with bilateral hydronephrosis and impaired renal function, catheterization leads to the development of a diuresis that may be considerable (6–12 L/ 24 hours) and prolonged (2–7 days). The mechanism is incompletely understood, but probably reflects maintained glomerular filtration in the context of inadequate tubular reabsorption. Careful monitoring of fluid balance and serum electrolytes is essential and fluid supplementation with intravenous fluids is often necessary.

Definitive treatment is usually by TURP, although ultimate bladder function is not always perfect as a consequence of the prolonged period of overdistension before diagnosis and treatment. Chronic retention of urine should never be treated by medication and/or catheter removal alone.

PROSTATIC CARCINOMA

INTRODUCTION, EPIDEMIOLOGY AND AETIOLOGY

In most Western countries, prostatic carcinoma (CaP) is the most commonly found malignancy in men and it is the second commonest cause of cancer deaths (after lung). However, 95% of all cases of CaP are diagnosed in men aged between 45 and 89 years of age, with the median age of diagnosis being 72 years. The condition varies significantly by geography and by race. For instance, it is rare in Japan, although in Japanese immigrants to the USA the incidence approaches that of native

North Americans. This may reflect some dietary factor that has aetiological importance. The highest incidence of CaP in the USA, however, is in the Afro-Caribbean population.

In the past 10–15 years, with increasing longevity of the ageing population, and with the increasing use of PSA testing as a quasi screening test, the incidence of prostate cancer, and particularly the early form of the disease, has increased. This almost certainly reflects increased detection, rather than a true increase in incidence.

The aetiology of CaP is not fully understood, but it is probably multifactorial. There are genetic factors, as alluded to by the varying racial differences in incidence. Furthermore, a positive family history for CaP is an important risk factor for the development of the disease. Dietary fat may be an important environmental risk factor via some alteration in sex hormone production.

There is current interest in the potential to prevent prostatic cancer, largely as a result of the Prostate Cancer Prevention Trial (PCPT) (Mellon 2005). This was a study of 18882 men, aged over 55 years, with a normal digital rectal examination and a PSA of 3.0 ng/mL who were randomized to treatment with finasteride or placebo for 7 years. The trial results suggested that while finasteride might prevent the development of prostate cancer, the proportion of those cancers that did develop that were high grade (and therefore more aggressive) was increased. Further studies with other 5α-reductase inhibitors, and indeed with other agents (such as selenium), are under way.

PATHOLOGY AND NATURAL HISTORY

The presence of histological prostatic cancer does not necessarily imply that the man will develop clinical cancer, or that he will die from CaP. For instance, in the USA, for a man aged 50 years of age, his lifetime risk of having histological CaP is 42%, while his risk of developing clinical CaP is 9.5% and risk of dying from CaP is only 2.9%.

What we know about the natural history of prostate cancer is crucial to the rationale for therapy of prostate cancer. The course of the disease is mainly affected by the stage and grade of the tumour at presentation. In general, the higher the stage and the less well differentiated the tumour, the greater the risk of metastasis, progression and

death. For instance, men with localized low-grade disease are unlikely to develop progression within 10–15 years while men with metastatic disease at presentation have a median survival of around 30 months. The most commonly used staging system is the TNM (Tumour, Node, Metastasis) system and the most widely used histological grading system is the Gleason grading system, which provides a number between 2 and 10 according to the degree of differentiation. The greater the number, the less well differentiated the tumour.

COMMON CLINICAL PROBLEMS

Localized prostate cancer

In elderly men the tumour will usually be identified by chance, either at TURP or following a needle biopsy in a man with a raised PSA. The PSA will typically be less than 20 ng/mL. Men with a small cancer within the prostate have a low risk of:

- Metastatic disease at the time of presentation
- Progression of the disease within 5 years
- Dying from prostate cancer within 10 years

Accordingly, aggressive local treatments are only appropriate in men with a life expectancy greater than 10 to 15 years. Local radical therapy is therefore offered to men up to the age of around 75 years, but in men over this age a policy of 'watchful waiting' is usually followed. At present there is some doubt as to the relative efficacy of the varying local treatments, and randomized controlled trials are in place to assess the relative merits of these therapies. The first of these to report has suggested a marginal advantage for radical prostatectomy over watchful waiting, although around 20 patients need to be treated in order to save a single life.

- *Radical prostatectomy.* An open surgical procedure with complete excision of the prostate and the pelvic lymph nodes. A 5–10% incontinence rate and a 50% impotence rate accompany mortality rates of around 1–2%.

- *Radical radiotherapy.* Delivered in one of two ways, either by external beam or by interstitial treatment (brachytherapy). Complications include impotence, proctitis, urinary retention and haematuria.

- *Watchful waiting.* Regular assessment and monitoring of the patient, by clinical assessment and PSA testing. PSA might not be a perfect diagnostic test for prostate cancer, but it is an excellent tumour marker and will usually identify disease progression. When there is significant disease progression as demonstrated by a rise in the serum PSA, endocrine therapy is the usual treatment (see later).

Table 33.4 The chances of detecting a prostatic cancer on biopsy	
Serum PSA (ng/mL)	Chance of detecting prostate cancer on biopsy
< 4	2%
4–10	25%
> 10	50–65%

Management of raised PSA

Prostate specific antigen is secreted by the normal prostate, but is secreted in increased amounts in men with prostatic disease or following instrumentation (Box 33.5). It also increases with age and with increasing prostate size. The normal range therefore is age dependent, and for men over 70 years of age a level greater than 4 ng/mL is usually considered important. At very high levels (> 60 ng/mL) and in the absence of recent prostatic surgery the underlying cause is nearly always prostate cancer, but at lower levels benign causes are possible (Table 33.4). Given what we know about the natural history of the disease, and given the current attitudes to the treatment of men with localized prostate cancer, a number of questions arise:

- *Which elderly men should have a PSA test?* The short answer is that it should be tested in men in whom it would alter management. It should be tested when there is a suspicion of metastatic disease, where endocrine therapy might help clinically. It should *not* be used as a screening tool in asymptomatic elderly men, since most cancers identified would not need treatment in the lifetime of the patient. It is now common practice to test PSA in all men presenting with LUTS, but this should be carefully considered in elderly subjects.

- *What is the appropriate management for an elderly man with a raised PSA?* The answer to this is again influenced by the attitudes to treatment. To make a diagnosis of prostate cancer a transrectal ultrasound scan and biopsy are needed, but there are complications, including bleeding and infection (in ~ 5–10% of cases), so it is not an investigation to be undertaken lightly. Accordingly, in an elderly man with a PSA in the approximate range of 4–20 ng/mL who has a life expectancy less than 10 years, most urologists would pursue an expectant policy. At the other extreme, an elderly man with a PSA over 100 ng/mL would usually be investigated. Clearly, there are a wide variety of clinical situations between these two extremes, but the general principles should be clear. In elderly patients, there is usually little point in striving to identify localized disease, because it probably would not be treated. In contrast, if there is a suspicion of metastatic disease, then urgent investigation is justified.

Box 33.5 Causes of a raised PSA

- Prostate cancer
- Benign prostatic hyperplasia
- Prostatitis
- Urinary tract infection
- Following cystoscopy or TURP
- Following catheterization
- Following prostate biopsy

Locally advanced prostate cancer

Prostate cancers that have penetrated through the prostatic capsule carry a much higher risk of progression, metastasis and death. Unless there are important co-morbid conditions treatment is usual, even in elderly subjects. Patients will typically present with lower urinary tract symptoms, a raised PSA (usually around 20–50 ng/mL), or an abnormal digital rectal examination. Staging of the disease is important by means of bone scan, PSA, full blood count and liver function tests. If

LUTS are present, then an ultrasound scan of the urinary tract and a flow rate are valuable. Optimal treatment is unclear, but external beam radiotherapy or hormone therapy or both treatments combined are options. With treatment, 5- and 10-year survival rates in this group of patients are around 50–60% and 20–30% respectively.

Metastatic prostate cancer

Assessment

Historically, around 40% of all patients with prostate cancer had metastatic disease at the time of initial assessment. With the increasing use of PSA testing, there has been a 'stage migration' with a consequential fall in the numbers with metastatic disease at presentation. Of the men with metastatic disease, half will have symptoms attributable to their prostate cancer, while the other 50% will be asymptomatic. Bone pain is the predominant symptom of metastatic disease, due to skeletal metastases. Renal failure (5%), pathological fractures, spinal cord compression and bone marrow infiltration are also occasionally seen. Constitutional symptoms of disseminated malignancy are usually present (e.g. lethargy, weight loss). The serum PSA is usually elevated over 50 ng/mL and may be over 1000 ng/mL. A transrectal ultrasound scan and biopsy may be needed to provide tissue for histology. Sclerotic deposits are typically found in the pelvic girdle and lumbosacral spine, and are usually identified by bone scan and/or X-rays. A full blood count might give circumstantial evidence of marrow infiltration and both serum calcium and liver function tests can be valuable.

Treatment

Most prostatic cancers are dependent for their growth upon testosterone and removal of testosterone leads to regression of most tumours. A small number of androgen insensitive cells are left, and some time later these cells proliferate and an androgen insensitive tumour again progresses. Around 90% of circulating androgens emanate from the testes and the remaining 10% come from the adrenal gland. Although there are several methods of androgen deprivation, there is no evidence that any are superior in efficacy. Currently available methods of hormone treatment for prostate cancer include:

- *Surgical castration.* There is a rapid fall of plasma testosterone levels to basal levels within 1 to 2 days. It can be performed under local anaesthetic and the side-effects are primarily immediate loss of libido, impotence and hot flushes. Its main role nowadays is in those cases where rapid response to treatment is needed (e.g. spinal cord compression, obstructive renal failure).

- *Luteinizing hormone-releasing hormone (LHRH) analogues.* These inhibit the secretion of LH from the pituitary gland which in turn leads to reduced testicular testosterone secretion. They take about 2 weeks to suppress testosterone to basal levels and initially they actually enhance testosterone secretion and can induce a 'flare reaction'. Skeletal metastases can become increasingly painful and may result in cord compression. This period should therefore be covered by a simultaneous administration of an anti-androgen. Side-effects include loss of libido, impotence and hot flushes. The drugs are given by depot injection every 1 or 3 months.

- *Anti-androgens.* These are direct competitive inhibitors of the androgen receptor and are of two types – steroidal (e.g. cyproterone acetate) and non-steroidal (e.g. flutamide, bicalutamide). All are taken orally each day and side-effects include hepatic dysfunction, lethargy, impotence (all cyproterone), diarrhoea and painful gynaecomastia (flutamide and bicalutamide).

- *Oestrogens.* Stilboestrol is still occasionally used, but because of the high incidence of cardiovascular related side-effects it is usually given in conjunction with aspirin.

Other situations

In the later stages of prostate cancer a number of complications can arise. A broad plan of management for patients with these is shown in Figure 33.2.

Ultimately the tumour becomes refractory to hormone therapy. Once present, hormone refractory prostate cancer usually leads to the death of the patient within 10 months. It manifests itself as a rising PSA while on endocrine therapy. Second-line treatments with the oestrogens, steroids and

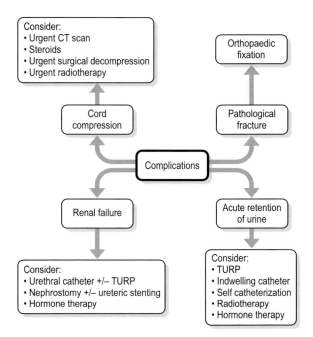

Figure 33.2 Complications of metastatic prostate cancer and their management.

cytotoxics have all been used with variable but minor efficacy. There is increasing interest in the use of taxols for hormone escape prostate cancer.

CONCLUSION

Prostate disease is essentially a disease of elderly men. With the increasing age of our population, the clinical situations outlined above will become more common. However, the principles of treatment are not too complicated. In the elderly patient, treatment must be tailored to the individual, always remembering the effect of other co-morbid conditions.

REFERENCES

McConnell J D, Roehrborn C G, Bautista O M et al 2003 The long-term effect of doxazosin, finasteride, and combination therapy on the clinical progression of benign prostatic hyperplasia. MTOPS Research Group. New England Journal of Medicine 349: 2387–2398

Mellon J K 2005 The finasteride prostate cancer prevention trial (PCPT) – what have we learned? European Journal of Cancer 41:2016–2022

RECOMMENDED READING

Benign prostatic hyperplasia

AUA Practice Guidelines Committee 2003 AUA guideline on management of benign prostatic hyperplasia 2003, Ch. 1: diagnosis and treatment recommendations. Journal of Urology 170:530–547

Berry S J, Coffey D S, Walsh P C et al 1984 The development of benign prostatic hyperplasia with age. Journal of Urology 132:474

Guess H A 1995 Epidemiology and natural history of benign prostatic hyperplasia. Urology Clinics of North America 22:247–261

Logan Y T, Belgeri M T 2005 Monotherapy versus combination drug therapy for the treatment of benign prostatic hyperplasia. American Journal of Geriatric Pharmacotherapy 3:103–114

McConnell J D, Roehrborn C G, Bautista O M et al 2003 The long-term effects of doxazosin, finasteride, and combination therapy on the clinical progression of benign prostatic hyperplasia. New England Journal of Medicine 349:2387–2398

Madersbacher S, Marberger M 1999 Is transurethral resection of the prostate still justified? British Journal of Urology International 83:227–237

Madersbacher S, Alvivizatos G, Nordling J et al 2004 EAU 2004 Guidelines on assessment, therapy and follow-up of men with lower urinary tract symptoms suggestive of benign prostatic obstruction (BPH Guidelines). European Urology 46:547–554

Oesterling J E, Jacobsen S J, Chute C G et al 1993 Serum prostate specific antigen in a community based population of healthy men. Establishment of age specific reference ranges. Journal of the American Medical Association 270: 860–864

Speakman M J, Kirby R S, Joyce A et al 2004 Guideline for the primary care management of male lower urinary tract symptoms. British Journal of Urology International 93:985–990

Wasson J, Reda D, Bruskewitz R et al 1994 A comparison of transurethral surgery with watchful waiting for moderate symptoms of benign prostatic hyperplasia. New England Journal of Medicine 332:75–79

Prostate cancer

Albertsen P C, Fryback D G, Storer B E et al 1995 Long-term survival among men with conservatively treated localized prostate cancer. Journal of the American Medical Association 274:626

Al-Booz H, Ash D, Bottomley D M et al 1999 Short term morbidity and acceptability of 125 iodine implantation for localised carcinoma of the prostate. British Journal of Urology International 83:53–56

Aus G, Abbou C C, Pacik D et al 2001 EAU guidelines on prostate cancer. European Urology 40:97–101

Bill-Axelson A, Holmberg L, Ruutu M et al 2005 Scandinavian Prostate Cancer Group Study No. 4. Radical prostatectomy versus watchful waiting in early prostate cancer. New England Journal of Medicine 352:1977–1984

Catalona W J 1995 Surgical management of prostate cancer. Cancer 75:1903–1908

Gann P H, Hennekens C H, Stampfer M J 1995 A prospective evaluation of plasma prostate-specific antigen for detection of prostate cancer. Journal of the American Medical Association 273:289–294

Mellon J K 2005 The finasteride prostate cancer prevention trial (PCPT) – what have we learned? European Journal of Cancer 41:2016–2022

Petrylak D P 2005 Future directions in the treatment of androgen-independent prostate cancer. [Review – 27 refs] Urology 65:8–12

Postma R, Schroder F H 2005 Screening for prostate cancer. European Journal of Cancer 41:825–833

Shipley W U, Zietman A L, Hanks G E et al 1994 Treatment related sequelae following external beam radiation for prostate cancer: a review with an update in patients with stages T1 and T2 tumour. Journal of Urology 152:1799–1805

Thompson I M, Goodman P J, Tangen C M et al 2003 The influence of finasteride on the development of prostate cancer. New England Journal of Medicine 349:215–224

Whitemore A S, Kolonel L N, Wu A H et al 1995 Prostate cancer in relation to diet, physical activity and body size in blacks, whites and Asians in the United States and Canada. Journal of the National Cancer Institute 87: 652–661

SELF-ASSESSMENT QUESTIONS

Are the following statements true or false?

1. Recognized complications of BPH include:
   a. Renal failure
   b. Acute retention of urine
   c. Transitional cell carcinoma of the bladder
   d. Prostate cancer
   e. Haematuria

2. Appropriate early assessment for a 78-year-old man in acute painful urinary retention, with a smooth prostate gland on rectal examination includes:
   a. Serum electrolytes
   b. Abdominal X-ray
   c. Catheter specimen of urine for culture
   d. Prostate specific antigen
   e. Ultrasound of the urinary tract

3. In the treatment of BPH:
   a. 5α-reductase inhibitors may take up to 6 months to produce symptomatic improvement
   b. α-adrenergic agonists are rapidly acting drugs for the treatment of BPH
   c. TURP commonly results in permanent urinary incontinence
   d. Erectile dysfunction is a recognized complication following TURP

4. Regarding carcinoma of the prostate:
   a. The incidence falls with increasing age
   b. Most cases never produce clinical symptoms
   c. Most cases that do present clinically never kill the patient
   d. The mortality can be reduced by population screening

5. Treatment options for a 78-year-old man with a localized prostate cancer and a PSA of 12 ng/ml include:
   a. Radical prostatectomy
   b. Prostatic brachytherapy
   c. α-adrenoceptor blockers
   d. Watchful waiting
   e. LHRH analogues

6. Treatment options for a 72-year-old man with metastatic prostate cancer and a PSA of 665 ng/mL include:
   a. Radical prostatectomy
   b. Prostatic brachytherapy
   c. α-adrenoceptor blockers
   d. Watchful waiting
   e. LHRH analogues

SECTION 5

Genitourinary

Chapter 34

Urinary tract infections

Rosaire Gray

Urinary tract infections (UTIs) are among the most common infections in humans. Although usually uncomplicated, they are often recurrent and can cause considerable morbidity. Both UTI and asymptomatic bacteriuria are common in elderly people (Table 34.1) and especially those in long-term care. About 40% of nosocomial infections are urinary in origin and these infections are a major cause of Gram-negative bacteraemia. Bacteraemic UTI in the elderly has a high mortality. In frail elderly patients with multiple pathologies and cognitive impairment, early recognition of bacteraemic UTI and prompt appropriate treatment are critical in reducing mortality.

Table 34.1 Prevalence of bacteriuria

	65–85 years	> 85 years
Women	15%	25%
Men	5%	15%

DEFINITION OF URINARY TRACT INFECTION

On the basis of the work of Kass in 1956 (Kass 1956), 10^5 colony forming units (CFUs) of a single species per mL in a mid-stream urine (MSU) specimen became established as 'significant' bacteriuria. This definition has a very low sensitivity, about 0.50, for detecting infection in some groups. While it still holds in asymptomatic patients, in other circumstances lower thresholds are considered 'significant' (Table 34.2). These criteria have specificities of about 85% and sensitivities of about 95% (Stamm 1988).

Asymptomatic bacteriuria is defined as clinically significant bacteriuria (10^5 CFUs per mL) in two consecutive cultures from a patient without symptoms attributable to the urinary tract. It may be intermittent and the clinical relevance, especially in the absence of pyuria, is unclear.

■ The prevalence increases with age in both sexes.

Table 34.2	Criteria for significant bacteriuria
$\geq 10^2$	CFU coliforms/mL in a symptomatic woman
$\geq 10^5$	CFU non-coliforms/mL in a symptomatic woman
$\geq 10^3$	CFU of a single species/mL in symptomatic men
$\geq 10^5$	CFU of a single species/mL on two consecutive specimens in asymptomatic individuals
$\geq 10^2$	CFU of a single species/mL in a specimen obtained by suprapubic aspiration in symptomatic patients

- Other than in pregnancy or in association with instrumentation of the urinary tract, there is no convincing evidence linking asymptomatic bacteriuria to the subsequent development of acute infection.
- Except in pregnancy, there is little evidence that treatment protects against subsequent renal damage.
- In patients with *indwelling catheters* bacteriuria is almost universal (Stamm 1991). Suprapubic catheters have a lower prevalence of bacteriuria than urethral catheters. Catheter-associated bacteriuria is an important source of Gram-negative bacteraemia. However, treating asymptomatic bacteriuria has no effect on the incidence of fever, new episodes of bacteriuria, or the number of bacterial strains identified in urine specimens. *Antibiotics should be avoided in catheterized patients unless they have symptomatic infection.*

SYMPTOMS OF URINARY TRACT INFECTION IN ELDERLY PATIENTS

The characteristic symptoms of lower UTI or cystitis include some combination of dysuria, frequency, urgency, haematuria and suprapubic discomfort. Acute symptomatic UTI can cause urinary incontinence. In the absence of other symptoms, the relationship between bacteriuria and incontinence is unclear. The overactive bladder, which is common in elderly subjects, involves some symptoms common to cystitis, and significant UTIs in old age may be painless. Overactive bladder symptoms such as frequency, urgency

and incontinence may therefore reflect genuine UTI, which may be undetected if the traditional threshold of 10^5 CFUs per mL is used. In a recent study, up to 60% of patients attending a continence clinic with frequency and incontinence had positive microscopy (see below) and leucocyte esterase tests. Pilot data indicate that treatment of infection is associated with symptomatic improvement and an ongoing study will evaluate this.

The elderly patient with a UTI may present atypically with falls, immobility, confusion or poor general health. Treatment of these patients with appropriate antibiotics generally results in a return to their previous state of health. Urine culture is indicated, as resistant organisms are not uncommon. While awaiting results, empirical treatment (see below) should be started and then altered appropriately. In patients with atypical symptoms, a positive urinary nitrite test (see below) is an immediate and reliable indicator for the presence of infection, with a 100% specificity and over 80% sensitivity.

DIAGNOSIS OF URINARY TRACT INFECTION

There are a number of diagnostic tests available for UTI (Box 34.1) but all have limitations as outlined below. Proteinuria alone is not a useful diagnostic test.

- *Urine microscopy* to detect leucocytes and/or Gram-stained organisms. Microscopy of fresh un-spun urine using a haemocytometer to count pus cells is the most reliable technique for the detection of pyuria. A threshold of $\geq 10^3$ white

Box 34.1 Diagnostic tests for UTI
■ Urine microscopy
– Pyuria
– Gram stain
■ **Urine culture**
■ **Rapid assay techniques**
– Leucocyte esterase
– Urinary nitrite
– Haematuria

Box 34.2   Indications for urine culture

- Doubt about the diagnosis
- History of recent urinary tract infection (within 3 weeks)
- Recent instrumentation of the urinary tract
- Diabetes mellitus
- Pyelonephritis suspected
- Recent antibiotic therapy
- Structural abnormalities of the urinary tract
- Immunosuppressed patients
- Suspected urinary tract infection in elderly patients with atypical presentation

Table 34.3   Accuracy of strip tests for diagnosis of UTI in elderly subjects

	Sensitivity (%)	Specificity (%)
Nitrite	83	100
Blood	67	66
Protein	72	66
Urinary leucocytes	72	81
Classical symptoms	28	59
Pyrexia	22	84

blood cells.mm^{-3} was identified in 1969 from leucocyte excretion studies and has been shown to identify significant infections with symptoms and a quantative culture of 10^2 CFUs per mL.

- *Macroscopic or microscopic haematuria* is present in about 50% of patients with UTI but on its own is not diagnostic of infection. In the absence of infection, haematuria should be further investigated. In those with infection, it is important to check that the haematuria resolves on treatment of the infection.

- *Urine culture* has been traditionally used to confirm or exclude the diagnosis of UTI but is no longer considered essential. Box 34.2 shows currently accepted indications for urine culture. Conventional culture techniques require about 24 hours to obtain an accurate colony count. Automated culture systems produce faster results but have limited value in detecting low colony counts and have a threshold of 10^4 CFUs per mL. An MSU may fail to detect nearly 50% of UTIs in symptomatic patients (especially young women) and false positive rates of up to 17% are reported.

- *Leucocyte esterase* is an enzyme found in leucocyte granules. It can be detected by the blue colour reaction with a chloracetate stain impregnated in a dipstick pad (Ames Multistix 8SG, Bayer Diagnostics). The test has been validated and the sensitivity is 75 to 96% and specificity 94 to 98% (Table 34.3) (Deville et al 2004, Pfaller & Koontz 1985).

- *Nitrite* in the urine is produced by the action of bacterial nitrate reductase on dietary nitrate. It can be detected by its action on an amine-impregnated pad on a urine dipstick to form a diazonium compound. This results in a pink colour reaction (Ames Multistix 8SG, Bayer Diagnostics). False negatives may result from insufficient dietary nitrate, or insufficient urinary nitrite levels due to diuretics. *Staphylococci, Enterococci* and *Pseudomonas* species do not produce nitrate reductase. Therefore, the sensitivity of this test is low (35 to 85%) but the specificity is high (92 to 100%) (Table 34.3) (Deville et al 2004, Pfaller & Koontz 1985).

INFECTING ORGANISMS

The microbiology of UTI in older people differs from that in younger patients (Nicolle 2001). The reasons for the altered microbiology probably include hospitalization, catheterization and instrumentation, urinary tract obstruction related to prostatic enlargement in men, bladder prolapse in women, neuropathic bladder in both sexes, and the greater use of antimicrobial agents. *Escherichia coli* is still the commonest infecting organism in community-acquired infection, but elderly patients are more likely to have infection with *Proteus, Klebsiella, Enterobacter, Serratia, Pseudomonas,* other Gram-negative organisms and *Enterococcus.* Polymicrobial infections account for up to 1 in 3 infections in elderly patients, especially in those with indwelling catheters or stents (Stamm 1991). The recent rise of antibiotic-resistant bacteria e.g. methicillin-resistant *Staphylococcus aureus* and vancomycin-resistant *Enterococcus,* and *Candida* species is a particular problem in certain populations, such as intensive care unit patients receiving broad-spectrum antimicrobials and those with indwelling catheters (Stamm 1991). Strict adherence to hygiene practices is necessary to prevent the spread of resistant organisms.

TREATMENT OF URINARY TRACT INFECTION

Symptomatic urinary infection must be treated with an antibiotic. Asymptomatic bacteriuria is generally a benign condition and is not an indication for antibiotic therapy. There is, unfortunately, no ideal antibiotic for treating UTI in elderly patients.

- *Nitrofurantoin* is a good choice in young patients but should be used with caution in elderly patients as it is ineffective in patients with a glomerular filtration rate of less than 30 mL/min. It may cause a partially reversible peripheral neuropathy in those with reduced renal function.

- *Sulphonamides* are effective against *Escherichia coli* but are associated with the emergence of resistant bowel flora.

- *Amoxicillin* is reasonably well absorbed from the gastrointestinal tract and excreted in the urine but affects vaginal flora and can lead to candida vaginitis in up to 25% of women.

- *Trimethoprim* used alone is as effective as the trimethoprim–sulfamethoxazole combination and is active against most common urinary pathogens. However, it has an effect on vaginal flora and resistance is not uncommon.

- *Cephalosporins* are effective against most urinary pathogens but they tend to be expensive. They also affect vaginal flora.

- The newer *fluoroquinolone* antibiotics (e.g. *ciprofloxacin*) are effective against urinary pathogens including *Pseudomonas aeruginosa* and are available orally. They are expensive and at present are used excessively as first-line therapy. Indications for their use are recurrent, complicated and nosocomial infections.

Box 34.3   Features indicating complicated UTI

- Instrumentation of the urinary tract
- Hospital-acquired infection
- Diabetes mellitus
- Immunosuppressed patients
- Failure of first-line therapy
- Symptoms lasting over 7 days
- Symptoms or signs of upper tract disease
- Structural anomalies of the urinary tract
- Urinary calculi

Antimicrobial agents can cause vulvovaginal candidosis, hypersensitivity reactions, rashes and gastrointestinal disturbances, all of which can increase morbidity. Limiting treatment to a minimum reduces adverse effects and cost while increasing compliance. Unfortunately the optimal treatment duration for uncomplicated symptomatic lower UTI remains to be determined as the available trials are methodologically poor. Recent reviews indicate that single dose antibiotic treatment is less effective, although better accepted by the patients, than longer treatment durations (3–14 days) (Lutters & Yogt 2002). In addition there was no significant difference in achieving a symptomatic cure between a short course (3–6 days) versus a longer course (7–14 days) of antibiotics, although the latter was more effective in obtaining bacteriological cure. Well-designed randomized controlled trials to test the effect on clinically relevant outcomes of different treatment durations of a given antibiotic in elderly women are needed. In men or when urinary tract infection is complicated (Box 34.3) then a 7-day course should be used. A useful approach in elderly patients with lower UTI is to prescribe trimethoprim 200 mg twice daily for 3 or 7 days or a cephalosporin as a first-line agent. Ciprofloxacin is a useful second-line agent but other agents may be chosen in the light of sensitivity tests on failure of first-line therapy. For pyelonephritis, the recommended duration of treatment is 14 days. Antibiotics for initial oral treatment include fluoroquinolones and oral cephalosporins (e.g. cefuroxime). For patients with community-acquired infections who have not received previous antibiotic treatment, a second-generation cephalo-

---

Box 34.4   Indications for further investigation of UTI

- Slow resolution of infection
- Recurrent infections
- Frank haematuria
- Persistent microscopic haematuria
- Acute pyelonephritis
- Suspected renal calculi
- Unusual infecting organism

Box 34.5   Further investigation of UTI
(see Box 34.4 for indications)

Initial

- Post-voiding residual and voiding cystogram
- Ultrasound of renal tract
- CT scan in selected cases
- Rectal examination (PSA if indicated)
- Cystoscopy (haematuria)

---

sporin (e.g. cefuroxime) covers most pathogens; for patients with nosocomial infections, a third-generation cephalosporin (e.g. cefotaxime, ceftazidime, ceftriaxone), a quinolone or an aminoglycoside are preferred.

RECURRENT URINARY TRACT INFECTIONS

The management of recurrent symptomatic UTIs depends largely on the frequency of recurrence. Recurrent infections may be a relapse or reinfection UTI. Relapse UTI is defined as an infection in which urine is rendered partially or temporarily sterile by antimicrobial therapy, with the subsequent recurrence of bacteriuria from the un-eradicated pathogen, usually within 2 weeks of completion of therapy. Reinfection UTI is defined as an infection that arises greater than 4 weeks after the previous infection has been cured and usually involves a different bacterial strain. Further investigation may be indicated as outlined in Boxes 34.4 and 34.5. If they are infrequent, each new episode should be treated with a short course of antibiotic therapy, remembering that recurrent infection is more likely to occur with organisms of increased resistance. In the case of frequent or incapacitating symptoms, long-term prophylactic therapy may be indicated. Trimethoprim 100 mg daily, nitrofurantoin 50–100 mg daily or cefalexin 125 mg daily are recommended. As a lack of oestrogen in elderly women causes marked changes in vaginal microflora, including loss of lacto-bacilli and increased colonization by *Escherichia coli*, intravaginal oestrogen replacement is recommended as a choice for the prevention of recurrent UTIs in post-menopausal women. Cranberry juice is often given to older people to prevent UTI but at present there is little evidence to support its use and further studies are required. Bacterial prostatitis is not uncommon in older men and the symptoms may be mistaken for UTI. Chronic bacterial prostatitis is probably the commonest cause of relapsed UTI in elderly men. The diagnosis is suggested when bacterial colony counts from urine or expressed prostate secretion are at least 10-fold greater than counts from the urethral urine sample. This requires at least 4 weeks of antibiotic treatment (e.g. trimethoprim or erythromycin) to penetrate tissues adequately.

In summary, bacteriuria is common in elderly patients. Asymptomatic bacteriuria is benign and is not an indication for antibiotic therapy. Urine culture is not essential for diagnosis before giving first-line therapy in patients with urinary symptoms. Newer diagnostic techniques including leucocyte esterase and nitrite strips and automated culture units are useful but have limitations, especially with lower colony counts.

REFERENCES

Deville W L, Yzermans J C, van Duijn N P et al 2004 The urine dipstick test useful to rule out infections. A meta-analysis of the accuracy. BMC Urology 4:4–18

Kass E H 1956 Asymptomatic infections of the urinary tract. Transactions of the Association of American Physicians 956:56–64

Lutters M, Yogt N 2002 Antibiotic duration for treating uncomplicated, symptomatic lower urinary tract infections in elderly women. Cochrane Database of Systemic Review 3. Art. No.: CD001535. DOI: 10.1002/14651858.CD001535

Nicolle L E 2001 Urinary tract pathogens in complicated infection and in elderly individuals. Journal of Infectious Diseases 183:55–58

Pfaller M A, Koontz F P 1985 Laboratory evaluation of leucocyte esterase and nitrite tests for the detection of bacteriuria. Journal of Clinical Microbiology 21:840–842

Stamm W E 1988 Protocol for diagnosis of urinary tract infection: reconsidering the criterion for significant bacteriuria. Urology 32(Suppl):6–12

Stamm W E 1991 Catheter-associated urinary tract infections; epidemiology, pathogenesis and prevention. American Journal of Medicine 91(Suppl 3B): 65S–71S

RECOMMENDED READING

Gray R P, Malone-Lee J 1995 Urinary tract infection in the elderly – time to review management? Age and Ageing 24:341–345

Matsumoto T 2001 Urinary tract infections in the elderly. Current Urology Reports 2:330–333

Pappas P G 1991 Laboratory in the diagnosis and management of urinary tract infections. Medical Clinics of North America 75:313–325

Stamm W E, Hooton T M 1993 Management of urinary tract infections in adults. New England Journal of Medicine 329:1328–1334

SELF-ASSESSMENT QUESTIONS

Are the following statements true or false?

1. Uncomplicated urinary tract infection in elderly people:
   a. May be present in elderly subjects in the absence of lower urinary tract symptoms
   b. Antibiotic therapy for > 5 days is more effective than 3 days of therapy
   c. Is an indication for investigation of the urinary tract
   d. Nitrofurantoin is a useful first-line antibiotic
   e. *E. coli* is the commonest infecting organism

2. In the diagnosis of urinary tract infection in old age:
   a. The detection of $\geq 10^3$ white blood cells per mm^3 is a reliable diagnostic tool
   b. Urinary nitrite has a high sensitivity and low specificity as a diagnostic test
   c. The threshold for diagnosis from culture of a mid-stream urine specimen is $\geq 10^4$ colony forming units of a single species/mL in symptomatic men
   d. Microscopic or macroscopic haematuria is frequently present
   e. Antibiotic therapy should be delayed until culture results are available

3. Recurrent urinary tract infections in old age:
   a. Always involve infection with a new organism
   b. Chronic bacterial prostatitis is a frequent underlying cause in men
   c. Cranberry juice is useful in prevention
   d. Intravaginal oestrogen is not recommended in post-menopausal women
   e. Is usually an indication for imaging of the urinary tract

4. Asymptomatic bacteriuria:
   a. Is defined as $\geq 10^5$ organisms of two species in three consecutive urine cultures
   b. Is more common in elderly men than women
   c. May lead to septicaemia in patients with long-term suprapubic catheters
   d. Antibiotic therapy reduces mortality in patients with long-term suprapubic catheters
   e. Is always associated with pyuria

SECTION 5

Genitourinary

Chapter 35

Sexuality and ageing

Karen M. Goodman

'(My) … Age is as a lusty winter
Frosty, but Kindly.'

(Shakespeare in *As You Like It*)

'… Do not let Sadness come over you,
for all your white hairs
You can still be a LOVER'

(De Beauvoir in *The Coming of Age*)

Sex, a subject that often generates interest, is generally taboo in clinical discussions. We should not ignore the fact that our patients are sexual beings.

'How is Billy going to manage with this in?' asked a female patient who had been catheterized in order to manage her incontinence. No one had discussed the sexual implications of the procedure with her.

Sexuality encompasses much more than the sexual act. It includes sexual attitudes, behaviour, practices and activity. Sexuality is an integral part of the whole person.

Sex is one of the four primary drives, along with thirst, hunger and avoidance of pain. The National Service Framework (NSF) for older people makes no direct reference to sexuality but Standard Two – 'Person-centred Care' – outlines the need to 'recognise individual differences and specific needs' (this should include expression of sexuality) (DoH 2001).

AGE–RELATED CHANGES IN SEXUAL FUNCTION

What happens to sexual activity with advancing age? Despite an age-related decline in sexual activity and drive (Table 35.1), many older couples continue to enjoy a healthy sex life. Surveys suggest that of married couples aged 60 years and over, 74% of men and 55% of women are sexually active (Diokno et al 1990). 63% of men and 30% of women aged between 80 and 102 years are sexually active (Bretschneider & McCoy 1988).

Table 35.1   Main age-related changes in sexual function

	Men	Women
Sexual drive	Reduced, less urgent	Reduced, less urgent
Arousal	Increased time to attain erection. Sometimes full erection is not attained until ejaculation occurs	Increased time to attain arousal. Reduced vasocongestive response. Lubrication response impaired
Ejaculation/orgasm	May take longer to achieve. Not consistent – may not occur in some encounters. Reduced seminal volume and force of discharge. Reduced sensation	May take longer to achieve. Reduced sensation. Less likelihood of multiple orgasms. Uterine contractions may be painful
Genital changes	Reduced angle of erect penis. Testicular activation reduced or lost	Atrophy of clitoral hood and labia. Reduced vasocongestion of vulval structures
Genital sensation	Reduced penile sensitivity	Clitoral sensitivity may be reduced. Occasionally increased causing pain on stimulation
Breast/ nipples	N/A	Reduced or absent vasocongestion. Nipple erection may not be impaired
Resolution	Rapid loss of erection	Accelerated
Refractory period	Prolonged	N/A

WHY DOES SEX STOP?

Alex Comfort (Comfort & Dial 1991) wrote: 'The things that stop you having sex with age are the things that stop you riding a bicycle!' That is:

- Bad health
- Thinking it looks silly
- No bicycle

Reasons why sex stops

1. *Sexual dysfunction:*	erectile disorder less sexual satisfaction less aroused
2. *Endocrine problems:*	less testosterone hypo/hyperthyroidism less oestrogen in women
3. *Systemic:*	heart disease hypertension liver disease anaemia
4. *Aesthetic considerations:*	not attractive deformities
5. *Depression (and treatment of)*	
6. *Pain:*	osteoarthritis dyspareunia
7. *Medication:*	antihypertensives tranquillizers
8. *Lack of a partner*	
9. *Use it or lose it:*	an active sex life reduces genital atrophy and delays the onset of sexual dysfunction

ERECTILE DYSFUNCTION

Erectile dysfuntion affects:

~ 52% of men aged 40–70 years
~ 95% of men aged > 70 years with diabetes mellitus

Its prevalence increases by 10% with each decade of life.

Causes

1. Vascular disease
2. Alcohol/smoking
3. Endocrine disease
4. Renal disease
5. Liver disease
6. Neurological disease
7. Psychiatric illness
8. *Medication:* NSAIDs, digoxin, H_2 blockers, diuretics, antihypertensives, anticonvulsants … to name but a few

Up to 16% of people on thiazide diuretics may experience erectile dysfunction.

VIAGRA (SILDENAFIL)

Over 30 years ago the Pill led the sexual revolution. In 1998 Viagra was approved by the Federal Drug Association. There is now 7 years of safety data in over 20 million men. Two new phosphodiesterase-5 inhibitors are now approved in Europe, vardenafil and tadalafil.

In the UK, Viagra is only available at NHS expense in certain cases, e.g. men with diabetes mellitus, renal failure, multiple sclerosis, Parkinson's disease (others are listed in the British National Formulary). Viagra promotes erections by relaxing the smooth muscle of the blood vessels (through inhibition of phosphodiesterase) thus increasing the blood flow to the penis in response to sexual stimulation.

There are contraindications to giving the drug, which has vasoconstrictive effects. It is inadvisable in pre-existing cardiac conditions where sexual activity would be harmful. A history of recent stroke, hypotension or severe hepatic impairment are also contraindications.

There is no reported increased risk of myocardial infarction or death in elderly men taking sildenafil, other than men with advanced cardiac disease or those taking nitrates.

SEX AND HEART DISEASE

What should we advise our patients? It is said that if patients can climb up and down two flights of stairs briskly (13 steps) without symptoms, they can have symptom-free sex. The exertion equates to ironing at the lower end to a round of golf at the more vigorous end.

Simple measures that we could institute might include the prophylactic use of nitrates, optimizing the treatment of heart failure with the addition of an ACE inhibitor and advising patients to avoid sex within 2 hours of a meal.

Less than 1% of sudden deaths from myocardial infarction occur during sex. Eighty percent of those that occur are due to extramarital sex!

When is it safe to resume sexual activity following a cardiac event? After a myocardial infarction the consensus is to wait a month; following a coronary artery bypass graft, when the patient is ready (this is usually limited by chest wall pain); after angioplasty, it is considered safe after 2–3 days.

AIDS AND THE OLDER PERSON

Since 1982, when reporting began, 59 497 people in the UK have been diagnosed as being HIV positive. 12 760 people were reported to have died with AIDS. Of those diagnosed with HIV, less than 7% (4083) were aged ≥ 50 years and less than 1% (400) were aged ≥ 65 years (statistics from the Terrence Higgins Trust [http://www.tht.org.uk]). The most common route of exposure is through heterosexual sex. Blood/tissue transfer accounts for less than 3% as a route of exposure.

The most common presentation as the AIDS index illness is progressive multifocal leucoencephalopathy dementia, which can be manifest by focal motor weakness, gait abnormalities, speech disorders and neuro-ophthalmic symptoms.

WHAT IS OUR ROLE AS HEALTH PROFESSIONALS?

- First we should be more open and knowledgeable in discussing the sexual needs of the older person.
- We should be aware of how our treatments will affect the sexual function of our patient, e.g. the prescription of medication and insertion of catheters.
- When we discuss the implications of the chronic illness of a patient we should consider including,

for example, the impact of their stroke or heart disease on their sex lives.

- Aside from the hospital setting, nursing/residential homes need to provide some privacy for their clients, e.g. private visiting areas where couples can be together, double rooms for resident couples.
- Exhibition of sexual acts should not be reprimanded but perhaps encouraged, possibly in a private room.

Finally remember that the need for love and intimacy does not decline with age but remains part of an older person's appreciation of him or herself as a total human being.

Key points

- Being old does not prohibit expression of sexuality.
- Remember to consider the implications of treatment and chronic illnesses on sexuality and try to approach these issues openly but sensitively.

REFERENCES

Bretschneider J G, McCoy N L 1988 Sexual interest and behaviour in healthy 80–102 year olds. Archives of Sexual Behaviour 17:109–129

Comfort A, Dial L K 1991 Sexuality and ageing – an overview. Geriatric Clinics 7:3–7

Department of Health 2001 National Service Framework for Older People. Modern Standards and service models. DoH, London

Diokno A C, Brown M B, Herzoq A R et al 1990 Sexual function in the elderly. Archives of Internal Medicine 150:197–200

RECOMMENDED READING

Brogan M 1996 The sexual needs of elderly people: addressing the issue. Nursing standard 10:42–45

Davidson S 1995 Sexuality in the elderly: what is the health professional's role? Perspectives 19:6–8

Ginsberg T B, Pomeranntz S C, Kramer-Feeley V 2005 Sexuality in older adults: behaviours and preferences. Age and Ageing 34:475–480

Inelman E M, Gasparini G, Enzi G 2005 HIV/AIDS in older adults: a case report and literature review. Geriatrics 60:26–30

Kaiser F E 1996 Sexuality in the elderly. Urologic Clinics of North America 23:99–108

Meston C M 1997 Ageing and sexuality. Western Journal of Medicine 167:285–290

Riley A 1999 Sex in old age. Geriatric Medicine. March: 25–28

SELF-ASSESSMENT QUESTIONS

Are the following true or false?

1. Which of these drugs has the potential to affect sexuality negatively?
   a. Antacids
   b. Antispasmodics
   c. Mild analgesics
   d. Anticoagulants
   e. Antihypertensives

2. You notice that two residents in the ward/home you work in seem to be striking up a liaison. You should:
   a. Encourage this
   b. Allow it to take its own course
   c. Put a stop to it before it goes too far
   d. Discuss it with the team to decide if it is suitable or not
   e. Report it to their next of kin and let them decide

SECTION 6

Bone and locomotor system

Chapter 36

Management of osteoporosis

Roger M. Francis

INTRODUCTION

Osteoporosis is a skeletal disorder characterized by compromised bone strength, which predisposes a person to an increased risk of fracture. These fractures generally occur after minimal or low trauma (defined as a fall from standing height or less). The three major osteoporotic fractures are those of the forearm, vertebra and hip, but fractures of the humerus, clavicle, pelvis and ribs are also common. The incidence of these fractures rises steeply with age: most occur above the age of 65 years, and are associated with increased mortality and morbidity (Tuck & Francis 2002).

IMPACT OF OSTEOPOROTIC FRACTURES

- The lifetime risk of asymptomatic fracture for a 50-year-old white woman in the UK is 16.6% for the forearm, 3.1% for the vertebra and 11.4% for the hip. The corresponding figures for a 50-year-old man are 2.9%, 1.2% and 3.1%.

- Excess mortality after hip fracture is 15–25%, mainly related to the fracture itself and to subsequent surgery. There is a similar excess mortality after symptomatic vertebral fracture, probably due to co-morbid conditions associated with the fracture.

- Up to 50% of patients are more dependent and less mobile after hip fracture, many requiring placement in a care home.

- The annual cost of osteoporotic fractures in the UK is estimated at £1.7 billion, most of which is attributable to hip fractures.

PATHOGENESIS OF OSTEOPOROSIS AND FRACTURES

The risk of fracture is determined not only by skeletal risk factors, such as bone mineral density (BMD), bone turnover, trabecular architecture, skeletal size and geometry and bone mineralization, but also by non-skeletal risk factors associated with a propensity to falling. BMD is influenced

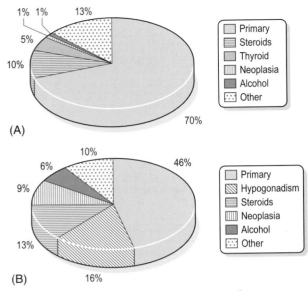

Box 36.1   Determinants of peak bone mass and subsequent bone loss

Peak Bone Mass	Bone Loss
Heredity	Menopause
Exercise	Smoking and alcohol
Dietary calcium	Physical inactivity
Age at puberty	Vitamin D insufficiency

Figure 36.1   Prevalence of secondary causes of osteoporosis in women **(A)** and men **(B)** with symptomatic vertebral fractures attending the Bone Clinic in Newcastle upon Tyne.

by peak bone mass at maturity and subsequent bone loss (Box 36.1). Bone loss starts between the ages of 35 and 40 years in both sexes, with an acceleration of bone loss in the decade after the menopause in women. Bone loss then continues into the ninth decade in both men and women (Tuck & Francis 2002).

There are a number of secondary causes of osteoporosis, which are found in 30% of women and 55% of men with symptomatic vertebral crush fractures (Fig. 36.1). Secondary causes of osteoporosis, such as oral glucocorticoid therapy, anticonvulsant treatment, thyroid disease and male hypogonadism have also been identified as risk factors for hip fractures. The risk of hip and other non-vertebral fractures is also increased by conditions predisposing to falls, such as stroke, Parkinson's disease, dementia, vertigo, alcoholism and visual impairment (Tuck & Francis 2002) (see Ch. 23 on syncope).

DIAGNOSIS OF OSTEOPOROSIS

Osteoporosis was previously a clinical diagnosis, based on the development of fractures after minimal trauma. Dual energy X-ray absorptiometry (DXA) bone densitometry has increased interest in the diagnosis of osteoporosis before fractures occur. BMD measurements may be expressed as standard deviation units above or below the mean value for normal young adults (T score). The World Health Organization (WHO) has defined osteoporosis as a BMD 2.5 standard deviations or more below the mean value for young adults (T score < –2.5). There are a number of other risk factors for fractures that are, at least in part, independent of low BMD, including advancing

age, previous low trauma fracture after the age of 50 years, parental history of hip fracture, current smoking, oral glucocorticoid therapy, alcohol intake > 2 units/day and chronic conditions such as rheumatoid disease. The WHO is currently using these risk factors to develop an algorithm for predicting the 10-year likelihood of fractures. This could then be used to identify patients at greatest risk of fracture, who would benefit most from osteoporosis treatment (Tuck & Francis 2002).

Although a number of indications for BMD measurements have been suggested, the relevance of these indications in older people remains uncertain. Spine bone density measurements may also be spuriously elevated in this age group, because of aortic calcification and spondylosis. Pragmatic suggestions on appropriate indications for bone density measurement in older people are provided in Box 36.2. BMD measurements may be of limited value in the assessment of older patients with low trauma fractures, as most are at high risk of further fracture and the results are unlikely to influence management. The National Institute for Health and Clinical Excellence (NICE) therefore advocates that osteoporosis treatment should be given to women above the age of 75 years presenting with a low trauma fracture, without the need for DXA bone density measurement (NICE 2005). Prolonged oral glucocorticoid therapy has also been excluded from the list of indications for bone density measurement, as the Royal College of Physicians recommended that all people over the age of 65 years on oral prednisolone for 3 months or more should be offered treatment for osteoporosis (BTS, NOS, RCP 2002).

INVESTIGATION

Specific treatment of underlying causes of secondary osteoporosis (such as male hypogonadism, primary hyperparathyroidism and hyperthyroidism) increases BMD by 10–20%, so these conditions should be sought in patients with osteoporosis and/or low trauma fractures by performing a careful history, physical examination and appropriate investigations (Table 36.1). Nevertheless, testosterone supplementation should be used with caution in older men with hypogonadism because of potential adverse effects on the prostate and cardiovascular system. Serum 25 hydroxyvitamin D (25 OHD) and intact parathyroid hormone (PTH) measurements may be useful in excluding vitamin D deficiency and secondary hyperparathyroidism in patients with limited sunlight exposure, previous gastric resection, malabsorption or anticonvulsant treatment. These measurements are probably unnecessary if calcium and vitamin D supplementation is planned, as the results are unlikely to influence management.

GENERAL MEASURES

All patients with osteoporosis and fractures should be given advice on lifestyle measures to decrease

Table 36.1   Investigations for secondary osteoporosis

Investigation	Finding	Possible cause
Full blood count	Anaemia	Neoplasia or malabsorption
	Macrocytosis	Alcohol abuse or malabsorption
ESR	Raised ESR	Neoplasia, multiple myeloma
Biochemical profile	Hypercalcaemia	Hyperparathyroidism or neoplasia
	Abnormal liver function	Alcohol abuse or liver disease
	Persistently high alkaline phosphatase	Skeletal metastases
Thyroid function tests	Suppressed TSH; high T_4 or T_3	Hyperthyroidism
Testosterone, SHBG, LH, FSH	Low testosterone or free androgen index with abnormal gonadotrophins	Hypogonadism
Serum and urine electrophoresis (Patients with vertebral fractures)	Paraprotein band	Myeloma

ESR, erythrocyte sedimentation rate; FSH, follicle stimulating hormone; LH, luteinizing hormone; SHBG, sex hormone binding globulin; T_3, triiodothyronine; T_4, thyroxine; TSH, thyroid stimulating hormone further bone loss and reduce the risks of falls, including eating a balanced diet rich in calcium, moderating tobacco and alcohol consumption and maintaining regular physical activity and exposure to sunlight.

DRUG TREATMENT

As bone loss continues into old age in both men and women, the need for specific treatment should be considered in all patients with osteoporosis or low trauma fractures. Although most studies of the treatment of osteoporosis have recruited few women above the age of 80 years, there is no evidence of an attenuated response to treatment with advancing age. Furthermore, treatment of osteoporosis is likely to be more cost-effective in older people, because of their higher fracture rate.

A number of treatments have been shown to increase BMD and decrease the risk of vertebral and hip fractures. The Royal College of Physicians has published guidelines on the management of osteoporosis (RCP, BTS 2000), grading their recommendations on the levels of evidence for each therapeutic intervention (Table 36.2). Grade A recommendations are based on randomized con-

trolled trials, whereas Grade B recommendations result from controlled studies without randomization, studies with a quasi-experimental design and epidemiological studies.

HORMONE REPLACEMENT THERAPY (HRT)

Small studies in post-menopausal women with osteoporosis show that HRT increases spine bone density by about 5% and decreases vertebral fractures by 60%. The large Women's Health Initiative Study shows that although HRT decreases the incidence of fractures in post-menopausal women, the benefits are outweighed by the increased risk of breast cancer, coronary heart disease, stroke and thromboembolism (Rossouw et al 2002).

Advantages: HRT reduces the incidence of vertebral, hip and other non-vertebral fractures. It controls climacteric symptoms and decreases the risk of colon cancer.

Disadvantages: These are vaginal bleeding and increased risk of breast cancer, coronary heart disease, stroke and thromboembolism.

Appropriate use: HRT may be useful in younger post-menopausal women with osteoporosis and severe climacteric symptoms.

Table 36.2 The effect of treatments on the incidence of vertebral, non–vertebral and hip fractures. Grading of recommendations adapted from the updated Royal College of Physicians Clinical Guidelines for Prevention and Treatment of Osteoporosis.

	Vertebral	Non–vertebral	Hip
HRT	A	A	A
Raloxifene	A	ND	ND
Etidronate	A	B	B
Alendronate	A	A	A
Risedronate	A	A	A
Ibandronate	A	A**	ND
Strontium ranelate	A	A	A**
Teriparatide	A	A	ND
Calcitonin	A*	B	B
Calcium and vitamin D	ND	A*	A*

A = Recommendations based on randomized controlled trials
B = Recommendations from controlled studies without randomization, a quasi-experimental design and epidemiological studies
ND = Not demonstrated, *indicates inconsistent results, **indicates *post-hoc* analysis

RALOXIFENE

Raloxifene (Evista) is a selective oestrogen receptor modulator (SERM), which has oestrogen agonist actions on the skeleton and lipid profile, but acts as an oestrogen antagonist on the breast and endometrium. The Multiple Outcomes of Raloxifene Evaluation (MORE) Study in post-menopausal women with osteoporosis showed that raloxifene increased lumbar spine and femoral neck bone density by 2–3%, reduced the risk of vertebral fractures by 30–50% and decreased the incidence of breast cancer by 76% (Cummings et al 1999, Ettinger et al 1999).

Advantages: Raloxifene causes no vaginal bleeding and decreases the risk of breast cancer.

Disdavantages: There is no evidence of reduction in non-vertebral fractures. There is increased risk of thromboembolism.

Appropriate use: It is useful in younger post-menopausal women with predominantly vertebral osteoporosis who are concerned about their risk of breast cancer.

BISPHOSPHONATES

Bisphosphonates have become the treatment of choice for patients with osteoporosis. Intermittent cyclical etidronate therapy (Didronel PMO) increases bone density and reduces the incidence of vertebral fractures, but there are no interventional studies investigating the effect of treatment on hip fracture incidence (RCP, BTS 2000). Alendronate (Fosamax) and risedronate (Actonel) have been shown in large studies to increase BMD and decrease the incidence of vertebral, hip and other non-vertebral fractures (RCP, BTS 2000). Ibandronate (Bonviva) has also been shown to improve BMD and decrease the incidence of vertebral fractures, but no reduction in hip fractures has been demonstrated.

Advantages: Alendronate and risedronate are available as daily or weekly preparations, whereas ibandronate is administered on a monthly basis. Alendronate and risedronate are effective in post-menopausal and glucocorticoid-induced osteoporosis. Alendronate is also licensed for the management of osteoporosis in men.

Disadvantages: Oral bisphosphonates have to be taken fasting before food, to ensure adequate absorption. They should also be taken with a glass of water and recumbency should be avoided for half an hour, to decrease the risk of oesophageal side-effects of treatment.

Appropriate use: They are the first-line treatment for most patients with post-menopausal and glucocorticoid-induced osteoporosis.

STRONTIUM RANELATE

Strontium ranelate (Protelos) is a dual action bone agent, which reduces bone resorption and increases bone formation. This leads to large increases in BMD, although this is partly spurious, because strontium has a higher atomic number than calcium. Strontium reduces the incidence of new vertebral fractures (Meunier et al 2004), but also decreases non-vertebral fractures by 16%. *Post-hoc* analysis in older women with a low femoral neck T score taking part in the TROPOS study showed a 36% reduction in hip fractures with strontium ranelate (Reginster et al 2005).

Advantages: Strontium is generally well tolerated, even in patients with upper gastrointestinal disease.

Disdavantages: It has to be taken in the middle of a 4-hour fast, to ensure adequate absorption. An unexplained small increase in thromboembolism was noted in clinical trials of strontium. There are no data on glucocorticoid-induced osteoporosis or osteoporosis in men.

Appropriate use: It is the second-line treatment in patients unable to take or tolerate bisphosphonate treatment.

TERIPARATIDE

Teriparatide (Forsteo) is recombinant human parathyroid hormone which has anabolic actions on the skeleton when administered by daily subcutaneous injection. Studies show a larger increase in BMD than that observed with bisphosphonates. Teriparatide decreases the incidence of vertebral and non-vertebral fractures, but no reduction in hip fractures has been demonstrated (Neer et al 2001).

Advantages: Teriparatide is the first licensed anabolic treatment for osteoporosis.

Disdavantages: It is ten times more expensive than bisphosphonates. The treatment course is limited to 18 months because of the theoretical risk of osteogenic sarcoma. The anabolic effect of teriparatide may be attenuated by previous bisphosphonate treatment.

Appropriate use: It is the second line treatment in patients with severe osteoporosis, who fail to respond to other treatments.

CALCITONIN

Calcitonin (Miacalcic) is an antiresorptive agent, with a rapid but short-lived effect on osteoclast function. In a study in women with established osteoporosis, there was a 36% reduction in new vertebral fractures with intranasal calcitonin 200 iu daily, but there was no significant decrease in fractures with 100 or 400 iu/day (Chesnut et al 2000).

Advantages: Calcitonin has a possible analgesic effect.

Disdavantages: There are inconsistent fracture data.

Appropriate use: It may be useful in the short-term management of acute vertebral fractures.

CALCIUM AND VITAMIN D

Calcium and vitamin D supplementation reduces the incidence of hip and other non-vertebral fractures in older people living in care homes (Chapuy et al 1992). In contrast, recent large studies show no benefit of calcium and vitamin D supplementation in the primary or secondary prevention of low trauma fractures in community-dwelling older people. Studies of vitamin D alone on fracture risk in community-dwelling older people (Grant et al 2005, Porthouse et al 2005) or care home residents have been inconsistent (Francis 2006).

Advantages: Calcium and vitamin D are the physiologically appropriate treatment for people with vitamin D deficiency and secondary hyper-parathyroidism.

Disdavantages: There is no clear benefit of calcium and vitamin D alone in community-dwelling people.

Appropriate use: They are useful in housebound or institutionalized older people, who are likely to have vitamin D insufficiency and secondary hyperparathyroidism. They are also advocated as an adjunct to other osteoporosis treatments.

REDUCING FALLS

Standard Six of the National Service Framework (NSF) for Older People aims to reduce the number of falls that result in serious injury and ensure effective treatment and rehabilitation for those who have fallen (DoH 2001). The NSF explicitly mentions osteoporosis assessment in the prevention of falls and fractures, and mandates the establishment of local integrated falls services. NICE has subsequently published a clinical guideline on falls, which recommends that older people who present for medical attention after a fall should be assessed for gait and balance and considered for multifactorial falls risk assessment and intervention (NICE 2004). Multifactorial intervention reduces the risk of falls, but studies with the statistical power to demonstrate effective fracture prevention have not yet been performed. Nevertheless, it is clearly appropriate that all patients with hip and other non-vertebral fractures should undergo a falls assessment.

DECREASING IMPACT OF FALLS

An alternative approach to fracture prevention is to decrease the impact of falls using external hip protectors, which are incorporated into specially designed underwear. A Cochrane Review found a marginally significant reduction in hip fractures with hip protector use in residential or nursing homes, but no benefit in older people living at home (Parker et al 2005). The disappointing results with hip protectors may reflect poor compliance.

MANAGEMENT OF THE INDIVIDUAL PATIENT

Measures to decrease bone loss and reduce the risk of falls should be advised in all patients with osteoporosis and low trauma fractures. The use of external hip protectors may be considered in those who continue to fall regularly, particularly in patients living in residential or nursing homes, where help and supervision is available.

NICE has published a Technology Appraisal of the secondary prevention of osteoporotic fragility fractures in post-menopausal women, which is being updated to include strontium ranelate. NICE guidance recommends bisphosphonate treatment in women over 75 years presenting with a low trauma fracture, without the need for DXA bone density measurement. In younger women presenting with a low trauma fracture, bone density measurements are recommended. Bisphosphonate treatment is then advised in women aged 65–74 years with a femoral neck T score < -2.5 and in women under the age of 65 with a T score < -3.0, or a T score < -2.5 and an additional risk factor for fracture. The NICE Technology Appraisal currently recommends raloxifene as a second-line agent, when bisphosphonates are contraindicated, not tolerated or ineffective. The respective roles of raloxifene and strontium ranelate in this situation should be addressed in the updated Technology Appraisal. Teriparatide is only recommended for the secondary prevention of fractures in women aged 65 years and above who have had unsatisfactory response to bisphosphonates, or intolerance to bisphosphonates *and* who have an extremely low BMD (< -4 or T score < -3, with multiple fractures and additional risk factors). Unless clinicians are confident that women who receive osteoporosis treatment have an adequate calcium intake and are vitamin D replete, NICE recommends that calcium and/or vitamin D supplementation should be provided.

NICE is currently performing a Technology Appraisal of the primary prevention of osteoporotic fragility fractures in post-menopausal women, which is likely to use risk factors incorporated in the WHO fracture risk prediction algorithm. NICE is also developing a clinical guideline on osteoporosis, which should include the management of glucocorticoid-induced osteoporosis, other secondary causes of osteoporosis and osteoporosis in men.

COMPONENTS OF AN OSTEOPOROSIS SERVICE

- Enthusiastic lead clinician (essential!)
- Osteoporosis specialist nurse (useful)
- Management protocols
- Biochemical and haematological support
- Good liaison with an orthopaedic department
- Access to DXA bone density measurements
- Access to a falls clinic with a tilt table

REFERENCES

Bone and Tooth Society of Great Britain, National Osteoporosis Society, Royal College of Physicians of London (BTS, NOS, RCP) 2002 Glucocorticoid-induced osteoporosis. Guidelines for prevention and treatment. Royal College of Physicians, London

Chapuy M C, Arlot M E, Duboeuf F et al 1992 Vitamin D_3 and calcium to prevent hip fractures in elderly women. New England Journal of Medicine 327: 1637–1642

Chesnut C H III, Silverman S, Andriano K et al 2000 A randomized trial of nasal spray salmon calcitonin in postmenopausal women with established osteoporosis: the prevent recurrence of osteoporotic fractures study. American Journal of Medicine 109:267–276

Cummings S R, Eckert S, Krueger K A et al 1999 The effect of raloxifene on risk of breast cancer in postmenopausal women: results from the MORE randomized trial. Multiple Outcomes of Raloxifene Evaluation. Journal of the American Medical Association 281:2189–2197

Department of Health 2001 National Service Framework for Older People. Department of Health, London

Ettinger B, Black D M, Mitlak B H et al 1999 Reduction of vertebral fracture risk in postmenopausal women with osteoporosis treated with raloxifene. Results from a 3 year randomised clinical trial. Journal of the American Medical Association 282:637–645

Francis R M 2006 Calcium, vitamin D and involutional osteoporosis. Current Opinion in Clinical Nutrition and Metabolic Care 9:13–17

Grant A M, Avenell A, Campbell M K et al; RECORD Trial Group 2005 Oral vitamin D3 and calcium for secondary prevention of low-trauma fractures in elderly people (Randomised Evaluation of Calcium Or vitamin D, RECORD): a randomised placebo-controlled trial. Lancet 365:1621–1628

Meunier P J, Roux C, Seeman E et al 2004 The effects of strontium ranelate on the risk of vertebral fracture in women with postmenopausal osteoporosis. New England Journal of Medicine 350:459–468

Neer R M, Arnaud C D, Zanchetta J R et al 2001 Effect of parathyroid hormone (1–34) on fractures and bone mineral density in postmenopausal women with osteoporosis. New England Journal of Medicine 344:1434–1441

NICE 2004 Falls: the assessment and prevention of falls in older people. Clinical Guideline 21. NICE, London

NICE 2005 Bisphosphonates (alendronate, etidronate, risedronate), selective oestrogen receptor modulators (raloxifene) and parathyroid hormone (teriparatide) for the secondary prevention of osteoporotic fragility fractures in postmenopausal women. Technology Appraisal 87. NICE, London

Parker M J, Gillespie W J, Gillespie L D 2005 Hip protectors for preventing hip fractures in older people. The Cochrane Database of Systematic Reviews, Issue 3. Art. No: CD001255. DOI: 10.1002/14651858. CD001255.pub3

Porthouse J, Cockayne S, King C et al 2005 Randomised controlled trial of calcium and supplementation with cholecalciferol (vitamin D3) for prevention of fractures in primary care. British Medical Journal 330:1003–1006

Reginster J Y, Seeman E, de Vernejoul M C et al 2005 Strontium ranelate reduces the risk of nonvertebral fractures in postmenopausal women with osteoporosis: Treatment of Peripheral Osteoporosis (TROPOS) study. Journal of Clinical Endocrinology and Metabolism 90:2816–2822

Rossouw J E, Anderson G L, Prentice R L et al; Writing Group for the Women's Health Initiative Investigators 2002 Risks and benefits of oestrogen plus progestin in healthy postmenopausal women: principal results from the Women's Health Initiative randomized controlled trial. Journal of the American Medical Association 288:321–333

Royal College of Physicians of London, Bone and Tooth Society of Great Britain (RCP, BTS) 2000 Osteoporosis: clinical guidelines for prevention and treatment. Royal College of Physicians, London

Tuck S P, Francis R M 2002 Best practice: osteoporosis. Postgraduate Medical Journal 78:526–532

Patient support

Information for patients and healthcare professionals is available from the National Osteoporosis Society, Camerton, Bath, BA2 0PJ (Tel: 01761 471771, Helpline: 0845 4500230, Online: http://www.nos.org.uk)

SELF-ASSESSMENT QUESTION

Are the following statements true or false?

1. Osteoporosis:
   a. Commonly causes back pain in the absence of vertebral fractures
   b. Costs the UK £1.7 billion annually
   c. Is characterized by impaired mineralization of osteoid
   d. Is an inevitable consequence of the ageing process

SECTION 6

Bone and locomotor system

Chapter 37

Painful shoulder

Christopher I. M. Price

SCHEME TO GUIDE BASIC MANAGEMENT OF A PAINFUL STIFF SHOULDER IN THE ABSENCE OF SYSTEMIC ARTHROPATHY OR TRAUMA

Shoulder pain is very common in the older population and can easily become a chronic condition, with a significant impact on quality of life. In the absence of a known systemic arthropathy or trauma, attempts should be made to identify aetiology according to the scheme in Figure 37.1. However, a single cause often cannot be identified, and management should be pragmatic, comprising analgesia and early mobilization.

PAINFUL STIFF SHOULDER AFTER STROKE

After stroke many patients with upper limb weakness complain of shoulder pain. Shoulder girdle weakness and immobilization increase the likelihood of developing the musculoskeletal problems described above. The additional motor and sensory effects of stroke can create a complicated clinical picture. A detailed examination is required to identify any features which inform an individual management strategy. The conditions in Table 37.1 may coexist, so you should consider treatment for each in turn as well as for a stiff shoulder. All management decisions should be made in conjunction with the attending physiotherapist.

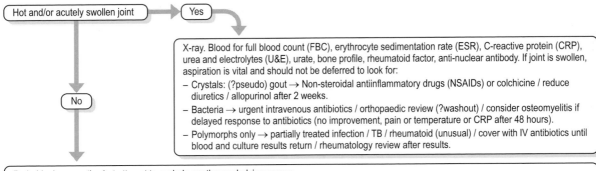

Hot and/or acutely swollen joint → Yes

No

X-ray. Blood for full blood count (FBC), erythrocyte sedimentation rate (ESR), C-reactive protein (CRP), urea and electrolytes (U&E), urate, bone profile, rheumatoid factor, anti-nuclear antibody. If joint is swollen, aspiration is vital and should not be deferred to look for:
– Crystals: (?pseudo) gout → Non-steroidal antiinflammatory drugs (NSAIDs) or colchicine / reduce diuretics / allopurinol after 2 weeks.
– Bacteria → urgent intravenous antibiotics / orthopaedic review (?washout) / consider osteomyelitis if delayed response to antibiotics (no improvement, pain or temperature or CRP after 48 hours).
– Polymorphs only → partially treated infection / TB / rheumatoid (unusual) / cover with IV antibiotics until blood and culture results return / rheumatology review after results.

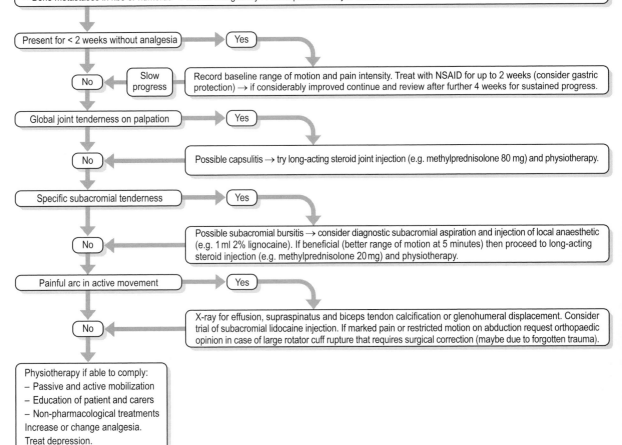

Probably degenerative but attempt to exclude another underlying cause:
– Cervical nerve root / brachial plexus entrapment → specific nerve root pain (shooting / tingling) or weakness (C3–C6) possibly with biceps or supinator reflex inversion (?lower limb spasticity). Consider magnetic resonance imaging (MRI) for nerve root compression and chest X-rays (Pancoast tumour). May respond to TENS, amitriptyline or gabapentin.
– Diaphragmatic radiation → little found at the shoulder. Consider abdominal exam / liver function tests (LFTs) / chest X-rays / ultrasound examination of abdomen.
– Polymyalgia rheumatica → inquire about morning stiffness and pelvic girdle symptoms / ?raised ESR.
– Bone metastases in ribs or humerus → known malignancy? / bone profile / X-rays / bone scan.

Present for < 2 weeks without analgesia → Yes

No ← Slow progress ← Record baseline range of motion and pain intensity. Treat with NSAID for up to 2 weeks (consider gastric protection) → if considerably improved continue and review after further 4 weeks for sustained progress.

Global joint tenderness on palpation → Yes

No ← Possible capsulitis → try long-acting steroid joint injection (e.g. methylprednisolone 80 mg) and physiotherapy.

Specific subacromial tenderness → Yes

No ← Possible subacromial bursitis → consider diagnostic subacromial aspiration and injection of local anaesthetic (e.g. 1 ml 2% lignocaine). If beneficial (better range of motion at 5 minutes) then proceed to long-acting steroid injection (e.g. methylprednisolone 20 mg) and physiotherapy.

Painful arc in active movement → Yes

No ← X-ray for effusion, supraspinatus and biceps tendon calcification or glenohumeral displacement. Consider trial of subacromial lidocaine injection. If marked pain or restricted motion on abduction request orthopaedic opinion in case of large rotator cuff rupture that requires surgical correction (maybe due to forgotten trauma).

Physiotherapy if able to comply:
– Passive and active mobilization
– Education of patient and carers
– Non-pharmacological treatments
Increase or change analgesia.
Treat depression.

Figure 37.1   Management of a new painful shoulder without trauma.

Table 37.1 Common shoulder problems after stroke

Clinical syndrome	Pain description	Clinical features	Simple management
'Subluxation' Usually inferior, but can be superior (possible rotator cuff tear) or anterior-inferior (possible pectoral muscle spasticity)	Mechanical ache Varies with (sleeping) position NB – subluxation without pain is common and may not require intervention other than careful handling	Palpable subacromial space Muscle tone may be low or high Indicates a shoulder susceptible to all causes of pain	Simple analgesia, carer education and careful positioning Chair arm supports (slings/cuffs restrict movement, may not alter position, and may impede recovery, but can be a last resort for difficult pain) Superior elastoplast strapping of glenohumeral joint (for stability, particularly at night) Electrical stimulation under supervision
'Spasticity'	Painful spasms Worse with cold, stress Upper limb position may make dressing and hygiene difficult	Increased resistance to passive elbow flexion/ shoulder abduction Hyperreflexia Classic hemiplegic posture may be adopted	Positioning, orthoses, warmth Consider anti-spasticity drugs if several muscle groups affected (but beware loss of muscle strength and mobility) Referral for botulinum injection if hygiene and dressing impeded
'Sudeck's atrophy' also known as: reflex sympathetic dystrophy syndrome (RSDS)	Constant deep discomfort May report limb flushing or freezing	Arm mottled/atrophic/ cold/flushed Tender metacarpopha-langeal joints on gentle compression	Trial of amitriptyline up to 75 mg and/or prednisolone 30 mg for 4 weeks Consider pain specialist review regarding sympathetic blockade
'Thalamic pain' also known as: central post-stroke pain (CPSP)	Ice burning. Worse with stress, light touch or repeated touch. Starts 1–3 months after stroke (but can be much later). Sometimes uncomfortable tingling rather than pain	Pain is within an area of pin-prick and/or temperature sensory loss (test simply with pin/finger and cold/ warm metal such as a spoon)	Trial of amitriptyline up to 75 mg for 4 weeks. If this fails try gabapentin 900 mg. Consider combination with opioids. Treat anxiety (often present) Local counter-stimulation, e.g. TENS or capsaicin. Consider specialist review

RECOMMENDED READING

*** Essential reading; ** recommended reading; * interesting but not vital

Management of shoulder pain

Daigneault J, Cooney L M 1998 Shoulder pain in older people. Journal of the American Geriatrics Society 46:1144–1151 ***

Green S, Buchbinder R, Glazier R et al 2000 Interventions for shoulder pain. Cochrane Database of Systematic Reviews Issue 2. Art. No.: CD001156. DOI: 10.1002/14651858.CD001156 ***

van der Heijden G J, van der Windt D A, de Winter A F 1997 Physiotherapy for patients with soft tissue shoulder disorders: a systemic review of randomised clinical trials. British Medical Journal 315: 25–30 **

van der Windt D A, Koes B W, Deville W et al 1998 Effectiveness of corticosteroid injection versus physiotherapy for treatment of painful stiff shoulder in primary care: randomised trial. British Medical Journal 317:1292–1296 *

Winters J C, Sobel J S, Groenier K H et al 1997 Comparison of physiotherapy, manipulation and corticosteroid injection for treating shoulder complaints in general practice. British Medical Journal 314:1320–1325 *

Shoulder pain after stroke

Ancliffe A 1992 Strapping the shoulder in patients following a CVA: a pilot study. Australian Journal of Physiotherapy 38:37–41 *

Gilron I, Bailey J M, Tu D et al 2005 Morphine, gabapentin, or their combination for neuropathic pain. New England Journal of Medicine 352:1324–1334 *

Leijon G, Boivie J 1989 Central post-stroke pain – a controlled trial of amitriptyline and carbamazepine. Pain 36:27–36 *

Morin L 1997 Strapping the hemiplegic shoulder: radiographic evaluation of its efficacy. Physiotherapy Canada (Spring):103–108 *

Price C I M 2003 Treatment of shoulder and upper limb pain after stroke: an obstacle course for evidence based practice. Reviews in Clinical Gerontology 13:321–333 **

Price C I M, Pandyan A D 1999 Electrical stimulation for preventing and treating post-stroke shoulder pain. Cochrane Database of Systematic Reviews 3. Art. No.: CD001698. DOI: 10.1002/14651858.CD 001698 **

Roy C W 1988 Shoulder pain in hemiplegia: a literature review. Clinical Rehabilitation 2:35–44 **

Royal College of Physicians 2004 National Clinical Guidelines for Stroke, 2nd edn. Online. Available: http://www.rcplondon.ac.uk ***

Smith S J, Ellis E, White S et al 2000 A double-blind placebo-controlled study of botulinum toxin in upper limb spasticity after stroke or head injury. Clinical Rehabilitation 14:5–13 *

Tepperman P S, Greyson N D, Hilbert L et al 1984 Reflex sympathetic dystrophy in hemiplegia. Archives of Physical Medicine and Rehabilitation 65:442–447 *

Wanklyn P 1994 The painful hemiplegic shoulder: pathogenesis, diagnosis and management. Reviews in Clinical Gerontology 4:245–251 *

Wiffen P, Collins S, McQuay H et al 2005 Anticonvulsant drugs for acute and chronic pain. Cochrane Pain, Palliative and Supportive Care Group. Cochrane Database of Systematic Reviews 4. Art. No.: CD 001133. DOI: 10.1002/14651858.CD001133 ***

Zorowitz R D, Idank D, Ikai T et al 1995 Shoulder subluxation after stroke: a comparison of four supports. Archives of Physical Medical Rehabilitation 76:763–771 *

SELF-ASSESSMENT QUESTIONS

What assessment would you undertake for each of the following scenarios:

1. An 84-year-old lady with dementia has been admitted from a nursing home with increasing agitation and poor oral intake for 24 hours. She requires assistance for all personal care and cannot provide a history. The nursing home staff have noticed that her left shoulder is swollen compared to the right side

2. A 72-year-old man suffered a right total anterior circulation stroke 2 weeks ago, causing flaccid left-side hemiparesis. He is sleeping poorly because of pain in his left shoulder overnight

3. A 75-year-old lady suffered a left lacunar stroke 6 weeks previously. She is able to walk with a stick but has increasing pain in the right arm, which has little residual function

SECTION 6

Bone and locomotor system

Chapter 38

Foot disorders

Barbara Wall

Foot problems should never be considered in isolation. The performance of the foot and lower limb is intimately related to normal functioning of proximal joints, an intact neuromuscular system and cardiovascular system.

A few facts:

- Each foot comprises 26 bones, 30 synovial articulations and over 100 ligaments
- During their lifetime, an individual will have walked approximately 115 000 miles
- With every step, mechanical forces exert the equivalent of five times the individual's body weight on their feet

It is easy to disregard the feet when assessing older people who have multisystem pathologies but this is a serious oversight. An elderly person with diabetes mellitus who has a neglected foot ulcer, or the older house-bound person with toenails that are too long to let them wear shoes, are examples familiar to podiatry. These situations are preventable and inexcusable.

> Pathology of the spine, hip, knee, ankle and proximal anatomical structures may compromise foot function during walking.

Ageing affects many structures important in normal foot function (Fig. 38.1). In the older person the protection afforded by the skin is diminished: the stratum corneum, the outermost layer of the epidermis, has an altered lipid content which reduces its normal barrier action. With ageing, abnormal elastic and collagen fibres occur in the dermis. Thus both the epidermis and dermis are prone to damage, and their normal protective functions are compromised.

Ageing alters the mechanical properties of bone: in the foot, pathological 'stress' fractures can occur when bones are subjected to abnormal stresses that result from altered gait, perhaps caused by osteoathrosis of the hip or knee.

Systemic diseases associated with advancing age have a direct impact on foot health and function. Some examples:

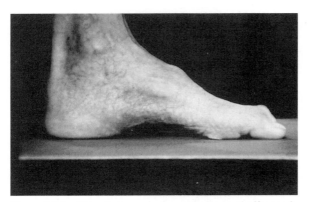

Figure 38.1 This photograph shows the general effects of the ageing process on the foot. Note the atrophy of the protective subcutaneous tissue which normally provides shock absorption under the metatarsal heads and heel. The epidermis is thin and liable to damage, and the toes are clawed and are prone to trauma. This foot is vulnerable and must be treated with respect.

1. Rheumatoid arthritis can produce deformed and painful joints of the hands and wrists, and it also affects joints of the feet. Rheumatoid disease may compromise tissue viability and wound healing. Consider the patient presenting with disease affecting the feet: involvement of the knee joint generates abnormal mechanical forces and exacerbates foot deformity. The disease process impairs tissue viability, so tissue necrosis and ulceration may follow unless treatment redirects abnormal mechanical stress away from the affected joints. Disease-modifying drugs can increase a person's susceptibility to infection and ulceration.

2. Reduced arterial blood supply may render the skin and soft tissues of the feet vulnerable to damage. Once damage has occurred, ischaemia impairs healing.

It is important to recognize the signs and symptoms indicative of lower leg and foot ischaemia so that the problem is identified early and preventative measures taken:

■ Absent foot pulses (dorsalis pedis and posterior tibial pulses)
■ The foot may be cool, and the skin appears atrophic with pallor of the foot and the leg developing on elevation of the limbs

■ Intermittent claudication and rest pain
■ Patches of gangrene and/or ulceration
■ Calculation of the ankle–brachial systolic pressure index (see Ch. 44)

DIABETES MELLITUS

Diabetes mellitus affects 2% of the population, and for every diagnosed person with diabetes there is another undiagnosed person with diabetic disease.

> There is no such person as one with mild diabetes regardless of the method of diabetic control.

Box 38.1 Foot–care advice for people with diabetes

■ Please look at your feet regularly (every day is best).
■ A hand mirror can help you examine under your feet.
■ Look for any areas of *discoloration* or *swelling*.
■ Also look out for any build-up of hard skin (callous and corns).
■ If you notice any of these consult your doctor/ nurse or a qualified podiatrist.
■ If you should notice any open cuts or sores, cover them with a sterile/clean dressing.
■ Please don't try and remove hard skin yourself.
■ If your toenails are very tough it is best to let a qualified podiatrist trim them for you.
■ If your skin is very dry, use a cream (for example E45 or aqueous cream) daily. The best time to apply cream is after washing your feet.
■ When you wash your feet, use a mild soap and check the water is not too hot (if your feet are numb a thermometer can be used to check the temperature of the water which should be no more than 40°C).
■ When drying your feet, be careful to dry between the toes, otherwise cracking may occur that can allow infection in.

If you have any worries or any problems concerning your feet, contact a qualified podiatrist, your doctor, nurse or other healthcare professional.

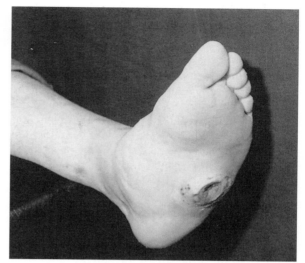

Figure 38.2   An example of a neuropathic joint (Charcot joint). The patient has sensory and autonomic neuropathy. The tarsal joints have collapsed and a large neuropathic ulcer has developed due to excessive pressure. Prevention is paramount in (a) preventing neuroarthropathy occurring or (b) if this fails, protecting the deformed joint from ulceration.

PREVENTABLE FOOT–RELATED PROBLEMS

In diabetes mellitus the majority of foot-related problems are *preventable*.

Diabetes mellitus directly affects the feet, and is a major cause of foot ulceration. The complications of diabetes that affect the feet are ischaemia, peripheral neuropathy and increased susceptibility to infection. Reduction in morbidity and mortality associated with diabetic foot disease requires education: this must involve patients, carers and health professionals. Its importance cannot be overemphasized.

Typical signs and symptoms of chronic ischaemia may not occur. In diabetes, associated neuropathy (neuroischaemia) can mask ischaemic pain, and calcification of arteries can make ankle–brachial systolic pressure ratios inaccurate and meaningless.

Peripheral neuropathy affects more than 50% of diabetic patients over 60 years of age and can cause motor, sensory and autonomic nerve dysfunction.

Motor nerve damage may cause deformity of the toes leading to altered mechanical forces and trauma to the skin and underlying tissues. If shoes are incorrectly fitted, deformed toes are traumatized. This can cause blistering and ulceration.

Sensory neuropathy reduces the person's ability to appreciate protective warning signs of damage. Autonomic neuropathy makes the skin dry because sweating is reduced. Arterio-venous shunting, associated with autonomic dysfunction, allows blood to be diverted through thermoregulatory arterio-venous shunts at the expense of perfusing superficial nutritive capillaries. A further effect of autonomic neuropathy is the development of a highly destructive arthropathy – Charcot neuroarthropathy (Fig. 38.2). This frequently results in severe destruction of the foot structure and ulceration.

Susceptibility to infection is a consequence of ischaemia, neuropathy and altered white blood cell function. Infection is serious in diabetic patients and must be treated urgently and aggressively.

Impaired vision may limit the person's ability to examine their feet for signs of infection and damage.

Frequently the aftermath of stroke affects the feet. Circumductory gait results in pressure areas and ulceration developing particularly under the lateral metatarsal heads. Additionally, immobility associated with stroke can subject the heels and malleoli to abnormal pressures, which may result in ulceration.

LOCAL FOOT PROBLEMS

TOENAILS

Changes in the structure of the nail are associated with advancing age. Over the years, mechanical forces alter the nail matrix and the nail bed: both these structures contribute to the growing nail plate. Nail plates can become hypertrophied and distorted (onychogryphosis). Unless reduced in thickness, the pressure exerted by the nail plate causes necrosis and ulceration of the underlying nail bed.

Fungal infection of the nail (onychomycosis) can also cause hypertrophy (Fig. 38.3). Once confirmed by laboratory tests, treatment can be initiated, either by applying fungicidal paints or sprays directly to the nail plate, or (unless contra-indicated) by systemic antifungal drugs. The nail plate must be reduced in thickness to allow penetration of any topical agent, and to help prevent sub-ungual necrosis and ulceration.

It is important that toenails are cut straight across and are not cut down the sides, as this will let splinters of nail damage the soft tissues of the nail sulcus. This allows infection to develop (onychocryptosis).

SKIN CONDITIONS

The skin responds to abnormal mechanical stresses by producing hypertrophied stratum corneum (hyperkeratinization) which presents clinically as corn and callosity (Fig. 38.4); if stresses causing these skin changes are not dissipated, tissue necrosis will occur under hyperkeratotic plaques, and ulceration will follow. Corn 'cures' are not recommended – they do nothing to address the cause. Additionally, corn 'cures' may contain acids

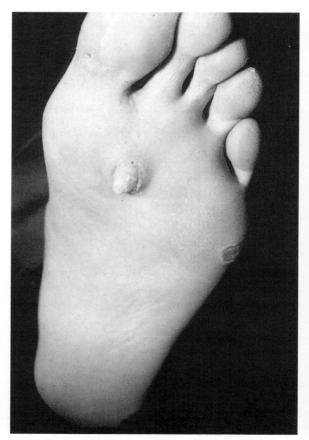

Figure 38.4 A large plantar corn under the 2nd metatarsal head. Another area of hyperkeratosis under the 5th metatarsal head has been reduced by a podiatrist.

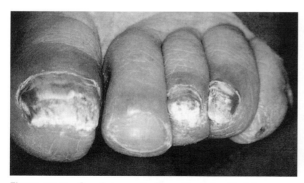

Figure 38.3 Onychomycosis. The affected nail plates appear thickened and friable. The bulk of the nail can cause necrosis of the underlying nail bed.

(e.g. salicylic acid) which macerate the epidermis allowing a portal of entry for microorganisms. Corn and callouses should be treated by a qualified podiatrist.

It is important that areas of very dry skin, for example around the heel, are not allowed to crack or fissure, otherwise pathogens can enter the dermis and cause infection (Fig. 38.5). Emollient creams should be used after bathing to rehydrate the skin. Before use, remember to check that emollients do not contain potential sensitizing agents such as lanolin. Maceration and fissuring can affect the skin between the toes. These 'wet' fissures are frequently infected by fungi, which can exacerbate the condition of the skin. After

washing, it is important to dry between the toes; surgical spirit painted between the toes can help treat maceration.

It is imperative to note the signs and symptoms of spreading infection – cellulitus, lymphangitis and lymphadenitis – and treat urgently. If the signs occur on the dorsal aspect of the foot, examine the interdigital spaces as they are often the site of the infection. Moles, particularly on the sole of the foot, should be inspected for signs of change (e.g. increase in size, uneven pigmentation, ulceration, bleeding or pain). Urgent dermatological referral is indicated in these circumstances.

TOE DEFORMITIES

Common toe deformities found in the older person include hallux abducto valgus, hammered, clawed and retracted toes. These conditions expose prominent joints to abnormal mechanical forces and the overlying skin develops corns and callosities. The joints may become so fixed by osteoarthrosis that the deformities are only amenable to surgical correction. If surgery is contraindicated, protective padding and orthoses can be used to deflect stresses away from the prominent areas, and to 'replace' the shock absorbing fibro-fatty tissue (normally found on the plantar aspect of the foot) which atrophies with age.

FOOTWEAR

Regardless of a person's age, and whatever structural changes have occurred in their feet, it is important that shoes fit properly. Ill-fitting shoes, particularly slippers, are important factors in contributing to falls (See Ch. 14).

Specialist footwear is sometimes needed to accommodate deformed joints, or to prevent trauma to neuropathic feet. In some cases, modifications can be made to 'off the shelf' shoes by a qualified podiatrist.

In summary, foot problems, especially those perceived as being relatively minor, such as corns and dystrophic toenails, can cause pain, immobility and lack of independence. Many foot problems are amenable to simple treatment. The podiatrist will be able to help and advise on all aspects of foot care.

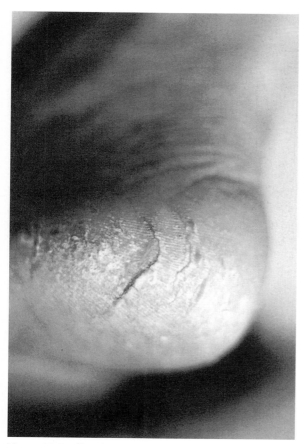

Figure 38.5 Fissuring around the periphery of the heel due to very dry skin and mechanical shearing stresses. Maceration can also cause fissures (particularly between the toes) these are treated by careful hygiene and astringents such as surgical spirit.

RECOMMENDED READING

Edmonds M E 1986 The diabetic foot: pathophysiology and treatment. Clinics in Endocrinology and Metabolism 15:889–916

Elton P J, Sanderson S P 1987 A chiropodial survey of elderly persons over 65 years in the community. The Chiropodist 42:175–178

Quaglino D, Bergamini G, Boraldi F et al 1996 Ultrastructural and morphometrical evaluation on normal human dermal connective tissue – the influence of age, sex and body region. British Journal of Dermatology 134:1013–1022

Rogers J, Harding C, Mayo A et al 1996 Stratum corneum lipids: the effect of ageing and the seasons. Archives of Dermatological Research 288:765–770

Saunders L, Frykberg R 1991 Diabetic neuropathic osteoarthropathy. The Charcot foot. In: Frykberg R G (ed.) The high risk foot in diabetes mellitus. Churchill Livingstone, New York, p 297–338

SELF-ASSESSMENT QUESTIONS

Are the following statements true or false?

1. Foot ulcers are:
   a. Unrelated to excessive mechanical forces
   b. Unrelated to the use of some 'corn cures' best treated using proprietary corn plasters
   c. Associated with morbidity or mortality
   d. Not associated with diabetes mellitus

2. Diabetes mellitus is:
   a. Uncommon in the older population
   b. Associated with serious foot complications
   c. Not associated with increased susceptibility to infection
   d. Unlikely to be associated with lower limb amputation

SECTION 6

Bone and locomotor system

Chapter 39

Contractures

Gudrun Seebass

CONTRACTURES

Contractures are fixed restrictions of the passive range of movement of a joint. They are associated with immobilization and inactivity. In the past, contractures were thought to be inevitable. Bed-ridden patients in a fetal position were a common sight on long-stay wards. Howell (1975) called contractures one of five 'dragons' of geriatrics, which carry a poor prognosis. Thirty years later, the National Care Standard Commission only lists Howell's other four dragons (mental confusion, incontinence, pressure sores and falls) in the health standards for older people in care homes (DoH 2003). Current US care standards include contractures, and the Grey Panthers are encouraging their members to take action against care homes in which contractures are not successfully prevented (National Citizens' Coalition for Nursing Home Reform). Has the British dragon been slain?

The emphasis of nursing care has shifted away from putting each joint through its full range of passive movement each time a patient is turned.

Instead, early active functional movement is encouraged. But what about those people who rely on hoists for transfer, and who are cared for in accordance with the latest moving and handling policy? Will they continue to use the functional range of their joints?

The dragon is still with us – a vignette

A lady is admitted to hospital from her home because of pressure sores and constipation. Both her legs are flexed at the hips and knees. Because of hip adduction, she tends to cross her shins. Both hands are clenched. She will extend her fingers just far enough to allow a glimpse of her palms. Passive extension of her legs causes pain before any resistance is met, even though her joints are neither tender nor inflamed. She takes strong opioid analgesia. Diagnoses in her case notes include cervical myelopathy, peripheral neuropathy, rheumatoid arthritis and Alzheimer's disease. Her husband confirms that she has spent

Continued

WHAT CONTRACTS?

The term 'contracture' implies restriction of joint movement due to shortening of tendons, muscles, the joint capsule or alterations of the cartilage. Scarring of the skin (most notably from burns) and bony fusion (ankylosis) can have a similar effect. Contractures develop as a result of a combination of intrinsic (illness or injury) and extrinsic (functional or external) risk factors (Table 39.1).

WHY DOES IMMOBILITY CAUSE CONTRACTURES?

An animal experiment by Akeson et al (1980) showed the following changes after 9 weeks of complete immobilization of a knee joint:

- A reduction of water and proteoglycan, rendering collagen fibres less mobile
- Fibro-fatty connective tissue proliferation within the joint space, leading to adhesions and scar tissue
- Fibroblasts transforming the contact areas of cartilage in line with increasing degree of immobility, rigidity and compression of the joint
- New collagen forming abnormal cross-links between connective tissue fibres, thus limiting the maximum length a bundle of fibres can reach on stretching

Metabolism and biosynthesis in muscle and soft tissue depend on their mechanical activity. When a muscle is immobilized in a shortened position, e.g. a paretic arm resting on a stroke patient's lap, a shortening of muscle fibre length occurs due to a loss of sarcomeres, accompanied by shortening of muscle connective tissue and increased muscle stiffness. At first, it is still possible to move the arm through its full functional range. However, increased force is needed to overcome the increased muscle tone (O'Dwyer et al 1996). Spastic muscles continuously contract and pull the limb into a deformed position. This active muscle shortening produces a greater loss of sarcomeres than immobility alone (Farmer & James 2001).

Pressure in a joint and tension on its surrounding structures depend on its position. Each joint has a position of minimum pressure: 30–45 degrees of flexion for the hip and knee and 15 degrees

Table 39.1 Risk factors for contracture formation

Intrinsic	Extrinsic
Joint:	Pain, leading to the individual resting the joint in the most comfortable
Infection	position (antalgic posture)
Inflammation	Splints, casts and fixation
Trauma	Bed rest
Compartment syndrome	Inactivity
Brain:	Immobility
Stroke, head injury, cerebral palsy	Deconditioning, 'learned helplessness'
Parkinson's disease	
Alzheimer's disease	
Spinal cord compression	
Polyneuropathy	
Peripheral nerve lesions	
Fear and lack of motivation to move	

plantar-flexion at the ankle. These positions are spontaneously assumed when the joint is painful ('antalgic posture'). A few weeks' rest in the position of comfort is sufficient for contracture formation to occur (Perry 1987).

Contractures are described by the degree of movement lost and the resulting position of the joint. Hence a '30-degree flexor contracture of the knee' means that the knee is bent and will only extend to a maximum of 150 degrees (equivalent to the position of comfort).

Exercise

- Walk across the room keeping your right knee bent 30 degrees.
- Now take another walk, this time with the left ankle in 15 degrees plantar-flexion. What do you find?

EFFECTS OF CONTRACTURES

Even a small degree of contracture greatly increases energy expenditure for walking, slows down walking speed and causes strain on compensating adjacent joints (e.g. hip, lumbar spine). If the patient is unable to compensate because of arthritis, muscular weakness or low stamina, immobility will result – starting a downward spiral of functional loss, dependence and further contracture formation, poor aesthetic appearance leading to social isolation, difficulties in seating, positioning and meeting hygiene needs, pain on forced movement, incontinence and pressure sores.

Do a mental ward round: How many of your current in-patients have contractures?

Assessment of contractures traditionally involved measuring joint angles with a goniometer. This requires identification of bony landmarks (not always easy in the presence of oedema or well-padded hip joints) and positioning of the patient with the adjacent joint in the neutral position. The range of movement will be less if the patient is tense, in pain, cold or unable to cooperate. In stroke patients, care and patience are

needed to differentiate contractures from high muscle tone and spasticity.

Three surveys of long-term care residents in the 1990s found the prevalence of contractures to be 27% (Rabiner et al 1995), 55% (Yip et al 1996) and 87% (Mollinger & Steffen 1993). These different figures do not necessarily reflect variations in the quality of care, because in each of the surveys contractures were measured and defined in a different way: Mollinger and Steffen documented any restriction in knee extension measurable on goniometry, Yip et al also used goniometry but defined contractures as restriction of more than 30 degrees in hip, knee, elbow, wrist or finger joints, and in the survey by Rabiner et al prevalence is based on any contracture mentioned in the residents' case notes. The presence of contractures correlated with disability and length of stay in long-term care (Yip et al 1996). Virtually all patients with knee contractures of more than 30 degrees were unable to walk (Mollinger & Steffen 1993, Yip et al 1996).

For practical purposes a simple screening of functional movements will be sufficient to identify clinically relevant limitations. American care homes covered by Medicaid regularly screen their residents as part of the Minimum Data Set (CMS) (Table 39.2). This instrument has been translated into several European and Asian languages and is increasingly used for comparative epidemiological research.

Use this screening on your next ward round:
- How many of your patients do indeed have contractures?

Treatment for contractures is an evidence-free zone. Most formal trials are small and limited to one joint with a contracture caused by one specific condition. The aim of any treatment is to maintain or increase contractile and connective tissue length while reducing stiffness and loss of elasticity. Animal studies have suggested the following principles (summarized from Farmer & James 2001):

- Sarcomeres are gained when muscle is held in a lengthened position, and these gains are increased with contractile activity, stretching and electrical stimulation.

Table 39.2	Screening for contractures (adapted from CMS Minimum Data)	
Neck	Sitting	Ask the patient to turn the head slowly from side to side Then try to reach each ear towards the shoulder
Arm	Sitting	Reach with both hands and touch palms to the back of the head Touch each shoulder with the opposite hand
Hand	Any position	Make a fist Then open the hand
Leg	Lying supine	Lift one leg, bending it at the knee Then extend the leg flat on the mattress
Foot	Lying supine	Pull the toes up towards the head Then push toes down, away from the head

■ Connective tissue accumulates with immobility. This is ameliorated by contractile activity.

■ When connective tissue is stretched continuously, it loses tension with time. Stretching with high force for a short duration at normal temperatures produces an elastic response (the connective tissue resumes its original length when the stretch is released). Prolonged low force stretch at high temperatures produces plastic deformation, especially if the tissue is cooled down before the tension is released.

According to these principles, the simplest and most effective contracture treatment consists of active exercises, which stretch shortened muscles and strengthen antagonists. These exercises can be combined with physical agent modalities (heat, cold, ultrasound, electrical stimulation). They are most effective if the patients regularly use the full range of their functional movement in between treatment sessions. Unfortunately, most patients with contractures are unable to use this approach.

Significant progress in contracture prevention and treatment has been made in areas where the causes for contracture formation are temporary – for instance in orthopaedic surgery. Historically, joint injuries were treated with absolute rest until complete healing was achieved, resulting in very restricted joint movement. Any attempt to maintain the range of a joint by allowing earlier active movement would lead to poor healing – the 'orthopaedic dilemma'. Internal fixation of fractures, antibiotics and antiinflammatory drugs, early controlled movement or continuous passive movement for joint replacement and septic arthritis have transformed contractures from an inevitable consequence of joint trauma to an avoidable complication (Perry 1987).

Table 39.3 summarizes treatment strategies for patients with established contractures, immobility and neurological illness. Most of these are cumbersome and laborious for both patient and therapist. They lead at best to a temporary increase in range of movement. This new range of movement may allow the patient to relearn a functional activity (e.g. feeding, walking). If the patient then carries out this activity frequently, some improvement may be maintained.

In a French case series on 12 older patients who failed to improve on physiotherapy, multiple tenotomies for lower limb contractures were done. Five patients regained the ability to walk, two were sitting more comfortably, two patients died and the remainder had no functional gain (Roger & Kirsch 1985).

Prevention of contractures is the key – and this should take place in most hospital and care facilities. Most of it is done subconsciously or as a by-product of treatment given for other reasons – encouragement of active movement during nursing care, positioning of patients in intensive care or on the acute stroke ward and physiotherapy are examples. Contracture prevention is much more difficult and controversial in situations where

Table 39.3 Strategies for contracture treatment (summarized from Farmer & James 2001, Perry 1987)

Treatment modality	Application	Use and evidence	Caveat
Passive movement	1. Intermittent (carried out by nurses, carers or physiotherapists)	Moving each joint through its functional range regularly has helped to maintain joint mobility in acute polio	May maintain range of movement but does not increase it
	2. Continuous (on a hinged splint which continuously alters its angle)	Helps maintain range of movement after total knee replacement and corrective surgery for paretic limbs	In the presence of spasticity, passive movement above a certain velocity causes a spastic contraction, which is detrimental
Passive stretch	Applied by a physiotherapist	A trial in spinal cord injury was inconclusive (Harvey & Herbert 2002). No scientific basis for frequency and duration	Difficult to counteract dynamic effects of spasticity
Serial plastering	The joint is immobilized in a stretched position. Regular changes of plaster are needed with the joint held at the new limit of range	Increases the range of movement in the short term. This may permit relearning of functional active movement. Persistent spasticity, high muscle tone and immobility will lead to recurrent contractures after plaster removal	Immobilization leads to atrophy of antagonist muscles and connective tissue accumulation. 'Drop-out' casts allow active movement in the direction opposite to the contracture and alleviate the effects of immobilization
Splinting	1. Static	Widely used for hemiplegic wrists despite conflicting trial results (Lannin & Herbert 2003). No scientific basis for frequency and duration of use	Often difficult to apply, leading to the joint not being held at the limit of its range. The effect of stretch on connective tissue diminishes over time
	2. Dynamic – the splint contains a coil which applies continuous stretch to the joint	A case study on nursing home residents with knee contractures failed to demonstrate benefit (Steffen & Mollinger 1995)	Compliance dependent
Electrical stimulation	Simulates active muscle contraction and can increase muscle volume and reduce atrophy in immobilized muscle, especially when combined with passive stretch	Increases the range of wrist extension in stroke patients (Pandyan et al 1997) and leg strength in children with cerebral palsy	Effects are not maintained when the treatment is discontinued
Botulinum toxin	Injected into spastic muscle	Temporarily relieves spasticity allowing the muscle to be stretched – either by its antagonist or by a carer, therapist, splint or cast	The contracture recurs when the effect of the injection wears off. Repeated injections can sometimes sustain improvement
Surgery	Tenotomies, surgical transfer of muscles	Mainly used in children with cerebral palsy or congenital contractures	Temporary lengthening of contracted muscle may help relearning of functional movement. If this fails the contracture will recur over time

active movement cannot be restored. Hence it is crucial to address any reversible factors contributing to immobility: musculoskeletal and neuropathic pain, high muscle tone and depression. Active movement and functional positioning must be encouraged by all members of the hospital or community team.

Joint movement is no different from any other human skill – if we do not use it, we will lose it.

REFERENCES

Akeson W H, Amiel D, Woo S L 1980 Immobility effects on synovial joints – the pathomechanics of joint contracture. Biorheology 17:95–110

CMS's RAI Version 2.0 Manual, p 3–107 to 3-109. Online. Available: http://cms.hhs.gov/Medicaid/mds20

Department of Health (DoH) 2003 Care homes for older people – national minimum standards, 3rd edn. HMSO, London

Farmer S E, James M 2001 Contractures in orthopaedic and neurological conditions: a review of causes and treatment. Disability and Rehabilitation 23:549–558

Harvey L A, Herbert R D 2002 Muscle stretching for treatment and prevention of contracture in people with spinal cord injury. Spinal Cord 40:1–9

Howell T H 1975 Old age, some practical points in geriatrics, 3rd edn. HK Lewis, London

Lannin N A, Herbert R D 2003 Is hand splinting effective for adults following stroke? A systematic review and methodological critique of published research. Clinical Rehabilitation 17:807–816

Mollinger L A, Steffen T M 1993 Knee flexion contractures in institutionalized elderly: prevalence, severity, stability, and related variables. Physical Therapy 73:437–446

National Citizens' Coalition for Nursing Home reform. Online. Available: http://www.nccnhr.org

O'Dwyer N J, Ada L, Neilson P D 1996 Spasticity and muscle contracture following stroke. Brain 119:1737–1749

Pandyan A D, Granat M H, Stott D J 1997 Effects of electrical stimulation on flexion contractures in the hemiplegic wrist. Clinical Rehabilitation 11:123–130

Perry J 1987 Contractures – a historical perspective. Clinical Orthopaedics and Related Research 219: 8–14

Rabiner A, Roach K E, Spielholz N I 1995 Characteristics of nursing home residents with contractures. Physical and Occupational Therapy in Geriatrics 13:1–10

Roger M, Kirsch J M 1985 Straightening of bedridden patients blocked in flexure (French). Revue de Geriatrie 10:379–382

Steffen T M, Mollinger L A 1995 Low-load prolonged stretch in the treatment of knee flexion contractures in nursing home residents. Physical Therapy 75: 886–897

Yip B, Stewart D A, Roberts M A 1996 The prevalence of joint contractures in residents in NHS continuing care. Health Bulletin 54:338–343

SELF–ASSESSMENT QUESTION

Are the following statements true or false?

1. Contracture prevention:
   a. Is included in the health standards for older people resident in care homes in the UK
   b. Involves encouragement of active movement through the full functional range
   c. Is more difficult in the presence of spasticity
   d. Is regularly done by orthopaedic surgeons
   e. Cannot be aided by medication

SECTION 7

Cancer

Chapter 40

Cancer in old age

Margot Gosney

Commonly asked questions about cancer in older people are:

- Is the epidemiology of cancer in older people changing?
- Is screening for cancer appropriate for older people?
- Should older patients with cancer be investigated and managed in a similar way to younger subjects?
- Can the survival differences seen in younger and older groups be explained?

The answer to all of these questions is 'yes'. Our knowledge about cancer and older people is patchy and incomplete. We do know that in considering older patients with cancer:

- There is more diagnosed co-morbidity (Turner et al 1999, Yancik & Ries 1991)
- They are less likely to participate in screening (Holmes & Hearne 1981)
- They are less likely to be investigated (Bennett et al 1991, Mor et al 1989)

- They are less likely to have a definitive histopathological diagnosis (Crawford & Atherton 1994)
- They are more likely to have advanced local disease at presentation (Goodwin et al 1986)
- They are more likely to have metastatic disease at presentation (Mor et al 1985)
- They are more likely to have delays in presentation (Smith et al 2005)
- They are less likely to undergo therapy, both palliative and curative (Bergman et al 1991, Greenfield et al 1987, Markman et al 1993, Samet et al 1986, Silliman et al 1989)
- Chemotherapy and radiotherapy have their own specific problems in older patients (Gosney 2000)
- They are less likely to enter into chemotherapy trials (Hutchins et al 1999)
- The only report of the elderly patient with cancer may be the death certificate
- They have reduced survival
- Cancer assessment scales have been poorly developed in older individuals (Gosney 2005)

Cancer is a main cause of death worldwide and as the incidence and prevalence of cancer increases it has overtaken heart disease as a leading cause of death in many countries. Of the 7 million cancer deaths worldwide in 2001 it has been estimated that 35% were attributable to nine potentially modifiable risk factors. Worldwide, smoking, alcohol use and low fruit and vegetable intake were the leading risk factors for deaths from cancer, and in high-income countries smoking, alcohol use and being overweight/obesity were the most important causes of cancer (Danaei et al 2005).

During the last decade the mortality from cancer has fallen by 17% in those aged 30–69 years and it has risen by 0.4% in those over 70 years (Murray & Lopez 1996, WHO 2002).

Over half of all cancer will occur in patients aged 70 years or above – a good reason for geriatricians to know about the investigation and management of such patients. In this chapter I will deal with five common tumours: colon and lung cancer (common tumours in both men and women), breast and ovary (as related to older women) and prostate cancer (specific to older men).

BREAST CANCER

Over half of all cases of breast cancer are diagnosed in women aged 70 or above.

In 1999, of the estimated 175 000 cases of breast cancer diagnosed in the USA, 46% occurred in women over 65 years. SEER (Surveillance, Epidemiology and End Results) data indicate that the incidence of breast cancer is 74.5 per 100 000 in those less than 65 years compared with 483 per 100 000 in those aged 65 years or above (Havlik et al 1994).

Some women who are elderly and frail, and who previously may have died from unrelated causes before the recurrence of their tumour, are now surviving.

SCREENING

Screening for breast cancer is important because of the positive relationship between the stage of disease and age at diagnosis (Holmes & Hearne 1981). The NHS breast screening programme was introduced in England and Wales in 1988 on the recommendations of the Forrest Committee (Forrest 1986). Until then, few mammograms were done on women aged 60 years or above (Robie 1989), despite the fact that early detection reduces mortality (Collette et al 1984) and mammography increases the proportion of early cancers detected (Tabar et al 1992). In 1992 the Department of Health set a target for a reduction in breast cancer mortality of 25% in the age group invited for screening by the year 2000 (DoH 1992). As the age of screening extended from 50–64 to 50–69 years, it was recognized that screening would not be expected to affect mortality in the 50–54 years age group because the average age at first screening for women in the programme is 51.5 years and in previously published trials there has been little or no effect of screening in the first 4 years. In England and Wales between 1971 and 1999, improvements in treatment and screening have had major roles in the reduction in mortality from breast cancer. A 6.4% reduction in mortality is attributable to screening and 14.9% to improvements in treatment and other factors (Blanks et al 2000).

Unfortunately, older women believe that they are at less risk of developing breast cancer than younger women (Harris et al 1991) and, because of this, consider self-examination to be adequate. Older women are less likely to have breast examinations performed by their doctors (King et al 1993) and doctors are less likely to send older people for screening (Weinberger et al 1991). A UK study (Edwards & Jones 2000) of 1604 women aged 65 years or above found only 8% had previously undergone breast cancer screening and rates were higher in those who were either presently or had previously been married than those who were single. Age influenced potential future attendance with only 27% of those aged over 80 years compared with 67% of those aged 65–69 years reporting they would attend if invited. As with many areas of screening, future attendees were significantly more likely to be from higher social classes and significantly less likely to be disabled or depressed (Edwards & Jones 2000).

A Swedish study comparing the cancer mortality rates in women aged 65–74 years found, when comparing a group who had undergone mammographic screening (21 925) with controls (15 344), at 13 years of follow up, that the relative breast cancer mortality in the screened group was 0.68, i.e. there was a third reduction which could potentially be ascribed to the screening process (Chen et al 1995). If screening results in early detection of potentially treatable tumours, then only quality of life and patient anxiety can outweigh the need for routine screening procedures. An increase in the percentage of older women to 80% undergoing mammography would result in a 30% reduction in mortality (Albert 1987).

TREATMENT

The primary treatment for all breast tumours is surgery. Much of the evidence-based practice rests entirely on evidence from younger women, since older women have been excluded from most clinical trials.

Several studies have demonstrated the equivalence of total mastectomy and partial mastectomy in combination with postoperative radiation in the management of primary breast tumours. Unfortunately, the tumour size varied within the reported trials from less than 2.5 cm to greater than 5 cm (Fisher et al 1995, Jacobson et al 1995, van Dongen et al 1992, Veronesi et al 1990). An important factor in the decision between two surgical procedures is patients' preference, which should be considered whenever possible. Quality of life appears equal following partial or total mastectomy (Kiebert et al 1991).

The receipt of radiation therapy among women undergoing breast-conserving surgery declines markedly with age irrespective of co-morbidity and stage of disease, with only 24% of women over the age of 80 years receiving radiotherapy despite the absence of co-morbidity (Ballard-Barbash et al 1996). This is not an isolated finding, with age often being negatively associated, not only with radiotherapy, but also any surgical treatment and non-conserving procedures (Newschaffer et al 1996).

Axillary dissection is done both for staging and to eliminate any residual disease. If axillary dissection results in lymphoedema, this is particularly troublesome for the older woman with already impaired upper limb function. Prolonged surgery lengthens the anaesthetic period therefore the sampling of a sentinel 'lymph node' will ensure that if the lymph node is free from tumour

the patient is spared axillary dissection (Giuliano et al 1994).

In a meta-analysis of 20 000 women, postoperative radiotherapy resulted in a reduction of about two-thirds for local recurrence, which was largely independent of the type of patient or the type of radiotherapy. The most common trials were mastectomy with axillary clearance (23) with 6 trials each of mastectomy with axillary sampling or breast conservation with axillary clearance and 5 trials of mastectomy alone. Unfortunately, less than 700 individuals were aged 70 years or above – although the evidence was that the underlying mortality rate from breast cancer in this age group depended strongly on nodal status and not on age (whereas death from other causes depended strongly on age and not on nodal status [Early Breast Cancer Trialists' Collaborative Group 2000]).

In the 1970s and 1980s some older patients with breast cancer who may or may not have been fit for surgery were treated with tamoxifen. While the majority of the primary tumours responded to tamoxifen, long-term local disease control was poor. However, there has until recently been little interest in the role of preoperative endocrine therapy, although there is evidence that a delay in surgery to administer 3 or 4 months preoperative endocrine therapy does not compromise long-term outcomes. Further work is required to ensure that older women with breast cancer are not treated suboptimally (Ellis 2000).

Adjuvant tamoxifen

It has been known since the 1990s that older women with early stage breast cancer have decreased recurrence and mortality rates if treated with adjuvant tamoxifen. A review of 133 randomized trials with a total population of 75 000 women (of whom 2500 were aged 70 years or above) found a 28% decrease in recurrence and 21% reduced mortality in patients with node-positive disease who were treated with tamoxifen (Early Breast Cancer Trialists' Collaborative Group 1992). Further work by this group found that patients with estrogen receptor (ER)-positive disease who were allocated to about 5 years of adjuvant tamoxifen had a reduced annual breast cancer death rate of 31% – largely irrespective of the use of chemotherapy, and/or age, ER status, or other tumour characteristics. Receiving tamoxifen for 5 years was significantly more effective than therapy for 1–2 years (Early Breast Cancer Trialists' Collaborative Group 2005).

As with hormonal therapy for prostate cancer, an initial flare of the disease may occur on commencing therapy. The side-effects of tamoxifen are generally mild, and include nausea and vomiting. Tamoxifen is highly protein bound and thus interacts with drugs such as warfarin.

An increased risk of deep vein thrombosis and endometrial cancer has been seen in patients on tamoxifen. In ER-poor disease, even 5 years of tamoxifen has little effect on recurrence or breast cancer mortality (Early Breast Cancer Trialists' Collaborative Group 1998). In ER-positive disease, tamoxifen is highly effective, though in both younger and older women, chemoendocrine therapy is significantly better than endocrine therapy alone (recurrence relative risk 0.85 for older women) (Early Breast Cancer Trialists' Collaborative Group 1998).

Adjuvant chemotherapy

In a meta-analysis of 75 000 women published in 1992, only 274 were aged 70 years or above and receiving adjuvant chemotherapy, and there was no definite proven efficacy of adjuvant chemotherapy in this small and often unrepresentative group (Early Breast Cancer Trialists' Collaborative Group 1992). However, in 2005 the same group reported a meta-analysis of 194 unconfounded randomized trials of adjuvant chemotherapy or hormonal therapy that had begun before 1995. They divided the data into those individuals < 40 years, 40–49, 50–59, 60–69 and > 70 years. When considering single-agent chemotherapy, those individuals > 70 years had a reduced ratio of annual events and reduced annual death rate when compared to those individuals not receiving chemotherapy. The benefits of polychemotherapy were also seen to be greater in this age group, with reduced events and overall death rate. However, few women older than 70 years and very few older than 80 years were randomized into chemotherapy trials. When considering all age groups together for single-agent chemotherapy (treatment vs control), the ratios were 0.86

for recurrence and 0.96 for breast cancer mortality, while for polychemotherapy they were 0.77 and 0.83 respectively. The polychemotherapy regimens predominantly involved 6 or 12 months of cyclophosphamide, methotrexate and 5-fluorouracil (CMF)-based treatments or about 6 months of anthracycline-based treatments with combinations such as FACE (fluorouracil, doxorubicin, cyclophosphamide) or FEC (fluorouracil, epirubicin and cyclophosphamide) (Early Breast Cancer Trialists' Collaborative Group 2005). Thus, allocation to about 6 months of anthracycline-based chemotherapy reduces the annual breast cancer death rate by about 38% for women < 50 years of age and about 20% for those aged 50–69 years, largely irrespective of the use of tamoxifen, ER status, nodal status or other tumour characteristics. Unfortunately, these data cannot be extrapolated to those aged 70 years or older since so few were entered into trials (though early data suggest that beneficial effects also exist in this age group).

Nearly all of the evidence on sequential chemoendocrine therapy involved older women among whom it appeared somewhat more effective than concurrent chemoendocrine (tamoxifen and chemotherapy at the same time) treatment, but the comparisons were indirect (different trials) and the difference failed to reach significance (Early Breast Cancer Trialists' Collaborative Group 2005).

There is concern about the administration of chemotherapy because of higher grades of toxicity in women aged 65 years or older. Older women receiving CMF chemotherapy had higher grades of toxicity and received less than their expected CMF dose. The subjective burden of treatment, however, was similar for both age groups when based on quality of life measures, which included performance status, coping, mood, appetite and physical well-being (Crivellari et al 2000).

METASTATIC DISEASE

Tamoxifen

Tamoxifen is often the first line of treatment, since it is easy to administer and well tolerated. About 30% of women with metastatic disease respond to tamoxifen, with the highest response rates in those who are ER positive, have soft tissue or bony metastases or who have had a long disease-free interval. If response to tamoxifen is not seen or if the patient relapses while on tamoxifen, megestrol acetate or aromatase inhibitors may be useful. Unfortunately, nausea, weight gain and fluid retention are common side-effects of megestrol and are troublesome in older women with coexisting cardiac disease or orthopaedic problems.

While megestrol may have the undesired effect of weight gain, in the presence of tumour cachexia it may stimulate appetite and cause palliative weight gain.

Chemotherapy

Many women who have been treated with hormone therapy for metastatic disease will fail to respond or will relapse subsequently (Marchei et al 1996). A decision must then be made about chemotherapy. Although, as with many younger women, a complete response is rare, partial responses lasting several months may be expected in up to half of the patients treated (Muss 1994).

Paclitaxel is licensed for the treatment of metastatic breast carcinoma when standard anthracycline-containing therapy has failed or is inappropriate. Studies of elderly women have found an overall response rate of only 23% with a median time to progression of 4 months. Patients in whom a consideration of paclitaxel is being made are often heavily pretreated and febrile neutropenia may occur in as many as 45% – far above that expected in a previously untreated group (Abrams et al 1995).

For the future

Reduced doses of chemotherapy are often seen in older patients, though the evidence for this is lacking. In a similar fashion, chemotherapy doses are often reduced when treating obese patients in an attempt to avoid overdosing. Colleoni and colleagues found that, for younger women with ER-absent or ER-low tumours, a reduction in chemotherapy dose should be avoided as a reduced dose during the first course of chemotherapy was detrimental (Colleoni et al 2005).

Further work must be undertaken in older subjects in whom dose reduction also occurs to ensure

that this seemingly compassionate act does not reduce efficacy. Febrile neutropenia occurs in many older subjects undergoing chemotherapy. Newer colony-stimulating growth factors (such as pegfilgrastim) can markedly reduce febrile neutropenia, associated hospitalizations and antibiotic use in patients receiving docetaxel. The pegfilgrastim study group included individuals up to the age of 88 years and was well tolerated. However, further data are required in the use of colony-stimulating growth factors during the administration of chemotherapy to older patients with breast cancer (Vogel et al 2005).

OVARIAN CARCINOMA

Although the aetiology of ovarian carcinoma is not known, both familial factors (which may be more important in younger patients) and uninterrupted ovulation (more evident in many older women) are associated factors. Ovarian cancer becomes increasingly common with advancing age. For women under 50 years, the incidence is 20 per 100 000 whereas over the age of 50 years it is 40 per 100 000 (Yancik 1993). In England and Wales there are more deaths due to ovarian cancer than all other gynaecology cancers combined. Despite current first-line management of surgical debulking followed by platinum-based chemotherapy, most women will relapse and the 5-year survival rate is only 20–30% (Morrison 2005).

SCREENING

As ovarian carcinoma has few specific symptoms, the role of screening to identify tumours must be considered. Two areas are currently under debate – serum CA125 estimations and transvaginal ultrasonography. CA125 is an epithelial marker which is elevated in more than 80% of patients with ovarian carcinoma. Its use is limited however, since although 90% of patients with stage III or IV disease have an elevated CA125, only 50% of those with stage I disease have raised levels. It is also raised in benign gynaecological conditions and may therefore be a cause of anxiety due to false positive results.

In a trial of over 21 000 women aged 45 years or older, subjects were randomized to three annual

Table 40.1	FIGO staging system for ovarian carcinoma (FIGO 1986)
Stage	Description
I	*Growth limited to the ovaries*
	A – One ovary; no ascites; capsule intact; no tumour on external surface
	B – Two ovaries; no ascites; capsule intact; no tumour on external surface
	C – One or both ovaries with either: surface tumour; ruptured capsule; or ascites or peritoneal washings with malignant cells
II	*Pelvic extension*
	A – Involvement of uterus and/or tubes
	B – Involvement of other pelvic tissues
	C – IIA or IIB with factors as in IC
III	*Peritoneal implants outside pelvis and/or positive retroperitoneal or inguinal nodes*
	A – Grossly limited to true pelvis; negative nodes; microscopic seeding of abdominal peritoneum
	B – Implants of abdominal peritoneum 2 cm or less; nodes negative
	C – Abdominal implants greater than 2 cm and/or positive retroperitoneal or inguinal nodes
IV	*Distant metastases*

screens that involved measurement of serum CA125, pelvic ultrasound if CA125 was > 30 U/mL and referral for gynaecological opinion if ovarian volume was 8.8 mL or more on ultrasound. This study showed that a large number of women were prepared to undergo screening and of the original 10 958 who were screened, 29 women underwent surgery, of whom six had an ovarian cancer and 23 had false-positive results associated with benign ovarian tumours or other pathology. While preliminary evidence suggests a survival benefit, this was not analysed by age and the results of larger screening trials are awaited (Jacobs et al 1999).

TREATMENT

It is important that patients are managed by specialists in ovarian cancer. Patients with stage I or II disease when treated by a gynaecological oncologist are more likely to undergo lymph node dissection (60%) than those treated by a general gynaecologist (36%) or a general surgeon (16%). Similar results are seen in patients with stage III and IV disease and this group are more likely to receive postoperative chemotherapy. Survival figures also confirm a reduced risk of death from any cause when the operation is performed by gynaecological oncologists (Earle et al 2006).

Table 40.2 Risk groups of patients with limited ovarian carcinoma	
Group	Characteristics
Low Risk	Grade 1 or 2 disease Intact capsule No tumour on external surface Negative peritoneal cytology No ascites Growth confined to ovaries
High Risk	Grade 3 disease Ruptured capsule Tumour on external surface Positive peritoneal cytology Ascites Growth outside ovaries

If any high-risk factors are present, the patient is considered high risk.

Limited disease

Laparotomy determines the extent of disease (Table 40.1). Those tumours confined to the ovary (stage I) or pelvis (stage II) are then assessed for risk of recurrence (Table 40.2). Those patients who undergo total abdominal hysterectomy, bilateral salpingo-oophorectomy and omentectomy alone, and are considered to have a low risk for recurrence, have a cure rate which exceeds 90%, whereas those considered to be at 'high risk' have a recurrence rate which may be as high as 40%. Ovarian cancer patients who have been optimally debulked survive longer, irrespective of the disease stage (Crawford et al 2005).

All patients with stage III or undiagnosed stage IV disease should have an exploratory laparotomy. The standard care for advanced epithelial ovarian cancer is six cycles of platinum-taxane. While some centres continue therapy for eight cycles there is no evidence that only six cycles provides inferior results (Dizon et al 2006). Two further cycles do not improve disease-free or overall survival and patients who do not enter remission after six cycles are unlikely to benefit from additional chemotherapy with the same agents (Dizon et al 2006). Cisplatin requires in-patient administration, usually every 3 weeks, and is very nephrotoxic. Carboplatin can be given as a day case, lacks nephrotoxicity but bone marrow suppression remains a problem, particularly in older women.

Unfortunately, many women relapse after initial therapy and further treatment is based on whether they are considered to be platinum sensitive or resistant. To be platinum sensitive, patients must have had an initial response to a platinum-based regimen and had a platinum-free interval of greater than 6 months before recurrence.

ICON 2 (1998) found when comparing single agent carboplatin with CAP (cyclophosphamide, doxorubicin and cisplatin) that single agent carboplatin is a safe, effective and appropriate treatment for women with advanced ovarian cancer. While only 30% of those studied were over 65 years of age, there was no evidence that CAP or carboplatin were more or less effective in different subgroups (though CAP resulted in more leucopenia, alopecia and nausea but less thrombocytopenia than carboplatin [ICON Collaborators 1998]).

Unfortunately, despite good first-line therapy, many patients develop recurrent disease within 3 years of diagnosis. A randomized controlled trial of 802 patients with platinum-sensitive ovarian cancer who had relapsed within 6 months of treatment were randomly assigned to paclitaxel plus platinum chemotherapy vs conventional platinum therapy. The survival curves favoured the addition of paclitaxel to platinum (hazard ratio 0.82) which provided an absolute difference in 2-year survival of 7% and a prolongation of the median survival by 5 months (Parmar et al 2003).

For the future

A variety of substances have been suggested to reduce the incidence of ovarian cancer. These include the use of non-steroidal antiinflammatory drugs (including aspirin) which, when administered within 5 years of the diagnosis, were found to be associated with a reduction in the risk of ovarian cancer (OR = 0.72) (Schildkraut et al 2006).

In a study of 61057 women aged 40–76 years in Sweden who were followed up for an average of 15.51 years, tea consumption was inversely associated with a risk of ovarian cancer after controlling for potential confounders. Each additional cup of tea per day was associated with an 18% lower risk of cancer. Although the authors do not postulate a reason for this, it may provide useful advice for the future management of older people (Larsson & Wolk 2005).

COLON

Colorectal cancer accounts for about 10% of all cancer registrations and is the second most common malignancy (after lung cancer). The cumulative lifetime risk of developing colon cancer is 1:40 for men and 1:48 for women. About 945000 people develop colon cancer worldwide each year and 492000 die (Weitz et al 2005). The incidence rises sharply with age, with rates of just 4 per 100000 of the population below 50 years rising to 380 per 100000 of the population over 80 years. Three-quarters of all cases occur in patients over 65 years and the age distribution is the most important factor determining the prevalence – the incidence doubles every decade reaching a peak between 75 and 80 years (Curless et al 1994). Overall, 60% of colorectal registrations are for colon cancer and the remainder due to rectal or multiple tumours. In older patients, colorectal cancer presentation is often atypical and symptoms are less specific than in younger subjects. The presence of anaemia or change in bowel habit is a 'textbook' rather than 'typical' presentation – the familiar symptoms of lethargy and abdominal pain making diagnosis more challenging.

In order to understand management and outcome studies the Dukes' classification must be understood:

Stage A: Tumour has not penetrated the entire thickness of the bowel wall – no nodes involved

Stage B1: Lesions up to, but not through, serosa

Stage B2: Lesions through the serosa with involvement of adjacent organs

Stage C1: Lesions up to, but not through, serosa plus regional lymph node metastases

Stage C2: Lesion through serosa with involvement of adjacent organs plus regional lymph node metastases

While Dukes did not describe stage D, this has not prevented us adding this later and the modified Astler-Coller classification is commonly used. Patients with metastatic disease to the liver and other distant sites are thus labelled Dukes' D in some series. With more advanced disease, both treatment and outcome will be affected.

SCREENING

If detected early, carcinoma of the large bowel is curable and screening is a way of detecting early tumours in the absence of any symptoms. There are three basic tools for screening: digital rectal examination, faecal occult blood testing and sigmoidoscopy.

Digital rectal examination can detect low rectal lesions and should be mandatory in the annual screening of elderly patients; however, it will detect only a few tumours, since most colorectal tumours are in the proximal colon.

The use of faecal occult blood results in the detection of earlier stage tumours (Mandel et al 1993) and the percentage of adenomas and carcinomas found in patients with positive tests increases with advancing age (Winawer et al 1980). Elderly people are no less likely to comply with this investigation than younger subjects. Why we are loath to perform this simple and often helpful test remains unexplained (Winawer et al 1983). While experimental at the present time, the

use of faecal DNA to identify colorectal cancers at an early stage remains a possible hope for the future (Müller et al 2004).

Flexible sigmoidoscopy provides a potentially greater yield but is more expensive than testing for faecal occult blood (UK Flexible Sigmoidoscopy Screening Trial Investigators 2002). Since 2000, the American College of Gastroenterology has issued guidelines recommending that adults over the age of 50 years should undergo flexible sigmoidoscopy every 5 years to reduce their risk of colorectal cancer. The findings from this initiative have been an overall response rate of 70% and an age range of cases that is very different from the United Kingdom (age 20–74 years in the US) (Newcomb et al 2003). It must also be remembered that a patient with a negative flexible sigmoidoscopy may, 3 years later, be found to have advanced adenomas or a carcinoma (Schoen et al 2003).

In November 2002 the then UK Minister of Health, Alan Milburn, announced that screening for colorectal cancer would be rolled out nationally (Milburn 2002). As with all screening programmes, follow-up data will take time and the results of the UK MRC flexible sigmoidoscopy trial are awaited (Scholefield & Moss 2003, UK Flexible Sigmoidoscopy Screening Trial Investigators 2002).

Cardin and colleagues (2005) report the outcome of 2014 colonoscopies in patients of whom 976 were aged over 65 years and 148 over 85 years. Colonoscopy was unsuccessful in 26% of older patients (and in 51% this was due to poor pre-procedure preparation). This is considerably greater than the 28% of a total of 12% unsuccessful colonoscopies in those less than 65 years of age. Increasing age was associated with a failed procedure and insufficient cleansing. Being female, an in-patient at the time of investigation, or having a colonoscopy for an indication other than follow-up of a colonic lesion were associated with a higher risk of failure. When studying the completed examinations in older patients, the factors that predicted a clinically important diagnosis were: being male (OR 1.85), out-patient status (OR 1.16), an indication of rectal bleeding or faecal occult bleeding (OR 2.15 and 2.47), further investigation of radiological findings (OR 3.7) or the presence of an abdominal mass on palpation

(OR 2.59). In this study, even without taking full bowel cleansing preparation, a 71.5% completion rate in older individuals was reported (Cardin et al 2005).

In a UK study of 247 colonoscopies performed on 225 patients aged 80 years or over, the main indication for colonoscopy was anaemia. This group found the overall carcinoma rate was 10.1% and numerous therapeutic procedures including polypectomies, metallic stent placement and argon plasma coagulation were also undertaken during colonoscopy. Only one serious complication occurred: the perforation of the sigmoid colon in a 92 year old (Syn et al 2005).

Controversy still exists about the role of CT colonoscopy for detection of colon polyps and cancer. In 2005, Rockey et al (2005) reported a low sensitivity of CT colonoscopy but others have suggested operator variables as a cause of their findings (Ferruci, Working Group on Virtual Colonoscopy 2005).

TREATMENT

Surgery

A meta-analysis using aggregate data broken down by age from 28 independent studies looking at 34194 patients (Colorectal Cancer Collaborative Group 2000a) found that elderly subjects:

- Have an increased frequency of co-morbid conditions
- Present with later stage disease
- Undergo emergency surgery
- Were less likely to undergo curative surgery than younger patients
- Had increased postoperative morbidity and mortality
- Had reduced survival

However, for cancer-specific survival, age-related differences were much less marked because the interrelationship between age and outcome from colorectal cancer surgery is complex. If older patients present with later stage disease and have pre-existing co-morbidity, they will require different surgical intervention.

In 2005, a study of 794 patients (mean age 69 years) showed that laparoscopic-assisted surgery for colorectal cancer is as effective as open surgery in the short term and is likely to produce similar long-term outcomes. While the duration of operation was shorter in the open surgery group, and time to first bowel movement and resuming normal diet were similar, the median hospital stay was 2 days shorter for those who underwent laparoscopic surgery. With further improvements in laparoscopic-assisted surgery, older patients may benefit from a procedure which enables earlier mobilization and return home without any increased morbidity and mortality (Guillou et al 2005).

A major advance in the surgery of rectal cancer has been the concept of total mesorectal excision, with resultant reduction in perioperative morbidity and local recurrence (Cecil et al 2004). Lymph node positive patients may have excellent results with such surgery without the need for postoperative radiotherapy (Simunovic et al 2003).

Adjuvant therapy

Older patients with Dukes' stage B2 or C disease benefit from adjuvant therapy. Elderly trials using 5-fluorouracil (FU) and levamisole showed no alteration in survival in those patients over 60 (Laurie et al 1989, Moertel et al 1995). There was concern that older patients receiving these two drugs may have increased toxicity, but this has not been confirmed. Using pooled data from 3302 patients with stage II and III colon cancer in a multivariate analysis, fluorouracil-based adjuvant therapy showed a beneficial treatment effect across all subsets. The benefits were consistent across gender, location, age, stage of disease and grade of tumour. Therefore older high-risk individuals benefit just as much as younger individuals from adjuvant chemotherapy (Gill et al 2004).

Radiotherapy

The aim of radiotherapy in patients with rectal cancer is to reduce local recurrence and improve survival. Adjuvant radio-chemotherapy is considered standard care for patients with stage II and III rectal cancer, though more recently neo-adjuvant methods have been advocated for stage

II and III patients to improve local tumour control and provide lower morbidity (Gunderson et al 2003). Sauer and colleagues (2004) compared preoperative and postoperative long-term radio-chemotherapy in over 800 patients with a resectable rectal carcinoma. The 5-year local recurrence rates were 6% vs 13% (p = 0.006), though distant recurrence rates and survival were similar in both groups. Preoperative radio-chemotherapy was less toxic than postoperative treatment and preoperative treatment resulted in a down-staging effect with more sphincter preserving procedures possible in this group (39% vs 19%, p = 0.004) (Sauer et al 2004). In 2004, Martenson and colleagues reported the premature termination of a study of adjuvant radiotherapy in colon cancer patients with high risk of local recurrence because of slow recruitment. The median follow up of 6.6 years revealed no difference in disease-free survival and therefore adjuvant radiotherapy cannot be recommended for colon cancer (Martenson et al 2004).

METASTATIC DISEASE

Unfortunately, many patients with colorectal cancer require palliative therapy during the course of their disease. This may be due to metastatic cancer at presentation, local relapse or late metastatic disease. A meta-analysis of 13 randomized controlled trials showed that, in a subset of trials, palliative chemotherapy was associated with a 35% reduction in the risk of death (Colorectal Cancer Collaborative Group 2000b). For an elderly patient, this translated into an absolute improvement in survival of 16% at both 6 and 12 months, and an improvement in median survival of 3.7 months. There is, however, little information on treatment toxicity, symptom control and quality of life. While prolongation of life is a fundamental issue, an extra 3.7 months' median survival must be weighed against the side-effects and inconvenience of palliative chemotherapy.

Newer cytotoxic drugs such as irinotecan or oxaliplatin have shown response rates between 39 and 55% and progression-free survival between 7 and 9 months. The addition of these drugs has resulted in an almost doubling of survival when compared with single-agent fluorouracil (> 20 months vs 11–12 months) (Tournigand et al 2004).

The UKCCCR (United Kingdom Co-ordinating Committee on Cancer Research) has worked hard to ensure that older patients are included in clinical trials of both palliative and curative therapy. Though we remain a long way from full inclusion, their position statement has highlighted the problems and possible solutions (UKCCCR 2000).

Most metastases from colorectal cancer are in the liver. Hepatic resection is useful in younger patients, but there is limited evidence on the tolerability of the procedure in older patients. The only evidence is retrospective and, though it showed no significant differences in morbidity and mortality in patients over 70 years, much of the data were collected in the late 1980s when there was a higher morbidity and mortality than is now acceptable (Fong et al 1995). The resection of both hepatic and/or pulmonary metastases can lead to a 5-year survival rate of 35–58% and a further 15% of patients with liver metastases initially judged to be unresectable will reduce sufficiently with systemic chemotherapy to become resectable and have excellent long-term survival (Fernandez et al 2004).

For the future

A systematic review of randomized controlled trials of the effects of dietary calcium has shown a moderate reduction in recurrent colorectal adenomas (OR 0.74) (Weingarten et al 2004). Data are lacking as to the effects of calcium intake on colorectal cancer but there is some evidence that the protective effect of calcium can be greater when serum levels of 25-hydroxyvitamin D are in the higher range (Grau et al 2003). In the future, older individuals on both calcium and vitamin D as part of a bone-strengthening regime may be reducing their risk of colorectal cancer, though side-effects have made some researchers cautious (Benamouzig & Chaussade 2004).

The most important and cheapest form of prevention of colorectal cancer is a change in lifestyle. Tobacco avoidance, an increase in physical activity and weight control can reduce risk. The role of aspirin and non-steroidal antiinflammatory drugs remains experimental but further data may influence geriatricians' prescribing (Asano & McLeod 2004, Weitz et al 2005).

LUNG

Bronchial carcinoma is a disease particularly of older people. The epidemiology of lung cancer is hampered by poor investigations and a high proportion of death-certificate-only cases reported to cancer registries. Despite this, cancer statistics for 2003 show 172 000 new cases, 157 000 deaths and a 5-year survival rate from 1992–1998 of only 15%. While some series have shown only 50% of cases to occur in patients over 60 years, a Royal College of Physicians lung cancer audit report showed a median age of 69 years for those investigated for suspected lung cancer within 51 participating hospitals. Furthermore, 29% of the men (oldest 92 years) and 27% of women (oldest 94 years) investigated were aged 75 years or above (RCP 1999). Thus the disease is common in the elderly population but doctors are not good at reporting cases. This ageist attitude is prevalent both in primary and secondary care and may partly stem from the poor investigation of patients suspected of having lung cancer (Gosney & Myerscough 1997).

A UK general practice study identified seven symptoms independently associated with lung cancer at the time of clinical presentation. These included haemoptysis, loss of weight, loss of appetite, dyspnoea, thoracic pain, fatigue and cough. In addition, the finding of finger clubbing or thrombocytosis and abnormal spirometry, as well as cigarette smoking, were all independently associated with a cancer diagnosis (Hamilton et al 2005). In this study undertaken in 21 general practices in Exeter and Devon, little data were provided that were different from the list that any undergraduate medical student would use to predict a symptom associated with lung cancer.

Using Royal College of Physicians' data, Peake and colleagues found an overall mortality at 6 months of 58% in those aged 75 years and above vs 42% in those under 65 years. This has been attributed to a lower number undergoing definitive treatment, despite having equivocal stage of disease and histological diagnosis (Peake et al 2003).

INVESTIGATION

Older patients are less likely to undergo bronchoscopy. Perhaps this may be due to a false belief by clinicians that elderly people do not want to be investigated for suspected cancer or they feel that such investigations are too invasive and risky to be undertaken (O'Hickey & Hilton 1987, Slevin et al 1990). The histopathology of tumours in older patients differs from younger subject in that:

- They are less likely to have small cell carcinoma and more likely to have a non-small cell carcinoma
- Older men have a greater than expected proportion of squamous carcinoma
- Older women have a greater than expected proportion of adenocarcinoma

Unfortunately, with increasing age there is less likely to be a histopathological diagnosis in patients suspected of having lung cancer (Watkin et al 1990). Without a definitive diagnosis, it is unlikely that the patient will be referred for definitive therapy. This is not only ageist but also prevents patients from being referred for palliative, as well as curative, treatment.

TREATMENT

Small cell carcinoma accounts for between 10–14% of investigated bronchial tumours but few elderly patients have chemotherapy. The lack of representation is true for both formal chemotherapeutic trials and those patients treated outside clinical trials. The exclusion of patients 65 years of age or above from cancer trials has been addressed (UKCCCR 2000). The pharmaceutical industry is still loath to include older patients in trials, arguing that few elderly patients are free from co-morbidity and that older patients are less likely to be treated in the 'real world'.

Chemotherapy

'Having chemotherapy is awful but having cancer is worse!' Unfortunately, most patients with small cell lung cancer (SCLC) have extensive disease and require palliation. Studies of elderly patients with SCLC receiving chemotherapy vs no therapy or radiation alone have shown that:

- Three-quarters of patients receiving chemotherapy require dose reduction
- Less than half the patients completed all six cycles of chemotherapy
- Chemotherapy is strongly correlated with survival (Shepherd et al 1994)

Since all drugs used in the treatment of SCLC are very toxic, factors such as oral vs IV (Carney & Byrne 1994) and the ability to administer in out-patients rather than the need for in-patient treatment must be considered. Neutropenia is a common side-effect of most agents and patients require careful follow up. There is no evidence that granulocyte-colony stimulating factor, though allowing dose escalations, improves survival and it should therefore not be routinely prescribed (Katakami et al 1996).

For both the limited and extensive stages, SCLC combination chemotherapy remains the cornerstone of treatment. Those individuals with good performance status and limited disease are generally treated with etoposide and cisplatin, plus chest radiotherapy. In general, this provides a 5-year cancer-free survival of 12–25% and a median survival of about 17 months (Janne et al 2002, Turrisi et al 1999). Unfortunately those individuals with extensive disease who received combination chemotherapy had only a median survival of 7 months.

There are many new drugs for the treatment of non-small cell carcinoma of the bronchus and, while any data are better than none, negative trials are seldom reported (Shepherd et al 1996).

Patients with stage IIIB or IV lung cancer who have not previously received chemotherapy were randomized to receive either docetaxel and cisplatin or gemcitabine and docetaxel. About one-third of all individuals responded and there was no difference in time to tumour progression or overall survival. Both groups received granulocyte colony-stimulating factor and despite such intensive therapy the median survival was only 10 months. The study did include some individuals over the age of 75 and the gemcitabine and docetaxel group showed a better toxicity pro-

file, suggesting the need for future work in this area (Georgoulias et al 2001).

The role of vinorelbine as a single agent in older patients with inoperable non-small cell lung cancer has been studied by several groups, but unfortunately despite being a well-tolerated and moderately active drug, the median survival was only 34 weeks (Buccheri & Ferrigno 2000).

Gefitinib has been used for a phase III study of locally advanced or metastatic non-small cell lung cancer. In a study of 1692 patients who received either gefitinib or placebo plus best supportive care, no significant improvement in survival was found for either group. This study is of particular interest, since individuals up to the age of 90 years were included (Thatcher et al 2005).

Surgery

The relative excess of non-small cell carcinoma in older patients should result in older patients being considered for surgical intervention. This may be the only chance of cure but older patients are still poorly represented in surgical series.

Cardiopulmonary complications account for most of the morbidity and mortality from lung resections (Shields 1994). When considering pulmonary reserve it must be remembered that there are age-related changes in forced expiratory volume in 1 second (FEV_1) and forced vital capacity (FVC). Many patients with a primary lung cancer have been or continue to be smokers and the coexistence of other cardiac and pulmonary diseases increases both morbidity and mortality. It is interesting, however, to consider 'what surgical mortality is acceptable in a disease that has a nearly 100% mortality rate?' (Burggen et al 1984). Given the choice, older people may be willing to accept risks that younger groups decline.

The staging of lung cancer is critical to ensure that older patients do not undergo unnecessary 'open and close' thoracotomy and conversely those with curable disease are not deprived of surgery. Many invasive surgical staging interventions such as mediastinoscopy have disadvantages including the need for hospital admission, general anaesthesia and the actual risk of operative complications which is not small. The use of endoscopic ultrasound (EUS)-guided fine-needle aspiration has been seen to prevent 70% of scheduled surgical procedures because of the demonstration of more advanced disease than initially considered. The majority of those procedures cancelled (52%) were due to the finding of lymph node metastases (Annema et al 2005).

Surgery gives the best hope of cure, despite 50% of tumours being unresectable at initial assessment. In older patients the presence of coexisting disease has not discouraged some groups from operating on selected octogenarians in whom the 1-year survival was 86% and the 5-year survival 43% (Pagni et al 1997). Morbidity and mortality have been addressed by groups who have looked particularly at the preoperative preparation of older patients using aggressive perioperative pulmonary toilet and video-directed limited resection. They have found postoperative mortality rates of 4.8% in contrast to 1.6% in the general population but with similar morbidity rates (17.9% vs 15%) (Knott-Craig et al 1997).

Radiotherapy

Most trials of palliative radiotherapy for non-small cell lung cancer (NSCLC) include few patients over 75 years. When elderly patients have been included in trials, the median ages of those studied are often under 70 years suggesting that elderly patients may have been included as a 'token gesture'. In a study by Patterson and colleagues (1998) of 149 patients aged 75–93 years who had had radiotherapy for lung cancer, older people seemed to benefit with 81% treated as outpatients, and haemoptysis and chest pain were well palliated. Although 18% of patients reported side-effects, these were usually mild and self-limiting (Patterson et al 1998). A further area where elderly patients may potentially be given radiotherapy is after resection of a NSCLC. A meta-analysis however, has shown that, whatever age one is, there is no role here for postoperative radiotherapy. Of interest is that the same number of patients were recruited over 65 years of age as those aged 55–59 years (PORT Meta-analysis Trialists Group 1998). This is the only example I know of which has included so many elderly patients in a trial – it is a shame that it showed the intervention to be hazardous!

SURVIVAL

The age of the patient influences survival, with the relative risk of death being greatest in the over-75s; however, these differences disappear after adjusting for case mix and treatment. This improved survival in older people after adjusting for treatment suggests that the lower treatment rates in the elderly group may be the cause of their poorer survival.

Three issues pertinent to lung cancer should also be considered in the management of all tumours in older patients. The first is collusion. The Royal College of Physicians' audit highlighted that 12% of patients were not told their diagnosis (RCP 1999). The reasons given were that the patient had dementia or that the family requested that the patient was not told. This is a trend that many geriatricians resist.

Second, should older patients be managed by geriatricians or by a specialist? Older patients with lung cancer are less likely to be managed by a lung cancer specialist (Muers & Howard 1996). In some cases this may be appropriate (because of poor functional performance, extent of disease and general condition of the patient). However, older patients with suspected lung cancer should not be excluded from high-quality management protocols because of reluctance of the geriatrician to refer or the specialist to take older patients.

The third issue concerns patients in whom a diagnosis of cancer is first made at the time of death. These are patients in whom cancer registry data are only provided at the time of death certification and such patients have generally not been investigated or received active management. While in some cases it may be appropriate that frail or demented patients are managed in primary care, some 'death-certificate-only' registrations will include patients for whom investigation and therapy would have been appropriate.

For the future

The possibility of screening for lung cancer has been considered within the prostate, lung, colorectal, ovarian (PLCO) cancer screening trial. Almost 150 000 participants were enrolled whose ages ranged from 55 to 74 years, and half were randomly assigned to the intervention arm who underwent a single view posterior–anterior chest radiograph. Overall 8.9% were suspicious for lung cancer and the highest rates were found in older individuals and for smokers. Of the 5991 with a positive screen, 206 underwent biopsy examination of which 126 were diagnosed with lung cancer. The positive predictive value was 2.1% and 1.9 cases of lung cancer were detected per 1000 screens. As is hoped with all screening, a high proportion were stage I (44%). The possible use of such screening in the future for older present or previous smokers remains under debate (Oken et al 2005).

PROSTATE CANCER

Prostate cancer is now the most common malignancy to affect older men (Anson & Kirby 1997) and it is the second most common cancer death in males (Kirby & Wager 1997). In England and Wales in 1997 there were 8519 deaths from prostate cancer (ONS 1997) and worldwide 180 000 new cases in 2002 (American Cancer Society 2000). While there was a rapid increase in prostate cancer incidence in the 1980s and early 1990s this has been followed by a decline: the peak probably due to early detection largely attributable to prostate-specific antigen (PSA) testing, and this figure has now reached a plateau (Cookson 2001). High risks for prostate cancer include age and being of African origin. A total of 10% of cancers are thought to be hereditary in nature. However, it is a slowly progressive disease (Harwood 1994) and consequently more men will die with the disease rather than from it (Wolfe & Wolfe 1997).

Newschaffer and colleagues (2000) found only 39% of patients in a prostate cancer cohort to have this as a registered cause of death. Thus older men should be reassured that in the presence of co-morbidity and advancing age, there are competing causes of death (Newschaffer et al 2000).

SCREENING

There is controversy as to whether screening for prostate cancer is worthwhile (Box 40.1). This is not because of problems with screening for early disease but, rather, whether or not active intervention alters patient outcome. Without evidence that radical prostatectomy vs watchful waiting reduces morbidity and mortality, screening may be a waste of valuable resources. However, the management of an elderly man with prostate cancer is expensive and quality of life issues must be considered.

There are only two proven interventions in prostate cancer screening. These are digital rectal examination (Catalona et al 1994, Richie et al 1993) and PSA measurements (Coley et al 1995). Digital rectal examination in older patients has been considered to be poorly received, although evidence shows otherwise (Morgan et al 1998). A review of several studies evaluating rectal examination as a diagnostic tool has shown that the detection rates of prostate cancer vary between 0.1% to 2.5% (Coley et al 1995).

PSA is found in both semen and serum. The levels in the former are much greater than in the latter and thus any process that allows PSA to leak into the blood will cause increased serum levels. Therefore, rectal examination, prostatic biopsy and malignancy may all result in elevated levels. PSA is a protein which is primarily manufactured by the prostatic epithelium. Unfortunately it is

Box 40.1 Controversy over prostate cancer screening

For screening
- Prostate cancer is very common in elderly men
- Allows early detection of cancer
- If the tumour is localized, curative treatment may be possible

Against screening
- Many men die with, rather than from, prostate cancer
- Some tumours may have similar results with watchful waiting rather than active therapy
- Other less differentiated tumours do badly, irrespective of therapy
- Prostate cancer tends to be a disease of older men, thus other causes of death often supervene
- The most cost-effective age group may be elderly men in whom co-existing morbidity prevents aggressive therapy

expressed in the serum in benign and malignant prostate tissue and is neither organ- nor cancer-specific. Inflammation of the prostate and urinary retention may result in elevated serum PSA estimations. Cystoscopy, Foley catheter placement and prostatic biopsy can falsely elevate PSA and therefore blood should not be taken immediately after such activities. There is also controversy about the normal range of PSA with increasing age. Laboratories that consider a higher level to be normal in older men may lead to an underestimation of prostate cancer or may provide false reassurance (Brawer 1995).

Patients on finasteride have an artificially lowered PSA (by an average of 50% after 6 months of therapy) and this must be considered during surveillance follow-up (American Cancer Society 2000).

Up to 20% of significant prostate cancers will have a level below 4.0 ng/mL (Catalona et al 1997). The positive predictive values (PPV) of digital rectal examination alone and PSA alone are 31.4 and 42.1% with a collective PPV of 60.6%, and therefore should be used in combination (Crawford 1997).

Transrectal ultrasound-guided biopsies may be performed under local anaesthetic with a quarter of all investigations being falsely negative (Rodriguez & Terris 1998), though the more biopsies taken the less this occurs.

It has been suggested that the PSA level on commencement of screening is a strong predictor of that individual's eventual risk of being diagnosed with prostate cancer. A PSA < 2.5 ng/mL equates to a 1% chance of being diagnosed with prostate cancer over the next 4 years compared to a 13% chance with a PSA between 2.6 and 4 ng/mL and a 38% chance among men with a PSA of 4.1–10 ng/mL (Smith et al 1996).

TREATMENT

The key to treatment is determining which tumours are safe to be treated by watchful waiting and which require radical therapy. This appears to depend primarily on the differentiation of the tumour, with very aggressive tumours requiring radical therapy and well-differentiated tumours that are slow growing benefiting from a watchful waiting philosophy.

The most common grading system used in prostate cancer is the Gleason system (Gleason 1966). Although this was first published in 1966, few systems have supervened that show superior predictive characteristics. In the Gleason system, there are two numbers: the first represents the primary tumour grade and the second the grading of the next most prevalent glandular area. Thus a combined score is obtained, with a low figure being found in well-differentiated tumours and a score of between 7 and 10 indicating a poorly differentiated tumour. Unfortunately, only 10–20% of prostatic tumours are well differentiated with most being moderately differentiated. A further 10% of patients have poorly-differentiated tumours.

There are four main treatment options:

- Watchful waiting
- Surgery
- Radiation therapy
- Hormonal therapy

Watchful waiting

Many men with a new diagnosis of cancer of the prostate are faced with a variety of treatment options. Patients with low-risk disease may be considered as suitable candidates for watchful waiting. Delays of up to 180 days before undergoing surgery have not been associated with a worse outcome (Freedland et al 2006) and longer periods of expectant management with a mean delay of surgical intervention of 26.5 months for small low-grade tumours have also not been seen to compromise curability (Warlick et al 2006).

Surgery

Radical prostatectomy may affect continence and result in a high incidence of impotence. As operative procedures improve and radical retropubic prostatectomy is replaced by radical peroneal prostatectomy, a shorter hospital stay is necessary. Full recovery is quicker without an abdominal wound, and early mobilization due to diminished postoperative pain is important in the very elderly man. Radical prostatectomy is rarely undertaken if the patient has an expected survival of less than 10 years and patients must be counselled since

50% of them will be rendered impotent by the operation and severe urinary incontinence can occur in up to 20%.

Radiation therapy

External-beam radiation therapy is a potentially curative treatment, particularly for patients with localized small volume tumours (Kish 2001). Radiation proctitis and cystitis occur as either acute or chronic side-effects, as can incontinence and impotence (Shipley et al 1994). There is one study comparing the efficacy of radical prostatectomy vs radiation therapy, though it was heavily criticized for selection bias (Frydenberg et al 1997).

Radiotherapy has a 0.2% treatment-related mortality with 1.9% of severe complications (Shipley et al 1994).

Brachytherapy (percutaneous transperineal placement of radioactive seeds into the prostate) shows excellent early results with T1 (cancer is small and completely inside the gland which feels normal on rectal examination) and T2 (cancer is inside the prostate gland, which is larger and has a lump or a hard area on rectal examination) disease patients with PSA concentrations returning to normal in 98% of cases (Kaye et al 1995).

There is now evidence that neoadjuvant hormonal deprivation in conjunction with external-beam radiation improves local control and survival. Patients with clinical stages I–IV in the absence of nodal disease were, in addition to their conventional external-beam radiation, administered goserelin subcutaneously every 4 weeks starting on the first day of pelvic irradiation and continuing for 3 years. Cyproterone acetate was used to block the initial tumour flare. The 5-year survival was 79% vs 62% for combined therapy vs radiation therapy alone and, of the surviving patients, 85% vs 48% were free of disease at 5 years (Bolla et al 1997).

Hormonal therapy

Hormone therapy has no role in the treatment of early localized prostate cancer. For disseminated disease, symptomatic relief may be provided by hormonal manipulation. Hormone therapy for prostatic cancer works in one of three ways, i.e.

blocking the various steps of androgen production, secretion or its action. Hormone therapy may be administered as the result of an orchidectomy (seldom done) or the administration of various chemical agents.

Luteinizing hormone–releasing hormone (LHRH) analogues

GnRH (gonadotrophin-releasing hormone) analogues reduce levels of testosterone through their action on the pituitary gland. They cause downregulation of GnRH receptors, resulting in the pituitary being refractory to further stimulation, as well as depleting pituitary leutinizing hormone. Current formulations of available GnRH agonists such as goserelin acetate and zoladex require monthly injections and may cause an initial increase in pain from metastases, as just before blocking testosterone production, they stimulate the testes to increase the output of testosterone. Particular care must be taken in patients with metastatic disease, as this flare phenomenon may result in pressure effects, particularly in sites where metastases may cause obstruction (such as the spinal cord). They do, however, avoid the potential increase in cardiovascular deaths, since no antithrombin III increase is seen with goserelin (Blackledge et al 1989, Varenhorst et al 1981). Goserelin, leuprorelin acetate and triptorelin are given by subcutaneous or intramuscular injection every 4 to 12 weeks. Gynaecomastia can be troublesome but testosterone levels should fall to near castration levels within 2 months (Moffat 1999).

Cyproterone acetate has both anti-androgenic and anti-progestogenic properties. It does not, however, suppress gonadotrophin release or androgen production completely.

Flutamide is a non-steroidal anti-androgen that blocks the effect of dihydrotestosterone on the cell nucleus. This, therefore, protects from the initial rise in testosterone levels, as well as permanently blocking the effects of adrenal steroids. Flutamide is given in combination with GnRH agonists, i.e. complete androgen blockade. As with most effective drugs, flutamide is not free from side-effects and diarrhoea may complicate its administration, a particular problem if proctitis is already present. A careful watch must also be made for hepatic dysfunction and a further problem for older patients is the tds dosage of flutamide. Sodium retention may result in oedema. Flutamide also has a high incidence of gynaecomastia (Moffat 1999).

The introduction of casodex (which has a once daily dosing) may further improve compliance in very elderly men and supervene the prescribing of flutamide.

Hormone manipulation results in hot flushes. While this diminishes with time, there are reports of megestrol acetate being used successfully in their obliteration (Loprinzi et al 1994).

In advanced prostate cancer there is evidence to suggest that maximum androgen blockade (MAB) is superior to androgen suppression by drugs or surgery. MAB is obtained by the further addition of an anti-androgen, such as flutamide or cyproterone acetate (Prostate Cancer Trialists' Collaborative Group 2000).

CONCLUSION

Older people account for many cancer cases but few of the treated ones. Ageism stems from many quarters and may even include geriatricians. Evidence for treatment effectiveness is sometimes contradictory. There is a lack of guidelines for the management of older cancer patients but work is now being undertaken to rectify this. Geriatricians must continue to strive to engage others who care for patients with cancer to look at our patients with interest and enthusiasm.

REFERENCES

*** Essential reading; ** recommended reading; * interesting but not vital

Abrams J S, Vena D A, Balz J 1995 Paclitaxel activity in heavily pretreated breast cancer: a National Cancer Institute Treatment Referral Centre trial. Journal of Clinical Oncology 13:2056–2065 *

Albert M 1987 Health screening to promote health for the elderly. Nurse Practitioner 12:42–58 *

American Cancer Society 2000 Cancer facts and figures 2000. American Cancer Society. Atlanta, Georgia *

Annema J T, Versteegh M I, Veselic M et al 2005 Endoscopic ultrasound-guided fine-needle aspiration in the diagnosis and staging of lung cancer and its impact on surgical staging. Journal of Clinical Oncology 23:8357–8361 *

Anson K, Kirby R 1997 Examine the prostate closely. Health and Ageing, March:38–39 *

Asano T K, McLeod R S 2004 Nonsteroidal anti-inflammatory drugs and aspirin for the prevention of colorectal adenomas and cancer: a systematic review. Diseases of the Colon and Rectum 47: 665–673 *

Ballard-Barbash R, Potosky A L, Harlan L C et al 1996 Factors associated with surgical and radiation therapy for early stage breast cancer in older women. Journal of the National Cancer Institute 88: 716–726 *

Benamouzig R, Chaussade S 2004 Calcium supplementation for preventing colorectal cancer: where do we stand? Lancet 364:1197–1199 *

Bennett C, Greenfield S, Avonow H et al 1991 Patterns of care related to age of men with prostate cancer. Cancer 67:2633–2641 *

Bergman L, Dekker G, van Leeuwen F E et al 1991 The effect of age on treatment choice and survival in elderly breast cancer patients. Cancer 67: 2227–2234 *

Blackledge G, Emtage L, Trethowan C et al 1989 'Zoladex' depo vs DES 3 mg/day in advanced prostate cancer: A randomised trial comparing efficacy and tolerability. Journal of Urology 141:347 *

Blanks R G, Moss S M, McGahan C E et al 2000 Effect of NHS breast screening programme on mortality from breast cancer in England and Wales, 1990-8: comparison of observed with predicted mortality. British Medical Journal 321:665–669 *

Bolla M, Gonzalez D, Warde P et al 1997 Improved survival in patients with locally advanced prostate cancer treated with radiotherapy and goserelin. New England Journal of Medicine 337:295–300 *

Brawer M 1995 How to use prostate-specific antigen in the early detection or screening for prostatic carcinoma. CA: A Cancer Journal for Clinicians 45: 148–164 *

Buccheri G, Ferrigno D 2000 Vinorelbine in elderly patients with inoperable nonsmall cell lung carcinoma. Cancer 88:2677–2685 *

Burggen H, Ekroth R, Malmberg R et al 1984 Hospital mortality and long term survival in relation to preoperative function in elderly patients with bronchogenic carcinoma. Annals of Thoracic Surgery 38:633–636 **

Cardin F, Barbato B, Terranova O 2005 Outcomes of safe, simple colonoscopy in older adults. Age and Ageing 34:513–515 *

Carney D N, Byrne A 1994 Etoposide in the treatment of elderly/poor-prognosis patients with small-cell lung cancer. Cancer Chemotherapy and Pharmacology 34:S96–100 *

Catalona W J, Richie J P, Ahmann F R et al 1994 Comparison of digital rectal examination and serum prostate specific antigen in the early detection of prostate cancer: results of a multicenter clinical trial of 6630 men. Journal of Urology 151:1283–1290 *

Catalona W J, Smith D S, Ornstein D K 1997 Prostate cancer detection in men with serum PSA concentrations of 2.6 to 4.0 ng/mL and benign prostate examination: enhancement of specificity with free PSA measurements. Journal of the American Medical Association 277:1452–1455 *

Cecil T D, Sexton R, Moran B J et al 2004 Total mesorectal excision results in low local recurrence rates in lymph node-positive rectal cancer. Diseases of the Colon and Rectum 47:1145–1150 *

Chen H-H, Tabor L, Faggerberg G et al 1995 Effect of breast screening after age 65. Journal of Medical Screening 2:10–14 *

Coley C M, Barry M J, Fleming C et al 1995 Should medicare provide reimbursement for prostate-specific antigen testing for early detection of prostate cancer? Part II: Early detection strategies. Urology 46:125–141 *

Colleoni M, Li S, Gelber R D et al 2005 Relation between chemotherapy dose, oestrogen receptor expression, and body-mass index. Lancet 366:1108–1110 *

Collette H J, Day N E, Rombach J J et al 1984 Evaluation of screening for breast cancer in a non-randomized study (the Dom project) by means of a case-control study. Lancet 1:1224–1226 *

Colorectal Cancer Collaborative Group 2000a Surgery for colorectal cancer in elderly patients – systematic review. Lancet 356:968–974 **

Colorectal Cancer Collaborative Group 2000b Palliative chemotherapy for advanced colorectal cancer – systematic review and meta-analysis. British Medical Journal 321:531–535 ***

Cookson M S 2001 Prostate cancer: screening and early detection. Cancer Control 8:133–139 *

Crawford E D 1997 Prostate Cancer Awareness Week: September 22 to 28, 1997. CA: A Cancer Journal for Clinicians 47:288–296 *

Crawford S M, Atherton F 1994 Lung cancer: histological aspects of diagnosis in England and the south east Netherlands. Journal of Epidemiology and Community Health 48:420–421 *

Crawford S C, Vasey P A, Paul J et al 2005 Does aggressive surgery only benefit patients with less advanced ovarian cancer? Results from an international comparison within the SCOTROC-1 Trial. Journal of Clinical Oncology 23:8802–8811 *

Crivellari D, Bonetti M, Castiglione-Gertsch M et al 2000 Burdens and benefits of adjuvant cyclophosphamide, methotrexate, and fluorouracil and tamoxifen for elderly patients with breast cancer: The international breast cancer study group trial VII. Journal of Clinical Oncology 18:1412–1422 *

Curless R, French J M, Williams G V et al 1994 Colorectal carcinoma: do elderly patients present differently? Age and Ageing 23:102–107 ***

Danaei G, Vander Hoorn S, Lopez A D et al 2005 Causes of cancer in the world: comparative risk assessment of nine behavioural and environmental risk factors. Lancet 366:1784–1793 *

Department of Health 1992 The health of the nation: a stategy for health in England. HMSO, London *

Dizon D S, Weitzen S, Rojan A et al 2006 Two for good measure: six versus eight cycles of carboplatin and paclitaxel as adjuvant treatment for epithelial ovarian cancer. Gynecologic Oncology 100:417–421 *

Earle C C, Schrag D, Neville B A et al 2006 Effect of surgeon specialty on processes of care and outcomes for ovarian cancer patients. Journal of the National Cancer Institute 98:172–180 **

Early Breast Cancer Trialists' Collaborative Group 1992 Systemic treatment of early breast cancer by hormonal, cytotoxic, or immune therapy: 133 randomised trials involving 31 000 recurrences and 24 000 deaths among 75 000 women. Part 1. Lancet 339: 1–15 *

Early Breast Cancer Trialists' Collaborative Group 1998 Tamoxifen for early breast cancer: an overview of the randomised trials. Lancet 351:1451–1467 *

Early Breast Cancer Trialists' Collaborative Group 2000 Favourable and unfavourable effects on long-term survival of radiotherapy for early breast cancer: an overview of the randomised trials. Lancet 355: 1757–1770 *

Early Breast Cancer Trialists' Collaborative Group 2005 Effects of chemotherapy and hormonal therapy for early breast cancer on recurrence and 15-year survival: an overview of the randomised trials. Lancet 365:1687–1717 *

Edwards N I, Jones D A 2000 Uptake of breast cancer screening in older women. Age and Ageing 9: 131–135 **

Ellis M J 2000 Preoperative endocrine therapy for older women with breast cancer: renewed interest in an old idea. Cancer Control 7:557–562 *

Fernandez F G, Drebin J A, Lineham D C et al 2004 Five-year survival after resection of hepatic metastases from colorectal cancer in patients screened by positron emission tomography with F-18 flurodeoxyglucose (FDG-PET). Annals of Surgery 240: 438–447 *

Ferrucci J, Working Group on Virtual Colonoscopy 2005 CT colonography for detection of colon polyps and cancer. Lancet 365:1464–1466 *

FIGO 1986 The new FIGO stage grouping for primary carcinoma of the ovary 1985. Gynecologic Oncology 25:383 *

Fisher B, Anderson S, Redmond C K et al 1995 Reanalysis and results after 12 years of follow-up in a randomized clinical trial comparing total mastectomy with lumpectomy with or without irradiation in the treatment of breast cancer. New England Journal of Medicine 333:1456–1461 *

Fong Y, Blumgart L H, Fortner J G et al 1995 Pancreatic or liver resection for malignancy is safe and effective for the elderly. Annals of Surgery 222: 426–437 *

Forrest P 1986 Breast screening. Report to the Health Ministers of England, Wales, Scotland and Northern Ireland by a working group chaired by P Forrest. HMSO, London **

Freedland S J, Kane C J, Amling C L et al 2006 Delay of radical prostatectomy and risk of biochemical progression in men with low risk prostate cancer. Journal of Urology 175:1298–1303 *

Frydenberg M, Stricker P D, Kaye K W 1997 Prostate cancer diagnosis and management. Lancet 349: 1681–1687 **

Georgoulias V, Papadakis E, Alexopoulos A et al 2001 Platinum-based and non-platinum-based chemotherapy in advanced non-small-cell lung cancer: a randomized multicentre trial. Lancet 357:1478–1484 *

Gill S, Loprinzi C L, Sargent D J et al 2004 Pooled analysis of fluorouracil-based adjuvant therapy for stage II and III colon cancer: who benefits and by how much? Journal of Clinical Oncology 22: 1797–1806 *

Giuliano A E, Kirgan D M, Gunther J M et al 1994 Lymphatic mapping and sentinel lymphadenectomy for breast cancer. Annals of Surgery 220:391–398 *

Gleason D F 1966 Classification of prostatic carcinomas. Cancer Chemotherapy Reports 50:125–128 *

Goodwin J, Sament J, Key C et al 1986 Stage at diagnosis of cancer varies with age of the patient. Journal of the American Geriatrics Society 34:20–26 **

Gosney M 2000 Cancer. In: Crome P, Ford G Drugs and the older population. World Scientific Publishing, Singapore **

Gosney M 2005 The assessment of older people with cancer. Lancet Oncology 6:790–797 ***

Gosney M, Myerscough R 1997 Investigation of suspected lung cancer in the elderly. Age and Ageing 26:47 **

Grau M V, Baron J A, Sandler R S et al 2003 Vitamin D, calcium supplementation and colorectal adenomas: results of a randomized trial. Journal of the National Cancer Institute 95:1765–1771 *

Greenfield S, Blanco V M, Elashoff R M et al 1987 Patterns of care related to age of breast cancer patients. Journal of the American Medical Association, 257:2766–2770 *

Guillou P J, Quirke P, Thorpe H et al 2005 Short-term endpoints of conventional versus laparoscopic-assisted surgery in patients with colorectal cancer (MRC CLASICC trial): multicentre, randomised controlled trial. Lancet 365:1718–1726 *

Gunderson L L, Haddock M G, Schild S E 2003 Rectal cancer preoperative versus postoperative irradiation as a component of adjuvant treatment. Seminars in Radiation Oncology 13:419–432 *

Hamilton W, Peters T J, Round A et al 2005 What are the clinical features of lung cancer before the diagnosis is made? A population based case control study. Thorax 60:1059–1065 *

Harris R P, Fletcher S W, Gonzalez J J et al 1991 Mammography and age: are we targeting the wrong women? A community survey of women and physicians. Cancer 67:2010–2014 **

Harwood R H 1994 Review: should we screen for prostate cancer? Age and Ageing 23:164–168 **

Havlik R J, Yancik R, Long S et al 1994 The National Institute on Aging and the National Cancer Institute SEER collaborative study on comorbidity and early diagnosis of cancer in the elderly. Cancer 74: 2101–2106 *

Holmes F, Hearne E 1981 Cancer stage-to-age relationship: implications of cancer screening in the elderly. Journal of the American Geriatrics Society 19:55–57 **

Hutchins L F, Unger J, Crowley J J et al 1999 Under-representation of patients 65 years of age or older in cancer-treatment trials. New England Journal of Medicine 341:2061–2067 *

ICON Collaborators 1998 ICON2: randomised trial of single-agent carboplatin against three-drug combination of CAP (cyclophosphamide, doxorubicin, and cisplatin) in women with ovarian cancer. Lancet 352:1571–1576 *

Jacobs I J, Skates S J, MacDonald N et al 1999 Screening for ovarian cancer: a pilot randomised controlled trial. Lancet 353:1207–1210 **

Jacobson J A, Danforth D N, Cowan K H et al 1995 Ten year results of a comparison of conservation with mastectomy in the treatment of stage I and II breast cancer. New England Journal of Medicine 332:907–911 *

Janne P A, Freidlin B, Saxman S et al 2002 Twenty-five years of clinical research for patients with limited-stage small cell carcinoma in North America. Cancer 95:1528–1538 *

Katakami N, Takada M, Negoro S et al 1996 Dose escalation study of carboplatin with fixed-dose etoposide plus granulocyte-colony stimulating factor in patients with small cell lung carcinoma. A study of the Lung Cancer Study Group of West Japan. Cancer 77:63–70 *

Kaye K W, Olson D J, Payne J T 1995 Detailed preliminary analysis of [125]Iodine implantation for localized prostate cancer using percutaneous approach. Journal of Urology 153:1020–1025 *

Kiebert G M, de Haes J C J M, van der Velde C J H et al 1991 The impact of breast conserving treatment and mastectomy on the quality of life of early stage breast cancer patients: a review. Journal of Clinical Oncology 9:1059–1070 *

King E S, Resch N, Rimer B et al 1993 Breast cancer screening practices among retirement community women. Preventive Medicine 22:1–19 *

Kirby M, Wager E 1997 Prostate ca: put quality of life first. Health and Ageing, March:42–44 *

Kish J A 2001 Neoadjuvant androgen ablation in localized carcinoma of the prostate. Cancer Control 8:155–162 *

Knott-Craig C J, Howell C E, Parsons B D et al 1997 Improved results in the management of surgical candidates with lung cancer. Annals of Thoracic Surgery 63:1405–1409 *

Larsson S C, Wolk A 2005 Tea consumption and ovarian cancer risk in a population-based cohort. Archives of Internal Medicine 165:2683–2686 *

Laurie J A, Moertel C G, Fleming T R et al 1989 Surgical adjuvant therapy of large bowel carcinoma: an evaluation of levamisole and the combination of levamisole and fluorouracil. Journal of Clinical Oncology 7:1447–1456 *

Loprinzi C L, Michalak J C, Quella S K et al 1994 Megestrol acetate for the prevention of hot flashes. New England Journal of Medicine 331:347–352 *

Mandel J S, Bond J H, Church T R et al 1993 Reducing mortality from colorectal cancer by screening for fecal occult blood. New England Journal of Medicine 328:1365–1371 **

Marchei P, Bianco V, Pignatelli E et al 1996 Adjuvant treatment for breast cancer in the elderly. Anticancer Research 16:911–913 *

Markman M, Lewis J L, Saijo P et al 1993 Epithelial ovarian cancer in the elderly: the Memorial Sloan-Kettering Cancer Center experience. Cancer 71: 634–637 *

Martenson J A, Willett C G, Sargent D J et al 2004 Phase III study of adjuvant chemotherapy and radiation therapy compared with chemotherapy alone in the surgical adjuvant treatment of colon cancer: results of intergroup protocol 0130. Journal of Clinical Oncology 22:3277–3283 *

Milburn A 2002 Winning the fight against cancer. Britain Against Cancer Conference, London, Nov 5. Online. Available: http://www.doh.gov.uk *

Moertel C G, Fleming T R, Macdonald J S et al 1995 Fluorouracil plus levamisole as effective adjuvant therapy after resection of stage III colon carcinoma: a final report. Annals of Internal Medicine 122: 321–326 *

Moffat L E F 1999 Therapeutic choices in prostate cancer. Prescribers' Journal 39:16–23 *

Mor V, Masterson-Allen S, Goldberg R et al 1985 Relationship between age diagnosis and treatments received by cancer patients. Journal of the American Geriatrics Society 33:585–589 **

Mor V, Guadagnoli E, Weitberg A et al 1989 Influence of old age, performance status, medical, and psychosocial status on management of cancer patients. In: Yancik R, Yates J (eds) Cancer in the elderly. Springer, New York, p 127–146 *

Morgan R, Spencer B, King D 1998 Rectal examinations in elderly subjects: attitudes of patients and doctors. Age and Ageing 27:353–356 ***

Morrison J 2005 Advances in the understanding and treatment of ovarian cancer. Journal of the British Menopause Society 11:66–71 *

Muers M F, Howard R A 1996 Management of lung cancer. Thorax 51:557–560 ***

Müller H M, Oberwalder M, Fiegl H et al 2004 Methylation changes in faecal DNA: a marker for colorectal cancer screening? Lancet 363:1283–1285 *

Murray C J L, Lopez A D 1996 The global burden of disease: a comprehensive assessment of mortality and disability from diseases, injuries, and risk factors in 1990 and projected to 2020. Harvard School of Public Health, on behalf of the World Health Organization and the World Bank, Boston *

Muss H B 1994 The role of chemotherapy and adjuvant therapy in the management of breast cancer in older women. Cancer 74:2165–2171 **

Newcomb P A, Storer B E, Morimoto L M et al 2003 Long term efficacy of sigmoidoscopy in reduction of colorectal cancer incidence. Journal of the National Cancer Institute 95:622–625 *

Newschaffer C J, Penberthy L, Desch C E et al 1996 The effect of age and comorbidity in the treatment of elderly women with nonmetastatic breast cancer. Archives of Internal Medicine 156:85–90 *

Newschaffer C J, Otani K, McDonald M K et al 2000 Causes of death in elderly prostate cancer patients and in a comparison nonprostate cancer cohort. Journal of the National Cancer Institute 92: 613–621 *

Office for National Statistics (ONS) 1997 Vital statistics – mortality statistics registered in 1997. England and Wales *

O'Hickey S, Hilton A M 1987 Fibreoptic bronchoscopy in the elderly. Age and Ageing 16:229–233 **

Oken M M, Marcus P M, Hu P 2005 Baseline chest radiograph for lung cancer detection in the randomized Prostate, Lung, Colorectal and Ovarian Cancer Screening Trial. Journal of the National Cancer Institute 97:1832–1839 ***

Pagni S, Federico J A, Ponn R B 1997 Pulmonary resection for lung cancer in octogenarians. Annals of Thoracic Surgery 63:785–789 *

Parmar M K, Ledermann J A, Colombo N et al 2003 Paclitaxel plus platinum-based chemotherapy versus conventional platinum-based chemotherapy in women with relapsed ovarian cancer: the ICON4/AGO-OVAR-2.2 trial. Lancet 361:2094–2095 *

Patterson C J, Hocking M, Bond M et al 1998 Retrospective study of radiotherapy for lung cancer in patients aged 75 years and over. Age and Ageing 27:515–518 ***

Peake M D, Thompson S, Lowe D et al 2003 Ageism in the management of lung cancer. Age and Ageing 32:171–177 ***

PORT Meta-analysis Trialists Group 1998 Postoperative radiotherapy in non-small-cell cancer: systematic review and meta-analysis of individual patient data from nine randomised controlled trials. Lancet 352:257–263 *

Prostate Cancer Trialists' Collaborative Group 2000 Maximum androgen blockade in advanced prostate cancer: an overview of the randomised trials. Lancet 355:1491–1498 *

Richie J P, Ratliffe T L, Catalona W J et al 1993 Effect of patient age on early detection of prostate cancer with serum prostate-specific antigen and digital rectal examination. Neurology 42:365–374 *

Robie P W 1989 Cancer screening in the elderly. Journal of the American Geriatrics Society 37:888–893 *

Rockey D C, Paulson E, Niedzwiecki D et al 2005 Analysis of air contrast barium enema, computed tomographic colonography, and colonoscopy: prospective comparison. Lancet 365:305–311 **

Rodriguez L V, Terris M K 1998 Risks and complications of transrectal ultrasound guided prostate needle biopsy: a prospective study and review of the literature. Journal of Urology 160:2115–2120 *

Royal College of Physicians 1999 Lung cancer: a core data set. RCP, London **

Samet J M, Hunt W C, Key C R et al 1986 Choice of cancer therapy varies with age of patient. Journal of the American Medical Association 255:3385–3390 ***

Sauer R, Becker H, Hohenberger W et al 2004 Preoperative versus postoperative chemoradiotherapy for rectal cancer. New England Journal of Medicine 351:1731–1740 *

Schildkraut J M, Moorman P G, Halabi S et al 2006 Analgesic drug use and risk of ovarian cancer. Epidemiology 17:104–107 *

Schoen R E, Pinsky P F, Weissfeld J P et al 2003 Results of repeat sigmoidoscopy 3 years after a negative examination. Journal of the American Medical Association 290:41–48 *

Scholefield J, Moss S 2003 Screening sigmoidoscopy for colorectal cancer. Lancet 362:1167–1168 *

Shepherd F A, Amdemichael E, Evans W K et al 1994 Treatment of small cell lung cancer in the elderly. Journal of the American Geriatrics Society 42:64–70 **

Shepherd F A, Burkes R, Cormier Y et al 1996 Phase I trial of gemcitabine and cisplatin in advanced non-small cell lung cancer: a preliminary report. Lung Cancer 14:135–144 *

Shields T W 1994 General features and complications of pulmonary resections. In: Shields T W (ed) General thoracic surgery, 4th edn. Williams and Wilkins, Baltimore, p 394–414 *

Shipley W U, Zietman A L, Hanks G E et al 1994 Treatment related sequelae following external beam radiation for prostate cancer: A review of an update in patients with stages T1 and T2 tumour. Journal of Urology 152:1799–1805 *

Silliman R A, Guadagnoli E, Weitgerg A B et al 1989 Age as a predictor of diagnostic and initial treatment intensity in newly diagnosed breast cancer patients. Journal of Gerontology 44:M46–50 *

Simunovic M, Sexton R, Rempel E et al 2003 Optimal preoperative assessment and surgery for rectal cancer may greatly limit the need for radiotherapy. British Journal of Surgery 90:999–1003 *

Slevin M L, Stubbs L, Plant H J et al 1990 Attitudes to chemotherapy: comparing views of patients with cancer with those of doctors, nurses and general public. British Medical Journal 300:1458–1560 **

Smith D S, Catalona W J, Herschman J D 1996 Longitudinal screening for prostate cancer with prostate-specific antigen. Journal of the American Medical Association 276:1309–1315 *

Smith L K, Pope C, Botha J L 2005 Patients' help-seeking experiences and delay in cancer presentation: a qualitative sythesis. Lancet 366:825–831 **

Syn W K, Tandon U, Ahmed M M 2005 Colonoscopy in the very elderly is safe and worthwhile. Age and Ageing 34:510–513

Tabar L, Fagerberg G, Day N E et al 1992 Breast cancer treatment and natural history: new insights from results of screening. Lancet 339:412–414 *

Thatcher N, Chang A, Parikh P et al 2005 Gefitinib plus best supportive care in previously treated patients with refractory advanced non-small-cell lung cancer: results from a randomized, placebo-controlled, multicentre study (Iressa Survival Evaluation in Lung Cancer). Lancet 366:1527–1537 *

Tournigand C, Andre T, Achille E et al 2004 FOLFIRI followed by FOLFOX6 or the reverse sequence in advanced colorectal cancer: a randomised GERCOR study. Journal of Clinical Oncology 22:229–237 *

Turner N J, Hayward R A, Mulley G P et al 1999 Cancer in older age – is it inadequately investigated and treated? British Medical Journal 319:309–312 **

Turrisi A T 3rd, Kim K, Blum R et al 1999 Twice-daily compared with once-daily thoracic radiotherapy in limited small-cell lung cancer treated concurrently with cisplatin and etoposide. New England Journal of Medicine 340:265–271 *

UK Flexible Sigmoidoscopy Screening Trial Investigators 2002 Single flexible sigmoidoscopy screening to prevent colorectal cancer; baseline findings of a UK multicentre randomised trial. Lancet 359: 1291–300 **

UKCCCR 2000 Position paper by the UKCCCR. Elderly Cancer Patients in Clinical Trials Working Group. British Journal of Cancer 82:1–3 ***

van Dongen J A, Bartelink H, Fentiman I S et al 1992 Randomized clinical trial to assess the value of breast conserving therapy in stage I and II breast cancer. EORTC 10801 trial. Journal of the National Cancer Institute Monographs 11:15–18 *

Varenhorst E, Wallentin L, Risberg B 1981 The effects of orchidectomy, oestrogens and cyproterone-acetate on the antithrombin-III concentration in carcinoma of the prostate. Urological Research 9:25–28 *

Veronesi U, Banfi A, Salvadori B et al 1990 Breast conservation is the treatment of choice in small breast cancer: long-term results of a randomised trial. European Journal of Cancer 26:668–670 *

Vogel C L, Wojtukiewicz M Z, Carroll R R et al 2005 First and subsequent cycle use of pegfilgrastim prevents febrile neutropenia in patients with breast cancer: a multicenter, double-blind, placebo-controlled phase III study. Journal of Clinical Oncology 23: 1178–1184 *

Warlick C, Trock B J, Landis P et al 2006 Delayed versus immediate surgical intervention and prostate cancer outcome. Journal of the National Cancer Institute 98:355–357 *

Watkin S W, Hayhurst G K, Green J A 1990 Time trends in the outcome of lung cancer management: a study of 9090 cases diagnosed in the Mersey Region, 1974–1986. British Journal of Cancer 61:590–596 *

Weinberger M, Saunders A F, Samsa G P et al 1991 Breast cancer screening in older women: practices and barriers reported by primary care physicians. Journal of the American Geriatrics Society 39: 22–29 **

Weingarten M A, Zalmanovici A, Yaphe J 2004 Dietary calcium supplementation for preventing colorectal cancer and adenomatous polyps. Cochrane Database of Systematic Reviews, Issue 1. Art. No.: CD 003548. DOI: 10.1002/14651858.CD003548 *

Weitz J, Koch M, Debus J et al 2005 Colorectal cancer. Lancet 365:153–165 **

Winawer S J, Andrews M, Flehinger B et al 1980 Progress report on a controlled trial of fecal occult blood testing for the detection of colorectal neoplasia. Cancer 45:2959–2964 *

Winawer S J, Baldwin M, Herbert E et al 1983 Screening experience with fecal occult blood testing as a function of age. In: Yancik R, Carbone P P (eds) Perspectives on prevention and treatment of cancer in the elderly. Raven Press, New York, p 265–274 **

Wolfe E S, Wolfe W W 1997 Discussion of the controversies associated with prostate cancer screening. Journal of the Royal Society of Health 117:151–155 **

World Health Organization 2002 World health report 2002: reducing risks, promoting healthy life. WHO, Geneva *

Yancik R 1993 Ovarian cancer: age contrasts in incidence, histology, disease stage at diagnosis, and mortality. Cancer 71:517–523 **

Yancik R, Ries L G 1991 Cancer in the aged. An epidemiologic perspective on treatment issues. Cancer 68:2502–2510

SELF-ASSESSMENT QUESTIONS

Are the following statements true or false?

1. Patients with a Dukes' A colonic carcinoma:
   a. Have the highest rate of recurrence
   b. Should have adjuvant chemotherapy
   c. Have no lymph nodes involved
   d. Are unlikely to be found on screening
   e. Account for most cases of colon cancer

2. Megestrol acetate:
  a. Is useful as adjuvant therapy after surgery for breast cancer
  b. Causes nausea and weight loss
  c. Can be used for patients with 'non-breast' malignancies
  d. Should be given before tamoxifen to patients with relapsing breast cancer
  e. Is a better option than surgery for older women

3. In older patients with lung cancer:
  a. Postoperative radiotherapy may be useful
  b. There is an increased incidence of small cell tumours
  c. Histopathological verification decreases with age
  d. There is no role for chemotherapy
  e. Chemotherapy drugs prolong life by at least 2 years

SECTION 8

Vision and hearing

Chapter 41

Ophthalmology

Paul Diggory and Wendy Franks

'The laughing leaves of the tree divide
and screen from seeing and leave in sight
the god pursuing, the maiden hid.'

(Swinburne)

SORE AND RED EYES

In elderly people, eyelid problems are the main cause of sore eyes.

BLEPHARITIS

Blepharitis is caused by blockage and scarring of the meibomian glands behind the lash margin, secondary to staphylococcal infection. These glands secrete an oily film, reducing tear evaporation. The tear film becomes unstable, exposing corneal nerve endings, which results in pain.

- It is the commonest cause of a chronically irritable eye at all ages
- There is reflex increased tear production in response to pain and so paradoxically the complaint may be of a watery eye

Features

Itchy red eye, burning sensation, often watery. Associated with acne rosacea.

Treatment

- Twice-daily cleansing of the lashes with cotton wool soaked in saline or dilute bicarbonate of soda. (Dilute baby shampoo is also effective and does not sting the eyes)
- A 1-month course of broad spectrum antibiotic cream applied twice daily by rubbing into the lashes is occasionally needed
- Tear film supplements
- In severe cases, oral tetracyclines for 3 months

CHALAZION

This is a painless pea-like granuloma of a meibomion gland in the upper or lower lid, secondary to blepharitis. Not to be confused with a stye, which is an acute painful abscess around the base of an eye lash that resolves spontaneously within 10 days.

Treatment
- Incision and curettage

ECTROPION

Ectropion is rolling outwards of the lower eye lid, usually medially.

- Tears pool in the lower lid
- Exposed conjunctiva on the out-turned lid becomes inflamed

Features
Irritable eye with discharge. Mild conjunctival hyperaemia.

Treatment
- Surgery

ENTROPION

Entropion is rolling in of the lower lid. (Upper lid entropion is rare, but may occur in people who have had trachoma.)

- Eye lashes rub against the cornea
- Watery eye
- Redness inferiorly
- Pain
- Corneal ulceration

Features
Mild conjunctival hyperaemia, gritty eye.

Treatment
- Micropore/sellotape eyelid to cheek while awaiting surgery

TEAR FILM PROBLEMS

Tear production

Tear production reduces in old age and in association with systemic disease. Eye closure may be incomplete because of nerve damage, e.g. Bell's palsy or stroke.

Features
Gritty, inflamed eyes.

Treatment
- Artificial tears such as hypromellose drops four to six times daily
- Surgery (tarsorraphy) if eye closure impossible

Blocked tear duct(s)

Features
Painless watery eyes with no discharge (except when an infected lacramal sac [dacrocystitis] causes a painful swelling).

Treatment
- Syringing
- Surgery if syringing is ineffective or there is recurrent dacrocystitis

CONJUNCTIVITIS

Conjunctivitis is usually bilateral and due to bacterial or viral infection.

Features
Very red eyes, often sticky or watery discharge. Generally minor irritation. Vision unaffected.

Treatment
- Simple eye care hygiene, as for blepharitis
- Topical antibiotics – broad spectrum (e.g. chloramphenicol ointment or drops)
- Refer if no improvement in a week to confirm/refute diagnosis

A unilateral red eye is rarely conjunctivitis.

CORNEAL ULCERS

Causes of corneal ulcers include:

- Eyelid abnormalities
- Trauma (demented patients may give no history)
- Dry eye
- Herpes zoster

Features

■ Painful eye with photosensitivity. Reduced vision. Perilimbal (round edge of iris) hyperaemia. Cloudy cornea. Hypopyon (pus in the anterior chamber forming a fluid level).

Treatment

■ Urgent ophthalmological referral for intensive antibiotics or antivirals to prevent scarring or perforation

UNCOMMON CAUSES OF RED EYE IN ELDERLY PEOPLE

IRITIS

If this presents for the first time in old age and is bilateral, it is likely to be associated with systemic disease, classically lymphoma.

Features

■ Painful eye with photophobia
■ Perilimbal hyperaemia
■ Small non-reactive pupil
■ Reduced vision

Treatment

■ Urgent ophthalmological referral
■ Treatment includes mydriatics, topical/systemic steroids and non-steroidal antiinflammatory drugs

ACUTE GLAUCOMA

Acute glaucoma results in sudden painful visual loss.

■ It is a rare condition
■ Pain may be very severe, often with vomiting; some patients, especially those with cognitive impairment, may be admitted with a diagnosis of gastrointestinal disease
■ Can be precipitated by taking anticholinergic drugs systemically or by having the pupil dilated with eye drops

Features

A fixed mid-dilated pupil differentiates acute glaucoma from other causes of red eye. The cornea is cloudy so that the red reflex and the fundus cannot be seen.

Treatment

■ Immediate ophthalmological referral whatever the time of day or night
■ Therapy is to reduce aqueous formation with intravenous acetazolamide (may cause or exacerbate hypokalaemia due to renal tubular actions and/or vomiting) and topical pilocarpine to open the angle and increase aqueous drainage
■ Once the intraocular pressure has fallen, laser iridotomy to both eyes prevents further attacks
■ After iridotomy, anticholinergic drugs and pupil-dilating drops can be prescribed without risk of precipitating further attacks

---

Precipitation of glaucoma by drugs

■ Only acute (narrow angle) glaucoma can be precipitated by anticholinergic drugs
■ Anticholinergic drugs are not contraindicated in chronic simple (open angle) glaucoma

---

BLINDNESS AND VISUAL DISABILITY IN OLD AGE

The four most important causes of blindness and visual disability are:

1. Cataract
2. Macular degeneration
3. Chronic simple (open angle) glaucoma
4. Diabetic eye disease

CATARACT

This is a reversible cause of visual loss but is still the commonest cause of blindness both worldwide and in the UK.

■ Routine ophthalmological referral if symptomatic
■ The results of surgery are so good and the procedure so safe that most ophthalmologists will consider surgery for anyone with symptomatic cataract, regardless of age or general health
■ Surgery is performed under topical anaesthetic drops in stoical patients or local anaesthetic injection in more difficult cases

- If the patient cannot or, because of confusion, will not lie still then surgery must be under general anaesthetic

Features

Slowly progressive opacification of the lens with distance vision loss preceding near vision loss. The lens looks cloudy, dial ophthalmosope to +9 to see spoke-like opacity or central haze. The fundus may be obscured and in severe cases the red reflex lost.

Treatment

- Surgical removal of the anterior capsule and cavity of the lens followed by implantation of a synthetic lens resting on the remaining posterior lens capsule
- Cataract does not recur but the posterior capsule may opacify, reducing visual acuity; laser capsulotomy opens a gap, along the visual axis, in the posterior capsule to restore vision

MACULAR DEGENERATION

'Dry' macular degeneration

- 'Dry' macular degeneration is due to atrophy of the pigment epithelium and the overlying retina
- Visual loss is gradual and predominantly a central scotoma
- Preservation of peripheral vision leaves navigational sight allowing mobility
- Distance vision is often quite good
- Reduced acuity causes difficulty reading and recognizing faces
- Visual prognosis is relatively good and patients should be reassured that they will not go 'completely blind'
- Routine opthalmological referral

Features

Large pale accumulations of debris, called 'drusen', are typically seen at the macula. They resemble hard exudates in appearance. In more severe cases atrophy of the choroid gives the appearance of a large pale round lesion. In some cases the retina at the fovea disappears leaving a macula hole. This can be associated with localized retinal detachment.

Treatment

The Age-Related Eye Disease Study Research Group (2001) produced some evidence that dietary supplements and the combination of high doses of zinc and antioxidant vitamins may slow progression of visual loss in patients with age-related macular degeneration in one eye only.

The daily doses used were:

Vitamin C 500 mg
Vitamin E 400 I
Beta carotene 15 mg
Zinc 80 mg

There is some evidence that lutein 10 mg daily may be beneficial either alone or in combination with antioxidants.

Vitrectomy with intra-vitreal gas injection may close macular holes with good visual recovery.

'Wet' macular degeneration

- This is the more severe form accounting for about 15% of cases
- It is due to the formation of a neovascular membrane underneath the retina. This may invade through the pigment epithelium (the light absorbent layer underneath the photoreceptors), distort the retina and cause scarring
- The membrane is prone to bleed usually causing a thrombosis beneath the retina but occasionally bursting into the vitreous causing sudden visual loss

Features

Visual loss may be rapid with visual distortion. Fundoscopy as for 'dry' but there may be haemorrhage.

Treatment

- Intra-vitreal injection of a monoclonal antibody of vascular endotheilial growth factor (VEGF) inhibitor is effective in producing regression of blood vessels and preventing and reversing visual loss in some cases. Injections need to be repeated every 4–6 weeks indefinitely
- If vitreous haemorrhage has occurred then vitrectomy (removal of the vitreous) may be required
- Surgical removal of the membrane is successful in some cases

■ Optical low visual aids are helpful for most
  cases
■ Visual distortion may herald wet macular
  degeneration of age-related macular
  degeneration – refer urgently

GLAUCOMA

Chronic simple (open angle) glaucoma affects
up to 5% of people over the age of 65 years and
is commoner with increasing age. There is an
increased incidence among family members. First-
degree relatives should be screened by optometrists, at least every 2 years after the age of
40 years.

Most cases are detected by optometrists at routine
sight tests by finding:

■ Raised intraocular pressure (IOP)
■ Visual field defects
■ Optic disc cupping (enlargement of the depres-
  sion in the centre of the optic disc)

'Low-tension glaucoma' with pressures within
the normal range of 10 to 21 mmHg is found in
15% of patients.

Features

Slow irreversible painless visual loss that is
asymptomatic in the early stages. In later stages
there is poor navigational vision despite good
central acuity.

Treatment

Treatment is palliative, not curative. It consists of:

■ Routine ophthalmological referral
■ Eye drops
■ Laser treatment or surgery

Treatment of low-tension glaucoma is difficult,
but if the pressure can be lowered to less than
14 mmHg then progression appears to be halted.
Lowering IOP may be difficult to achieve even
with surgery and/or multiple eye drops. A compromise may have to be made between side-effects
of treatment and ideal IOP.

The choice of drug depends on the type of
glaucoma, response to treatment and systemic
and local side-effects. Polypharmacy and combination preparations are common.

Classes of topical therapy

■ Prostaglandin receptor agonist, e.g. latanoprost
■ Beta antagonists, e.g. timolol
■ Alpha adrenergic agonists, e.g. brimonidine
■ Carbonic anhydrase inhibitors, e.g. dorzolamide
■ Anticholinergics, e.g. pilocarpine

Side-effects of eye drops

■ Eye drops may produce local allergy even after
  months of use. If a red eye develops the drops
  should be stopped or substituted.
■ Absorption from the nasal mucosa, reached via
  the nasolacrimal duct, avoids first pass
  metabolism. Systemic side-effects of any eye
  drop should be considered.
■ Topical beta antagonists are absorbed
  systemically. Many elderly people prescribed
  topical beta antagonists develop respiratory
  impairment, heart failure or bradycardia.

DIABETIC EYE DISEASE

The risk of developing diabetic eye disease
increases with duration of the diabetes mellitus.
Retinal changes are rare before 10 years of disease.
Diabetic patients should receive screening for retinopathy. Sight loss occurs in three ways:

1. *Macular oedema* – Capillaries in the central
   retina leak fluid into the extravascular space
   due to endothelial dysfunction. This causes the
   appearance of hard exudates and swelling of
   the retinal layers. Treatment with laser is successful in reversing and preventing visual loss
   in many cases
2. *Macular ischaemia* – If the macula is ischaemic
   with loss of the capillaries, laser treatment is
   ineffective in preserving sight
3. *Neovascularization* – The formation of new
   blood vessels on the retina and iris can lead to
   haemorrhage, retinal detachment and secondary glaucoma. Visual loss may be complete. If
   neovascularization is detected before complications develop, laser treatment is effective in
   producing regression and preventing sight loss

Fluorescein angiography is used to visualize the
state of the capillaries in diabetic eye disease and
to reveal the extent of neovascularization.

Diabetic eye disease and myocardial infarction

Diabetic retinopathy, with or without neovascularization, is not a contraindication to thrombolytic therapy.

SUDDEN SEVERE LOSS OF VISION

- Temporal arteritis
- Acute anterior ischaemic optic neuropathy
- Central retinal artery occlusion
- Central retinal vein occlusion

Other causes

- Retinal detachment
- Vitreous haemorrhage

TEMPORAL ARTERITIS

Also known as giant cell or cranial arteritis, this is an inflammatory process that occludes small and medium-sized arteries, classically the ophthalmic artery.

Features

Headache, raised erythrocyte sedimentation rate (ESR) (but not always), tenderness of affected arteries, sudden visual loss. Diagnosis may be confirmed by temporal artery biopsy but, because only sections of arteries are affected, diagnosis is generally made without histology.

Treatment

- High-dose steroids (1 mg/kg). Gradual reduction over 1–2 years according to symptoms and ESR
- Concurrent antiosteoporotic drugs should be given (calcium and vitamin D as well as a bisphosphonate)

ACUTE ANTERIOR ISCHAEMIC OPTIC NEUROPATHY

This is a rare, non-inflammatory occlusion of the ophthalmic artery. It is more common in elderly people.

Features

Sudden painless loss of vision, sometimes. No rise in inflammatory markers.

Treatment

- There is no treatment for the condition, which is usually bilateral
- Refer to ophthalmologist for diagnosis, blind registration and low visual aids

CENTRAL RETINAL ARTERY OCCLUSION

Features

Sudden total loss of light perception. Painless unless associated with temporal arteritis. The fundus is pale with a cherry red spot at the macula. The cause is either embolic or associated with temporal arteritis.

Treatment

- Management is as for a stroke
- If embolic, immediate lowering of IOP and ocular massage may rarely dislodge the embolus

CENTRAL RETINAL VEIN OCCLUSION

Features

Sudden painless loss of vision but perception of light retained. Massive haemorrhages can be seen within the retina. Associated with atherosclerosis, hypercoagulability states and raised IOP.

Treatment

- Laser photocoagulation of the retina may prevent further complications such as vitreous haemorrhage or secondary glaucoma
- Antiplatelet/anticoagulant therapy to reduce risk to opposite eye

REFERRAL TO AN OPHTHALMOLOGIST

When making a referral to an ophthalmologist include:

History

- Time course
- Effect of visual loss on function and well-being
- Rate of visual loss
- Other medical problems
- All medication – not just eye drops

Findings

■ Check visual acuity with distance spectacles
■ Describe conjunctiva/cornea/iris/pupil and reactions as appropriate
■ Fundoscopy

WHO NOT TO REFER TO EYE CLINICS

■ *Neurological defects:* Strokes, homonymous field defects (unless for blind registration or visual aids), headaches, migraine and other neurological conditions, which are best assessed by neurologists
■ *Spectacle prescription:* Optometry services in the community provide free eye tests for people over 65 years. The health authority lists optometrists who will do domiciliary visits

Visual acuity (measure in both eyes)

■ Snellen chart line at 6 metres; use distance glasses if appropriate
■ Alternatively 'large newsprint', 'small newsprint', 'count fingers' (CF), 'hand movements' (HM), 'perception of light' (PL), 'no perception of light' (NPL); use reading glasses for near vision
■ A pinhole corrects for refractive error

LOW VISUAL AIDS

These are optical visual aids dispensed by optometrists both in hospital ophthalmology departments and opticians' shops.

Local authorities have a visual impairment team and may assess needs at home.

Aids include:

■ Hand magnifiers
■ Stand magnifiers
■ Scanners linked to computer screens with large fonts
■ Large digit telephone number labels
■ Large digit watches and clocks
■ 'Talking' clocks
■ Templates for cheque or pension book signature placement

FITNESS TO DRIVE

The Driving and Vehicle Licensing Authority visual acuity standard for driving is to be able to read a number plate at 25 yards with or without spectacles and in good light. This equates to a vision of about 6/12 or better on a standard Snellen acuity chart.

If there are visual field defects within 120 degrees horizontally and 40 degrees vertically the Driving and Vehicle Licensing Authority will withdraw the licence to drive regardless of the visual acuity. This typically occurs with glaucoma but may also apply after extensive laser treatment for diabetic retinopathy and in cases of quadrantianopia or hemianopia.

REGISTRATION OF VISUAL IMPAIRMENT OR SEVERE VISUAL IMPAIRMENT

To qualify for registration as visually impaired both eyes must have poor sight.

Visual impairment
Visual acuity in the better eye should be 6/24 or worse. A better visual acuity may be considered if there is a visual field defect.

Severe visual impairment
Visual acuity should be 6/60 or less in the better eye, or the visual field should be restricted to 10 degrees or less.

Benefits and help available

Social services
A visual impairment team assesses need automatically once registered. Benefits available vary between councils, as may time between registration and assessment.

Royal National Institute for the Blind
The Royal National Institute for the Blind has an excellent catalogue of optical and non-optical aids.

Guide dogs
Both the cost of the provision and the keep of the dog are free.

REFERENCES

Age-Related Eye Disease Study Research Group 2001 A randomised, placebo-controlled, clinical trial of high dose supplementation with vitamin C and E, beta carotene, and zinc for age-related macular degeneration and vision loss. Archives of Ophthamology 119:1417–1436

RECOMMENDED READING

Anonymous 2006 Nutritional supplements for macular degeneration. Drug and Therapeutics Bulletin 44: 9–11

Drivers Medical Group 2006 At a glance guide to the current medical standards of fitness to drive. Driver and Vehicle Licensing Agency (DVLA), Swansea. Online. Available: http://www.dvla.gov.uk

Elkington A R, Khaw P T 2004 ABC of eyes. British Medical Association Publications, London

USEFUL ADDRESSES

Driver and Vehicle Licensing Agency (DVLA), Swansea, SA99 1TU. Tel: 01792 783686.
  Website: http://www.dvla.gov.uk
Guide Dogs Association.
  Website: http://www.guidedogs.org.uk
Royal National Institute for the Blind.
  Website: http://www.rnib.org.uk

SELF-ASSESSMENT QUESTIONS

1. Are the following true or false?
   a. Conjunctivitis is a common cause of a painful red eye in elderly people
   b. Patients should be referred for visual impairment registration once one eye has a visual acuity of less than 6/60
   c. Deterioration in visual acuity following cataract extraction may be due to opacification of the posterior lens capsule
   d. Entropion always needs surgical correction
   e. In suspected acute glaucoma, a clear view of the fundus excludes the diagnosis

2. Are the following true or false?
   a. In patients with chronic open-angle glaucoma, nebulized ipratropium bromide should be avoided
   b. Topical beta antagonists for glaucoma should be stopped immediately, without waiting for ophthalmic advice, if a patient has bronchospasm
   c. Patients with severe cardio-respiratory disease should not be referred for cataract surgery
   d. Photodynamic therapy (PDT) is used to treat 'dry' macular degeneration
   e. Patients with macular degeneration should still be considered for cataract extraction to improve peripheral vision

SECTION 8

Vision and hearing

Chapter 42

Hearing disorders

T. A. Roper

'*Foreclosing a conversation which cannot be heard is like foreclosing a mortgage which cannot be paid. The deaf are evicted from the social world as the debtor is evicted from his home.*'

(Bernard Isaacs)

FAMOUS PEOPLE WITH HEARING IMPAIRMENT

Bill Clinton	Former President of the USA
Ronald Reagan	Former President of the USA
Ludwig van Beethoven	Composer
Lou Ferrigno	The Incredible Hulk (TV series)
Leslie Nielson	Actor/Comedian (Naked Gun/Police Squad)
Arnold Palmer	Golfer
Thomas Edison	Inventor

Thomas Edison claimed, with regard to his inventing prowess, that his hearing difficulties helped him concentrate on the task in hand without fear of distraction.

Sadly, not everybody's experience of hearing impairment is as positive as Thomas Edison's. Many people with hearing impairment experience:

- Difficulty following conversation, particularly in noisy environments
- Poor relationships with family and friends
- Problems hearing TV and radio
- Problems enjoying concerts/cinema/theatre
- Anxiety and depression
- Social isolation

PREVALENCE OF HEARING LOSS

The prevalence of hearing loss varies according to the type of survey used. Survey methods have included self-reporting, interview, audiometry or a combination of these. The national study of hearing found that about 16% of the adult population of the UK have hearing loss. The researchers used audiometry and chose a level of hearing loss of 25 decibels (dB) or greater in the better ear as their cut-off point. The prevalence rises with age so that 80% of people aged 75–79 years have hearing impairment according to the above criteria. The RNID report 'A Simple Cure' (RNID 2004) found that 42% of deaf/hearing impaired people found it difficult to communicate with NHS staff. 24% of deaf/hearing impaired people missed at least one appointment due to poor communication and, in 19% of cases, this happened on more than five occasions.

NHS providers have an obligation to make reasonable adjustments to ensure that their services are fully accessible to disabled people under the 1995 Disability Discrimination Act (DDA) which came into force in 2004. If they do not, they risk legal action. The RNID's report demonstrates how vulnerable the NHS is to litigation.

CAUSES OF HEARING LOSS

Sensorineural	Conductive
Presbycusis	Wax
Noise	Otitis externa
Drugs	Otitis media
Ménière's syndrome	Perforated ear drum
Acoustic neuroma	

Presbycusis and wax are the most common problems in old age and so only these will be discussed.

PRESBYCUSIS

(Presbus = old   akoustikos = hearing)

Presbycusis describes the decrease in hearing that occurs with ageing. It is the commonest cause of bilateral sensorineural loss in old age. The exact cause is unknown but a number of mechanisms have been proposed (Willott 1991):

Neural: degeneration of cochlear neurons, particularly in the basal section of the cochlea (the area responsible for high frequency)

Sensory: degeneration of the sensory cells (the organ of Corti) of the cochlea

Vascular: atrophy of the blood supply to the inner ear (striae vascularis)

Mechanical: loss of elasticity of the basilar membrane (the part of the cochlea that vibrates when sound reaches the inner ear)

All the above changes have been demonstrated pathologically, but which ones are primary changes of 'ageing' and which are secondary consequences of these changes is unknown. Further problems exist in studying the aetiology of hearing loss associated with ageing. It is difficult to separate environmental influences such as noise, illness or toxins from changes due to 'ageing' over a lifetime.

WAX

The role that wax plays in hearing impairment has been controversial. Some authorities suggest that wax causes little hearing loss (Gregg 1985, Sharp et al 1990) while others claim that wax can cause clinically significant impairment (Nassar 1980, Warwick-Brown 1986). The studies that show little impact on hearing used audiometry and demonstrated hearing loss of only 5–10 dB. However, as most elderly people have some form of hearing loss, it is reasonable to postulate that the additional burden of impairment caused by impacted wax can be sufficient to increase disproportionately the social handicap to the patient (Hanger & Mulley 1992).

In the UK about 4 million ears are syringed each year (Guest et al 2004). Impacted ear wax may be asymptomatic but may cause other symptoms such as earache, dizziness, vertigo, reflex cough or tinnitus. Despite its high prevalence, the optimal method of dealing with ear wax has not been the subject of rigorous randomized controlled trials. A small percentage can resolve spontaneously, while others may respond to the use of cerumenolytics (wax softeners). A recent Cochrane review highlighted the lack of good trial data and could not recommend any of the many agents outright (Burton & Doree 2003).

If softeners fail, the next step is a mechanical method of removal. A survey in primary care showed that 95% of GP practices use syringing as the treatment of choice (Sharp et al 1990) and 4% used curettage with a Jobson Horne probe, a technique that requires ENT training. Syringing with a metal syringe is no longer recommended, as it is now recognized that the pressures developed by the syringe can be sufficient to perforate the ear drum (particularly if the ear drum is atrophic as a result of ageing). Modern irrigation machines allow a more controlled pressure to be applied in a precise manner. They also deliver this water at the correct temperature to prevent the caloric effect and the precipitation of vertigo. Other complications of syringing include otitis externa, damage to the ear canal and perforation of the eardrum. If syringing fails, patients are usually referred to secondary care. At this stage, cerumen has usually been softened and can be removed by microsuction. Occasionally probes or forceps are used for more stubborn wax.

TINNITUS

Tinnitus is the perception of a sound (or sounds), e.g. whistles, ringing, buzzing, hums, in the ears or head, which are not caused by an external environmental source.

It should be distinguished from auditory hallucinations, where there is synthesis by the brain of sound into recognizable words or music in the absence of an external source. Sometimes, patients are aware of their own physiological processes, such as vascular hums or bruits (called autophony). These sounds should still be called tinnitus until the sound is identified as part of the bodily process.

FAMOUS PEOPLE WITH TINNITUS

William Shatner	Captain Kirk (Star Trek)
Leonard Nimoy	Spock (Star Trek)
Jack Straw	Cabinet Minister, Labour Government
Charles Darwin	British Naturalist
Phil Collins	Vocalist/Drummer
Pete Townshend	Musician (The Who)
Danny McNamara	Vocalist (Embrace)

PREVALENCE OF TINNITUS

Tinnitus is common, despite being relegated to a footnote in many textbooks of geriatric medicine. In a UK national survey, 1 in 3 adults had experienced tinnitus and 1 in 10 of the population had experienced tinnitus that lasted for 5 minutes or more (Davis 1989). Its prevalence increases with age and it is present in 21% of people in the 60–79 year age group. It is associated with (but not the cause of) hearing loss and the degree of distress it causes correlates with the amount of hearing loss.

EFFECTS OF TINNITUS

People with tinnitus complain about:

■ Lack of sleep
■ Inability to concentrate on their work
■ Altered mood, ranging from anxiety to depression
■ Concern that the tinnitus will damage their hearing (which is untrue). Tinnitus may be a marker of hearing loss and some people who present with this symptom are unaware that they have some hearing deficit

CAUSES OF TINNITUS

Physiological	Temporary	Permanent
Vascular hums	Spontaneous	Chronic noise
Exercise	Noise induced,	exposure
Occlusion of	e.g. disco	Ototoxic drugs
ear, e.g.	Drugs, e.g.	Ménière's
by pillow	alcohol,	syndrome
	caffeine,	Acoustic
	aspirin	neuroma
	Hypertension	

Physiological causes (autophony) are usually heard by healthy people when there is silence, especially around bedtime. Temporary causes are those that have been experienced by most people at some time in their lives, e.g. after a loud concert. Alcohol in small doses can relieve tinnitus because of its sedative effects but large binges can cause reversible tinnitus. Aspirin can cause tinnitus but only in high doses. (This was seen commonly in the past when aspirin was used to treat rheumatic fever.)

Any cause of deafness can cause tinnitus.

Occasionally, tinnitus may have a true environmental cause (pseudotinnitus). Suspect this if the noise is only heard in a particular location and especially if someone else can hear the noise as well. You may need to enlist the help of your local environmental officer to confirm that a sound is coming from the environment, e.g. overhead cables, transformers, rumbles from underground pipes, etc.

AURAL REHABILITATION

Most elderly people have sensorineural hearing loss and/or tinnitus which is irreversible. Therefore, as with any rehabilitative process, the aim of aural rehabilitation (in the absence of cure) is to minimize disability and reduce handicap as a result of hearing loss and/or tinnitus. This process has many elements and I will discuss those of tinnitus in more detail than hearing loss (because hearing loss is well covered elsewhere).

HEARING LOSS

1. *Treat a specific disease* if possible, e.g. otitis media, otitis externa with antibiotics, remove obstructive wax.

2. *Amplification*
   'A cheap hearing aid is like a cheap newspaper. It magnifies and distorts but does not discriminate.'
   (Bernard Isaacs)

   Many models of hearing aid exist, including:
   - Body-worn aids
   - Behind-the-ear aids
   - In-the-ear aids
   - Spectacle aids
   - Programmable digital aids

They all have their advantages and disadvantages (for a description of aids, see Corrado 1988, Weinstein 1998). Despite the choice of aids available (they are more limited in the NHS), there are still people who do not use their aids. In a recent MRC trial, 40% of hearing aid users did not use their hearing aid regularly (Smeeth et al 2002). Many people try to use miniature aids (compare with the visually impaired who choose to use contact lenses rather than spectacles). For many people, a hearing aid still stigmatizes them. Interestingly, spectacle users still retain a positive image, e.g. they are regarded as intelligent or 'boffins', whereas the hearing aid user may be regarded as being stupid.

'The miniature hearing aid is the triumph of vanity over utility.'
(Bernard Isaacs)

There are many other reasons why hearing aid users may not comply with their aid, e.g. unrealistic expectations of 'perfect hearing', or the amplification of unwanted sounds. These should be addressed during counselling.

3. *Counselling:* in this context, is to educate patients to let them know how to use their aids and what their limitations are. They will hear sounds that need to be relearned and integrated into the background once more (e.g. fridge noises, clock ticking). In the UK many people's rehabilitation is restricted to the prescription of a hearing aid, because of cost and time restraints.

4. *Lip-reading skills:* can be enhanced to improve the ability to follow a conversation.
   'The patient who says I can't hear you doctor I need my spectacles, teaches the role of vision in hearing.'
   (Bernard Isaacs)

5. *Environmental aids:* these include:

Vibrating clock alarms	Loop systems in banks, concerts, cinemas, etc.
Doorbells that flash	Teletext/ceefax subtitles on TV
Telephone/TV amplifiers	Typetalk – telephone relay service

6. *Joining a support group:* support, information and advice can be gained from the RNID (Tel: 0171 296 8000).

TINNITUS

1. *Treat specific disease* if possible, e.g. Ménière's syndrome with β-histine (Serc), and hypertension with antihypertensive drugs.

2. *Avoid situations* which will aggravate tinnitus, e.g.:
   - loud noises – keep volume low on walkman stereos, wear ear protection in noisy occupations
   - 'absolute silence' as tinnitus sounds are more likely to emerge; try to have gentle background music from a radio or TV and try to keep the mind occupied, e.g. reading, as this will distract the mind from the tinnitus
   - caffeine
   - large amounts of alcohol

3. *Drugs:* these have been disappointing. Lidocaine has been given intravenously or via a grommet into the ear with some short-term relief (from less than 1 hour to several days). Anticonvulsants and tranquilizers have also been tried with limited success. In some cases the tinnitus worsened, or their side-effects made the cure worse than the disease. Sedatives may have a short-term role when insomnia is a problem because they can break the vicious circle of tinnitus (see Fig. 42.1).

4. *Surgery:* this has helped where it has been performed for specific conditions such as otosclerosis. However, when it has been performed purely to cure tinnitus (e.g. dividing the VIIIth nerve), the results are unpredictable and can make the situation worse. It is not recommended.

5. *Masking:* this is the cancelling out of one sound by another, e.g. when you drown out somebody's words by shouting over them. This property is used in tinnitus by employing a noise generator, which can be incorporated into a range of aids (e.g. behind-the-ear, in-the-ear) to blot out the tinnitus. A crude bedside test to see if masking may be of benefit is to tune a radio in between stations so that only static is heard. If the static reduces the loudness of the tinnitus, then masking may be effective. A similar test can be performed by turning a water tap full

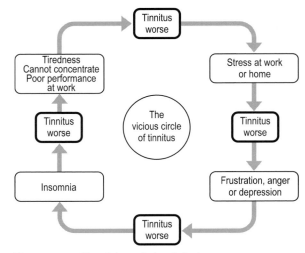

Figure 42.1 The vicious circle of tinnitus.

on. However, audiologists will need to assess patients carefully so that they can prescribe a noise generator at the appropriate loudness and pitch.

6. *Correct hearing loss:* as tinnitus is associated with hearing loss, correcting the hearing by amplification may help through a number of factors:
   - improving the hearing gives a psychological boost
   - background noise, which may mask tinnitus, is also amplified
   - it lessens the attention given to the hearing problem and the tinnitus
   - if proper counselling is given during fitting of the aid this may also improve the tinnitus

> If tinnitus is particularly bad, hearing aids combined with sound generators are available.

7. *Counselling:* this is a major component of rehabilitating the tinnitus sufferer. Education about the condition and what to expect is vital. It aims to get the patient to break the vicious circle that perpetuates tinnitus and to get the brain to reduce its perception of tinnitus so it is perceived as less of a problem (this is called tinnitus retraining therapy)

Part of counselling may involve relaxation, or stress reduction techniques. Some people advocate, for example, hypnotherapy and yoga, and these probably work by diverting the patient's attention from the tinnitus and also by facilitating relaxation.

8. *Joining a support group:* joining a tinnitus support group will help provide support and information for sufferers. There is the British Tinnitus Association (Tel: 0114 279 6600, Website: www.tinnitus.org.uk), which has local branches, and the RNID also has plenty of information.

REFERENCES

Aung T, Mulley G P 2002 10 minute consultation; removal of earwax. British Medical Journal 325:27

Burton M J, Doree C J 2003 Ear drops for the removal of ear wax. The Cochrane Database of Systematic Reviews 3. Art. No.: CD004326. DOI: 10.1002/14651858.CD004326

Corrado O J 1988 Everyday aids and appliances: hearing aids. British Medical Journal 296:33–35

Davis A C 1989 The prevalence of hearing impairment and reported hearing disability among adults in Great Britain. International Journal of Epidemiology 18:911–917

Gregg J B 1985 Ruminations upon cerumen. South Dakota Journal of Medicine 38:23–27

Guest J F, Greener M J, Robinson A C et al 2004 Impacted cerumen: composition, production, epidemiology and management. Quarterly Journal of Medicine 97:477–488

Hanger H C, Mulley G P 1992 Cerumen: its fascination and clinical importance: a review. Journal of the Royal Society of Medicine 85:346–349

Nassar A 1980 Hearing impairment and mental state in the elderly living at home. British Medical Journal 281:1354

Royal National Institute for Deaf People (RNID) 2004 A simple cure. RNID, London

Sharp J F, Wilson J A, Ross L et al 1990 Ear wax removal: a survey of current practice: British Medical Journal 301:1251–1253

Smeeth L, Fletcher A E, Ng E S et al 2002 Reduced hearing, ownership and use of hearing aids in elderly people in the UK – the MRC trial of the assessment and management of older people in the community: a cross-sectional survey. Lancet 359:1466–1470

Warwick-Brown N P 1986 Wax impaction in the ear. Practitioner 230:301

Weinstein B E 1998 Disorders of hearing. In: Tallis R C, Fillit H M, Brocklehurst J C (eds) Brocklehurst's textbook of geriatric medicine and gerontology, 5th edn. WB Saunders, Philadelphia

Willott J F (ed.) 1991 Aging and the auditory system. Whurr, London

RECOMMENDED READING

*** *Essential reading;* ** *recommended reading;* * *interesting but not vital*

Hull R (ed.) 1992 Aural rehabilitation. Chapman and Hall, London ***

Kerr G A (ed.) 1987 Scott-Brown's otolaryngology, 5th edn. Butterworth, Somerset ***

Lysons K 1996 Understanding hearing loss. Jessica Kingsley, London ***

Mackenzie I J 1999 Adult aural rehabilitation. Reviews in Clinical Gerontology 9:73–75 *

Roper T A, Setchfield N 1998 Diagnosis and management of impaired hearing. Geriatric Medicine 28:49–52 **

Roper T A, Setchfield N 1999 Effective rehabilitation in older people with hearing loss. Geriatric Medicine 29(6)19–22 **

SELF–ASSESSMENT QUESTIONS

Not all answers can be found in the text; some can be found from further reading.

1. Are the following true or false?
   a. Presbycusis is the commonest cause of conductive deafness
   b. Wax should be removed prior to assessment of hearing loss with pure tone audiometry
   c. 24% of deaf/hearing impaired people find it difficult to communicate with NHS staff
   d. Ménière's syndrome is not a cause of sensorineural deafness
   e. Tobramycin is a recognized cause of deafness

2. An elderly man says he cannot hear properly and the problem has been worsening for a few months. He now has difficulty conversing and watches television at high volumes. Normally he is a sociable man so he is frustrated and depressed (Aung & Mulley 2002). You find that both external ear canals are occluded with hard wax. Are the following statements true or false?

a. Removal of the impacted wax with a metal syringe is an acceptable method
b. Cough is a symptom of impacted ear wax
c. Perforation of the tympanum is an absolute contraindication to syringing the ear
d. In-vitro, oil-based softeners are superior to water-based softeners
e. Deafness is a recognized complication of cerumen removal

3. Tinnitus. Are the following statements regarding tinnitus true or false?
   a. Tinnitus is an auditory hallucination
   b. Tinnitus is a cause of hearing loss
   c. Low-dose aspirin is a cause of tinnitus
   d. William Shatner (Captain Kirk) and Leonard Nimoy (Spock) suffered tinnitus as a result of an explosion on the set of Star Trek
   e. Masking of the ear is an effective therapy for tinnitus

SECTION 9

Skin

Chapter 43

Pruritus

Michael J. Cheesbrough

*'Tis better than riches to scratch when it itches.'
(Anon.)*

Dermatology has its own language and the terminology used in the field of pruritus is particularly confusing, not only for non-dermatologists but also for practising dermatologists! This chapter will therefore begin with some essential definitions.

DEFINITIONS

The word *pruritus* (Latin past participle of *prurire*, to itch) is used to denote both the symptom of itching, which may be found in many skin conditions, and also as a provisional diagnosis in which itching is the only manifestation.

Itch is more difficult to define. It is generally regarded as a sensation eliciting the desire to scratch. However, as Savin (1998) has pointed out this definition is not entirely satisfactory as there are situations where there is itch without the desire to scratch and conversely where there is scratching without itch.

Prurigo is another imprecise term that is used to refer to intensely itchy papules without an obvious local cause. When qualified it is used more specifically, however, to indicate several itchy skin diseases, e.g. Besnier's prurigo (atopic eczema), prurigo nodularis and subacute prurigo. Prurigo nodularis is a chronic condition producing hemispheric nodules 5.0 to 30 mm in diameter. Subacute prurigo produces smaller lesions. Both are linked to atopic eczema but patients may not show any signs of eczema at the time they present.

Lichenification refers to thickened hyperkeratotic skin and accentuated skin creases which appear as a result of repeated scratching. However, this may occur in the absence of any recognized stimulus when it is called *lichen simplex*. When stimulated by an itchy dermatosis such as atopic eczema it is called *secondary lichenification*.

MECHANISM OF ITCHING

Itching is a common and often very unpleasant symptom which may be socially disabling and adversely affect quality of life. Yet it is not well understood and has not received as much scientific investigation as it merits. Difficulties of investigation include lack of standardized itch stimuli and lack of adequate measurement techniques.

There are many chemical mediators of itching, of which histamine is the most well known. Others include opioid peptides, serotonin, proteases and cytokines. Antihistamines are only likely to be effective treatment where histamine is the pathogenic mediator, e.g. urticaria.

It is thought that there are no specific itch receptors but that itch and pain are detected by unspecialized nerve endings found close to the dermo-epidermal junction.

The traditional view is that itch sensations are passed to the brain by pain fibres but this does not explain certain observations such as the facts that pain and itch can be experienced at the same time, morphine can alleviate pain yet induce itch (see Ch. 16) and itching stimulates scratching, whereas pain induces withdrawal. Recently this view has been challenged and the presence of separate itch and pain fibres has been suggested. It is now thought that itch is transmitted to the spinal cord by a specific group of slow conducting C fibres.

Itch sensations are relayed to the cerebral cortex and positron-emission tomography suggests that itch is perceived in the anterior cingulate cortex and that the premotor and supplementary motor areas are responsible for initiating scratching. There is much room for research into the pathophysiology of itching.

CLINICAL ASPECTS

There are many conditions in which itching is perceived and for practical purposes these can be divided into skin diseases in which there is a visible eruption and other conditions where there is no rash. Often it is easy to decide which category patients fit into but confusion may arise because of secondary signs of scratching (such as excoriations and staphylococcal infection) which may occur in the latter.

Examples of itchy skin conditions are eczema, scabies, urticaria, insect bites and pemphigoid. This chapter will confine itself to those conditions in which there is no rash and these include medical diseases such as liver and kidney failure, polycythaemia rubra vera and lymphomas. Also discussed will be pruritus as a symptom of senescence, psychogenic pruritus and various miscellaneous disorders.

Causes of pruritis

1. Dermatoses, e.g. eczema, scabies, pemphigoid, insect bites and urticaria
2. No visible skin disease:
   - Medical, e.g. uraemia, liver failure, lymphoma, polycythaemia rubra vera and drugs
   - Non-medical, e.g. pruritus of senescence

MEDICAL CAUSES OF PRURITUS

Chronic renal failure
Itching is commonly found in chronic, but not acute, renal failure and is well recognized in dialysis patients. The skin may be dry but may often be visibly quite normal. The pathogenesis is uncertain but suggested factors include attenuation of sweat and sebaceous glands, sprouting of nerve fibres in the skin, raised serum parathyroid hormone, aluminium overload and essential fatty acid deficiency. There appears to be little new work on its pathogenesis in the last 10 years.

The most effective therapy is kidney transplantation.

Cholestasis
As with uraemia, the pathogenesis of cholestatic pruritus has not been elucidated. There is no clear correlation with levels of bile acids. There may be an unknown pruritogenic factor. There is a notion that there may be an inappropriate response to central opioids and this belief is supported by an improvement on taking naloxone, a specific opioid antagonist.

It may be obvious in most patients with cholestatic pruritus that they have liver disease but patients with primary biliary cirrhosis may present with pruritus before they develop jaundice.

Polycythaemia rubra vera

Itching may precede polycythaemia rubra vera or coincide with it. Often the itching may appear when the skin is in contact with water and is sometimes called 'bath-time itch' or 'aquagenic pruritus' and it can be very distressing. The mechanism is not fully known but it may be due to histamine release and the absence of visible skin signs has been attributed to the slow release and low levels of histamine insufficient to cause urticaria but yet adequate to stimulate nerve endings.

Iron deficiency

This is a well-known association of pruritus but is not found in subjects made iron deficient by venesection, and itching may be caused by other factors, such as an underlying disease.

Thyrotoxicosis

Hyperthyroidism causes pruritus without visible signs of skin disease whereas hypothyroidism is thought to cause itching as a result of drying out of the skin.

Diabetes mellitus and malignancy

These conditions are often thought to sometimes present with pruritus without visible skin lesions but the evidence for this is weak.

Pruritus of senescence

This can be almost intolerable to many afflicted patients, yet the cause is usually elusive. In some patients it may be due to dry skin shown by fine scaling and cracking and symptom-relief by emollients. In others, investigation may reveal an underlying medical condition and specific therapy can be offered. An adverse drug reaction should be considered.

Psychogenic pruritus

Scrotal and vulval itching is commonly psychogenic in origin although a burning sensation (as in the 'burning scrotum' syndrome and vulvodynia) are perhaps more common psychogenic genital manifestations. A rare psychogenic form of pruritus is parasitophobia (delusions of parasitic infestation of the skin). Such patients are convinced that they have insects or mites creeping about

---

> **Box 43.1   Investigation of pruritis**
>
> 1. Full history and examination
> 2. Urinalysis
> 3. Blood: urea and electrolytes, liver function tests, full blood count and plasma viscosity, thyroid function tests, ferritin
> 4. Chest X-ray

their body and usually bring 'evidence' in the form of debris contained in a matchbox or other small container. This condition does not respond well to treatment.

Miscellaneous causes

Other causes of pruritus not discussed here include acquired immunodeficiency syndrome, hydroxyethyl starch-induced pruritus, notalgia paraesthetica, and brachioradial pruritus.

INVESTIGATION OF PRURITUS

A full history, examination and investigation are required for patients with pruritus but only simple basic investigations as shown in Box 43.1. If these turn up any pointers, more detailed investigations can be performed.

TREATMENT OF PRURITUS

This is usually only partially successful and most therapies are not evidence based; they are used as a result of custom and practice. If a cause can be identified, treatment of this should be addressed. For symptomatic relief, emollients such as bath oil and rub-on preparations, e.g. petroleum jelly or oily cream, should be applied, particularly if there are signs of dry skin. Low-sedating antihistamines are not usually of any benefit but sedating antihistamines such as chlorphenamine (short-acting) or promethazine (long-acting) may be helpful, particularly at night, mainly due to sedative rather than antihistamine properties. Doxepin sometimes gives effective symptomatic relief; this is generally known as an antidepressant but it also has strong antihistamine properties and is also used as a topical preparation for localized pruritus of any cause. However, there is the danger of excessive drowsiness and drug interactions in elderly patients.

Simple measures such as keeping the home environment cool, application of cold flannels or taking a cool shower can give relief and are clearly safer than drugs. Also alternative therapy such as acupuncture, hypnosis, aromatherapy and massage may be considered.

Empirically I occasionally give a patient with intractable pruritus a short reducing course of oral prednisolone and this may give dramatic relief for a short or prolonged time.

Recent publications record successful treatment for pruritus with rifampicin, ondansetron, ciclosporin and naloxone but these are not yet mainstream therapies.

Lastly, phototherapy with ultraviolet radiation, preferably UVB (ultraviolet B) but sometimes PUVA (psoralen ultraviolet A), can be effective for all forms of pruritus including renal and hepatic disease.

SCOPE FOR RESEARCH

It can be seen from the above account that there are lots of gaps in our knowledge in the subject of pruritus. Further work is needed on the neural pathways of itching, mechanisms of renal and cholestatic pruritus, and the causes of pruritus of senescence. New therapies are needed to provide safe but more effective relief. A geriatrician could well make significant contributions in this field!

Key points

1. Pruritus can mean either the symptom of itching or a diagnosis in which itching is present without any visible skin sign.
2. Medical conditions including uraemia, liver disease and polycythaemia rubra vera are common causes of pruritus.

3. The mechanisms of itching are not well understood, and particularly in pruritus of senescence.
4. Treatments for itching leave much to be desired.
5. There is much scope for research in the pathophysiology and treatment of pruritus.

REFERENCE

Savin J A 1998 How should we define itching? Journal of the American Academy of Dermatology 38:268–269

RECOMMENDED READING

*** *Essential*

Greaves M W 2004 Pruritus. In: Burns D A, Breathnach S M, Cox N et al (eds) Rook's textbook of dermatology, 7th edn. Blackwell Science, Oxford
Johnson G, Sladden M 2005 Scabies: diagnosis and treatment. British Medical Journal 331:619–622
Lapsley P 2005 Itching for a solution. British Medical Journal 330:522
Rees J, Murray C J 2005 Itching for progress. Clinical and Experimental Dermatology 30:471–473
Wojnarowska F, Kirtschig G, Highet A S et al 2002 Guidelines for the management of bullous pemphigoid. British Journal of Dermatology 147:214–221 ***

SELF–ASSESSMENT QUESTION

1. Pruritus: are the following true or false?
   a. Renal transplantation is a common cause of pruritus
   b. Senile pruritus may be psychogenic
   c. The sensation of itch is transmitted by pain fibres
   d. Topical steroids are the first-line treatment for pruritus
   e. Topical steroids are contraindicated in the treatment of pruritus

SECTION 9

Skin

Chapter 44

Leg ulcers

Michael J. Cheesbrough

INTRODUCTION

Leg ulcers affect about 1% of all adults and up to 3.6% of people over the age of 65 years. They can cause deterioration of general health and impairment of quality of life through pain, social isolation, depression and reduced mobility.

Geriatricians usually see leg ulcers as an incidental finding rather than as a presenting problem. However, leg ulcers are a challenge of holistic medicine rather than simply a problem of wound care. Geriatricians can contribute much to the care of their leg ulcer patients as they have the skills to assess *all* the health problems of the elderly patients and plan comprehensive care.

WHAT SKILLS DO GERIATRICIANS NEED TO TREAT PATIENTS WITH LEG ULCERS?

Geriatricians should be able to assess patients with leg ulcers, start treatment, deal with aspects of general health and know when to refer to dermatologists or vascular surgeons.

ASSESSMENT

Leg ulcers are often badly treated and generally this is because of inadequate assessment. Many doctors are bewildered by the large number of dressings available; they may assume that a detailed knowledge of wound care is a prerequisite for dealing with leg ulcers and so shy away from involvement.

In fact, expertise and knowledge of dressings are much less important than the ability to perform a meticulous assessment.

A leg ulcer is both a symptom and a sign, not a disease. In every case, therefore, the underlying aetiology must be evaluated before rational treatment can be planned.

90% of leg ulcers are vascular in origin of which about 70% are venous, 5% arterial and 15% mixed. The remaining 10% include such causes as skin cancers (e.g. basal cell carcinoma and squamous carcinoma), pyoderma gangrenosum, vasculitis, trauma and infection (Box 44.1).

Secondary factors such as immobility, leg oedema, anaemia and sleeping in a chair instead of going to bed are important contributory causes.

Box 44.1   Main causes of leg ulcers

90% vascular of which:
    70% venous
    15% mixed
    5% arterial
10% non-vascular

A competent assessment should produce a primary diagnosis, e.g. venous or arterial, and relevant secondary diagnoses, and doctors should commit themselves to a diagnosis. This simply involves taking a history and doing a full medical examination. Investigation and treatment then follow logically; all too frequently common sense and good medicine disappear at the sight of a leg ulcer!

Venous ulcers are due to ambulatory hypertension which means that the hydrostatic pressure in the leg veins is higher than normal and there is no reduction in pressure on exercise of the leg muscles. Venous hypertension is transmitted from the veins to the capillaries and produces skin damage. The precise mechanism of ulceration is not known and there are various theories (Box 44.2).

The cause of venous hypertension is either venous obstruction (usually post-thrombotic) or reflux (regurgitation) due to valvular dysfunction. Ulceration can occur as a result of reflux in either the deep or superficial veins or a combination of both. Before operating on incompetent superficial (varicose) veins it is essential that the surgeon checks that the varicose veins are the cause of the ulcer and not a consequence of deep vein obstruction; in the latter case the varicose veins are an essential route for venous return!

Arterial ulcers are usually caused by arteriosclerosis in large and medium arteries which produces ischaemia in the limb. Classically, arterial ulcers are described as occurring distally, in the foot, but in fact they may be found in the lower third of the leg which is where venous ulcers are found. Diabetics may develop small vessel disease, as well as medium and large vessel ischaemia (Box 44.3).

As venous disease is the commonest cause of leg ulceration most of this chapter will concentrate on this. Diagnosis of venous ulceration should be based on positive clinical features (see Box 44.2) supplemented by non-invasive testing e.g. hand-held Doppler, duplex scanning and plethysmography. Details of these methods will be found in the Recommended Reading at the end of the chapter.

The hand-held Doppler instrument is a clinical tool for checking venous and arterial flow. It is used to measure the systolic arterial pressure in the foot and it is also useful in skilled hands to assess venous obstruction and reflux. Duplex scanning (ultrasonography) is now the standard non-invasive tool for venous assessment and with plethysmography is normally found in a vascular laboratory. With colour coding it can show veins and arteries, whether there is flow, in which direction, and with what velocity.

These and other tools are mainly employed for pre- and post-surgical assessment to clarify anatomy and pathophysiology. However, where there is doubt as to the diagnosis, such as whether the patient's symptoms and signs can be explained by the clinical diagnosis, it may be helpful to refer patients to the vascular laboratory, even if surgery is not contemplated.

Box 44.2   Signs of venous disease

1. Gaiter area of the leg
2. Eczema
3. Ankle flare
4. Lipodermatosclerosis (thickening of the dermis and subcutis due to fibrosis)
5. Varicose veins
6. Atrophie blanche (white shiny scar tissue with stippled telangiectasia within)

Box 44.3   Signs of arterial ulcers

1. 'Punched out' appearance
2. Deep ulceration, sometimes down to tendons
3. Poorly perfused ulcer bed
4. Cold legs
5. Shiny taut skin
6. Dependent rubor
7. Pale or blue feet, white on elevation
8. Gangrenous toes

Venography has very little part to play in the diagnosis of venous disease as it is invasive and only shows anatomy; it provides little information about function.

The CEAP Classification (Porter & Moneta 1995) takes into account the clinical features (C), aetiology (E), anatomical distribution (A) and pathophysiological dysfunction (P). The clinical classification is based on clinical signs of chronic venous disease in increasing severity of disease. These include:

- Class 0: No signs of venous disease
- Class 1: Telangiectases or reticular veins
- Class 2: Varicose veins
- Class 3: Oedema
- Class 4: Skin changes, e.g. pigmentation, venous eczema, induration (lipodermatosclerosis)
- Class 5: Healed ulceration
- Class 6: Active ulceration

WHAT ARE THE COMPLICATIONS OF LEG ULCERS?

Pain

It was thought that only arterial ulcers were painful, but in fact all ulcers, including venous, can be painful and patients should be offered analgesia appropriate to their suffering. This often includes opiates.

Anaemia

This should be suspected in every leg ulcer as ulceration itself can cause the anaemia of chronic disease. Also some ulcers cause anaemia due to bleeding. Elderly patients are often anaemic for other reasons and since anaemia can cause fatigue, cardiac failure and contribute to oedema, it should be investigated and treated where possible. Contrary to long-held belief there is no evidence that normovolaemic anaemia retards wound healing, unlike poor perfusion (Jonsson et al 1991).

Depression

This may be characterized by apathy and self-neglect and such patients may need anti-depressants.

Dermatitis

Leg ulceration may lead to dermatitis (eczema). This may be localized around the wound due to irritation from exudate or may be more extensive. The usual explanation for the latter is 'secondary sensitization' though the mechanism is speculative.

Therefore the non-ulcerated skin requires care and attention by the use of simple emollients (e.g. yellow soft paraffin) or a paste (e.g. Lassar's paste) around the ulcer edge and topical steroids to heal active eczema. However, patients may become sensitized to their dressings and this should be considered whenever dermatitis develops. Contact allergy can be minimized by using non-sensitizing dressings. If suspected, it needs investigation by patch testing.

Ankle stiffness

Chronic leg ulceration often leads to stiffness and immobility of the ankle. The precise mechanism is uncertain, but efforts should be made to prevent and treat this. In particular, patients must be advised to walk properly and not hold their ankle rigid, as this reduces or abolishes the calf muscle pump. This pump is essential for venous return.

TREATMENT OF LEG ULCERS

> 'It's not what you do with the ulcer that's important, it's what you do with the leg.'
>
> (Mortimer & Burnand 2004)

Once a diagnosis has been made treatment is usually straightforward. Thus, venous ulcers require reduction of venous pressure by compression or postural drainage; patients with arterial ulcers should be referred to a vascular surgeon and anaemia needs investigating and correcting. The reason for sleeping downstairs in a chair should be investigated so that patients can be enabled to lie flat at night.

Risk factors for poor healing
■ Large ulcer (> 10 cm)
■ Long-standing ulcer (> 1 year)
■ Immobility of the patient
■ Immobile ankle joint

Compression and postural drainage are the basic tools for treating venous ulcers. The purpose of postural drainage is to reduce gravitational oedema. It may be used before compression or as adjuvant therapy. Whatever the cause of leg ulcers, they will not heal if waterlogged. It is important in the initial assessment to determine whether oedema is peripheral (gravitational), which should respond to postural drainage or compression, or central in origin (e.g. heart failure or hypoprotein-aemia), in which case diuretics or more specific therapy may be needed.

The simplest way of arranging postural drainage is to put the patient to bed. This reduces the venous pressure and reverses the hydrostatic forces causing the oedema. Geriatricians are often reluctant to recommend this because of the known hazards of bed rest. However, I usually prescribe *modified bed rest* which allows the patient up for the toilet and meals and exercise but ensures the horizontal posture for about 20 out of every 24 hours. Standing and sitting are strongly discouraged. If this regimen is hard for patients to follow at home I would admit them to hospital. Usually only a few days of postural drainage are required to clear the oedema, after which compression therapy can be introduced and the patient sent home.

Sometimes compression therapy alone will clear leg oedema, in which case postural drainage is not required (other than sleeping flat at night). However, compression bandaging will need changing daily at first until the oedema resolves. After this, once-weekly therapy is usually all that is necessary. Bandages are sometimes changed too frequently; this causes wastage of nursing time and material costs as well as damage to delicate new epithelium.

Compression therapy reduces venous hypertension, reduces healing times and increases healing rates. How it works at the microscopic level is uncertain but at the macroscopic level it improves venous haemodynamics.

There are several methods of achieving compression therapy; all are effective if applied correctly. Four-layer bandaging is the most well known. Other methods include use of long-stretch bandages, short-stretch bandages, Unna's boot

(an American expression indicating a non-elastic casing), intermittent pneumatic compression and elastic stockings over a primary dressing.

Important points to consider with compression therapy are:

■ It should be applied by trained personnel; these are usually nurses but may be relatives, carers or patients themselves.

■ Short-stretch bandages are easier to apply than long-stretch bandages and are less likely to cause ischaemia at night.

■ It should not be applied to ischaemic legs. The arterial circulation to the limb should be assessed first by clinical history and examination, and calculation of the ankle–brachial pressure index (ABPI). To do this, the systolic blood pressures in the arm and foot (usually measured with a hand-held Doppler machine) are compared.

$$ABPI = \frac{\text{Foot systolic BP}}{\text{Brachial systolic BP}}$$

In a normal individual the ABPI will be about 1.1. If the ABPI is less than 0.8 extreme caution should be exercised when considering the application of compression therapy because of the risk of aggravating arterial ischaemia. The worst case scenario is the development of iatrogenic gangrene.

■ If the ABPI is more than 1.5 do not assume that the arterial circulation is satisfactory; it means that the arteries are non-compressible, possibly calcified, and the limb may actually be ischaemic. This situation is usually found in diabetics.

■ All doctors and nurses treating leg ulcer patients should know how to use the hand-held Doppler machine.

■ The degree of compression achieved is proportional to the number of compression layers.

■ Compression is accentuated over bony prominences and reduced in hollows, so padding (e.g. orthopaedic wool which is applied under plaster of Paris) is required to even out the degree of compression.

- The amount of compression is inversely proportional to the size of the leg so there is a danger of too much compression on thin legs and too little on large limbs.

What should I put on the ulcer itself?

The dressing applied to the ulcer is called the primary dressing and all the other pads and bandages are called secondary dressings. There is no evidence to show that the choice of primary dressing affects healing rates and choice is therefore determined by other considerations.

In the original 4-layer system a simple non-adherent (NA) dressing was applied directly on to the ulcer, followed by orthopaedic wool and a light cotton bandage to hold it in place. These were chosen as they were cheap, easily accessible, non-sensitizing, not painful to remove, easily removed, and absorbent. The two elastic layers cover these dressings.

Wounds heal best if kept moist and warm and disturbed as little as possible. Unless wound discharge is heavy, dressings can be left in place for 2 weeks at a time. Unfortunately, many are changed too often to the detriment of the ulcer and the nurse's time.

It is possible to manage with only NA dressings and absorbent wool. However, a small range of primary dressings allows more flexibility. If the wound discharges a lot, the normal surrounding skin should be protected with paste, e.g. ichthammol or Lassar's paste. If there is secondary eczema a topical steroid may be used. For dry skin on the leg, liquid paraffin or yellow soft paraffin will protect and hydrate the affected skin.

What if the ulcer is infected?

A lot of money is wasted taking and analysing bacteriology swabs. All ulcers will be contaminated with bacteria and it is not possible or desirable to achieve a sterile ulcer bed.

Topical antibiotics should be avoided as they encourage bacterial resistance, sensitize and cause contact dermatitis. They do not aid healing.

If cellulitis develops, systemic antibiotics are required. Since the cause is usually *Staphylococcus aureus* or β-haemolytic *Streptococcus*, oral or intravenous flucloxacillin is required in most cases.

Almost more important than antibiotics for tissue infection is *elevation of the affected limb*. This simple but essential measure is sadly often neglected. It is a well-known surgical principle that infected limbs should be elevated and this reduces pain and oedema. It is the author's experience that a patient with cellulitis of the leg who is nursed in a chair may fail to resolve despite appropriate antibiotic therapy, only to get better on elevation of the limb. There does not, however, appear to be any published evidence to support this intervention.

How should I deal with slough?

The first task is drainage of oedema. If this is not eliminated and controlled, removal of slough is almost impossible. I presume this is because natural elimination of slough is promoted by autolysis which is an oxygen-dependent process. Once the oedema is drained, slough can be removed in one of several ways, e.g. surgical debridement, autolysis aided by an interactive dressing (such as an alginate or hydrocolloid), or lastly larval (maggot) therapy. A combination of methods can also be used.

Larva therapy is efficient, quick-acting and cost-effective (Thomas et al 1998). It is well tolerated by most patients though some are squeamish. The larvae can be ordered from Bridgend (The Surgical Materials Testing Laboratory, Bridgend and District Trust, Prince of Wales Hospital, Coity Road, Bridgend, CF31 1RQ) and arrive within 48 hours. They are applied carefully to the ulcer bed and the surrounding skin is covered and protected with a hydrocolloid dressing cut to the shape of the ulcer in order to confine the larvae to the ulcer bed. The wound is covered with gauze padding and a light bandage. It is important that the coverings are breathable otherwise the maggots die. The dressings are normally removed after 3 days by which time they will have visibly grown. They are then easily removed from the wound manually or by irrigation and placed in a yellow bag for disposal.

The sterile blow-fly maggots chosen for wound therapy are harmless to living tissue and do not metamorphose into flies in the time between application and disposal.

WHAT ARE THE GENERAL HEALTH ISSUES?

A holistic assessment of leg ulcer patients will reveal factors that affect the ability to heal and that can be ameliorated. Examples are:

■ Anaemia: this may be secondary to the ulcer itself and may require blood transfusion but may also be due to coincidental causes such as poor diet or bleeding. Appropriate investigation and correction will aid healing of the ulcer.
■ A poor diet may result from apathy, immobility, dementia, poverty or ignorance.
■ Immobility is common in leg ulcer patients and may be due to arthritis, obesity, stroke or an assumption that 'rest' is good for the healing of ulcers.
■ One textbook states that all patients with leg ulcers should have a rectal examination! This may seem extreme but abdominal palpation is desirable since pelvic tumours can cause venous obstruction and are potentially treatable.

Causes of non-healing

■ Inadequate assessment
■ Inadequate compression
■ Persistent oedema
■ Calcification in the ulcer bed; causes a mechanical barrier to vascularization

---

WHEN SHOULD I REFER A PATIENT WITH A LEG ULCER?

If initial assessment suggests a leg ulcer is venous in origin, with no complications, treatment can be instituted immediately via district or practice nurses. Indications for referral to a dermatologist would include non-healing after 3 months of compression therapy, development of dermatitis or doubt as to the diagnosis. All patients with

arterial ulcers should be referred to a vascular surgeon for assessment and possible surgical intervention (e.g. angioplasty, arterial bypass or arterial reconstruction).

SURGERY FOR VENOUS LEG ULCERS

Generally surgeons do not like operating on legs with active ulcers so it is better to try and heal the ulcer by compression and then consider a surgical referral. In theory, operating on incompetent major superficial and perforating veins should help with preventing recurrence and there is some evidence to support this (Barwell et al 2004). However, surgery to deep veins is still experimental. If you think a patient with a healed leg ulcer is medically fit for and prepared to consider surgery, I suggest referral to a vascular surgeon with an interest in veins for an opinion in the first instance. Normally duplex scanning will be required before undertaking venous surgery.

HOW SHOULD LEG ULCER SERVICES BE ORGANIZED?

This is controversial but the trend is towards more patients with leg ulcers being assessed and treated at home or in locality clinics and referral to hospital only for those patients with complicated problems or who fail to respond to therapy.

There is agreement in the need for training and some universities offer courses that cover the theory and practice of leg ulcer management (ENB N18). A nurse leg ulcer specialist would be expected to have this qualification.

One successful model of care is the setting up of three or four locality clinics staffed by nurse specialists, where patients are assessed and their treatment planned. This is then implemented by district or practice nurses. The skills of the community nurses are developed and enlarged by systematic training carried out by the nurse specialists.

Key points

1. Full assessment is the priority in the management of patients with leg ulcers.

---

2. 90% of leg ulcers are vascular in origin and 70% are venous. Therefore a vascular diagnosis should be made in these cases.
3. Most patients with leg ulcers can be managed by geriatricians, as part of a multidisciplinary team.
4. Patients with arterial ulcers should be referred to a vascular surgeon, and those without a diagnosis, those who fail to improve with treatment, and those with a non-vascular cause should be referred to a dermatologist.
5. The mainstay of therapy for venous ulcers is compression therapy.

REFERENCES

Barwell, Davies C E, Deacon J et al 2004 The ESCHAR venous ulcer study: a randomized controlled trial assessing venous surgery in 500 leg ulcers. Lancet 363:1854–1859

Jonsson K, Jensen A, Goodson W H et al 1991 Tissue oxygenation, anaemia, and perfusion in relation to wound healing in surgical patients. Annals of Surgery 214:605–613

Mortimer P S, Burnand K G 2004 Diseases of the veins and arteries: leg ulcer. In: Burns T, Breathnach S, Cox N et al (eds) Rook's textbook of dermatology. Blackwell Science, Malden, MA, p 50.41

Porter J M, Moneta G L 1995 Reporting standards in venous disease: an update. International Consensus Committee on Chronic Venous Disease. Journal of Vascular Surgery 21:635–645

Thomas S, Andrews A, Jones M 1998 The use of larval therapy in wound management. Journal of Wound Care 7:521–524

RECOMMENDED READING

*** Essential reading; ** recommended reading; * interesting but not vital

Ruckley C V, Fowkes F G R, Bradbury A W 1999 Venous disease: epidemiology, management and delivery of care. Springer-Verlag, London ***
This is a 270 page text covering every aspect of venous disease and essential reading for every clinician concerned with the management of venous leg ulcers.

Lunt M J 1999 Review of duplex and colour Doppler imaging of lower-limb arteries and veins. Journal of Tissue Viability 9(2):45–55 ***
Ultrasonic imaging is the mainstay of non-invasive imaging of the venous and arterial systems and this article describes the theory, techniques, strengths and limitations of ultrasonography.

Royal College of Nursing 1998 Clinical practice guidelines: the management of patients with venous leg ulcers. Recommendations for assessment, compression therapy, cleansing, debridement, dressing, contact sensitivity, training/education and quality assurance. RCN Institute, Centre of Evidence-Based Nursing, University of York and the School of Nursing, Midwifery and Health Visiting, University of Manchester ***
This booklet gives straightforward guidelines for the management of all aspects of venous leg ulcers with comprehensive references and evidence tables. It also includes the 'Effective Health Care' bulletin on compression therapy.

International Task Force 1999 The management of chronic venous disorders of the leg: an evidence-based report of an international task force. Phlebology 14(Suppl 1):1–126 **
This is more comprehensive than the clinical practice guidelines (RCN 1998 above) and deals with epidemiology, economic outcomes, clinical outcomes and quality of life, diagnosis and treatment as well as highlighting priorities for research.

Mortimer P S, Burnand K G 2004 Diseases of the veins and arteries: leg ulcers. In: Burns T, Breathnach S, Cox N et al (eds) Rook's textbook of dermatology. Blackwell Science, Malden, MA, Ch. 50 *
This is a good overview of pathology, diagnosis and management of leg ulcers.

SELF-ASSESSMENT QUESTIONS

Are the following statements true or false?

1. Leg ulcers are mostly venous in origin
2. Compression is the first-line treatment for all leg ulcers
3. Skin cancers do not present as leg ulcers
4. Biopsy should be considered in all patients with leg ulcers
5. Lipodermatosclerosis is a sign of arterial disease

SECTION 10

Infection

Chapter 45

Preventing infections
Clostridium difficile infection, methicillin–resistant *Staphylococcus aureus*, influenza and pnuemococcal bacteraemia

Rhian Jones, Mark Wilcox, Oliver J. Corrado, Sheldon Stone

INTRODUCTION

Healthcare-associated infections (HCAIs) are a common, often serious and increasing problem, that particularly affect older people. The term HCAI refers to infections acquired during or as a result of an episode of healthcare (usually an in-patient admission). They are often caused by microorganisms that are resistant to multiple antibiotics. HCAI is associated with excess morbidity and mortality and may affect up to 10% of hospital in-patients, and up to 17% of elderly medical in-patients. Each case of HCAI triples the cost of a hospital admission, mainly due to an increased length of stay in hospital that averages 11 days per case.

In 2003 a report by the Chief Medical Officer entitled *Winning Ways* was published (Chief Medical Officer 2003). This aimed to reduce HCAIs and to curb the proliferation of antibiotic-resistant organisms by the strengthening of basic infection control practices, emphasizing hygiene and cleanliness, surveillance of HCAI and antimicrobial resistance, and prudent use of antibiotics. The

Department of Health has recently required all trusts to sign up to 'Saving Lives', a programme that will embed into clinical governance five 'high impact' interventions intended to reduce HCAIs. These are urinary catheter care, intravenous line care, wound care, aseptic technique and ventilator care. There is now national mandatory reporting by all NHS trusts of methicillin-resistant *Staphylococcus aureus* (MRSA) bloodstream infections (bacteraemias) and *Clostridium difficile* infections (CDIs), both of which are especially common in elderly patients.

Prevalence rates of MRSA infection increased markedly during the 1990s, but have plateaued at a high level in the last few years. In the UK, 7212 cases of MRSA bacteraemia were reported in 2004/2005. MRSA is now responsible for up to 70% and 50% of staphylococcal wound infections and bacteraemias, respectively. Reports of CDI continue to increase. In 1990 there were < 1000 cases of CDI reported each year, in 2002 about 28000, and in 2004 there were 44488 (Health Protection Agency 2003, 2005, Health Protection Agency Communicable Diseases Surveillance

Centre for the Department of Health 2006). This alarming increase may in part be explained by improved voluntary and now mandatory reporting of cases.

MRSA and CDI are particularly relevant to the older population, with most of these infections occurring in those aged over 65 years. Both pathogens are associated with the use of antibiotics. Methicillin-susceptible *Staphylococcus aureus* (MSSA) strains rarely mutate to become MRSA, however the selective pressure imparted by antibiotic use encourages MRSA growth and spread. *Both organisms are carried on the hands of healthcare workers, and this remains the most important route of spread. Meticulous hand hygiene is vital to eliminate cross infection and is the most effective single infection control measure.*

Hospital admissions for pneumonia and flu are 12 times and 25 times more common, respectively, in elderly subjects. Morbidity and mortality are also higher in this age group. In the UK, it is policy to vaccinate 70% of those over 65 years with the influenza vaccine. Targeted immunization against *Streptococcus pneumoniae,* starting with those aged over 80 years, was also introduced in a stepwise fashion in 2003.

CLOSTRIDIUM DIFFICILE

Clostridum difficile is an anaerobic, spore-forming bacterium that is the major identifiable cause of antibiotic-associated diarrhoea. CDI is a serious condition often affecting frail elderly subjects with a reported mortality of up to 25% (although directly attributable mortality, which is often difficult to calculate, is probably about 3%). The clinical manifestations of CDI range from asymptomatic carriage and mild diarrhoea to severe fulminant colitis, pseudomembranous colitis and toxic megacolon. Why some develop more serious disease than others is probably the result of a complex interaction between host factors and the infecting organism.

The pathogenesis of CDI involves a triad of factors. The first step is the disruption of the protective intestinal microflora, leaving this niche susceptible to colonization by potential pathogens. Antibiotics are strongly implicated in this process,

---

Box 45.1   Risk factors identified in the development of CDI

- Increasing age
- Severe underlying illness
- Multiple antibiotics
- Long duration of antibiotic course
- Long hospital stay
- Presence of a nasogastric tube
- Non-surgical gastrointestinal procedures
- Intensive care stay
- Anti-ulcer medications
- Chemotherapy and immunosuppressants

---

as they alter the intestinal flora – thus creating conditions favouring the acquisition and proliferation of *C. difficile. Almost any antimicrobial has the potential to cause CDI, but clindamycin, cephalosporins and aminopenicillins are particularly implicated. Crucially, the risk of CDI increases with the use of multiple antibiotics and prolonged administration.* Other factors, which may disrupt the intestinal microflora also pose a risk for CDI and are outlined in Box 45.1.

Individuals predisposed to CDI are typically exposed to the bacterium in hospital. Asymptomatic and symptomatic patients shed *C. difficile,* which can be found as resistant spores in hospitals and care homes. The spores are resistant to heat and chemicals and can remain in the ward for many months, providing a reservoir for further infection. The hands of healthcare workers provide an important means of exposure; *C. difficile* can be recovered from hands after contact with patients or their immediate surroundings.

Once the bowel flora have been disrupted and *C. difficile* ingested, patients can become colonized and subsequently develop disease manifestations. Not all develop symptoms of infection: some will remain asymptomatic. Three per cent of the healthy adult population and 20–30% of those in hospital are asymptomatic carriers.

CDI is associated with the production of two toxins, A and B. These toxins are responsible for the inflammation, fluid and mucus secretion and mucosal damage. Toxin A is an enterotoxin that loosens the tight junctions between the epithelial cells while toxin B is a potent cytotoxin. The progression to clinical disease depends on the presence of a toxigenic strain, but this alone does not guarantee disease as asymptomatic carriage of these strains is known. The presence of certain host factors, in particular those relating to the immune response, plays an important role in influencing disease severity. The ability of the host immune response to produce high levels of a protective antibody against toxin A can reduce the likelihood of infection and protect against recurrence. The high prevalence of debilitating disease and the use of immunosuppressants in older patients probably further reduces the efficacy of the *C. difficile*-specific immune response.

A VIRULENT STRAIN

The recent emergence of a new virulent strain of *C. difficile* (referred to as type 027 or NAP1) is causing great concern. Epidemics in Canada, parts of the USA, the UK and Netherlands have occurred. This particular strain of *C. difficile* has been associated with higher rates of CDI, especially in elderly subjects, and has a greater propensity to cause serious disease. Directly attributable mortality is higher (7%) and this rises with age (10% in the 81–90 years age group and 14% in the over-90s). The virulence of this strain may result from increased toxin production (Loo et al 2005, Pépin et al 2005).

The acquisition of fluoroquinolone resistance has been observed in this strain and may be implicated in its emergence. Fluoroquinolones are widely prescribed in hospitals, and this increased use may well have provided a selective advantage for this strain. However, not all studies concur that fluoroquinolones are a risk factor for CDI: broad-spectrum antibiotics in general can select for this and other *C. difficile* strains.

TREATMENT

First infection

Antiperistaltic agents should be avoided in acute cases, as theoretically they may exacerbate toxin-mediated disease and precipitate toxic megacolon. The offending antibiotic should be stopped if at all possible, as up to 25% of patients with mild disease recover spontaneously with this alone. However, because of practical difficulties in predicting who will respond to this simple measure, and the need to continue antibiotics in patients, many receive specific antimicrobial therapy for CDI.

Studies comparing oral metronidazole and vancomycin indicate equal efficacy, for a 10–14 day treatment course, with a response rate of 97% and a similar relapse rate (Teasley et al 1983, Wenisch et al 1996). Metronidazole is associated with slightly slower (1–2 day) response time, but is usually recommended as first-line treatment; vancomycin is considerably more expensive and there are concerns about the potential risk of vancomycin-resistant enterococcus (VRE) and vancomycin intermediate resistant *Staphylococcus aureus* (VISA).

Recurrence

Recurrence is a difficult problem, occurring in up to 30% of patients. In patients who have had more than one recurrence, the risk of additional recurrences increases to 50–65%. Recurrence was initially thought to be due to failure to eradicate *C. difficile* resulting in a relapse of symptoms. However, about 50% of recurring symptoms are due to re-infection with a different strain.

Most recurrences respond to another course of the original therapy, with response ranging from 70–90%. Further recurrences pose a difficult challenge.

Strategies have been tried with some success and include: (1) a longer duration of therapy, (2) vancomycin in combination with rifampicin alone, (3) in pulsed doses or (4) tapered regimens given over 4–6 weeks. Tapered or pulsed doses of antibiotics were thought to gradually clear *C. difficile* by eradicating cells as spores germinate. It is more likely, however, that such prolonged therapy is acting as prophylaxis against reacquisition of *C. difficile*.

There are case reports of successful treatment of recurrent relapse by administration of normal faeces, donated by a spouse or family member, either as an enema or through a naso-jejunal tube. Its success is probably due to the restoration of normal bowel organisms, in particular anaerobes.

An alternative – and perhaps more refined strategy – is the oral administration of a non-toxigenic strain of C. *difficile*.

Alternative therapies

Alternative regimens for the treatment and prevention of CDI have focused on the restoration of the normal colonic microflora and improving the immune response. Probiotics, often described as 'harmless' bacteria, can affect the intestinal microflora. Their role in the prevention and management of CDI is controversial. A recent systematic review concluded that there was no convincing evidence for the routine use of probiotics to prevent or treat CDI in adults (Dendukuri et al 2005). A few studies have found a beneficial effect of probiotics in recurrent or severe disease when used in conjunction with antimicrobial therapy. This requires further evaluation with randomized controlled trials. There have been reports of fungaemia in patients given the most widely studied probiotic, *Saccharomyces boulardii*.

Another treatment strategy has been to bind the toxins of C. *difficile* using adsorbents within the colonic lumen. Studies with cholestyramine and similar non-specific binding agents have not shown any superiority over standard agents. In addition, such adsorbents can bind to vancomycin, thus reducing colonic drug levels and so limiting their use further.

The observation that some patients with recurrent CDI have low levels of antibodies to toxin A has postulated a role for immunoglobulins. Pooled human immunoglobulin has been used with success in recurrent CDI and requires further evaluation (McFarland 2005, Wilcox 2004).

Treatment of CDI

- Stop the inciting antibiotic
- Fluid and electrolyte replacement
- First-line treatment: metronidazole 500 mg tds for 7 to 10 days. Use vancomycin 125 mg qds if allergic or intolerant
- Recurrent episode: repeat full course of initial antibiotic

- For multiple recurrences: consider tapered or pulsed vancomycin, the addition of probiotics or immunoglobulins
- For all: isolation (if possible) and strict adherence to infection control precautions

PREVENTION

Antibiotic restrictive policies

Cephalosporins in particular have been implicated in the development of CDI, especially in elderly patients. A crossover study comparing empirical use of cefotaxime and piperacillin-tazobactam for moderate to severe infection in the elderly found that the former was associated with a seven-fold greater risk of CDI (Settle et al 1998).

The use of antibiotic policies restricting the use of cephalosporins can be successful. A well-designed, controlled before and after, study showed that in three acute elderly wards a narrow spectrum antibiotic policy, reinforced by carriage of a laminated antibiotic policy card and regular feedback to doctors of CDI rates and antibiotic usage, not only reduced broad-spectrum usage (cephalosporins and co-amoxyclav) and increased narrow-spectrum antibiotic use (benzylpenicillin, trimethoprim and amoxicillin) but substantially reduced CDI. These benefits did not appear to be outweighed by an increase in mortality. Other studies have illustrated the successful role that alternative antibiotic policies have played in reducing the incidence of CDI (McNulty et al 1997). However, a recent systematic review on interventions to change antibiotic prescribing, and their effects on microbiological outcomes including CDI, have concluded that most studies are flawed in their design, provision of data and analysis (Davey et al 2006). Restrictive antibiotic policies need to be reinforced, as the rates of CDI can increase markedly if antibiotic restriction is lost (Fig. 45.1) for example, in a California hospital, rates of CDI doubled once a cephalosporin restrictive policy was relaxed.

In light of such evidence, the use of cephalosporins in elderly patients has to be questioned. A recent randomized controlled trial (RCT) reported that the beta-lactamase inhibitor piperacillin with

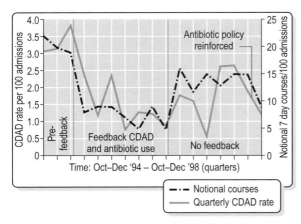

Figure 45.1 Effect of discontinuing feedback of *Clostridium difficile*-associated diarrhoea (CDAD) rates and antibiotic use on CDI infection rates and cephalosporin usage in an acute elderly unit.

tazocin was as effective as cephalosporins in intra-abdominal sepsis but without the risk of CDI. *There are no RCTs to support the use of cephalosporins rather than common alternatives in the treatment of pneumonia, infective exacerbations of chronic obstructive pulmonary disease, urinary tract infections or Gram-negative sepsis.*

Isolation and contact precautions

Transmission of *C. difficile* occurs from patient to patient via the hands of healthcare workers and from the environment, with up to 60% of healthcare workers having same-strain contamination of their hands by *C. difficile* after contact with *C. difficile* patients – even if the contact is simply handling the drug chart. *Hands must be washed with liquid soap and water after contact with patients (or their immediate environment) who have proven or suspected CDI, as alcohol gel does not kill the spores,* which are predominant in faeces and the environment. Isolating patients – especially those with faecal incontinence (which is associated with increased transmission) – is of paramount importance to prevent further spread.

Much of the evidence on the use of infection control measures is observational; however, some higher quality studies have demonstrated that the use of gloves and hand washing with an antiseptic soap reduced the rate of CDI (Bettin et al 1994, Johnson et al 1990, Jones & MacGowan 1998).

Environmental

Consistent and adequate environmental cleaning is a vital measure in preventing CDI, as spores can survive for many months. There is a correlation between environmental contamination and *C. difficile* infection rates. Commodes, bed frames, sluice and toilet floors are most frequently contaminated but call bells, window sills and light switches are also implicated. Studies on the optimal cleaning agent are limited, but there is some evidence to suggest that hypochlorite-containing disinfectants are preferable to detergents (Mayfield et al 2000, Wilcox et al 2003). The dedication of single-use items to infected individuals is an important infection control measure, as transmission of CDI can be via equipment such as stethoscopes, thermometers and blood pressure cuffs.

Immunization

Immunization aims to produce neutralizing antibodies to toxins A and B in order to prevent symptomatic infection. Vaccines against *C. difficile* toxins have been successful in animals and early safety trials in humans, producing levels of antibody to toxin A associated with protection against CDI. There is concern about its efficacy in elderly subjects as response to vaccination in this age group is often limited.

Clinical governance

Until vaccination becomes available, the focus on prevention and control of CDI must remain within the remit of antibiotic and infection control measures. These simple measures should be part of everyday clinical practice. Ensuring compliance is a challenge, but it is a key component of any strategy if it is to be successful. The Health Care Commission (http://www.healthcarecommission.org.uk) reported in 2005 that nearly 40% of NHS trusts had no restrictions on broad-spectrum antibiotic use and that 20% had no system of audit of antibiotic use. This is likely to be addressed through regular audit and clinical governance, as all NHS trusts are required to report all cases of CDI as an extension of the national hospital-associated infection surveillance initiatives. Through this and regular feedback, we should start to see a decline in the rate of CDI and its associated mortality.

MRSA

MRSA was first detected in the UK within a year of the introduction of flucloxacillin (a meticillin-like antibiotic). It was uncommon in the 1970s until the mid 1990s and the last 10 years have seen a major rise in the number of infections caused by MRSA. The outcome of MRSA infection is likely to be the result of the interaction between the virulence and epidemicity of some MRSA strains, the patient case mix or risk group, and the effectiveness of infection control approaches (including hand-washing compliance, antibiotic use, staff–patient ratios, and detection and isolation of cases).

VIRULENCE

MRSA causes a spectrum of diseases similar to that of MSSA, ranging from asymptomatic carriage, soft tissue infection to life-threatening bacteraemia. In the UK, two clones (EMRSA 15 and EMRSA 16) account for most of the infections. Most people who encounter MRSA will not become infected. For example, EMRSA 16 causes asymptomatic colonization in 80% of patients – usually of wounds, throat, nose and perineum.

The virulence of MRSA varies with the strain. It remains controversial whether MRSA is more virulent than MSSA. A recent meta-analysis revealed that patients with MRSA bacteraemia had an increased risk of mortality when compared to MSSA. In addition to the excess mortality, patients with MRSA infection had a more protracted hospital stay. The excess mortality could be attributed to the delays in commencing appropriate antibiotic therapy that may occur if MRSA is not suspected. However, vancomycin, the usual treatment for MRSA, has poor pharmacokinetics and pharmacodynamics. Vancomyin and teicoplanin are less efficacious than flucloxacillin at treating (susceptible) staphylococcal infections and incur higher costs.

Virulent strains of MRSA acquired in the community have been emerging. These strains are genetically distinct from the hospital-associated MRSA and do not share the multiple antibiotic resistant traits and are therefore more susceptible to antibiotics. These strains produce a toxin that is associated with skin infections and pneumonia. These can be severe, and (particularly skin infections) can spread throughout institutions.

The prevalence of these community-associated strains is unknown in the UK and, although not typically associated with the older adult, could pose a threat to those in care.

There is increasing evidence that antibiotics provide a selection pressure that encourages MRSA to multiply (Eveillard et al 2002, Hori et al 2002, Sax et al 2005). Fluoroquinolones and third-generation cephalosporins have been particularly implicated. Cephalosporin-restrictive antibiotic policies can reduce MRSA in pre- and post-intervention studies. However, intervention studies designed to reduce antimicrobial prescribing – and therefore the prevalence of MRSA – are lacking.

Vancomycin and teicoplanin are often used as first-line treatment of MRSA. However, the emergence of strains with low-level resistance to the glycopeptides (termed vancomycin intermediate resistance *Staphylococcus aureus* [VISA]) may compromise therapy. More worryingly, a small number of fully vancomycin resistant strains (VRSA) have been reported in the USA. The genetic events resulting in the phenotypic expression of vancomycin resistance appear to be different between VISA and VRSA. The genetic mechanisms of VISA are not fully understood, but it is thought that changes to the bacterial cell wall (the site of action of glycopeptides) may be key. VISA has a thick cell wall in comparison to vancomycin susceptible isolates. VRSA strains are resistant as a result of the acquisition of the van A gene from enterococci.

UK guidelines published in 2006 for the treatment of MRSA infection have emphasized that older antibiotics may be useful in some cases; for example, depending on susceptibility results, tetracyclines can be used in urinary tract infection, and tetracyclines, clindamycin or combined rifampicin/fusidic acid can be used in mild to moderate soft tissue infection. For bacteraemia, severe cellulitis or wound infection, or pneumonia, vancomycin or linezolid are recommended; and for bone infection vancomycin with rifampicin or fusidic acid can be used. Linezolid can be given orally and still achieves high tissue levels, which may be particularly useful in elderly patients if intravenous access is a problem. Protracted linezolid therapy should be used with caution because of the potential for haematological toxicity and neuropathy.

The cornerstone of MRSA management in hospital is reduction of transmission. This may be achieved by isolation in a single room, cohort bay or, occasionally, an isolation unit or ward. MRSA is transmitted by direct contact, mainly via the hands of healthcare workers. Staff dressing MRSA-infected wounds have an 80% chance of carrying the organism for up to 3 hours. Immediate hand-washing virtually eradicates carriage. The value of screening for asymptomatic carriage as a control measure for MRSA in the endemic setting remains contentious. The UK guidelines advocate screening of high-risk patients and those in high-risk units. (High-risk patients are those in whom MRSA is more likely to be present and comprise those with a past history of MRSA, recent hospitalization, or residence in a care home.) Elderly people therefore frequently fall into this group. High-risk units comprise those serving patients at particular risk of deep-seated invasive and hard to treat infection such as ITU, neurosurgical, orthopaedic and major surgery wards or units. The guidelines also advocate isolation and cohorting of MRSA-positive patients according to the risk to the patient group and, notably, the availability of isolation facilities. Decolonization of patients with nasal mupirocin, and chlorhexidine baths and shampoos is also advocated in selected patient groups (such as preoperative patients).

The evidence base for these recommendations is largely unsound. A systematic review found many inadequacies in the design of studies, the reporting and analysis of outcome and the assessment and adjustment of potential confounders. Nonetheless the review found evidence in some higher quality studies that a package of measures – including isolation – can reduce endemic levels of MRSA. Intensity of screening or the isolation capacity can reduce the endemicity of MRSA, provided neither is the limiting factor. The larger the isolation capacity or ward and the sooner it opens, the lower the endemic level of MRSA. Current pressure on beds in the NHS means that infection control teams often have to struggle to secure isolation facilities. A recent study showed that almost a quarter of cases that require isolation in a single room, often because the patient is MRSA positive, cannot be isolated (Wigglesworth & Wilcox 2006).

A systematic review of eradication therapy concluded that there was no definite evidence that it cleared MRSA or prevented infection (Loeb et al 2003). Similarly, the systematic review of isolation could not provide definitive interventions for the control of MRSA, but considered that both the modelling and the better quality studies provided hypotheses worth testing – either in cluster randomized controlled trials or high-quality non-randomized studies. As there is little evidence that the current isolation guidelines are ineffective, they should continue to be applied (Cooper et al 2003).

Although most MRSA occurs in elderly people, patients on general medical elderly wards are considered to be at intermediate risk and those in rehabilitation or long-stay wards at low risk. Side-room isolation may be detrimental; depression may occur because of social exclusion, and rehabilitation is more difficult in isolation wards. Nevertheless, low-risk patients may act as a reservoir for MRSA, which may be transmitted to higher-risk individuals following transfer or re-admission to acute settings.

RISK IN ELDERLY PATIENTS

Although MRSA is predominately a problem of older patients, deep-seated, invasive and hard-to-treat infection is probably relatively rare in elderly subjects. The elderly population is particularly at risk for MRSA carriage, probably because of frailty and debility, multiple co-morbidities and frequent contact with healthcare services.

Concerns about the prevalence of healthcare-associated MRSA in the community have arisen in the UK as early discharge of patients with MRSA forms part of our national guidelines. The community prevalence of MRSA in older people living at home is less than 1% (Maudsley et al 2004).

The hospitalized elderly patient

Elderly in-patients have higher MRSA carriage rates. The prevalence of MRSA carriage on admission to hospital may be high and studies have attempted to clarify this in addition to identifying specific risk factors associated with MRSA carriage (Eveillard et al 2002, Lucet et al 2005, Sax et al 2005). The reported prevalence of non-documented MRSA carriage on admission ranges from 5.8 to 13.6%. Risk factors are numerous but include: previous hospitalization (up to 2 years), transfer from other hospitals or nursing homes, recent antibiotics and the presence of wounds/decubitus ulcers (see Ch. 20). The identification of such risk factors could alert us to the potential of MRSA colonization, allowing for infection control measures to prevent transmission and cross-infection.

Further MRSA colonization is acquired by older people in hospital. In Nottingham, the prevalence of MRSA carriage 3 weeks after hospital admission was about 16%, though an unknown proportion of these were MRSA positive on admission (Hori et al 2002). Risk factors for MRSA acquisition during hospitalization include: longer duration of stay, previous surgery, poor functional status, presence of skin lesions, use of invasive devices, prior antibiotic exposure – especially ciprofloxacin and cephalosporins, severe co-morbidity and proximity to an already infected/colonized patient.

Once again, these risk factors could potentially allow elderly patients to be stratified into low- and high-risk groups for nosocomial infection, thereby allowing preventative steps to be taken.

Colonization with MRSA increases the risk of subsequent infection by as much as 30% in acute care. Should all patients or those with the highest risk of colonization be screened on admission? Perhaps not: in the elderly population, MRSA carriage may occur without infection.

In contrast to acute care, MRSA in elderly patients in rehabilitation wards or in long-term care may be of less importance, however the transfer or readmission of these patients into acute wards makes them a potential reservoir for further spread.

Rehabilitation units

One study of patients on a rehabilitation ward revealed an 11.8% MRSA colonization rate with 14% of those developing clinical infection. There was no difference in rates of functional decline or mortality but there was an increased length of stay in MRSA-positive patients (Morrison & Stolarek 2000). This may be because of isolation and the limitations this creates for rehabilitation. Depression is twice as common (75%) in elderly patients isolated in side-rooms on a rehabilitation ward than in non-isolated patients (Tarzi et al 2001).

Elderly rehabilitation patients seem to be at lower risk of MRSA infection. MRSA should not be a barrier to access to rehabilitation, but guidelines do not offer advice on how this can be achieved.

Long-term care

MRSA in long-term care is an increasing problem. Nursing home residents constitute a large proportion of the MRSA reservoir and may be responsible for introducing MRSA into the acute wards (Cookson 1999, Cox & Bowie 1999, Garibaldi 1999, Hori et al 2002, Lucet et al 2005, O'Sullivan & Keane 2000, Talon & Bertrand 2001). A study of Northampton nursing homes showed a 4% prevalence of MRSA (Cox & Bowie 1999). In 1994 a study in Birmingham revealed a prevalence of 17% (Fraise et al 1997). In a large study of 39 care homes in Leeds in 2005, 22% of residents who were able to give informed consent were MRSA nasal carriers (Wilcox et al 2006).

Nursing home residents are predisposed to acquiring MRSA because of their likely history of recent hospitalization, general fragility and advanced age – increasing age and colonization are connected. The increased prevalence of other risk factors associated with MRSA acquisition also contribute to the high prevalence in long-term care. Other risk factors are outlined in Box 45.2.

> **Box 45.2   Risk factors for MRSA acquisition within the nursing home**
>
> - Male gender
> - Over 80 years old
> - Resident for less than 6 months
> - Decubitus ulcers
> - Functional disability
> - In-dwelling catheters
> - Gastrostomies
> - Prior antibiotic exposure

Although colonization with MRSA is relatively common in care homes, rates of infection and directly attributable mortality appear low in comparison to the acute units. Infection rates of 5–15% have been quoted in colonized residents of long-term care facilities in the USA compared to 30–60% in hospital (Bradley et al 1991, McNeil et al 2002, Muder et al 1991, Strausbaugh et al 1991). This suggests that MRSA may not be as virulent here as in acute care.

Nevertheless, MRSA transmission and cross-infection do occur. A study in six nursing homes in Ireland reported a prevalence of 1–27% in individual homes with about 10% of residents carrying MRSA (O'Sullivan & Keane 2000). Over a 6-month period, as many residents lost MRSA (6%) as gained it, with most transmission occurring in the home. This implies that infection control measures could have an impact on the prevalence of MRSA in nursing homes.

MRSA SCREENING

Screening for MRSA can permit the early identification of MRSA carriage or infection and allow the implementation of isolation precautions to prevent cross-transmission and spread. Similarly, secondary infection in carriers may also be prevented by focused infection control measures. In intensive care units the implementation of a voluntary strategy involving screening has controlled the spread of MRSA (Girou et al 1998).

Similar results might be achieved in hospitals.

Arguments against screening involve the extra cost and resources needed by the health service, as well as the additional infection control measures needed by this expanding population (in particular the high proportion of single to multi-bed rooms that are required). Selective screening strategies based on the profile of high-risk patients could help resolve this dilemma, but require that easily available risk factors are clearly established. MRSA transmission may occur during the period of identifying who is colonized. New, rapid screening techniques that can give a same day answer may be helpful here.

Given the additional morbidity and mortality associated with MRSA in acute care, and the emergence of more virulent and glycopeptide-resistant strains, implementing a screening programme as part of an infection control policy may have to be the way forward.

OTHER MRSA INFECTION CONTROL MEASURES

Current UK guidelines allow for local flexibility according to patient group and resources available.

In many hospitals, especially large tertiary referral hospitals, which have many patients with severe underlying disease, strict isolation polices are applied, with, as a minimum, side-room isolation of MRSA-positive patients. Side-rooms and isolation units are often unavailable. Such resources should be made available, as the cost of not controlling MRSA (e.g. extended length of stay, theatre closure and antibiotic budgets) is higher than that of control (isolation units, eradication, cleaning, etc.).

Eradication of MRSA is particularly difficult if skin lesions such as wounds or ulcers are present. Only short-term eradication may result if MRSA contact once again occurs.

These measures are not a substitute for basic infection control procedures, which are paramount to the success of infection control. *As MRSA is primarily transmitted via the hands of healthcare workers, meticulous hand hygiene is essential and probably constitutes the single most important infection control measure.*

Small (10%) increments in hand-washing frequency could have major effects upon MRSA prevalence, although once compliance reaches 60% there may be little further gain in terms of reducing MRSA by increasing compliance further. The universal availability of and compliance with alcohol-based hand gel preparations, which forms the centre of the *cleanyourhands* campaign, is an important step forward.

FOOD FOR THOUGHT

Some believe that these infection control measures are poorly effective, as the rates of MRSA have continued to rise despite their implementation. However, in countries such as Denmark where patients are screened, there are strict isolation policies, high-quality basic hygiene is achieved and MRSA has been controlled. A fundamental difference, however, is that MRSA is endemic in the UK healthcare system, and therefore piecemeal implementation of control measures is unlikely to be very effective.

The UK's rising figures may reflect our less fastidious approach to MRSA.

FLU AND PNEUMONIA

The risk of complications, hospitalization and death from influenza is particularly great among those over 65 years. One in four suffers complications and each year in the UK 3000–4000 deaths are attributed to influenza (more in epidemics). Pneumonia is also common in old age, with infection from *Streptococcus pneumoniae* accounting for the majority of cases.

About 50 000 cases of pneumococcal pneumonia occur each year with a 20% mortality. Mortality is even greater in those with invasive disease associated with bacteraemia. Despite advanced treatment and critical care, the mortality associated with pneumococcal infection has remained unchanged for many years. An additional worry is the emergence of *S. pneumoniae* strains that have reduced susceptibility to penicillin and other beta-lactam antibiotics. Community-based European data show that the national prevalence of

S. pneumoniae with reduced susceptibility to penicillin correlates with the extent of prescribing of antibiotics such as amoxicillin (Goossens et al 2005).

The use of vaccination to control both diseases has therefore assumed great importance. It is now national policy that everyone over the age of 65 years is considered for annual immunization against influenza. In 2003 the Department of Health introduced a programme for pneumococcal vaccination. This is now recommended for all individuals over 65 years.

HOW EFFECTIVE IS VACCINATION?

Influenza vaccine

The effectiveness of the influenza vaccine depends on the age and immuno-competence of the individual and the degree of similarity it has to the prevalent virus strain.

Vaccination may offer less protection against infection in elderly people. However, it significantly reduces the incidence of pneumonia, hospital admissions and mortality. A RCT of non-institutionalized people over 60 years reported a vaccine efficacy of 58% in preventing infection, but indicated that this was probably lower in those over 70 years (Govaert et al 1994). Vaccination may prevent hospital admission in 30–70% of adults over 60 who do not live in care homes (Mullooly et al 1994, Nichol et al 1998).

Of those living in nursing homes, vaccination is particularly effective at preventing secondary complications and death. It is only effective in 30–40% of residents in preventing infection but more effective in preventing pneumonia/hospital admissions and death (Arden et al 1986, Monto et al 2001, Patriarca et al 1985). Annual influenza vaccination of all older people is cost-effective (Mullooly et al 1994, Nichol et al 1998).

Pneumococcal vaccine

Systematic reviews indicate that pneumococcal vaccine is about 53% effective in preventing invasive disease but has little impact upon pneumonia per se (Dear et al 2003). Evidence from

Europe suggests that it is cost-effective (Ament et al 2000).

There are two types of pneumococcal vaccine. The 23-valent vaccine contains a mixture of capsular polysaccharides from 23 serotypes of pneumococci, and is the type that should be used in older children and adults. This provides protection against 96% of the isolates that cause serious infection in the UK. It is relatively poorly immunogenic, however, which may explain lack of complete protection. The effectiveness of the 23-valent vaccine in preventing invasive pneumococcal infection (e.g. septicaemia, meningitis and pneumonia complicated by septicaemia) is about 50–70%. This, coupled with the emergence of drug-resistant pneumococci, has stimulated research into new vaccine strategies.

Uptake of vaccination

National targets for influenza vaccination have been met over the last few years (68.6% were vaccinated in 2002/3, 71% in 2003/4 and 71.4% in 2004/5). Little is known about the uptake of influenza immunization in residential and nursing homes in the UK. One study, before the government initiatives, found a mean uptake of 67%. This was higher in nursing home residents (82%) than in those in residential care (65%). Individuals who had more than one risk factor were no more likely than those without to have been immunized (Evans & Wilkinson 1995).

TREATING INFLUENZA

Although vaccination remains the cornerstone of disease prevention, guidance on the use of antivirals for the treatment and prevention of influenza has been issued (NICE 2003, NICE 2003).

Amantadine is only effective against influenza A and has adverse effects. Resistance can occur rapidly and this drug is no longer recommended for the treatment or prophylaxis of influenza.

Zanamivir and oseltamivir (Tamiflu) are neuraminidase inhibitors that prevent the release of virons from infected cells. They are effective against both influenza A and B. In a recent meta-analysis, zanamivir has been shown to reduce the duration of influenza symptoms by 2 days (NICE 2003, Turner et al 2003). Further evaluation is required of its impact upon complication rates, hospitalization and mortality – especially in the 'high-risk' elderly population. Zanamivir is administered as an inhaled preparation, which some elderly patients have found difficult.

Tamiflu is licensed for the treatment and prophylaxis of influenza. Meta-analysis suggested that it probably reduces the duration of flu symptoms (not statistically significant) as well as reducing lower respiratory tract complications (statistically significant) (NICE 2003, Turner et al 2003). It is uncertain whether Tamiflu is effective in reducing serious complications, hospitalization or death.

Tamiflu is licensed for the prophylaxis of influenza A and B if an at-risk person is not immunized and comes into contact with an infected person, within 48 hours when influenza is circulating in the community. For those living in care homes, it is recommended for all residents, regardless of vaccination status. Tamiflu is 90% effective in preventing influenza in people aged 64–96 years living in residential care (NICG 2003). 80% of these residents had been vaccinated.

Key points

- Introduction of a cephalosporin-restrictive antibiotic policy is associated with a 50% reduction in CDI in acute elderly wards with no increase in infection-related mortality.
- Novel non-antibiotic mediated approaches to the treatment of CDI are under evaluation. They are especially attractive in view of the antibiotic-associated aetiology of CDI and the concern that antimicrobial resistance may develop.
- The elderly population form a heterogeneous group and MRSA infection and colonization reflect this. While the clinical impact of MRSA appears less in subacute and long-term care, these patients constitute a large proportion of the MRSA reservoir with potential to introduce MRSA into acute care.

- MRSA can be controlled by screening, eradication, isolation and strict attention to basic hygiene.
- MRSA and *C. difficile* are transmitted primarily via the hands of healthcare workers. Meticulous hand hygiene is essential and is probably the single most important infection control measure.
- The battle against antimicrobial-resistant organisms continues and poses a major threat. New antibiotics are not the answer, as resistance to these will appear too. Strict adherence to infection control policies incorporating basic hygiene, prudent use of antibiotics, surveillance, feedback and audit remains the way to curb the proliferation of such 'superbugs'.

REFERENCES

Ament A, Baltussen R, Duru G et al 2000 Cost-effectiveness of pneumococcal vaccination of older people: a study in 5 western European countries. Clinical Infectious Diseases 31:444–450

Arden N H, Patriarca P A, Kendal A P 1986 Experiences in the use and efficacy of inactivated influenza vaccine in nursing homes. Options for the control of influenza. Alan R Liss, New York

Bettin K, Clabots C, Mathie P et al 1994 Effectiveness of liquid soap vs chlorhexidine gluconate for the removal of *Clostridium difficile* from bare hands and gloved hands. Infection Control and Hospital Epidemiology 15:697–702

Bradley S F, Terpenning M S, Ramsey M A et al 1991 Methicillin-resistant *Staphylococcus aureus*: colonization and infection in a long-term care facility. Annals of Internal Medicine 115:417–422

Chief Medical Officer 2003 Winning ways – working together to reduce healthcare associated infection in England. Report from the Chief Medical Officer. Department of Heath, London

Cookson B D 1999 Nosocomial antimicrobial resistance surveillance. Journal of Hospital Infection 43(Suppl): S97–S103

Cooper B S, Stone S P, Kibbler C C et al 2003 Systematic review of isolation policies in the hospital management of methicillin-resistant *Staphlococcus aureus*: a review of the literature with epidemiological and economic modelling. Health Technology Assessment 7:1–194

Cox R A, Bowie P E S 1999 Methicillin-resistant *Staphylococcus aureus* colonization in nursing home residents: a prevalence study in Northamptonshire. Journal of Hospital Infection 43:115–122

Davey P, Brown E, Fenelon L et al 2006 Systematic review of antimicrobial drug prescribing in hospitals. Emerging Infectious Diseases 12:211–216

Dear K B G, Andrews R R, Holden J et al 2003 Vaccines for preventing pneumococcal infection in adults. The Cochrane Database of Systematic Reviews. Art. No.: CD000422. DOI: 10.1002/14651858.CD000422

Dendukuri N, Costa V, McGregor M et al 2005 Probiotic therapy for the prevention and treatment of *Clostridium difficile*-associated diarrhoea: a systematic review. Canadian Medical Association Journal 173:167–170

Evans M R, Wilkinson E J 1995 How complete is influenza immunization coverage? A study in 75 nursing and residential homes for elderly people. British Journal of General Practice 45:419–421

Eveillard M, Ernst C, Cuviller S et al 2002 Prevalence of methicillin-resistant *Staphylococcus aureus* carriage at the time of admission in two acute geriatric wards. Journal of Hospital Infection 50:122–126

Fraise A P, Mitchell K, O'Brien S J et al 1997 Methicillin-resistant *Staphylococcus aureus* (MRSA) in nursing homes in a major UK city: an anonymized point prevalence survey. Epidemiology and Infection 118:1–5

Garibaldi R A 1999 Residential care and the elderly: the burden of infection. Journal of Hospital Infection 43(Suppl):S9–18

Girou E, Pujade G, Legrand P et al 1998 Selective screening of carriers for control of methicillin-resistant *Staphylococcus aureus* (MRSA) in high-risk hospital areas with high level of endemic MRSA. Clinical Infectious Diseases 27:543–550

Goossens H, Ferech M, Vander Stichele R et al 2005 Outpatient antibiotic use in Europe and association with resistance: a cross-national database study. Lancet 365:579–587

Govaert T M, Thijs C T, Masurel N et al 1994 The efficacy of influenza vaccination in elderly individuals. A randomized double-blind placebo-controlled trial. Journal of the American Medical Association 272:1661–1665

Health Protection Agency 2003 *Clostridium difficile* England, Wales and Northern Ireland: 2000–2002. CDR Weekly 13:2 Oct

Health Protection Agency 2005 Results of the first year of *Clostridium difficile* mandatory reporting: January to December 2004. CDR Weekly 15:25 Aug

Health Protection Agency Communicable Disease Surveillance Centre for the Department of Health 2006 MRSA surveillance system results. 7 Mar 2005 (updated 6 Feb 2006)

Hori S, Sunley R, Tami A et al 2002 The Nottingham *Staphylococcus aureus* population study: prevalence of MRSA among the elderly in a university hospital. Journal of Hospital Infection 50:25–29

Johnson S, Gerding D N, Olson M M et al 1990 Prospective, controlled study of vinyl glove use to interrupt *Clostridium difficile* nosocomial transmission. American Journal of Medicine 88:137–140

Jones E M, MacGowan A P 1998 Back to basics in management of *Clostridium difficile* infections. Lancet 352:505–506

Loeb M, Main C, Walker-Dilks C et al 2003 Antimicrobial drugs for treating methicillin-resistant Staphylococcus aureus colonization. Cochrane Database of Systematic Reviews, issue 4. Art. No.: CD003340. DOI: 10.1002/14651858.CD003340

Loo V G, Poirier L, Miller M M et al 2005 A predominantly clonal multi-institutional outbreak of *Clostridium difficile*-associated diarrhoea with high morbidity and mortality. New England Journal of Medicine 353:2442–2449

Lucet J C, Grenet K, Armand-Lefevre L et al 2005 High prevalence of carriage of methicillin-resistant *Staphylococcus aureus* at hospital admission in elderly patients: implications for infection control strategies. Infection Control and Hospital Epidemiology 26:121–126

McFarland L V 2005 Alternative treatments for *Clostridium difficile* disease: what really works? Journal of Medical Microbiology 54:101–111

McNeil S A, Mody L, Bradley S F 2002 Methicillin-resistant *Staphylococcus aureus*: management of asymptomatic colonization and outbreaks of infection in long-term care. Geriatrics 57:16–27

McNulty C, Logan M, Donald I P et al 1997 Successful control of *Clostridium difficile* infection in an elderly care unit through use of a restrictive antibiotic policy. Journal of Antimicrobial Chemotherapy 40:707–711

Maudsley J, Stone S P, Kibbler C C et al 2004 The community prevalence of methicillin-resistant *Staphylococcus aureus* (MRSA) in older people living in their own homes: implications for treatment, screening and surveillance in the UK. Journal of Hospital Infection 57:258–262

Mayfield J L, Leet T, Miller J et al 2000 Environmental control to reduce transmission of *Clostridium difficile*. Clinical Infectious Diseases 31:995–1000

Monto A S, Hornbuckle K, Ohmit S E 2001 Influenza vaccine effectiveness among elderly nursing home residents: a cohort study. American Journal of Epidemiology 154:155–160

Morrison L, Stolarek I 2000 Does MRSA affect patient outcomes in the elderly? A retrospective pilot study. Journal of Hospital Infection 45:169–171

Muder R R, Brennen C, Wagener M M et al 1991 Methicillin-resistant staphylococcal colonization and infection in a long-term care facility. Annals of Internal Medicine 114:107–112

Mullooly J P, Bennett M D, Hornbrook M C et al 1994 Influenza vaccination programs for elderly persons: cost-effectiveness in a health maintenance organization. Annals of Internal Medicine 121:947–952

National Institute for Clinical Excellence (NICE) 2003 Guidance on the use of zanamivir, oseltamivir and amantadine for the treatment of influenza. No 58. Nice, London

National Institute for Clinical Excellence (NICE) 2003 Guidance on the use of oseltamivir and amantadine for the prophylaxis of influenza. No 67. NICE, London

Nichol K L, Wuorenma J, von Sternberg T 1998 Benefits of influenza vaccination for low-, intermediate-, and high-risk senior citizens. Archives of Internal Medicine 158:1769–1776

O'Sullivan N P, Keane C T 2000 The prevalence of methicillin-resistant *Staphylococcus aureus* among residents of six nursing homes for the elderly. Journal of Hospital Infection 45:322–329

Patriarca P A, Weber J A, Parker R A et al 1985 Efficacy of influenza vaccine in nursing homes. Reduction in illness and complications during an influenza A (H3N2) epidemic. Journal of the American Medical Association 253:1136–1139

Pépin J, Valiquette L, Cossette B 2005 Mortality attributable to a nosocomial *Clostridium difficile*-associated disease during an epidemic caused by a hypervirulent strain in Quebec. Canadian Medical Association Journal 173:1037–1042

Sax H, Harbarth S, Gavazzi G et al 2005 Prevalence and prediction of previously unknown MRSA carriage on admission to a geriatric hospital. Age and Ageing 34:456–462

Settle C D, Wilcox M H, Fawley W N et al 1998 Prospective study of the risk of *Clostridium difficile* diarrhoea in elderly patients following treatment with cefotaxime or piperacillin-tazobactum. Alimentary Pharmacology and Therapeutics 12:1217–1223

Strausbaugh L J, Jacobson C, Sewell D L et al 1991 Methicillin-resistant *Staphylococcus aureus* in extended-care facilities: experiences in a Veterans Affairs nursing home and a review of the literature. Infection Control and Hospital Epidemiology 12:36–45

Talon D R, Bertrand X 2001 Methicillin-resistant *Staphylococcus aureus* in geriatric patients: Usefulness of screening in a chronic-care setting. Infection Control and Hospital Epidemiology 22:505–510

Tarzi S, Kennedy P, Stone S et al 2001 Methicillin-resistant *Staphylococcus aureus*: psychological impact of hospitalization and isolation in an older adult population. Journal of Hospital Infection 49:250–254

Teasley D G, Gerding D N, Olson M M et al 1983 Prospective randomized trial of metronidazole versus vancomycin for *Clostridium difficile*-associated diarrhoea and colitis. Lancet 2:1043–1046

Turner D, Wailoo A, Nicholson K et al 2003 Systematic review and economic decision modeling for the prevention and treatment of influenza A and B. Health Technology Assessment 7:1–170

Wenisch C, Parschalk B, Hasenhundl M et al 1996 Comparison of vancomycin, teicoplanin, metronidazole, and fusidic acid for the treatment of *Clostridium difficile*-associated diarrhoea. Clinical Infectious Diseases 22:813–818

Wigglesworth N, Wilcox M H 2006 Prospective evaluation of hospital isolation room capacity. Journal of Hospital Infection 63:156–161

Wilcox M H 2004 Descriptive study of intravenous immunoglobulin for the treatment of recurrent *Clostridium difficile* diarrhoea. Journal of Antimicrobial Chemotherapy 53:882–884

Wilcox M H, Fawley W N, Wigglesworth N et al 2003 Comparison of the effect of detergent versus hypochlorite cleaning on environmental contamination and incidence of *Clostridium difficile* infection. Journal of Hospital Infection 54:109–114

Wilcox M H, Barr B, Brady A et al 2006 Prevalence and risk factors for methicillin resistant *Staphylococcus aureus* (MRSA) carriage in care home residents. 6th International Conference of the Hospital Infection Society, Amsterdam

RECOMMENDED READING

*** *Essential reading; ** recommended reading; * interesting but not vital*

General

Chief Medical Officer of the Department of Health 2003 Winning ways. Report by the Chief Medical Officer. Department of Health, London **

Clostridium difficile

Aslam S, Hamill R J, Musher D M 2005 Treatment of *Clostridium difficile*-associated disease: old therapies and new strategies. Lancet Infectious Diseases 5:549–557 ***

Berrington A, Borriello S P, Brazier J et al 2004 National *Clostridium difficile* Standards Group: Report to the Department of Health. Journal of Hospital Infection 56(Suppl 1):1–38 **

Bignargi G E 1998 Risk factors for *Clostridium difficile* infection. Journal of Hospital Infection 40:1–15 *

Bouza E, Muñoz P, Alonso R 2005 Clinical manifestations, treatment and control of infections caused by *Clostridium difficile*. Clinical Microbiology and Infection 11(Suppl 4):57–64 ***

McFarland L V 2005 Alternative treatments for *Clostridium difficile* disease: what really works? Journal of Medical Microbiology 54:101–111 ***

Pépin J, Valiquette L, Cossette B 2005 Mortality attributable to nosocomial *Clostridium difficile*-associated disease during an epidemic caused by a hypervirulent strain in Quebec. Canadian Medical Association Journal 173:1037–1042 *

Stone S, Kibbler C, How A et al 2000 Feedback is necessary in strategies to reduce hospital acquired infection. British Medical Journal 321:302 *

Sunenshine R H, McDonald L C 2006 *Clostridium difficile*-associated disease: new challenges from an established pathogen. Cleveland Clinic Journal of Medicine 73:187–197 ***

Wilcox M, Freeman J, Fawley W et al 2004 Long-term surveillance of cefotaxime and piperacillin-tazobactam prescribing and incidence of *Clostridium difficile* diarrhoea. Journal of Antimicrobial Chemotherapy 54:168–172 **

MRSA

Coia J E, Duckworth G J, Edwards D I et al 2006 The Joint Working Party of the British Society of Antimicrobial Chemotherapy, the Hospital Infection Society, and the Infection Control Nurses Association. Guidelines for the control and prevention of methicillin-resistant *Staphylococcus aureus* (MRSA) in healthcare facilities. Journal of Hospital Infection 63(Suppl 1):1–44 ***

Cosgrove S E, Sakoulas G, Perencevich E N et al 2003 Comparison of mortality associated with methicillin-resistant and methicillin-susceptible Staphylococcus aureus bacteraemia: a meta-analysis. Clinical Infectious Diseases 36:53–59 **

Davis K A, Stewart J J, Crouch H K et al 2004 Methicillin-resistant *Stapylococcus aureus* (MRSA) nares colonization at hospital admission and its effect on subsequent MRSA infection. Clinical Infectious Diseases 39:776–782 **

Stone S P, Beric V, Quick A et al 1998 The effect of an enhanced infection-control policy on the incidence of *Clostridium difficile* infection and methicillin-resistant *Staphylococcus aureus* colonization in acute elderly medical patients. Age and Ageing 27:561–568 **

Wilcox M H 2005 Treating MRSA infections: what every consultant should know. British Medical Journal Learning. 'Just in time' module ***

Influenza and pneumonia

Hedlund J, Christenson B, Lundbergh P et al 2003 Effects of a large-scale intervention with influenza and 23-valent pneumococcal vaccines in elderly people: a 1-year follow-up. Vaccine 21:3906–3911 *

Jackson L A, Neuzil K M, Yu O et al 2003 Effectiveness of pneumococcal polysaccharide vaccine in older adults. New England Journal of Medicine 348:1747–1755 **

Jefferson T, Rivetti D, Rivetti A et al 2005 Efficacy and effectiveness of influenza vaccines in elderly people: a systematic review. Lancet 366:1165–1174 **

Prodigy Guidance 2006 Immunizations – pneumococcal vaccine. Online. Available: http://www.cks.library.nhs.uk/immunizations_pneumococcal/view_whole_guidance **

Prodigy Guidance 2006 Immunizations – influenza. Online. Available: http://www.cks.library.nhs.uk/immunizations_influenza/view_whole_guidance **

SELF-ASSESSMENT QUESTIONS

1. Are the following statements true or false?
   a. *Clostridium difficile* has a mortality of up to 25% in the frail elderly
   b. The spores of *Clostridium difficile* are easily killed
   c. Cefotaxime is associated with a seven-fold greater risk of CDI than piperacillin-tazobactam

2. Are the following statements true or false?
   a. Staff dressing wounds with MRSA have a 60% chance of carrying the organism for 3 hours
   b. Colonization with MRSA increases the risk of subsequent infection by 30% in the acute care setting

3. Are the following statements true or false?
   a. Healthcare-associated infection affects up to 10% of elderly medical in-patients
   b. Older antibiotics such as tetracyclines and clindamycin have a role to play in the treatment of MRSA
   c. Pneumococcal vaccination is effective in preventing pneumonia

SECTION 11

Nutrition and feeding disorders

Chapter 46

Nutrition

Anita J. Thomas and Fiona Boyd

INTRODUCTION

'When I am old I will …
… eat three pounds of sausages at a go
Or only bread and pickle for a week'
(*Warning* by Jenny Joseph)

Nutrition, like geriatric medicine, is a multi-professional discipline. In evaluating the nutritional state of a patient, you should explore the appropriateness of nutritional support and intervention. Generational, ethnic and cultural differences can affect intake On examination of the evidence base for practice, you will find a knowledge base compiled by dieticians, nurses, clinical scientists, biochemists, geneticists, epidemiologists and doctors. Working effectively within a clinical team will enable you to formulate and implement a management plan for a patient.

In this chapter we will:

1. Describe UK nutritional surveillance studies relevant to older people
2. Review why old people are particularly at risk of malnutrition
3. Introduce you to methods of nutritional assessment
4. Refer to current national guidelines for older people
5. Highlight some topical subjects in nutrition
6. Summarize methods of nutritional support
7. Provide a general reference list as an introduction to the discipline

We will not cover the areas of obesity, parenteral nutrition, diet in the aetiology of disease or factors affecting food selection.

NUTRITIONAL ASSESSMENT
(Passmore & Eastwood 1986)

NUTRITIONAL SURVEILLANCE IN THE UK

The annual National Food Survey undertaken by the Department for the Environment, Food and Rural Affairs (DEFRA) samples 6000 households with a 7-day record of food expenditure and consumption broken down by region, income group and type of household. This shows trends in intake and consumption, not information about individuals.

National Diet and Nutrition Surveys (NDNS) are large detailed dietary studies of individuals undertaken by the Food Standards Agency. Groups of up to 2000 people are studied and information obtained on quantitative intake, anthropometric and biochemical measures of nutritional status, socioeconomic and demographic characteristics. The NDNS of people aged 65 years and over (NDNS 1998) reported findings in 1275 people living at home and 412 living in residential and nursing homes, and included an oral health examination. Mean nutrient intakes were generally satisfactory but some figures gave cause for concern.

> Vitamin D intakes were low and a third of institutionalized subjects studied had biochemical evidence of vitamin D deficiency, with a quarter also showing indices for folic acid, riboflavin, ascorbic acid and iron in the range associated with deficiency (NDNS 1998).

Previous studies in the UK by the Committee on Medical Aspects of Food (COMA) had suggested a 7% incidence of malnutrition in well older people living in their own homes, the figure doubling for those aged 80 years and over. The EPIC study revealed different patterns of diet in northern and southern Europeans (Bamia et al 2005).

The National Service Framework (NSF) for Older People (DoH 2001) sets standards for health service provision; relevant domains in the NSF include access to services, the single assessment process, disease prevention and personal care. The Health Care Commission (HCC) quality assures healthcare provision in public and private sectors using reference standards entitled Standards for Better Health (DoH 2004). The Royal College of Physicians has recently published an authoritative guide to the primary responsibility of doctors in patient care regarding nutrition (RCP 2002).

OLDER PEOPLE AT RISK

Even in the absence of disease, older people are at risk of malnutrition because:

1. They are more likely to live in an institution, alone, or be housebound
2. Income and expenditure decline
3. Average intake of energy falls with advancing age

> 'Boiled myself an egg on the ring and had it with a slice of Ryvita ...
> Eat less now. A buttered scone goes a long way'
> ('Soldiering On' from *Talking Heads* by Alan Bennett)

4. Quality of intake is then more important, yet often suboptimal
5. Access to shops may be difficult
6. Ingesting food may be harder with ill-fitting dentures and age-related oesophageal motility changes
7. Age-related physiological changes may mean inefficient gut function, nutrient metabolism and utilization
8. Previous experiences may influence nutritional status, e.g. fetal and childhood nutrition, gastrointestinal (GI) surgery

> In 1992, retired couples who were mainly dependant on the state pension spent about £15 per week on food*
> (Central Statistical Office expenditure survey on family spending. 1992 London, HMSO)
> (*as quoted by Webb & Copeman 1996)
>
> 'Have the men had enough?
> Never mind the men.
> Which men?
> Hurry up, the potatoes will be cold.
> I'd love a potato.
> Then take one, Grandma.
> Have the men had enough?'
> ('Have the men had enough?' by Margaret Forster)

9. Many of the diseases of later life themselves predispose to malnutrition, such as dementia, Parkinson's disease and stroke

The added insult of disease may unmask subclinical malnutrition, resulting in impaired immunity, repair and recovery. The following may significantly increase or change nutritional requirements:

1. Trauma
2. Infection
3. Hypercatabolic states, e.g. fever
4. Drug therapy, e.g. anticonvulsants

METHODS OF NUTRITIONAL ASSESSMENT (Gibson 1990)

Nutritional deficiency can be conceptualized as beginning with:

1. A predisposition to the development of deficiency, e.g. dietary inadequacy revealed by diet assessment
2. Followed by subclinical deficiency, revealed by biochemical or anthropometric tests
3. Culminating in clinical disease

ADEQUATE FOR WHAT?

Assessing whether dietary intake is adequate invites the question 'Adequate for what?' Estimates of nutrient requirements have used different methodology and outcomes for different nutrients, e.g. prevention or cure of deficiency states, biochemical or enzymatic indices of status, or function to metabolic balance studies. International approaches may differ; the UK estimate of vitamin C requirement is based on experiments in 1952 where volunteers deprived themselves of vitamin C in varying amounts and clinical signs of scurvy were the outcome measure (whereas in the USA isotopic studies were the basis for establishing a different requirement). For some nutrients much information is available, but for others, data may be sparse. Less information is available for the older age group, and extrapolation from younger groups is often invalid.

The same observations apply to anthropometric measures. The standard against which measurements of skin-fold thickness and mean arm circumference (as measures of total body fat and protein) were calibrated employed a latter-day version of the ducking stool to immerse subjects in water. Body weight in air and in water with volume of displacement and known density of fat allowed the calculation of mass. Unsurprisingly, there were few elderly volunteers!

The rationale for using a particular method for an individual nutrient is challenged by new methodology, which can also give insight into new physiological concepts. A good example here would be the use of labelled amino acids to study protein metabolism, in addition to the 'black box' approach of the conventional nitrogen balance study.

The objective of nutritional assessment should dictate choice of method. Three main aims are to:

1. Characterize the type and severity of malnutrition
2. Identify those at risk
3. Monitor response to nutritional support

Gariballa and Sinclair (1998) give an authoritative and full account of the subject in an excellent summary of nutrition, ageing and ill health.

DIETARY ASSESSMENT

1. Qualitative, e.g. diet history, food frequency questionnaire
2. Quantitative, e.g. dietary recall, written or weighed food record
3. Duplicate meals and metabolic balance

> Explore the limitations of the methods. Can you remember what you ate for breakfast 3 days ago? If asked to weigh and record the constituents of everything you ate for a week you might decide not to indulge in that seafood risotto, choosing something simpler that you would normally not eat. How would you feel about a metabolic balance study; an exact duplicate of everything you ate and drank being prepared and analysed together with your left-overs, the subtraction giving an accurate picture of intake? Worse to come, the output side of the metabolic balance requires collection of all urine, faeces and in some cases sweat and seminal fluid. Conducted in a laboratory, it might be technically easier but studying a subject in their own home would be preferable. Would you volunteer?

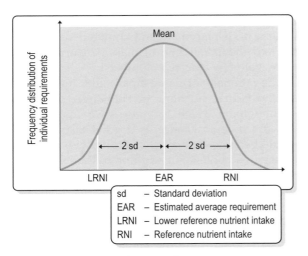

Figure 46.1 Dietary reference values.

Dietary reference values (DRVs) formulated by COMA assist in assessment of diet in groups. Figure 46.1 shows the derivation of the estimated average requirement (EAR – the notional mean requirement), the lower reference nutrient intake (LRNI – mean minus two standard deviations) and the reference nutrient intake (RNI – mean plus two standard deviations). Intakes at or above the RNI 'will almost certainly be adequate' while intakes at or below the LRNI will 'almost certainly be inadequate for most individuals'.

A Department of Health publication (DoH 1991) summarizes current recommendations, with a background summary and comprehensive reference list for each nutrient. A later publication (DoH 1992) deals specifically with recommendations for the older population.

BIOCHEMICAL TESTS

These may be tests of status, such as the blood level or tissue level of a nutrient, e.g. serum iron, or of function, such as activity of a dependent enzyme, e.g. red cell transketolase. Some measures are affected by disease and non-nutritional factors. Serum albumin is a good example, being affected by changes in the balance between synthesis and degradation (liver disease and hypothyroidism), by increases in plasma volume (heart failure), and by intra/extravascular shifts: in stress and trauma the shift results in a fall in serum albumin while in

semi-starvation, serum albumin levels may be artificially elevated by a shift from the extravascular to intravascular compartment. Serum albumin has a relatively long half-life (14–20 days) and is not sensitive to short-term changes in protein status. Serum proteins with a short half-life (e.g. thyroxine-binding prealbumin) may be of use when age- and gender-specific reference ranges are available. Informed selection of biochemical tests of status and function is critical.

ANTHROPOMETRY

Translation of the measurement of body weight into an estimate of body fatness has resulted in the formulation of a series of anthropometric indices. Body mass index (BMI = weight in kg divided by height in m^2) is the most familiar. Substitution of demi-span for height and the adoption of particular formulae for an older population may improve the relevance of these measures, and standards from a UK study of healthy older people are available. Demi-span is the distance measured from the sternal notch to the finger web with the arm outstretched (DoH 1992).

35 years ago, researchers used hydrodensitometry (underwater weighing), with an assumed lean body mass density of 1.10, and correction for lung volume, to calculate body volume and percentage fat. In a younger population these measures correlated with skin-fold thickness measurements. Measuring the circumference of the arm and applying a formula allowed calculation of fat-free mass. Body composition changes with age, there being less fat-free mass and less subcutaneous fat than earlier in life. Many assumptions about anthropometric measurements may not apply to the older population, though there are published reference data for the body mass indices specifically adapted for use in an older population.

Newer methods, such as MRI and electric conductivity, are research tools at present.

CLINICAL HISTORY AND EXAMINATION

The cachexia of protein-calorie malnutrition is sometimes overlooked in an older person, and the pathognomonic features of specific nutrient deficiencies are rarely seen. The proximal myopathy of osteomalacia and sheet haemorrhages of scurvy are notable when seen, but uncommon.

Screening tools should be used as intended since specificity and sensitivity are limited by the effect of non-nutritional factors. The British Society of Enteral and Parenteral Nutrition (BAPEN 2004) have developed the Malnutrition Universal Screening Tool (MUST) for use in hospitals and the community, and examples of others are mentioned below. The 'Subjective Global Assessment' is a method for extracting information (such as weight loss over the preceding 6 months, gastrointestinal symptoms, dietary changes, and examination findings) from the conventional history and examination. These factors are ranked for severity and considered in clinical context. The 'Mini Nutritional Assessment' (MNA) combines anthropometric, dietetic and subjective global measures. A future challenge is to validate non-invasive measures of nutritional assessment for the older person in clinical practice, whether unidimensional (such as measures of body composition) or multidimensional (such as nutritional assessment scores).

NUTRITIONAL SUPPORT

'Thousands are annually starved in the midst of plenty for want of attention to the ways which alone make it possible for them to take food.'

(Florence Nightingale)

SUPPLEMENTING THE NORMAL DIET

Supporting access to food (whether assistance with shopping, financial help or assistance with the physical act of getting food to the mouth) are all of obvious importance.

Oral disease and dysphagia are common in the older population, particularly in association with stroke, dementia and Parkinson's disease. A proper assessment of swallowing, made by a speech and language therapist, with video fluoroscopy where possible, is often a neglected part of the assessment of disability and represents a lost opportunity to improve personal well-being and clinical outcome.

Modification of volume, consistency and content of oral diet by a dietician can improve intake

sufficiently. The use of commercially prepared, nutrient dense supplements does not appear to reduce overall voluntary intake. Four cartons of milk-type supplements provide about half the daily energy and three quarters of the daily protein requirement of a bed-bound patient, but patients usually tolerate less than this. Other types of supplement include fortified juice-type supplements, fortified puddings and modular supplements (containing one or two macronutrients). Further details of types of enteral supplement are available (Thomas & Gill 1998).

ENTERAL FEEDING

If the above measures fail or are contraindicated, enteral support may be necessary. A fine bore nasogastric tube to provide overnight feeding may be adequate but a percutaneous endoscopic gastrostomy (PEG) may be needed for more prolonged support. Time spent with the patient and carers explaining the process involved in the placement and the use of the PEG is of vital importance. Defaecation may only occur once a week due to the lack of dietary fibre and patients need reassurance that constipation is not developing.

Most commercial general-purpose feeds are made up from a variety of protein sources, including casein, soya, and mixtures of amino acids with glucose polymers and triglycerides added to increase energy content. Typically, such a feed would provide about 1 kcal/mL and have an osmolality of 280–420 mmol/kg.

Elemental feeds contain hydrolysed proteins/amino acids as a protein source with little added fat. As a result they are easily absorbed, but their osmolality is high and they are rarely used today. Special feeds can be formulated for patients with hepatic or renal disease. Appropriate positioning of the tube should be confirmed radiologically before feeding is commenced. Hygienic precautions in the preparation, storage and administration of the feed should reduce bacterial contamination, though it is important to allow the feed to reach room temperature before administration. Floating islands of ice-cold feed do not encourage tolerance!

Bolus feeding is associated with diarrhoea, distension and nausea and delivering the feed at a defined rate using a pump delivery system overnight is better, also allowing the patient mobility during the day. Cyclical feeds with 'feed-free' periods reduce the risk of bacterial colonization by allowing a fall in gastric pH, reduction of sodium and water retention, and reduction of fat accretion caused by continuous stimulation of insulin release.

Some clinical situations in which to consider enteral feeding*

- Evidence of protein-energy malnutrition or cachexia
- Inability to eat or swallow
- Hypercatabolic states, e.g. sepsis, fever, burns
- Anorexia, e.g. prolonged illness (> 5 days), chronic or malignant disease
- Neurological disease with dysphagia or loss of gag reflex
- Pre- or post-major surgery

*Gut function is preserved; extensive gastrointestinal disease may mean that the patient requires parenteral feeding.

Here we do not deal with the ethical issues around the decision to commence or withhold nutritional support, but these are weighty matters that demand your attention and authoritative accounts in the major texts and journals are readily accessible (e.g. Lennard Jones 1999). The British Geriatrics Society offers helpful advice for common clinical situations (BGS 2003) (see Ch. 7).

The optimal time to start PEG feeding in the stroke patient is certainly within 1 week to 10 days though some would delay for 2 weeks and the decision must take account of individual factors. In some circumstances, nutritional support will not alter the eventual outcome or patient comfort and is then futile. In other cases, early support will hasten recovery and reduce eventual disability. There are problems associated with the procedure though recent studies indicate that PEG is well tolerated in post-stroke patients, and that quite late recovery of swallowing can occur (even after 6 months). Recent publications have greatly improved the evidence base (FOOD Trial Collaboration 2005a,b) (see Ch. 47).

Nutritional supplementation improves outcome (morbidity and mortality) after fractured femur but also in groups of patients with a variety of clinical conditions. A recent meta-analysis reviews protein and energy supplementation in adults of all ages (Potter et al 1998).

Some complications of tube feeding (see Ch. 47)

- *Aspiration pneumonia* – check tube position on X-ray, sit the patient up to 30 degrees during feed, and observe for problems
- *Wound infection*
- *Tube problems* – blockage (use a dispersible feed and flush the tube), leakage, breakage, dislodgement
- *Pneumoperitoneum*
- *Metabolic problems* – hyperglycaemia, low K, low P, low Zn, low RBC folate, low prothrombin, essential fatty acid deficiency
- *Hyperosmolar syndrome* – due to excess Na absorption, may also cause volume overload
- *Oesophagitis* is rare but can be caused by tube trauma or reflux
- *Diarrhoea and intestinal discomfort* – multi-factorial; iso-osmolar feed given too fast or hyperosmolar solution sometimes with excess lactose. Review the feed formula and administration, check for bacterial contamination of infusion, review medication, especially antibiotics

ENDPIECE

Here are some patient and carer subjects in the popular and scientific press to whet your appetite! Space does not allow a discussion here but all the subjects mentioned below have been headline news in the major journals over the last 5 years.

1. Antioxidants – the link between epidemiological studies, dietary manipulation and the incidence of cancer and vascular disease
2. Effect of early nutrition on adult disease (the Barker hypothesis) – how could programming in early life affect the incidence of disease in middle and late life?

3. Functional foods, e.g. the physiological effects of plant sterols and phyto-oestrogens
4. Food supplements and fortification (e.g. folic acid) – the public health benefits, risk assessment and the consumer's choice

REFERENCES

*** Essential reading; ** recommended reading; * interesting but not vital

Bamia C, Orfanos P, Ferrari P et al 2005 Dietary patterns among older Europeans: the EPIC-Elderly study. British Journal of Nutrition 94:100–113

British Geriatrics Society (BGS) 2003 Nutritional advice in common clinical situations. BGS, London. Online. Available: http://www.bgs.org.uk

British Society of Enteral and Parenteral Nutrition 2004 Malnutrition Universal Screening Tool (MUST). BAPEN, London. Online. Available: http://www.bapen.org.uk/must_tool.html

Department of Health 1991 Dietary reference values for food energy and nutrients for the United Kingdom. Reports on Health and Social Subjects, No 41. HMSO, London ***

Department of Health 1992 The nutrition of elderly people. Reports on Health and Social Subjects, No 43. HMSO, London ***

Department of Health 2001 National Service Framework for Older People. TSO, Norwich. Online. Available: http://www.dh.gov.uk

Department of Health 2004 Standards for better health. TSO, Norwich. Online. Available: http://www.dh.gov.uk

FOOD Trial Collaboration 2005a Routine oral nutritional supplementation for stroke patients in hospital: a multicentre randomized controlled trial. Lancet 365:755–763

FOOD Trial Collaboration 2005b Effect of timing and method of enteral tube feeding for dysphagic stroke patients (FOOD): a multicentre randomized controlled trial. Lancet 365:764–772

Gariballa S E, Sinclair A J 1998 Nutrition, ageing and ill health. British Journal of Nutrition 80:7–23 ***

Gibson R S 1990 Principles of nutritional assessment. Oxford University Press, New York *

Lennard Jones J E 1999 Giving or withholding fluid or nutrients: ethical and legal aspects. Journal of the Royal College of Physicians of London 33:39–45 **

National Diet and Nutrition Survey 1998 People aged 65 years and over. Report of the diet and nutrition survey. The Stationery Office, London

Passmore R, Eastwood M A 1986 Davidson and Passmore human nutrition and dietetics. Churchill Livingstone, London *

Potter J, Langhorne P, Roberts M 1998 Routine protein energy supplementation in adults: systematic review. British Medical Journal 317:495–501 *

Royal College of Physicians 2002 Nutrition and patients; a doctor's responsibility. RCP, London

Thomas A J, Gill C 1998 Malnutrition in elderly people. Prescribers Journal 38:249–254 *

Webb G P, Copeman J 1996 The nutrition of older adults. Arnold/Age Concern, London ***

SELF-ASSESSMENT QUESTIONS

Are the following statements true or false?

1. Serum albumin:
   a. Is a good measure of short-term protein status
   b. Is affected by changes in atmospheric humidity
   c. Is increased in patients suffering major trauma by shifts of albumin from the extravascular to intravascular compartment
   d. Is increased in patients suffering from semi-starvation by shifts of albumin from the extravascular to the intravascular compartment
   e. Has a half-life of 7–10 days

2. The following are recognized complications of enteral feeding by PEG or fine bore nasogastric tube:
   a. Diarrhoea
   b. Secondary lactase deficiency
   c. Hypercatabolic state
   d. Hirsutism
   e. Hypokalaemia

SECTION 11

Nutrition and feeding disorders

Chapter 47

Percutaneous endoscopic gastrostomy (PEG) feeding

Helen Terry and Alex Brown

*'It's good food that keeps me alive and not
fine words'*

(Molière 1672 from
Les Femmes Savantes)

The formation of a gastrostomy using a percutaneous endoscopic technique was first described in 1980 (Gauderer et al 1980). Until then, formation of a gastrostomy required laparotomy and usually general anaesthesia, but many patients in need of enteral feeding were too ill to undergo this procedure. In most cases, feeding via a nasogastric tube was attempted. Percutaneous endoscopic gastrostomy (PEG) provided an alternative to surgical gastrostomy which was simple, could be carried out under local anaesthesia, and was well tolerated even by sick elderly patients (Raha & Woodhouse 1994). It quickly gained in popularity and is now the main method of providing long-term enteral nutrition.

WHO SHOULD BE CONSIDERED FOR PEG FEEDING?

If the gut works, use it! Where possible, enteral nutrition is preferable to parenteral nutrition as it helps to maintain the integrity of the local defence barrier of the intestinal wall and prevents colonization and systemic invasion by gut bacteria. Enteral feeding is also cheaper and easier to monitor. All patients who have a functional gastrointestinal tract, but are not able to take food safely by mouth, should be considered for enteral feeding. Those who can swallow safely, but are unable to eat enough, may also benefit from enteral feeding to supplement their nutritional intake. Feeding via a gastrostomy tube may be considered as an interim measure in those who are expected to recover the ability to eat, as a means of providing long-term nutrition, or it may be palliative in those with incurable disease. These groups include those with:

- Neurological dysphagia
  - stroke
  - motor neuron disease
  - Parkinson's disease
  - multiple sclerosis
- Obstructing neoplasms
  - larynx, oesophagus, bronchus
- Severe facial trauma
- Severe catabolic conditions
  - post surgery
  - sepsis
  - pancreatitis
  - severe burns

PEG OR NASOGASTRIC FEEDING?

A nasogastric tube can be inserted on the ward and is often used as the initial means of providing enteral nutrition. It may be adequate if enteral feeding is a short-term measure. However, over recent years there has been a move towards earlier PEG feeding. This has come about partly as experience with PEG has increased and it has been shown to be a relatively simple and safe procedure. PEG feeding delivers a greater percentage of prescribed nutrition (mainly because of the frequency with which nasogastric tubes fall out), is generally more acceptable to patients than nasogastric tube feeding, and interferes less with rehabilitation (Norton et al 1996, Park et al 1992). However, recent work on enteral feeding in stroke patients with dysphagia has challenged this trend towards very early use of PEG feeding (see the section on PEG feeding after stroke).

CONTRAINDICATIONS TO PEG FEEDING

Some contraindications to PEG insertion are listed in Box 47.1. Most clinicians consider that PEG is contraindicated if a patient has a very limited lifespan or is likely to have a very poor quality of life. (See the section on ethical considerations.) When PEG is contraindicated for technical reasons, it may be possible to insert a gastrostomy tube by a radiological or operative method, or to consider feeding via a jejunostomy.

Box 47.1 Contraindications to PEG tube insertion

Absolute contraindications to PEG insertion

- Patient unfit for endoscopy, e.g. severe pneumonia with respiratory failure
- Inability to pass the scope through the oesophagus
- Gastric outlet obstruction
- Total gastrectomy
- Uncorrected bleeding disorders

Relative contraindications to PEG insertion

- Massive ascites
- Hepatomegaly or splenomegaly
- Portal hypertension with oesophageal or gastric varices
- Severe obesity
- Large hiatus hernia
- Active peptic ulcer
- Neoplastic or infiltrative diseases of stomach
- Partial gastrectomy

TEAM APPROACH

Well-coordinated interdisciplinary teamwork improves the care, and reduces the complication rates and cost, in patients receiving enteral nutrition. Speech and language therapists, dietitians, specialist nutrition nurses, ward nurses, doctors and pharmacists are all involved. Most hospitals now have a nutrition team responsible for enteral feeding. Team members may be directly involved with patient care, but also have a role in educating and supporting ward-based staff. A patient being considered for PEG feeding should have a nutritional assessment and a swallowing assessment (see below). The points for and against PEG feeding, the procedure itself, the practicalities of tube feeding and potential complications should be discussed with the patient and carer in advance.

Once feeding has started, the team must monitor the patient and, if appropriate, prepare the patient and carer for the transition to PEG feeding at home. This will include education about the use of the PEG, and advice on how to deal with any complications that arise. Some teams arrange home visits and have a telephone 'hot-line' for emergency advice. Once the patient is on a stable regimen, their clinical condition, nutritional status and ability to swallow should be assessed every 3–6 months.

SWALLOWING ASSESSMENT

Many patients who are fed via a PEG tube will have initially presented with difficulty swallowing. It is essential to identify swallowing problems promptly because, if they are overlooked, patients may be at risk of aspiration of food or fluids. The initial assessment is usually a bedside screening test conducted by ward nurses who are appropriately trained. The Standardised Swallowing Assessment (SSA) described by Ellul and colleagues is an example of a validated bedside screening tool (Ellul et al 1997), but consult your hospital protocol for information on the screening tool used locally. The first step of each test is to ensure that the patient:

■ Is awake and alert enough to be tested
■ Can be positioned upright and has some head control

Then certain clinical features are observed which are designed to highlight swallowing dysfunction such as:

■ A weak cough
■ Poor control over saliva
■ A wet or gurgly voice

If appropriate the patient then undergoes a water swallow test. They are given a teaspoon of water and their swallow is observed. If there are no problems, this step is repeated twice and then the patient is asked to drink about 50 mL of water from a glass. The test is abandoned if at any stage:

■ The patient makes no attempt to swallow
■ Water leaks straight out of the patient's mouth
■ The patient coughs, chokes or becomes breathless
■ The patient has a wet or gurgly voice afterwards
■ You are unhappy about the swallow

If no problems are identified the patient may eat and drink with supervision and this prevents unnecessary dietary restrictions while waiting for

more detailed assessment. If there is concern, this is an indication for keeping the patient 'nil by mouth' and referring on for a full clinical assessment of swallowing, which is usually conducted by a speech and language therapist. If the therapist finds that the patient has an unsafe swallow and cannot even manage thick fluids or a modified diet, they will suggest consideration of enteral feeding. They may recommend a dynamic assessment of swallowing using videofluoroscopy or a fibre-optic endoscopic evaluation of swallowing. These investigations may be helpful in detecting silent aspiration, where foreign material enters the trachea or lungs without an outward sign of coughing or respiratory difficulty by the patient.

MOUTH CARE

Do not forget about the mouth! In patients who are taking nothing by mouth, good mouth care is essential for their comfort and oral hygiene. Optimum mouth care includes twice daily brushing of the patient's teeth (or dentures), gums and tongue (if it is coated). The patient should rinse his mouth with water as often as is necessary to keep the mouth moist and clean. Alternatively the carer may clean the patient's mouth with a gauze sponge dipped in water or a mouth wash solution, and use Vaseline for the lips and pineapple for the coated tongue.

PERCUTANEOUS ENDOSCOPIC GASTROSTOMY – THE PROCEDURE

There are several endoscopic techniques for inserting a gastrostomy tube (Box 47.2). The 'pull' method is most widely used. It is usually performed by two operators, takes about 20 minutes, and is successful in 98% of cases. In some units it is policy to give a dose of a broad-spectrum antibiotic (e.g. cefotaxime) to cover the procedure. The patient is sedated and the endoscopist insufflates the stomach so that the anterior wall of the stomach meets the anterior abdominal wall. The best site for insertion of the gastrostomy tube is identified by transillumination from within and external indentation with a finger. The assistant infiltrates local anaesthetic into the abdominal wall and

---

> **Box 47.2 Procedures for inserting a gastrostomy tube**
>
> **Endoscopic gastrostomy procedures**
> - Pull method
> - Push method
> - Introducer method
>
> **Non-endoscopic gastrostomy procedures**
> - Percutaneous radiological gastrostomy
> - Laparoscopic gastrostomy
> - Open surgical gastrostomy

passes a cannula through the skin into the stomach. A thread is then passed through the cannula into the gastric lumen. The endoscopist grasps this with biopsy forceps or a snare and pulls the endoscope along with the thread out through the mouth. The PEG tube is attached to the thread and the assistant pulls it through the mouth, down into the stomach and out through the abdominal wall. An inner bumper or balloon retains the tube in the gastric lumen. The assistant applies gentle traction on the tube and then secures it with an external fixation device. It is important that there is not excess tension between the internal bumper and the external fixation device because of the risk of necrosis of the gastric mucosa and skin.

In some hospitals most gastrostomy tubes are put in by a radiologist using a non-endoscopic technique. The choice of insertion method will depend on local expertise. However, the endoscopic method has the advantage of allowing diagnosis of concurrent upper gastrointestinal disease, which is present in up to 20% of patients. The radiological procedure may be attempted in patients in whom it is not possible to pass an endoscope. If neither endoscopic nor radiological placement of a gastrostomy tube is possible, a surgical approach may be considered. The use of laproscopic gastrostomy is becoming popular as an alternative to open gastrostomy. The technical aspects of the different procedures for gastrostomy placement, and evidence of their relative merits, are well reviewed by Safadi and others (Safadi et al 1998).

A PEG tube may need to be removed when it is no longer needed for feeding, or if it deteriorates and needs replacement. The procedure will depend on the type of tube. Some require endoscopic removal; some can be cut off at skin level, allowing the inner crossbar to pass in the stool; and some may be pulled out through the stoma.

STARTING FEEDING

The position of the PEG tube should be checked before the first feed and gastric contents aspirated and checked with pH indicator paper. The patient should be propped up at 45 degrees. Several trials have shown that early tube feeding (as soon as 3 hours after the procedure) is safe, and that full strength feed can be used from the start, and the rate built up steadily. The dietitian will advise on this and on the type of feed that is appropriate for each patient's nutritional, metabolic and fluid requirements. Extra water may be needed. There are different feeds for use in renal, hepatic and cardiac disease. Further details on the content of enteral formulas and delivery of feed may be found in the article by Drickamer and Cooney (1993).

There are different patterns of feeding:

- Continuous infusion via a pump with a 4-hour break each 24 hours
- Bolus feeding using a syringe to deliver 250–400 mL of feed several times a day
- Intermittent gravity feeding, where a bag of 250–500 mL feed runs in over 30–60 minutes
- Cyclical feeding using a pump

Continuous feeding is used while feeding is being established, and then patients are often switched to bolus or intermittent feeding for their convenience. Cyclical feeding may be useful in patients in whom PEG feeding is supplementing oral nutrition or who are being weaned off PEG feeding. They can be fed by infusion overnight and take food by mouth in the day.

30–50 mL flushes of tap water are used before and after bolus feeding, and every 4 hours in continuous feeding. Table 47.1 gives a guide to the type of monitoring of patients that is required after PEG insertion and while starting feeding. The enteral feed may affect the absorption and metabolism of certain drugs (e.g. warfarin, digoxin, theophylline, carbamazepine). The pharmacist will be able to advise on dose modification and monitoring of levels.

Table 47.1 Aspects of initial monitoring of patients on PEG feeding	
Parameter	Frequency
Temperature, pulse and respirations	4–hourly first few days
Fluid balance	Daily
Stool chart	Daily
Weight	2 × weekly
Urea, electrolytes, phosphate	Daily. Once stable 2 × weekly
Glucose	Regular BMs or daily blood glucose
Liver function tests and albumin	2 × weekly
Trace elements	Weekly with long-term feeds for severely catabolic patients

COMPLICATIONS ASSOCIATED WITH PEG

The procedure itself has a mortality rate of less than 1% – mostly related to aspiration pneumonia or peritonitis. Some of the complications that have been reported after PEG are shown in Box 47.3. Major complications occur in only about 3% of patients. Minor complications are more common, but usually resolved easily. Retrospective studies have shown a high 30-day mortality rate, but most of these deaths are related to the underlying poor clinical condition of the patients, rather than to complications arising from the procedure. Careful selection of patients is critical.

EARLY LEAKAGE AROUND THE TUBE

A small amount of leakage is common and can be reduced by antisecretory treatment to lessen the gastric contents. Increased leakage may be an early sign of tube dislodgement or gastric necrosis. Attempts to adjust the tube on the ward have in some cases led to fatal peritonitis. The feed should be stopped and the gastroenterological team contacted. The position of the PEG may need to be checked by endoscopy.

ASPIRATION AND PNEUMONIA

Feeding via a PEG, rather than a nasogastric tube, does not eliminate the risk of aspiration and pneumonia (Cogen & Weinryb 1989). There is wide variation in reported prevalence rates of

---

Box 47.3   Complications associated with PEG

Major

- Aspiration with severe pneumonia
- Perforation of oesophagus
- Peritonitis due to:
  - early tube removal
  - unrecognized migration of catheter into the abdominal wall
  - necrotizing fasciitis
- Upper gastrointestinal haemorrhage
- Gastrocolic fistula
- Internal migration of catheter and intestinal obstruction

Minor

- Wound infection
- Stomal leakage and skin irritation
- Haematoma at gastrostomy site
- Transient ileus
- Transient pneumoperitoneum
- Diarrhoea or constipation
- Nausea and vomiting
- Tube blockage
- Late tube removal

---

aspiration in PEG fed patients (figures range from 3% to 90%). This reflects the underlying differences in populations studied, and the lack of an agreed definition of aspiration. Some studies have used a clinical definition while others have used videofluoroscopy. Some include aspiration of orpharyngeal secretions as well as of feed. Risk factors for aspiration pneumonia include swallowing difficulties, previous aspiration, previous pneumonia and reflux oesophagitis. Measures that may help to reduce the chance of aspiration during PEG feeding include:

- Ensuring that the patient is propped up at 30 to 45 degrees during feeding and for 30–60 minutes afterwards
- Checking that the position of the tube is correct
- Checking gastric residual volumes regularly and slowing the feed if they are high (in bolus feeding, the residual should be less than 100 mL before the next feed and in continuous feeding less than twice the hourly rate)
- Changing from bolus feeding to continuous feeding
- Trying an agent to promote gastric motility (e.g. metoclopramide)
- Converting to a jejunostomy feeding tube

A feeding tube may be placed in the jejunum surgically, radiologically via the stomach or by using a percutaneous endoscopic technique. A PEG-J tube can be inserted via a gastrostomy tube, which allows simultaneous jejunal feeding and gastric drainage, with the aim of avoiding aspiration of feed. Researchers have tried to determine whether this does reduce aspiration and pneumonia in comparison to PEG feeding, but results have been contradictory. The studies were mostly small, retrospective, used different methods and looked at very different populations. Further work is needed to clarify this issue.

DIARRHOEA

Diarrhoea often occurs in PEG-fed patients. The formula feed is frequently blamed, but there are other more common causes to exclude:

- Medications (e.g. antibiotics, sorbitol-based elixirs, magnesium-containing preparations)
- Infective causes (including *Clostridium difficile*)
- Constipation with overflow
- Too rapid delivery of feed
- Feed too cold
- Feed contamination
- Feed composition (osmolality, presence of lactose, fibre content)

Once an infective cause has been excluded, loperamide or codeine may help to control symptoms. A dietitian will advise on changes in the type of feed that might help.

TIPS FOR UNBLOCKING A BLOCKED PEG

A PEG tube may become blocked with feed residue or precipitated medications, particularly if it is not flushed with water before and after each use. Gently alternating aspiration and flushing with warm water for a few minutes may unblock it – use a 50 mL syringe, as a smaller one may cause the tube to collapse. Undoing the connections to remove the 90 degree bend before flushing may help. If this does not work the following may be tried:

1. Gently flushing with 30 mL of warm water and leaving for 30 minutes
2. Flushing with 30 mL of soda water or cola and leaving for a further 30 minutes
3. Try instilling 30 mL of pineapple juice. This contains an enzyme that may dissolve the material blocking the tube
4. Breaking open a pancreatic enzyme capsule and dissolving the contents with one sodium bicarbonate tablet (324 mg) in 10 mL of water. Leave this solution to activate for 5 minutes then flush this down the tube and leave for 30 minutes
5. If the above fail, contact a gastroenterologist who may be able to unblock the tube with endoscopic brushes or guide wires. Do not be tempted to poke wires down the tube yourself

If these measures are unsuccessful, the tube will have to be replaced.

WHAT TO DO IF A PEG TUBE FALLS OUT

If a PEG tube falls out soon after insertion, a mature tract will not have formed and there is a risk of leakage of gastric contents leading to peritonitis. (The tract is usually established within a week, but this may be delayed for up to 3 weeks in patients who are malnourished or on steroids.) Start intravenous antibiotics (e.g. cefotaxime and metronidazole), and a proton pump inhibitor to reduce the acidity of the leaking gastric fluid. Watch closely for signs of peritonitis and be prepared to seek a surgical opinion. Contact a gastroenterologist promptly – he or she may be able to use a guide-wire technique to re-establish the tract if this is done quickly enough. Otherwise, the gastrostomy tube will need to be replaced under endoscopic guidance – usually after a delay of 1–2 weeks.

If a PEG tube comes out once a fistula is established, it is important to put in a replacement tube within a few hours to keep the stoma open. A 16 or 20 French Gauge Foley urinary catheter may be used as a temporary measure. It should be carefully inserted into the stoma, the balloon inflated, gentle traction applied, and the catheter taped securely to the abdominal wall. A gastroenterologist will then be able to insert a replacement PEG tube or button gastrostomy without the patient having to go through the full endoscopic procedure again.

A confused patient is at particular risk of pulling out his PEG tube. Ensure that the tube is well secured and hidden by a dressing or bandage. Consider converting to a button gastrostomy once a mature tract is formed. This is less bulky, so attracting less attention from the patient, and is not as easy to pull out.

PEG FEEDING AFTER A STROKE

Swallowing problems in acute stroke are common, occurring in up to 45% of patients within the first 48 hours. About a third of these have resolved by the end of the first week, and swallowing difficulties persist in only 2% of survivors at 1 month. It is often unclear in the first few days which patients are going to regain a safe swallow quickly (Smithard 1999).

Many elderly patients with a stroke are already malnourished on admission to hospital, and if unable to take adequate food their nutritional status will quickly decline. Reduced muscle strength and lowered resistance to infection may result in a poorer outcome. Some clinicians have fed patients via a nasogastric tube, within a few days of their stroke, to maintain nutrition while waiting to see if swallowing recovers. Some have

arranged early insertion of a PEG tube because of the practical difficulties associated with nasogastric tubes. Others considered that the complications of early tube feeding outweighed the benefits and delayed feeding for 2 weeks or more. Stroke patients with dysphagia are in a poor prognostic group in terms of survival and functional recovery. Studies of long-term follow up of stroke patients with PEG have shown a high in-hospital mortality rate and a high level of disability in those who do leave hospital (James et al 1998, Wanklyn et al 1995). This raised concern that early PEG feeding was only prolonging imminent death for some patients, or increasing the chance of others being kept alive with severe disability and a poor quality of life.

This clinical uncertainty and variation in practice reflected the lack of evidence from prospective randomized controlled trials on feeding after stroke, and was addressed by the International Stroke Trials Collaboration in their FOOD Study (Feed Or Ordinary Diet) (FOOD Trial Collaboration 2005). They investigated whether early tube feeding increases the proportion of stroke patients surviving without severe disability, and if feeding via a PEG rather than a nasogastric tube affects the outcome. They found no significant difference between early (less than a week) and later enteral feeding. There was an absolute difference in the risk of death in favour of early feeding, but an excess of survivors with a poor outcome in this group.

The authors conclude that in stroke patients with dysphagia we should:

- Feed via a nasogastric tube within the first few days, unless there is a strong indication to delay enteral feeding
- Use nasogastric tube feeding for 2–3 weeks unless there is a strong practical reason to use a PEG tube

ETHICAL CONSIDERATIONS

Difficult decisions about PEG feeding usually arise when there is uncertainty about prognosis and whether PEG feeding is in patients' best interests. Patients may not be capable of making an informed choice about their care. In these cases, the team needs to consider the circumstances of each individual, and take into account any previously expressed wishes of the patient, and the views of family and carers, before deciding whether to start PEG feeding. It is often helpful to involve the general practitioner, who may know the patient well. It is important to be realistic about prognosis, but if in doubt it is better to feed the patient while further assessment and treatment of the underlying condition occur. The British Medical Association and General Medical Council have given helpful guidance on this difficult area.

Key points

- Consider PEG feeding in all patients with a functional gastrointestinal tract who are not able to take sufficient food by mouth and who have a reasonable life expectancy.
- In carefully selected patients PEG insertion has a less than 1% procedure-related mortality and a low rate of major complications.
- The high 30-day mortality rates reported after PEG insertion mainly reflect the underlying poor clinical condition of the patients who require PEG feeding.
- Successful PEG feeding requires an interdisciplinary approach involving doctors, nurses, dietitians, speech therapists, pharmacists and carers.

REFERENCES

*** *Essential reading; ** recommended reading; * interesting but not vital*

Cogen R, Weinryb J 1989 Aspiration pneumonia in nursing home patients fed via gastrostomy tubes. American Journal of Gastroenterology 84:1509–1512 *

Drickamer M, Cooney L 1993 A geriatrician's guide to enteral feeding. Journal of the American Geriatrics Society 41:672–679 **

Ellul J, Barer D, Fall S 1997 Improving detection and management of swallowing problems in acute stroke: a multicentre study. Cerebrovascular Disease 7(Suppl 4):18 **

FOOD Trial Collaboration 2005 Effect of timing and method of enteral tube feeding for dysphagic stroke patients (FOOD): a multicentre randomized controlled trial. Lancet 365:764–772 ***

Gauderer M W, Ponsky J L, Izant R J 1980 Gastrostomy without laparoscopy; a percutaneous endoscopic technique. Journal of Paediatric Surgery 15:872–875 *

James A, Kapur K, Hawthorne A B 1998 Long-term outcome of percutaneous endoscopic gastrostomy feeding in patients with dysphagic stroke. Age and Ageing 27:671–676 **

Norton B, Homer-Ward M, Donnelly M T et al 1996 A randomised prospective comparison of percutaneous endoscopic gastrostomy and nasogastric tube feeding after acute dysphagic stroke. British Medical Journal 312:13–16 **

Park R H R, Allison M C, Lang J et al 1992 Randomised comparison of percutaneous endoscopic gastrostomy and nasogastric tube feeding in patients with persisting neurological dysphagia. British Medical Journal 304:1406–1409 **

Raha S K, Woodhouse K W 1994 The use of percutaneous endoscopic gastrostomy (PEG) in 161 consecutive elderly patients. Age and Ageing 23:162–163 *

Safadi B Y, Marks J M, Ponsky J L 1998 Percutaneous endoscopic gastrostomy: an update. Endoscopy 30(9):781–789 **

Smithard D G 1999 Dysphagia following stroke. Reviews in Clinical Gerontology 9:81–93 ***

Wanklyn P, Cox N, Belfield P 1995 Outcome in patients who require a gastrostomy after stroke. Age and Ageing 24:510–514 ***

RECOMMENDED READING AND SOURCES OF INFORMATION

British Association for Parenteral and Enteral Nutrition. (BAPEN). Online. Available: http://www.bapen.org.uk

British Medical Association 2007 Withholding and withdrawing life-prolonging medical treatment: guidance for decision making, 3rd edn. BMA, London

General Medical Council 2002 Withholding and withdrawing life-prolonging treatments: good practice in decision making. GMC, London. Online. Available: http://www.gmc-uk.org/guidance/current/library.asp#supplementary.guidance

Royal College of Physicians 2004 National clinical guidelines for stroke, 2nd edn. Online. Available: http://www.rcplondon.ac.uk/pubs/brochure.aspx?e=130

SELF-ASSESSMENT QUESTIONS

Are the following statements true or false?

1. A PEG tube may be:
   a. Helpful in a patient with gastric outlet obstruction
   b. Unblocked using the dissolved contents of a pancreatic enzyme capsule
   c. Temporarily replaced with a urinary catheter if it falls out the day after insertion
   d. Used to deliver three bolus feeds of 800 mL a day

2. The risk of aspiration in a PEG-fed patient may be reduced by:
   a. Lying the patient on their left-hand side during feeding
   b. Nasogastric tube feeding
   c. Converting from bolus to continuous feeding
   d. Prescribing metoclopramide to promote gastric motility

PART 4

Personal and professional skills

Chapter 48

Education

Keren Davies and Gerry C. J. Bennett (Deceased)

Medicine involves lifelong learning. The General Medical Council (GMC) has stated that 'high quality patient care depends on sound education and training' and 'you must maintain the standard of your performance by keeping your knowledge and skills up to date throughout your working life'. In 2003, the plan to reform postgraduate medical education, 'Modernising Medical Careers' (MMC) was published (NHS Executive 1998). This chapter was written during the initial stages of MMC when some uncertainty still existed over the structure of postgraduate medical training in the UK.

In August 2005, newly qualified doctors entered the new 2-year foundation programme, which has replaced the preregistration house officer and first-year senior house officer posts. The foundation programme is designed to give a planned programme of supervised clinical training, with a published curriculum of competencies to be attained across a range of specialties. It includes a regular formal assessment of trainees and a commitment to careers counselling and advice. It is assumed that on completion of the foundation programme, trainees will move into specialty training.

The present specialist registrars (SpR) have a structured training programme supported by regular appraisal and assessment (SCOPME 1996). The Royal College of Physicians' curricula list those competencies required during SpR training. Assessment methods will alter to mirror those adopted in foundation programme training.

Many of the present consultant body did not have appraisal and assessment during training and until recently had little knowledge of these areas. There has recently been great emphasis on training consultants in techniques of assessment and appraisal. The introduction of the new Consultant Contract in 2003 allows the recognition of consultants' educational roles. There is a requirement for trainers to teach foundation programme trainees professional skills, team working and communication skills in addition to traditional clinical skills. Consequently, there has been much to learn by all those involved in postgraduate education.

In this chapter we look at adult learning, discuss the learning cycle and educational needs assessment, describe appraisal and assessment and discuss communication skills.

ADULT LEARNING

Why do adults learn? The motivation to learn may be due to external pressure (e.g. the need to pass an examination) or arise from a personal desire to learn more about a subject – perhaps because a problem area has been identified.

Adults learn best when:

- They are actively involved in the educational process
- Learning is relevant, with clear aims and objectives that are realistic and, hence, likely to be achieved

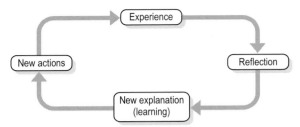

Figure 48.1   Experiential learning: experiences as a source of learning and development.

■ They are able to reflect on their own practice and obtain constructive feedback
■ Learning is non-threatening and fun

THE LEARNING CYCLE AND EDUCATIONAL NEEDS ASSESSMENT

The learning cycle (Fig. 48.1) builds on these principles and relies on individuals reflecting on their own practice and also receiving feedback (Joint Centre for Education in Medicine 1997).

EDUCATIONAL NEEDS ASSESSMENT

To determine learning needs it is necessary to:

■ Identify current knowledge, skills and attitudes – the foundation programme requires all trainees to undertake a self-assessment before discussing their learning needs
■ Compare this baseline assessment with what is required, either for the particular post or guided by the foundation programme or Royal College of Physicians' curricula
■ Identify specific areas for learning and set objectives
■ Identify the methods to achieve these objectives

Learning needs will change during a doctor's career, therefore the continual cycle of reflection on practice and setting new objectives is important.

Examples

1. A year 1 foundation programme trainee identifies a need to be able to insert a central venous line. This might be achieved by understanding the anatomy and principles of line insertion, observing a senior colleague insert a line, learning the procedure under supervision and then practicing under supervision.
2. A third year specialist registrar identifies learning needs as management skills in team leadership and budget management. This might be achieved by attending a course or shadowing a consultant colleague, the clinical director or business manager.

Practical point

Setting objectives on clinical skills and technical skills is often easier than those relating to attitudes and behaviour.

SETTING EDUCATIONAL OBJECTIVES

There is no accepted definition of an educational need. Learning needs and educational objectives are identified and assessed in terms of *knowledge, skills* and *attitudes*. Not all learning is specifically based on identified needs. Some learning will be aimed at developing or reinforcing previously learnt skills and knowledge.

HOW DO WE IDENTIFY LEARNING NEEDS?

This may be increasingly difficult with career progression. A first-year foundation programme trainee has many skills and a lot of knowledge to gain, while an experienced consultant may have very specific learning needs.

Table 48.1 lists examples of ways used to identify learning needs. Those requiring more information should study *The Good CPD Guide* (Joint Centre for Education in Medicine 1999). Learning objectives should be set by agreement between trainee and clinical or educational supervisor during appraisal sessions. A learning contract can be drawn up which documents what needs to be learnt and which describes the learning programme to achieve it, identifying the resources and support required. The foundation programme training portfolio requires all trainees to complete a personal development plan and an educational agreement (DoH 1998).

Table 48.1	Ways of identifying learning needs
Method	**Examples**
Own experience of patient care	Identify areas of ignorance, problems arising from complaints, comparison with competence standards
Clinical team working	Clinical educational meetings, departmental service plans, interdisciplinary working practice
Non-clinical activities	Grand rounds, conferences, research, teaching
Quality activities	Audit, critical incidents, morbidity and mortality meetings
Appraisal and assessment	Meetings with educational supervisor, annual review

Foundation programme trainees

Having obtained a medical degree, foundation programme trainees have some knowledge, skills and basic professional values. They need to become competent in dealing with clinical problems and to develop appropriate professional attitudes. All foundation programme doctors will follow the national Curriculum for the Foundation Years in Postgraduate Training and Education, which describes the competencies required at year one and two (DoH 2003).

Methods of achieving the objectives set out in the curriculum might include:

- Observation and questioning of more experienced colleagues
- Lectures, tutorials, journal clubs
- Discussion of clinical cases with peers
- Video and audio material, text books and journals
- Computer-assisted learning
- Appraisal with an educational supervisor
- Reflection on one's own practice and performance

Senior house officers (SHO)

At present, trainees in SHO posts develop generic skills, a career direction and some basic specialist skills. Learning is rooted in clinical service, in which the doctor should develop knowledge and skills in specialty areas, train for diplomas and examinations, and possibly gain experience in research and audit. In August 2006, the SHO post was included in foundation programmes (DoH 2004a). The future of the remaining SHO posts is still to be decided. It is clear that all trainees will be expected to follow defined curricula, complete a training portfolio and undergo similar assessments (as detailed in the foundation programme portfolio).

Both foundation programme training, and at present SHO training, should include a comprehensive curriculum-based educational programme and there should be opportunities for study leave.

Specialist registrars

The learning needs of specialist registrars are based on developing knowledge and skills in the specialty. The goal is to become a competent independent practitioner and holder of a Certificate of Completion of Training (CCT).

Learning needs are identified by reviewing previous experience and examining the training requirements of the college curriculum. The methods of achieving needs will include those discussed above and be further informed by the annual review and Record of In-Training Assessment (RITA).

Consultants

There is a requirement for consultants to ensure that their medical education continues throughout their professional life. Continuing professional development (CPD) first came to prominence through the initiative of clinical governance and the publication of *A First Class Service* in 1998 (DoH 1998). Clinical governance is now used to describe continuing medical education (CME) and other areas where consultants need to attain and develop skills, e.g. management skills, appraisal and assessment, information technology, audit and risk management. The Royal Colleges have systems for monitoring CME and CPD. All consultants must take part in a yearly appraisal and have a personal development plan which records their educational and training needs, the CPD to be undertaken, the resources required to meet their needs and the potential benefit to the clinical service.

APPRAISAL AND ASSESSMENT

Both appraisal and assessment are educational tools. Their meanings are often confused. There is some overlap as assessments may be used in appraisals, but educationalists would emphasize they should be considered and performed separately (DoH 2005a).

APPRAISAL

Definition

The Standing Committee on Postgraduate Medical and Dental Education defines appraisal as a dialogue focusing on the personal, professional and educational development needs of one of the parties concerned, which produces agreed outcomes.

There are different models of appraisal but the commonest is 'top down' (trainer to trainee). Alternative models do exist such as 'bottom up' (trainee appraises trainer), 'peer review' (e.g. consultant and medical director) and team review. The discussion here is confined to trainer to trainee appraisal.

Appraisal is designed to assist personal and career development. It seeks to improve performance through the setting of mutually agreed objectives.

Features of appraisal

Appraisal:

■ Should be continuous and part of day-to-day practice, not an 'event'
■ Is confidential between trainer and trainee
■ Involves constructive feedback
■ Focuses on the trainee's needs

■ Consists of planned non-threatening meetings between trainee and trainer
■ Is concerned with setting personal learning goals and agreeing how to achieve those goals
■ Involves periodic review of personal, educational and professional achievements

How to appraise

1. Hold an induction session:
   ■ Inform the trainee of the process and agree the purpose of the appraisal, i.e. to review performance and to plan the future by discussing individual career developments
   ■ Set a date for the first meeting with the chosen trainer or educational supervisor

2. Arrange the first meeting early in the post:
   ■ Set out the process and agree the rules for appraisal. These should include:
     – confidentiality/honesty
     – secured time
     – a suitable environment
     – setting dates for meetings
     – ensure trainee understands role in self-appraisal and involvement in discussion (ideally the trainee should talk most)
     – agree sources of feedback to inform process (e.g. the ward sister)
     – agree a method of record keeping

3. The trainee prepares for the first formal appraisal meeting:
   ■ By self-appraisal, looking at strengths and areas for development – knowledge, skills, responsibilities and attitudes
   ■ Reviews ways of realizing training needs

4. First formal meeting:
   ■ The trainee explains learning needs perhaps with reference to training record
   ■ The trainer responds using experience and knowledge of training requirements
   ■ The trainee and trainer agree educational objectives
   ■ The trainee and trainer agree ways of achieving objectives

5. Subsequent appraisal meetings at 2 to 3 month intervals:
   ■ The trainee reviews progress
   ■ The trainer collects information from agreed sources

Discussion of progress. Give positive feedback first, then discuss areas for improvement. Review of learning objectives and ways of achieving them.

Before any session, planning is required to complete any documentation. Give enough notice of the meeting, choose a suitable venue, ensure there will be no interruptions and allow adequate time for the meeting.

During the meeting, be comfortable! Agree the agenda, follow the agreed format, and allow the trainee to speak first and for most of the time. When giving feedback, always start with positive comments. Set mutually agreed objectives and take notes of the discussion.

After the meeting, record the main points of discussion and conclusions. Ensure that the trainee has agreed with the written record as a summary of the meeting.

There is debate about the nature of appraisal records. Some consultants feel the only documentation of appraisal should be the learning objectives and a confirmation that the appraisal meeting took place. Others believe records should be kept by the trainer and trainee.

Why do appraisal?

Proving that appraisal is beneficial is difficult. There is little published confirmatory evidence. The perceived benefits are listed below.

Benefits to the trainee
- Learning needs are identified early.
- Learning opportunities can be identified early.
- The trainee develops self-appraisal and reflective practice skills needed throughout his or her career.
- Progress should be reviewed and remedial action taken if there are problems.
- There is an opportunity to give feedback on the quality of training received.
- It can improve morale, motivation and confidence.
- It assists career planning.

Benefits to the trainer
- It is an opportunity to receive feedback on training.

- It allows familiarity with day-to-day issues affecting trainees.
- It is an opportunity to develop communication and negotiating skills.
- It is an opportunity to develop team building and working.
- It allows reflection on one's own abilities and practice.

Overall benefits
Overall, the benefits appear to be:

- Improved delivery of training
- More effective and efficient training
- Improvement of morale and motivation
- Development of team working
- Improvement of communication
- Better patient care

Problems with appraisal

- There is confusion in what constitutes appraisal and assessment (see Table 48.2).
- There is lack of training for trainers in appraisal – particularly in giving constructive feedback that concentrates on behaviours and actions, not personalities.
- There is a lack of awareness of the need to support trainees day to day in achieving learning objectives, through lack of time or resources.
- Ensuring the most appropriate person is the appraiser and that rapport is established can be a problem.
- Different grades need different types of appraisal.
- The process may provide evidence of problems involving the health, conduct or competence of the trainee and raise issues of patient safety. If such issues arise, stop the appraisal and address the problems through appropriate avenues, e.g. occupational health, counselling or disciplinary procedures.

ASSESSMENT

Assessment is a process whereby a doctor's performance is measured and compared with known criteria. Assessments have always taken

Table 48.2 Features of appraisal and assessment		
	Appraisal	**Assessment**
Purpose	Educational	Career regulation
Participants	Appraiser and trainee 1:1	Panel and trainee
Topics	Educational, personal, professional development	Generic skills, clinical and management skills, competence
Standards	Individual	National and local
Confidential	Yes	No
Documentation	Learning contract	National documents
	Confirmation of meeting	RITA forms
Outcome	Enhanced development	Career progression

place, formally, as examinations, and also informally with observation of clinical practice leading to trainers forming opinions expressed in references.

The purpose of assessment in specialist registrar training is to judge progress against defined criteria based on the curriculum. Trainees have to meet agreed standards to proceed from year to year and to obtain the CCT.

Why do we need assessment?

We need it to:

- Measure academic achievement
- Maintain standards
- Motivate trainees
- Identify trainees' problems
- Evaluate effectiveness of training programmes and trainers

The new foundation programmes include a formal requirement for regular trainee assessment to ensure the programmes produce doctors who are competent in all domains of the curriculum (DoH 2005b).

The Foundation Learning Portfolio describes the methods of assessment required to demonstrate competence. These include:

- Direct observation of procedural skills (DOPS), e.g. catheterization, intravenous cannulation, arterial gas sampling
- The Mini-Clinical Evaluation Exercise (Mini-CEX) – assessing a trainee/patient interaction in a clinical setting (e.g. history taking in outpatients)

- Multi-source feedback or the Peer Assessment Tool (Mini PAT) – the trainee nominates members of the clinical team to provide feedback on their performance in a number of areas
- Case-based discussion – trainees discuss a recent case they managed to demonstrate clinical skills in a number of areas, e.g. use of investigations, treatment planning

The purpose of assessment is to:

- Communicate to trainees what is important
- Motivate the trainee to learn
- Identify deficiencies and areas for further learning
- Identify where the training programme is weak

Features of assessment

Assessment:

- Is judgmental
- Is measured against defined criteria
- Must strive to be objective
- Should be reproducible
- Should be evidence based

Assessment of competence

When examining structured medical training, it is important to ensure that trainees are competent to practice. Assessment of competence is problematic as it is necessary to develop methods to assess performance at all levels of competence. To ensure that national standards are maintained, the methods used must be valid, reliable and sensitive to the task involved.

When measuring performance, there should be a clearly specified and shared understanding of good practice. The four levels of competence described in Miller's pyramid (DoH 2005c) are as follows:

1. *Knowing* – knowledge a trainee must possess. Methods of assessment – multiple choice questions, essay questions or vivas.

2. *Knowing how* – items a trainee must know how to do but not necessarily be able to do at this stage of training. Methods of assessment – patient management problems, case-based discussions, modified essays and orals.

3. *Showing how* – items trainees must be able to do. This can only be assessed by observing the trainee. Methods of assessment – Mini-CEX, practical examinations, Objective Structured Clinical Examinations (OSCEs).

4. *Doing* – the way the trainee practises in day-to-day work. The usual method of assessment is to observe the trainee at work; direct observation of procedural skills (DOPS).

Previously, most assessments in medical training looked at levels 1 and 2, while Royal College examinations looked at some aspects of level 3. Following the introduction of MMC, assessments will cover all the above levels.

Standards for assessment

Assessment involves observing performance in carrying out a pre-specified task in order to compare performance with a fixed standard. Tasks may be real-life service tasks or tests and examinations.

- The standard may be other people's performance – peer or norm referenced, e.g. written examinations. Candidates are ranked by the marks obtained. This is unnecessary when looking at competence: either you are competent or you are not.
- Alternatively, pre-specified criteria are used in a criterion-referenced system, e.g. the Advanced Life Support (ALS) course or foundation programme curriculum. The criteria necessary to prove competence are clearly defined. This may be the ideal, but is still problematic in medicine

Table 48.3	Methods of assessment
Method	Examples
Written examination	Multiple choice questions, essays, extended matching items, dissertation
Patient-based examination	Long cases, short cases, vivas, objective structured clinical examinations, Mini-CEX, DOPS
Non-clinical cases	Case note review, audit, critical incident review, review of log books
Assessment panels	Annual review

as the higher functions of medicine do not lend themselves to simplistic descriptions.

- The Limen referenced assessment – assessors use their expert understanding of the minimum standard required to practise safely, for example judging when a new SHO should be on the on-call rota. It has been used as part of fitness-to-practice procedure.

Methods of assessment

Examples of assessment (DoH 2003, 2004a,b, 2005a,b,c) are given in Table 48.3.

Problems with assessment

- Assessment, particularly examinations, may drive learning but often there is little or no feedback on performance. Therefore, there is no opportunity to reflect on the learning experience to gain a direction for further development.
- Assessment based on an assessor's opinion will inevitably be subjective and therefore variable. It may not be reliable.
- There are difficulties in setting appropriate criteria or standards.
- Most assessments are costly in time and people.

The annual review of specialist training and RITA

The Royal Colleges publish a curriculum of training for each specialty. On entry to the specialist registrar grade, the trainee applies for a training record that gives details of the curriculum, expected levels of achievement and the necessary documentation.

An annual review takes place at which the specialist registrar's progress is reviewed by a small panel of specialists on behalf of the regional specialty training committee. The assessment used must be valid, reliable, nationally agreed with minimum competence levels, specialty-specific and feasible. Remedial action can be taken if necessary. This process is managed by regional postgraduate deans.

At the annual review, the training record and the trainers' reports are reviewed. The results of the review are recorded on the appropriate documentation. The penultimate year assessment (PYA) is similar to the annual review in previous years but includes an external representative of the specialty nominated by the Joint Committee on Higher Medical Training (JCHMT). The PYA is important as it provides independent assurance that the trainee's progress is satisfactory and aids setting the final CCT date.

The record of in-training assessment (RITA) provides a record of the annual review and therefore of the trainee's progress through specialist training. It is available for review if any queries are raised at the completion of training. This regulatory form of assessment is for the benefit of patients as it is intended to ensure that doctors who provide medical care unsupervised are competent to do so.

It is likely that there will be changes to this system following the introduction of the 'run through' grade, a managed training grade immediately following foundation programme training and leading to specialist training and to the award of the Certificate for Completion of Satisfactory Training (CCST). The methods of assessment introduced for foundation programmes will be used for assessment of all trainees.

COMMUNICATION SKILLS

This section contains:

■ Introduction
■ Principles of communication
■ Avoiding pitfalls
■ Special aspects of communication skills: breaking bad news
■ Presentations

INTRODUCTION

Medical education does not have an illustrious past when it comes to communication skills. The consultant ward round could exemplify all that was wrong with an aspect of medicine that was not seen as crucial to being a good and effective doctor as it now is. Medical students suffered the worst, often learning by humiliation. Patients fared little better. They were objects to answer questions, be examined by innumerable people and to be consoled with a transient tap on the back of the hand.

Communication skills are now recognized as essential tools. Good communicators may be born but few of us have all the essential elements innately. We can all be taught many of the core components necessary to elicit a comprehensive and accurate history, feed back the results of an examination to our peers, seniors and, most importantly, the patient. Communication skills result in the practice of better medicine, but they also facilitate a more mutually satisfying clinical relationship between patient and doctor (and hopefully a less litigious one). Some clinicians will always have more obvious skills: empathy, a gift with words, the common touch. We can all learn the basic principles and improve in areas we may find stressful, such as breaking bad news.

The golden rule is treat your patients as you would want to be treated. Communication skills start with our responsibilities as a human being directed by the Hippocratic oath and focused by ethics and learned skills. Common humanity is an excellent starting place.

PRINCIPLES OF COMMUNICATION

A useful model for understanding the medical interview is that of Cohen-Cole and Bird described in *The Medical Interview: The Three-Function Approach* (Cohen-Cole 1991). The three functions of their model are:

■ Data gathering
■ Rapport and relationship building
■ Education and motivation

There is inevitably some overlap between these, but within each, particular behaviours or skills serve to fulfil the goals of the interview.

After qualification many doctors feel confident about their clerking skills. If given a checklist however, how many of us use all the skills described and to good effect?

Communication objectives are to:

- Introduce oneself and explore the patient's problems
- Use verbal and non-verbal skills that help build a rapport and put patients at their ease. Create an atmosphere of trust, respect and comfort in terms of physical ambience and personal interaction
- Identify and share with the patient their concerns, understanding, expectations and background
- Identify and share with the patient the goals of the interview and purposes of the procedures or examination undertaken
- Elicit accurate information by closed and open questions, reflection, clarification and summarizing
- Understand and use relationship skills that facilitate the expression of information, emotions and provide emotional support to the patient
- Recognize your reactions to patients
- Appropriately interrupt only when absolutely necessary and direct the discussion while still maintaining a logical and systematic flow of the interview
- Deal sensitively with the patient's questions, give relevant information simply and clearly, avoiding jargon and checking understanding
- Close the patient encounter
- Reflect on one's strengths and weaknesses

Developing the above list into an effortless, consistent communication tool can take a professional lifetime.

AVOIDING PITFALLS

Introductions are crucial and the bedrock of what follows. They should be straightforward, relatively formal and include eye contact, a greeting, an outstretched hand (expecting a returned handshake) and your name. Remember vision, hearing and comfort. You are often judged by what you write. Remarks such as 'difficult, vague historian' or even 'rambling old buffer' written in case notes tell us more about the attitudes and behaviour of the doctor than the patient. Hearing is crucial in many ways.

SPECIAL ASPECTS OF COMMUNICATION SKILLS: BREAKING BAD NEWS

This special area of communication skills is now a routine part of medical undergraduate learning. As with all communication, it is a life-long learning process. It may be helpful to refresh one's memory of the standard teaching techniques used to prepare students (and ourselves) for these emotionally difficult situations. The skills training is usually broken down into three sessions which build upon each other. The sessions involve the use of role-play and the use of feedback from peers and teachers to facilitate learning.

Role-play can be an excellent tool. An orientation session indicates how the session will be conducted. The teacher highlights what to look for; gives ground rules for participating (safe environment, confidentiality, etc.) and gives the rules of feedback. Before observers give feedback the 'learner' role-player says how they feel the interview went. Then it is the 'patient's' turn. The observers, who have usually been asked to observe behaviours, comment next. *Remember that feedback is not the same as criticism; it is part of building a trusting and learning climate.*

The first session involves introduction skills and the gathering of accurate data – this involves an analysis of:

- Questioning styles
- Facilitation
- Checking
- Summarizing
- Non-verbal behaviour
- Organizational skills of goal setting, orientation, direction and closure

The second session involves the exploration of the patient's reactions to bad news and demonstrates the skills of emotional support; these include:

- Empathy – acknowledging feelings and showing they are understood

- Ventilation – allowing patients to discuss emotions
- Respect
- Reassurance

The third and final session shows how a practitioner can talk and educate a patient about their illness and its management and demonstrates the skills of:

- Achieving understanding through explanations, instructions and checking
- Motivation through positive attribution and praise

The above pointers are simply a framework on which to hang learned experiences. The emotions generated within these discussions can be stressful. Recognizing that you may need de-briefing as a clinician either by colleagues, a mentor or someone specially provided for that purpose is important.

Even though the situations feel difficult, it is often the thought of a hard job done well that gives the most satisfaction. I once spent an hour with a patient and her daughter in a follow-up clinic explaining the results of an endoscopy (which revealed gastric cancer) and the process that would follow (referral to a gastric surgeon). The interview was stressful with many tears and obvious fear by both patient and daughter. Many tissues were used, diagrams drawn, tea drunk summaries repeated and questions asked. I started with discussing abnormal cells and moved gently into a discussion of cancer and the particular difficulties when it occurs in the stomach. As they left, the clinic nurse said she felt 'drained'. A few weeks later I received a call from the surgeon. He had left the patient and her daughter both hysterical with anxiety and anger in his room as he had used the word 'cancer' and they both reacted with adamant denial that this had ever been mentioned. Another lesson learned; they had both stopped listening, through anxiety and fear, after my opening words about abnormal cells. Nothing else had registered and I had missed it.

PRESENTATIONS

Giving presentations can instill fear and trepidation. A little nervousness is said to be a good thing

by ensuring a sparkling, witty and informative delivery. For many, the result is a dry mouth, stumbling speech and an overwhelming desire to use the toilet. These are some tips for the would-be presenter:

- Know the subject matter and rehearse a delivery for timing and difficult areas
- Only use technology you are comfortable with – PowerPoint is fine if you can use it (but be prepared if it goes wrong)
- Use aide-memoire cards if you need to
- Keep overheads/slides simple and embellish with spoken words
- Face the audience. If you glance at a slide or point to an overhead, remember to turn back or else your voice is lost and the talk becomes one between you and the screen
- Try not to rush – a slower delivery is usually much more effective
- Anecdotes, historical facts, and occasionally jokes can go down very well and make for a memorable performance (but beware)
- For a 'big' event prepare carefully. Have the information you need in another format and on disc
- Audiences like to take things home – handouts usually go down well and you can embellish the information orally
- Be prepared for questions. In the event of a nasty one try not to get defensive. If you had not thought of it, say so and ask to meet the questioner later to discuss it further. If it is an opinion (and you disagree with it) ask the rest of the audience what they think – thereby hoping to isolate your attacker!
- If someone disproves your results or shows that you made the wrong diagnosis, either thank them or feign a heart attack
- Before your presentation remember to empty your bladder and either zip your flies or make sure you are all tucked in

REFERENCES

Cohen-Cole S A 1991 The medical interview: the three-function approach. Mosby Year Book, St Louis

Department of Health 1998 A first class service: quality in the new NHS. HMSO, London

Department of Health 2003 Modernising medical careers. HMSO, London. Online. Available: http://www.MMC.nhs.uk

Department of Health 2004a Modernising medical careers: the next steps. HMSO, London. Online. Available: http://www.MMC.nhs.uk

Department of Health 2004b Modernising medical careers: the foundation programme. HMSO, London. Online. Available: http://www.MMC.nhs.uk

Department of Health 2005a Curriculum for the foundation years in postgraduate training and medical education. The Foundation Programme Committee of the Academy of Medical Royal Colleges, in co-operation with Modernising Medical Careers in the Departments of Health. Online. Available: http://www.MMC.nhs.uk

Department of Health 2005b Operational framework for foundation training. TSO, London. Online. Available: http://www.MMC.nhs.uk

Department of Health 2005c Foundation learning portfolio. Online. Available: http://www.MMC.nhs.uk

Joint Centre for Education in Medicine 1997 The good assessment guide. Joint Centre for Education, London

Joint Centre for Education in Medicine 1999 The good CPD guide. Joint Centre for Education, London

NHS Executive 1998 A guide to specialist registrar training. Department of Health, London

Standing Committee on postgraduate medical and dental education (SCOPME) 1996 Appraising doctors and dentists in training. SCOPME, London

RECOMMENDED READING

Cohen-Cole S A 1991 The medical interview: the three-function approach. Ch. 15: Understanding emotional responses of patients: 'normal responses'. Ch. 16: Understanding emotional responses of patients: 'maladaptive reactions'. Mosby Year Book, St Louis

Cushing A 1993 Communication skills course, tutors handbook. Department of Human Science and Medical Ethics, St Bartholomew's and the Royal London School of Medicine and Dentistry, London

Maguire P 1984 The way we teach … interviewing skills. Medical Teacher 6:128–133

SELF-ASSESSMENT QUESTIONS

Are the following statements true or false?

1. Features of assessment:
   a. Should be confidential
   b. Should be objective
   c. Should be non-judgmental
   d. Should not affect career progression
   e. Can be used to identify trainees in difficulty

2. Recognized methods of assessment include:
   a. Multiple choice examinations
   b. Direct observation of procedural skills (DOPS)
   c. Clinical audit
   d. Complaints
   e. Journal club presentations

Chapter 49

All you need to know about management in one chapter

Peter Belfield

WHAT THIS CHAPTER IS ABOUT

This chapter is a beginner's guide to management and covers a wide range of topics. The aim is to provide knowledge and understanding, useful tips and some resources. It is not an alternative to going on a management course but hopefully will encourage the reader to do some management training. The following topics will be covered:

- Clinicians working as managers
- Models of clinical management
- The NHS today
- Clinical governance
- Appraisal, personal development and managing yourself

CLINICIANS WORKING AS MANAGERS

Geriatricians frequently end up as managers and, during their training, trainees are likely to work with at least one geriatrician who is a manager. Two features of management that the geriatrician finds easy are team working and an interest in service development. There is an overlap between the role of a clinician and a manager (Fig. 49.1). Both clinicians and managers must make decisions and be effective planners, developers and leaders. For a doctor, this may be leading a group of juniors or an interdisciplinary team, making key decisions about patient care, and developing and training staff. Developing good leadership skills is essential and the successful doctors are the ones who understand and appreciate their staff. The manager has to make difficult decisions about resource allocation or competing bids for service development and also think of career development for colleagues. Both groups have a common agenda of setting and maintaining standards; some of these may be professional, others managerial. This quality assurance underpins clinical governance (see the section on clinical governance later).

Not all consultants need to be clinical managers but modern doctors achieve more if they have a better understanding of the managerial world (Fig. 49.2).

The manager (and increasingly the clinician) has to juggle many balls at once. We have to obtain best value, with limited resources, while carrying out the latest political imperative under the glare of media attention. An example of this

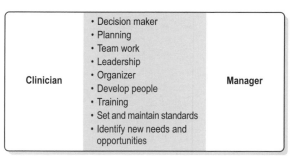

Figure 49.1 Overlap between the role of a clinician and a manager.

Clinician | Manager

- Decision maker
- Planning
- Team work
- Leadership
- Organizer
- Develop people
- Training
- Set and maintain standards
- Identify new needs and opportunities

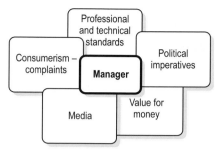

Figure 49.2 The managerial world.

would be managing waiting list targets and the winter bed crisis, with the local and national press wanting a 'good story'.

Doctors increasingly get drawn into the managerial world and some management training and understanding will increasingly be needed. As a consultant, you may be asked to give interviews to the local media about the flu epidemic or patients 'stuck' in hospital waiting for social services. The following highlights some practical tips for handling the media.

Beware of the media:

- Use your hospital's public relations department
- Go on a media skills day
- Only agree to interviews on your terms, e.g. in your office rather than the studio
- Give live interviews to avoid editing
- Avoid controversy!
- Say no if you feel uncomfortable

MODELS OF CLINICAL MANAGEMENT

There is no perfect system of NHS clinical management. Each trust has developed its own style but most arrangements are based on specialties and then aggregation of groups of these, e.g. geriatric medicine within a medical unit. Good descriptions of potential models can be obtained from either the British Association of Medical Managers (BAMM) or the British Medical Association (BMA). The commonest clinical managerial roles are those of clinical director, specialty lead or lead clinician. These terms are often interchangeable but there is variation in responsibility for

matters such as finance and performance management (management of 4-hour trolley waits in A&E, etc.).

All departments of elderly medicine should have a clinical manager, although in small district general hospitals the role might be combined with integration with general medicine. In larger departments, the work might be split between a number of individuals but there should always be clarity in who is doing what.

At some stage in your career as a consultant, it is likely that you will have the opportunity to take on such a role; if this occurs, ask for a job description and be clear what the job entails. The roles vary in responsibilities; time needed to do the job properly and the rewards given.

Doctors are better at some aspects of management than others, e.g. service planning rather than financial control. What is required are doctors who are clinical managers who work in partnership with managers and who complement each other's strengths and weaknesses. Successful organizations are built on such teamwork. Doctor-managers must take the lead managerial role for clinical governance.

THE NHS TODAY

The reforms of the Labour Government since the late 1990s have moved the NHS into new, less well-charted territory. What is clear, however, is that the political spotlight will always be on the NHS and consultants must learn to use this in a proactive way rather than just reacting to the next set of 'bad news'.

The internal market of the Thatcher era is now long gone but has been steadily replaced by a more complex agenda which offers many similar features, e.g. patient choice, payment by results and practice-based commissioning (see Useful websites and links at the end of the chapter). In addition we will all have to work to defined standards of National Service Frameworks (NSFs) and be regularly monitored by the Healthcare Commission.

The NSF for Older People was published in England in March 2001 (the Welsh NSF was released in 2006) and most of the milestones in the NSF were to have been achieved by early 2005.

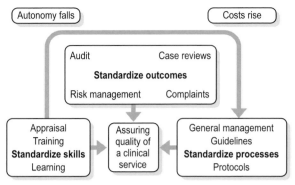

Figure 49.3   Clinical governance – key themes and their likely impact on individual autonomy and costs.

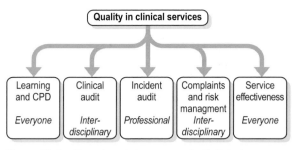

Figure 49.4   Departmental assessment of clinical governance. CPD, continuing professional development.

This far-reaching document sets standards and promotes improved care of older people. A key aim of the NSF was to achieve greater consistency in the availability and quality of services for a range of problems such as stroke, falls and mental health. This work was promoted by an older people's 'Czar', Professor Ian Philp, and the Department of Health website has a large range of resources, e.g. papers on improving stroke services and better health in old age.

Other standards and guidance are provided by the National Institute for Clinical Excellence (NICE), which gives a strong lead on clinical and cost-effectiveness of treatments. It draws up new guidelines that are evidence based. In 2005, it caused great controversy by questioning the cost and clinical effectiveness of some dementia treatments.

Standards and the performance of the NHS will be monitored by a number of means, most notably by the Healthcare Commission. This is an independent body for England and is at arms length from government but with statutory functions. In Scotland, as with many health matters, there are separate arrangements: the Clinical Standards Board for Scotland operates in a broadly similar way. The Healthcare Commission has an analogous position to the schools inspectorate; it can visit or be called in. All hospitals complete a declaration about how they comply with national standards and will get a visit at least every 4 years.

Change and reform are natural processes within the NHS, but the current sets of changes are more radical and far reaching. The move to a primary care-led NHS continues and will affect the way we all work by promoting joint working between health and local authorities. A consequence of this is that there will be an inexorable trend towards geriatricians having input into community services. Such patterns of activity will give us the challenge of working in a dispersed organization, but will also offer new opportunities to reinvent our specialty.

CLINICAL GOVERNANCE

Clinical governance focuses attention on improvements in quality in the NHS. It encompasses a number of initiatives which should improve the care we give to patients. The British Geriatrics Society (BGS) has produced a number of useful documents on this, e.g. from guidelines on delirium to an overall approach within the specialty.

Clinical governance can be challenging to individual doctors as autonomy will be reduced, transparency will increase and convergence to a particular way of doing things will be required (Fig. 49.3).

This framework highlights all the elements that make up clinical governance with professional development, appraisal and learning being required by the individual, a focused review of outcomes and the standardization of the way we will work in the future. Importantly, it recognizes that, to make improvements in quality, costs will inevitably rise.

In elderly care, a departmental assessment of clinical governance can occur with a systematic review of serious untoward incidents, deaths, complaints and service effectiveness. Figure 49.4 schematically shows such an approach.

Quality is something we all aim for in everyday practice but defining quality of care in elderly services can be difficult. Numerous national and local initiatives highlight the need for evidence-based practice, clinically effective services, use of guidelines and the move towards clinical governance. Much has been written and presented about these initiatives but as yet there is little that relates to everyday experience in a busy clinical department. The main concern expressed by clinicians is about finding time and resources to fit this quality assurance into busy working lives.

We all have different perspectives on quality – the patient may have a different view to their carer, the doctor a different view to the nurse. What is clear is that the new agenda of putting quality first puts the same value on patient experience as on a clinical result. Public consultation on the clinical safety of acute care in small hospitals reminds us that patients often prefer care in local accessible services in comparison to bigger centres some distance away (even though clinical outcome data show that larger units generally provide better care).

The key groups of staff in any drive to measure and improve quality are consultants – clinical governance will not work if managers force it onto doctors! Management support is required to help the administrative processes, e.g. to produce reports and records and to ensure that management action follows any lesson learned.

Interdisciplinary audit of selected topics and themes can provide a rich learning environment that promotes joint working. It is surprising that, in a specialty where multidisciplinary working is perceived to be the hallmark of good care, so little true clinical (as opposed to medical) audit has been carried out. Therapists and nurses bring fresh perspectives on problems. A different focus on topics such as falls and readmissions can be good for patients and staff and for improving the quality of the service.

Audit of deaths and serious untoward incidents (SUIs) is more sensitive. Most hospitals have a reporting mechanism for SUIs but doctors rarely use them. Nursing staff keep good records of drug errors, falls and the like, but doctors infrequently report adverse events. A regular focus on quality does, however, lead to a greater sharing of 'learning' from difficult cases in an informal way – usually at the start or end of a clinical meeting.

Mortality audit is rare in geriatric medicine, which is somewhat surprising in a specialty with high mortality rates. Regular mortality and morbidity meetings have become an everyday part of surgical practice, and initiatives such as the National Confidential Enquiry into Patient Outcome and Death (NCEPOD) are well regarded as drivers for improvement. Mortality rates for acute elderly care are around 15–20% and this could potentially mean that many deaths need review. The first step is to produce a regular mortality report with the names of patients, ward, consultant's name, coded cause of death and whether they were referred to the coroner. This in itself can be contentious, with individual consultants having a 'bad' month. Access to the report should be restricted to the relevant manager and all consultants. A system of self-referral by individual consultants of 'worrying cases', coroner referral, all postmortems, in-hospital falls, postsurgical cases and deaths in intermediate care or community hospitals will provide many cases to discuss review. Cases should be reviewed using a standardized format. Notes should be kept of meetings with an action plan for follow-up action. It is important that we collect accurate mortality data as these are part of the national performance measures and appear in guides such as Dr Foster (http://www.drfoster.co.uk) by which we are judged.

Complaints are another accessible measure of our services (see Ch. 52). There is a direct relationship between the likelihood of a complaint with length of stay and poor outcome. It is therefore no surprise that services for older people deal with large numbers of complaints. In most cases, the focus is on the investigative process. Responses are often in writing and the whole process can be threatening to staff and unsatisfactory to the complainants. Complaints can be reviewed at regular multidisciplinary meetings and allowing lessons to be learned can have a high educational value.

Dos and don'ts of complaints

- Do not bury your head in the sand – get on and respond
- Seek help and support from a colleague – talking about complaints helps

Continued

> **Dos and don'ts of complaints** *(Cont'd)*
>
> - Stick to the facts
> - Offer to meet the complainant: written responses often prolong the process
> - Most complainants want information and wish to avoid the situation recurring
> - Write notes of conversations with members of staff – you will forget otherwise
> - If the service failed or you did wrong – apologize

Complaints are usually handled locally within the trust. If things are not adequately resolved, a small number go on to independent clinical review (ICR). The ICR process is time consuming and involves external review – it should be avoided if at all possible by local resolution. Since 2004, ICRs have been coordinated by the Health Care Commission (http://www.healthcarecommission.org.uk). Historically less than 1% of complaints have gone to ICR but the number is steadily rising. A final port of call is available to complainants, the Health Service Ombudsman, who deals with a relatively small number of complaints a year (around 3000) and investigates the complaints-handling procedure. This process is lengthy and time consuming. The Ombudsman publishes a regular report, which is educationally valuable and is readily available.

As a fourth component of this practical approach to clinical governance, one can look at service effectiveness. There is a lot of information on this with reports from the Audit Commission on fractured neck of femur and regular national audits of stroke.

Clinical governance is about doing things better, working in a truly interdisciplinary way and changing the culture from one of blame to one of support and learning.

APPRAISAL, PERSONAL DEVELOPMENT AND MANAGING YOURSELF

Critical to your success and development is appraisal. Over the last 5 years, all groups of doctors (including consultants) have had an annual appraisal. It is likely that appraisal will provide the basis of information required for revalida-

tion. A key theme will be continuing professional development, and the appraisal and assessment systems that are now used for doctors in training (http://www.jchmt.org.uk) are being adapted and are likely to be used throughout all doctors' careers.

> **Useful resources for appraisal**
>
> Peyton J W R 2000 Appraisal and assessment in medical practice. ISBN: 1 900887 06 1
> *This is an excellent short book.*
>
> Chambers R, Wakley G, Field S et al 2003 Appraisal for the apprehensive. ISBN: 1 85775 982 6
> *The title of this book says it all.*
>
> BAMM 2003 Appraisal in practice: hints and tips for hospital consultants and staff grades and associate specialists. ISBN: 1900 120 356
> *This is an excellent publication from the British Association of Medical Managers (BAMM).*
>
> BAMM 2003 Appraisal: a guide for medical practitioners. ISBN: 0 7279 1848 6
> *This is a British Medical Association (BMA) publication.*

The key to managing yourself is to manage your time, manage personal stress and to set clear objectives for what you want to achieve (see Ch. 51). Many management courses focus on personal management. There is much to be gained by taking time out and reflecting on the way in which one works, but what is important is that weaknesses identified are corrected. Too many courses allow you to see where you are going wrong, but do not come up with new ways of working that are sustainable. Appraisal needs to be effective and about you – ensure you do most of the talking.

There are many courses for trainees and consultants on management training (see Useful websites and links at the end of the chapter).

> **Key points**
>
> - The NHS is changing at a faster pace than ever before.
> - Understanding what managers do is helpful.
> - Working together with managers is desirable and delivers better care for patients.

- The best way to keep up with what is happening in the NHS is the Department of Health and other related websites.
- Clinical governance will be time consuming but should mean improvements in quality for patients and staff.
- Think about your personal development, get appraised and manage your time well.

RECOMMENDED READING AND USEFUL CONTACTS

Books and journals

Books

Simpson J (ed.) 1995 Management for doctors. BMJ Publishing Group, London

Rosenthal M, Mulcahy L, Lloyd-Bostock S (eds) 1999 Medical mishaps. Open University Press, Buckingham

Young A (ed.) 1999 The medical manager. A practical guide for clinicians. BMJ Publishing Group, London

Journals

Clinicians in Management. Published quarterly. Journal of the British Association of Medical Managers. Website: http://www.bamm.co.uk

Health Service Journal. Published weekly and available electronically at http://www.hsj.co.uk

Useful organizations

British Association of Medical Managers. Tel: 0161 474 1141; website: http://www.bamm.co.uk

British Geriatrics Society. Website: http://www.bgs.org.uk

British Medical Association. Contact your local office; website: http://www.bma.org.uk

Providers of management courses

The King's Fund provides all types of management training. Website: http://www.kingsfund.org.uk

BAMM also organizes a number of management courses. Website: http://www.bamm.co.uk

The Open University provides Managing Health and Social Care. Website: http://www.open.ac.uk

Useful websites and links

How to obtain information about the NHS

The Department of Health has an excellent website: http://www.dh.gov.uk

It includes a What's New section, press releases, Chief Medical Officer page and an excellent search engine.

Key publications from the Department of Health

Heath Service Ombudsman. Online. Available: http://www.health.ombudsman.org.uk

Healthcare Commission. Online. Available: http://www.healthcarecommission.org.uk

Scottish Executive health matters on the web. Online. Available: http://www.scotland.gov.uk/health or Scottish Health on the web. Online. Available: http://www.show.scot.nhs.uk

NHS improvement plan: putting people at the heart of public services. June 2004

National Institute for Clinical Excellence. Online. Available: http://www.nice.org.uk

NSF for Older People. Online. Available: http://www.dh.gov.uk/PublicationsAndStatistics

Patient choice. Online. Available: http://www.dh.gov.uk/PolicyAndGuidance

Payment by results. Online. Available: http://www.dh.gov.uk/PolicyAndGuidance

Practice-based commissioning. Online. Available: http://www.dh.gov.uk/PolicyAndGuidance

SELF–ASSESSMENT QUESTIONS

Are the following true or false?

1. Features of a good clinician or manager include:
   a. Leadership
   b. Team working
   c. Prevarication
   d. Realizing that professionals always know best
   e. Developing people

2. Clinical governance is:
   a. A systematic approach to quality
   b. A disciplinary procedure
   c. A government fad
   d. Just for doctors
   e. A way of building on audit

Chapter 50

Preparing for a consultant post

Chris Patterson and Alex Brown

Preparation for being a consultant in geriatric medicine begins during the first year as a specialist trainee. This chapter deals with those factors, which assume importance as trainee time begins to run out and a consultant post beckons.

WHEN TO APPLY

Since January 1997, it has been a legal requirement for doctors to be on the General Medical Council (GMC) Specialist Register before taking up a consultant appointment. After specialist registrar or locum appointment-training (LAT), you should enrol with the Joint Committee on Higher Medical Training (JCHMT) at the Royal College of Physicians. They are supposed to send out a Certificate of Completion of Training (CCT) application form 2 months in advance of the date of completion of training. Do not assume this will happen so phone the college 3 months before the expected date.

The process should occur as set out in Figure 50.1.

WHERE TO APPLY

Personal considerations:

- Spouse's job
- Schools
- Travel
- City vs rural

Most locations have good schools and information is now freely available and league tables and Ofsted reports are accessible on the Internet. Rural areas have the benefit of less traffic, better access to scenery and more community involvement. Public transport is better developed in cities.

TEACHING HOSPITAL OR DISTRICT GENERAL HOSPITAL (DGH)

Potential differences are summarized in Table 50.1.

Remember that nowhere will be perfect. Hospitals in the south of England may have more private practice; in the north and west and in Wales, much of Scotland and Northern Ireland, living expenses are lower. Jobs in DGHs may be more 'hands-on' because there may be fewer junior staff. Doing a locum is a useful way of testing hospitals and departments, and confers an advantage when applying.

AGE-RELATED OR INTEGRATED OR NEEDS-RELATED?

It is simplistic to believe there are three models of geriatric care. Integration exists in many forms, but in general will involve looking after younger patients. Most consultant posts are now integrated. In practice, most departments are suited to local need, and experience should be gained in different models of care to compare and contrast styles of working.

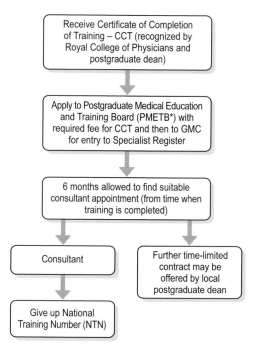

Figure 50.1 Application process. *The PMETB replaced the Specialist Training Authority in September 2005. Address: Hercules House, Hercules Road, London SE1 7DU. E-mail: info@pmetb.org.uk. For CCT inquiries: cct@pmetb.org.uk. Tel: 0871 220 3070 (8.30 a.m. to 4.30 p.m. UK time) and +44 (0)20 7160 6187.

HOW TO APPLY

Although the *British Medical Journal* classified and *Hospital Doctor* are worth keeping an eye on, the bush telegraph will warn of imminent job vacancies.

When the advertisement appears, ring for an application form and go and see the contact person. Speak to as many people as you can when visiting, as a well-informed, interested candidate creates a good impression. The hit list should include the clinical director, medical director, chief executive and directorate manager. Shrewd candidates would also seek out senior nursing and rehabilitation staff and perhaps the primary care trust chief executives. Prepare questions on accommodation, house prices, removal expenses as well as trust policy, strategic direction and potential hospital mergers. Time spent on Google checking out hospital star ratings, annual reports and any adverse publicity is recommended.

Make the most of informal visits – many decisions are made before the interview comes around.

WRITING YOUR CURRICULUM VITAE (CV)

WHY BOTHER?

A good CV will not get you a job; you have to do that yourself. However a poorly presented CV may only get a cursory inspection before landing in the bin. So first impressions count.

Do not make the mistake of dusting off your old CV, updating it and hoping that it will do. Use it as a template to produce something which is appealing, informative and above all relevant to the post on offer.

Table 50.1　Potential differences between the teaching hospital and the district general hospital (DGH)

	Teaching hospital	DGH
Specialization	May be highly specialized with little exposure to common complaints	Broad spectrum of disease. Opportunity for subspecialization
Research	Well-developed structures	Fewer opportunities but no escape, with clinical governance
Teaching	Much opportunity for teaching medical students and trainees	Opportunity for educating other disciplines. More fulfilling?
Competition for job	Likely to be hotly contested	Perceived to be less attractive but rumours usually historical
On call	Infrequent but intense	Frequent but less intense (especially in age-related units)

WHAT NEEDS TO BE IN IT?

Brief personal details, qualifications, management, audit, medical and research experience need to be in your CV (Table 50.2). Do not include any irrelevancies. Who cares about your GCSE grades and subjects? Make it pertinent to the post; check that you address the person specification. This should come with the information pack after your initial enquiry about the job. It will list both the professional and personal qualities needed to be a successful candidate. If an interest in orthogeriatrics is essential, do not relegate this to page 3, after hobbies and interests. There is bound to be a compromise between brevity and detail. Ask others to read it, and for their constructive comments.

WHICH FORMAT?

Management books list three basic formats – chronological, functional and combined.

Chronological

This is the most popular. It follows your work history (usually backwards) and is particularly useful if your career structure has been stable and logical. If you have had gaps, or a change in career direction, then these become all too obvious.

Functional

This concentrates on skills and responsibilities, and is usually grouped under the general headings of management, audit, medical, etc. It tends to ignore dates and is useful if your experience is scattered. However, it is difficult for the reader to pull out exact details and is of limited use for Calman trainees (specialist registrar [SpR]) who have had a structured training. (This grade was created in December 1995 in order to meet European models of training at the recommendation of a working party set up by Kenneth Calman, then Chief Medical Officer.)

Combined

As the name suggests, this is a mix of the functional and chronological formats. Appointments are listed by date and specific areas are highlighted under separate headings.

CV CHECKLIST

Type: Chronological
Functional (limited value)
Combined

Further action

Read your CV and ask others for comments. Put it away for a few days, then structure it again. Check grammar and spelling. Is it tailor-made for the job? Could the layout be improved?

Do not accept your first draft!

Table 50.2 Information for CV preparation	
Areas to cover	Notes
Personal history and contact data	Brief. Use date of birth, rather than age (will not get out of date)
Exam results and institutions	Highlight most relevant. Note honours and awards. Include any courses that strengthen your application
Work history and experience	Layout depends on format selected. Try and tailor to job specification. Do not forget management, audit, research, presentations, IT skills, teaching, special interests. Emphasize achievements
References	Let the referee know. Tell them about the job. Ensure they are likely to give a good reference. Let them know how you got on at interview

THE INTERVIEW

It is a sobering thought that a 45-minute interview can dictate the next 20–30 years of your life. Interviews are not an efficient form of personnel selection. However, inefficient or not, interviews are how candidates are usually selected, so do not blow your chances by poor interview technique.

HOW TO IMPROVE MATTERS

Preparation

- Know the hospital and department. Speak to key people.
- Review your experience for the job:
  - Prepare thoughts to broad questions
  - Try not to give 'pat' answers – they sound contrived
  - Look out for 'hot topics', whether they be medical, political, ethical or organizational
- Review your CV.
- Prepare any presentation you have been asked to give:
  - Check what presentation aids will be available, e.g. overheads, slide projectors. If you are going 'high-tech' (PowerPoint) have you a fall back if it goes wrong on the day? It is best to keep things simple
  - Stick to the topic
  - Ensure that it has a beginning, a middle and an end
  - Do not run over time
  - Rehearse, rehearse and rehearse
- A five-minute talk is much more difficult to do than an hour's presentation.
- Practice an interview with friends or colleagues.
- Arrive in good time.

Personal appearance

- *Well groomed* – a professional, confident smart appearance.
- *Dress appropriately* – also for pre-interview visits.
- *Dress rehearsal* – that old suit may not fit, and those new shoes might hurt.

Do not forget

Be yourself. Do not try to be someone you are not. A consultant appointment is usually for many years and you cannot keep up a façade for ever.

Finally

Prior preparation and planning reduce the risk of poor performance. Time and effort invested before the interview will seldom be wasted.

ASSESSING A JOB DESCRIPTION

Consultants are now working harder than ever due to changes in workload, lack of resources and raised public expectations. Increased admissions and reduction of bed numbers have contributed to more stressful working.

Strong recommendations have been made by the Royal College of Physicians in their report 'Consultant Physicians Working for Patients' which specifies conditions and facilities that ought to be provided to allow consultants to work optimally. Some of these of particular importance to geriatric medicine (often with the added duties of acute medicine) are given below:

- Acute on-call rota no more than one in five
- No single-handed consultants
- One consultant per 50 000 population (in elderly care) or per 4000 people over the age of 75 years
- Clinics after acute on-call should be cancelled
- Consultant-led post-take ward rounds with staff who have managed the patients
- All consultants should have their own office and a secretary
- A realistic job plan should be provided
- Adequately funded study leave
- Effective information technology

Job plans are detailed descriptions of duties and responsibilities, and the facilities needed to carry them out. Work is quantified in terms of notional half days (NHDs) or 'sessions'. The Royal College of Physicians provides guidance on job plans to physicians and managers for all specialist physicians. Considerations include patient care (clinics, ward rounds, rehabilitation) and supporting activities (teaching, training, audit, research, management).

When assessing a job description, consider the number of ward rounds and clinics expected (and the number of patients expected to be seen in clinics). Doing five ward rounds per week in three different hospitals leaves little time for other activities. Ensure there is adequate time for administration and subspecialty interests. Timetables tend to get more congested with time with development of services – it is much easier to take on new responsibilities than to offload existing ones!

STARTING A NEW JOB

It is often said that clinical practice is the easiest part of being a consultant. This is true.

Before starting, concentrate on domestic arrangements – housing, schools, crèches. Find out if you need to live within a certain radius of the hospital. Get on to mailing lists. Consider renting a house until you know the local areas. Remember that most crèches have long waiting lists.

Make sure the British Medical Association (BMA) checks the contract and job plan. They may have helpful suggestions. Check out the position regarding secretaries and an office. Offices should be adequately equipped with a desk, two chairs, telephone, shelves, filing cabinet and computer.

Tips when starting:

- Travel expenses ⎫
- Telephone rental ⎬ Find out how to claim
- Domiciliary visit payments ⎭
- Clarify managerial and administration responsibilities
- Agree on diary system with secretary
- Filing system
- Use e-mail where possible
- Find out who is who
- Try and avoid the first weekend on call
- Let people know of holidays early

Most importantly, politely say no to offers of being on committees – unless they are of interest and importance to you.

RECOMMENDED READING

*** *Essential reading; * interesting but not vital*

British Medical Association 1995 Model workload document for consultants in geriatric medicine: general notes for guidance. British Medical Association, London ***

Clarke J 1999 Write your own CV. Elliott Rightway, Kingswood *

Eggert M 1999 The perfect interview. Random House, London *

Eggert M 1999 The perfect CV. Random House, London *

Royal College of Physicians 1999 Consultant physicians working for patients: geriatric medicine and general internal medicine. Royal College of Physicians, London ***

Various authors 2005 Career focus. British Medical Journal Careers 331(7513):65–79 ***

An excellent collection of brief articles about preparation, dressing the part and the interview itself.

Useful information and key organizations

OFSTED reports on local schools: http://www.ofsted.gov.uk

NHS performance ratings: http://www.healthcarecommission.org.uk

General Medical Council: Tel:0845 357 3456. Website: http://www.gmc-uk.org

Postgraduate Medical Education and Training Board (PMETB), Hercules House, Hercules Road, London SE1 7DU. Tel: 0871 220 3070. Website: http://www.pmetb.org.uk. E-mail: cct@pmetb.org.uk

Royal College of Physicians, 11 St Andrews Place, Regents Park, London NW1 4LE. Tel: 020 7935 1174 (same number for JCHMT queries). Website: http://www.rcplondon.ac.uk

SELF-ASSESSMENT QUESTION

1. At the end of the interview, you are asked if you have any questions for the panel. Do you:
   a. Politely say 'No thank you, all my queries were answered at my pre-interview visit'
   b. Heave a huge sigh of relief, saying 'No' while already half way through the door
   c. Ask just one pertinent question about an area not covered during the interview (e.g. opportunities for research or sub-specialization)
   d. Produce a scribbled list of 20 questions from your pocket and proceed through each one in painstaking detail?

Chapter **51**

Time management and organizing paperwork

Rowan H. Harwood

JOB PLANS

An NHS consultant's working time should be determined by his or her job plan. The 2003 NHS consultant's contract:

- Is intended to provide flexibility, and to match remuneration to work done, by identifying 'programmed activities' or PAs
- Defines each PA as 4 hours' work during the 'normal working day' and 3 hours during 'premium time' (7 p.m.–8 a.m. weekdays, and all day weekends). It is possible to work three or more PAs in a single day, and in specialties such as anaesthetics, surgery and intensive care, full-time (10–12 PA) working weeks are sometimes delivered in 4 days

In a job plan, time is divided between:

- Direct clinical care (DCC): clinics, ward rounds, multidisciplinary meetings, day hospital, seeing relatives, admissions unit work, clinical administration, and procedures such as endoscopy or tilt testing. Some posts have 'community sessions', supporting home rehabilitation or intermediate care, doing peripheral clinics, domiciliary or care home consultations, and liaising with community matrons (chronic disease case managers). Most of us will expect DCC to take up most of our time
- Supporting professional activities (SPA): teaching, research, postgraduate supervision, junior doctor assessment and appraisal, continuing education, audit and governance, non-clinical administration
- Additional responsibilities (AR): usually managerial or educational roles (clinical director, director of postgraduate education, director of research and development, committees)
- External responsibilities (ER): some Royal College or Department of Health roles, journal editorship

Initial guidance from the Department of Health was that the starting point should be 7.5 DCCs and 2.5 SPAs. There is provision for hospital trusts to buy extra time, if you want to offer it, in the form of additional PAs, for extra clinical or other work. However, the European Union has ruled that a working week over 48 hours is potentially deleterious to health and safety, and can therefore be done only on a voluntary basis. Many hospital trusts interpret this as meaning they will not agree contracts of more than 12 PAs. Instead, some (mainly educational) roles attract an additional 'honorarium' outside of the PA system.

In practice, proper job planning has proven quite difficult:

- Consultants necessarily work flexibly to accommodate many different roles and responsibilities, and these may change week to week, and over a career.
- People work at different speeds and in different ways. This can lead to feelings of inequity and unfairness. Managers are suspicious about

variation, and are sometimes seduced by crude statistics about 'productivity'. Do you spend a lot of time in clinic sorting out a problem, then discharge the patient with a one-stop-shop philosophy? Or do you half sort it out, order some tests and bring the patient back for review? Which is more 'productive'? What is the effect on throughput of your particular case mix? Can you negotiate 'risky' discharges with patients and families? Will your therapists give defensive or pragmatic advice? Variation may be both reasonable and necessary.

■ There has been considerable reluctance to use the full extent of flexibility at the expense of clinical work.

■ Many valuable roles (e.g. examining, MRCP or foundation programme teaching, junior doctor appraisal and assessment, mentoring nurse-prescriber students, formal teaching or lectures, writing books) are not adequately accounted for in job plans.

■ Research time is particularly badly provided for, although large teaching hospitals will notionally have a large income supporting research.

■ Most undergraduate clinical teaching is done by NHS staff. Proper time allocation is contentious (how much extra time does it take having students in clinic or on a ward round?). Increasingly, the funding for teaching (the Service Increment for Teaching [SIFT]) is being identified, and matched with specific consultant time. Along with this comes increased accountability. Teaching must actually be delivered, and done properly.

■ If a full working week is being worked, time worked at weekends or 'out of hours' should be compensated, by time off in lieu (a weekend on-take will require 3 or more 3-hour PAs). Some job plans have a 'half day' scheduled in to take account of this.

■ Hospital trusts cannot afford to employ consultants for all the things they would like them to do, which it is reasonable to expect a consultant to do, and which consultants would like to do. With new mechanisms for hospitals

being paid ('payment by results') this is likely to get worse.

■ Be sympathetic towards your clinical director! Juggling interests, demands, different working styles, working and personal capacities, with a limited budget, and while trying to keep a large group of colleagues happy may be tricky. Bullying is unacceptable, but he or she will probably be trying their best in good faith.

■ A job plan should be agreed, not imposed. If you cannot agree, there is an appeals procedure – you must appeal in writing to the chief executive within 2 weeks and the chief executive will then convene an appeal panel

The problem is that a flexible 'professional' job is being accommodated to a 'line-managed' timetable. This arose because of alleged abuses ('surgeons on the golf course'). However, consultants are expected (and want) to do a lot of other interesting and valuable activities. In practice they are 'fitted in', or done in the evenings and weekends.

Keeping a work diary is an interesting occasional exercise. It is not easy (how exactly do you classify 'answering e-mails' or going to a meeting to discuss a proposed trust merger?). You may find that time spent varies from week to week if you rotate between activities. However, you may identify some 'dead time' that could be re-allocated. And if you think your job plan is seriously out of step with what you actually do, a diary may help inform discussions about how to change it.

Keep up your non-clinical activities if they are worthwhile and keep you eager. But do make sure that you concentrate on making sure you are good at the clinical job you are employed to do during your first 2 years as a consultant at least, before getting too involved in other things.

MAKING THE BEST USE OF YOUR TIME

Alternatives to the ongoing struggle to fit things in include:

■ Get more done by making better use of your time

- Agree that you are not going to do some things
- Delegation

Break up big tasks into achievable chunks. Get important things done first. Making lists is a way of giving you an overview of things you would like to achieve, even if some are nebulous and distant (e.g. 'finish MD thesis'). Some things have to be done before others. Other things you will want to do first because you enjoy them. There is a skill in getting the right balance.

How do you work best? Long sessions to complete the job, or short bursts to keep concentration? Early mornings or late nights? In office hours or later when you can do it undisturbed? A lot depends on how much you enjoy the task (or fear the consequences of failing to do it). The interests of efficiency will not be served by your trying to do things that you have little stake in or concern about. If you have to do them yourself, these tasks are best despatched with a minimum of time, cost and attention.

Two important skills are:

- Awareness of time requirements for a job
- Appropriate allocation of time

Neither is easy. You cannot plan (or manage) your time if you have no idea how long a task is going to take. The problem often presents the other way round. You have a fixed amount of time to complete a task. The issue is then how thorough or definitive a job you can do. If something is good enough for its purpose, get on with the next task. If possible, make sure that you get things right first time. Endless iterations are time consuming, and for some tasks (like answering complaints), the time consequences of not getting it right first time can be considerable.

You must have a diary – paper or electronic. I use both. Make sure they are kept synchronized. Some computer systems have schedulers, which can be helpful. Decide whether to carry your diary yourself, or if your secretary keeps it. Either way, you must tell her what you are doing when. Decide if your secretary can make appointments for you. If so, ask for a range of possible times for meetings, from which you can choose. Electronic scheduling makes this somewhat easier to man-

age. I prefer to vet requests first, and often find that enquiries from patients or relatives can be dealt with quicker and more efficiently by telephone than by meetings (but remember to write down what you have discussed).

Message books also help. Take them seriously, especially returning phone calls when asked. Mobile phones and e-mail make you more accessible than ever before. You may spend a lot of quality time (first thing in the morning) on very low quality work (sorting through e-mails). Work out how you can set limits. Who is allowed to call you on your mobile phone? Can your secretary deal with your e-mails? Ask your secretary for advice on what works and what does not, and if she has any ideas about improvements.

RELINQUISHING RESPONSIBILITIES

Some problems you can do something about yourself, some need an organizational response, and others you are probably stuck with for the time being.

Relinquishing responsibilities yourself may have an impact on other people – your department or the whole organization. If you do not do a job, either someone else has to or the organization stops providing it. The mechanism for redesigning your timetable is the job plan review, which should take place with your clinical director annually. The negotiation centres around how best to use your time.

Not doing clinics or procedures will have income repercussions. Not doing ward work may endanger patients, increase length of stay, or at least diminish the quality of their experience. This will be a particular problem in geriatric medicine, where staffing is often stretched.

Remember that hospital trusts are also paid for undergraduate and postgraduate teaching. Audit, clinical governance, and continuing medical education are professionally necessary, and with the introduction of 're-validation' of specialist status, will become less optional. Some individuals have the ability and motivation to make a contribution to research and service development. Try not to allow these activities to be squeezed out. Your time is not limitless. If you want to do other things as well as clinical work, you have to be somewhat hard-headed about it. Try not to upset anyone in the process.

The only way you can regulate time spent on discretionary activities is to say 'no'. The catch is that every request for you to do something is an opportunity as well as a burden. Most (if not all) of us do geriatric medicine because we think that maintaining the well-being of elderly people is worth doing. We have a responsibility to ourselves, patients and the profession, which may be greater than that to our hospital managers and political masters. We may, for example, welcome the opportunity to go to an after-hours meeting where we can hear what other people have to say, and meet colleagues and potential collaborators for service development or research; but not one which is simply a pharmaceutical company promotional event. A request to sit on the advocacy scheme steering group may be worthy, but not warrant a commitment of your time. However, you might welcome the opportunity to influence a national body, or contribute to a local policy on your sub-specialty. Many of us find teaching enjoyable and worthwhile. How much time you can spend on it depends on your other priorities and competing commitments.

You need an overall strategy. You need to know:

■ Where you are
■ Where you want to be
■ How you might get there
■ What might stop you
■ What problems will arise if you neglect other aspects of your job

A development of the 'just say no' theme is to deflect responsibilities. Management thinkers tell the story of the monkey, which has to sit on someone's back. The monkey is a problem, which has to be looked after, and no one wants it. When someone brings you a problem, if you say 'I'll sort it out' the monkey jumps onto your back, and is now your responsibility. If you say 'search the literature for possible solutions and make me some recommendations' the monkey remains with the original host. You are not abrogating all responsibility, but you are not going to do all the work either. You have to be subtle. There may be an important counselling element. The individual may need help to define the problem, or to be pointed in the direction of someone or some way of finding solutions. If simply left with the monkey, he or she may feel unsupported. If correctly 'managed', a problem represents an opportunity for empowerment and development.

DELEGATION

You should not do tasks that you do not need to do, and which someone else can do for you. Consultants are highly educated and experienced, scarce, overworked, and relatively highly paid. Therefore it is sensible that they should be supported by other people.

The organization supports you to a degree. Someone collects notes for your clinic, and makes sure that the right drugs are delivered to the ward. Unfortunately, however, the amount of delegation you can do is limited. The business model of line management does not really apply. Most of the people you work with are not directly responsible to you for what they do (usually only a secretary and a couple of junior doctors). And people who work for you are often also answerable to others, such as the regional training committee for specialist registrars.

NHS consultants work in teams, but these are not teams that the management theorists would recognize. Nurses, therapists and social workers each have their own professional responsibilities and management arrangements. This has implications for how the 'team' is cultivated and managed. Delegation is rather more a matter of negotiation and persuasion than giving orders. Common purpose is the main motivator. On a rehabilitation ward, for example, responsibility for information gathering and first-line communication with patients, families and other agencies may be delegated to nurses or therapists. But they will need your back up when things get difficult.

The key to this kind of teamwork is to ask what is the special and particular skill that you bring to the team, and try to get someone else to do the bits that you do not need to do. Extra responsibilities can make others' jobs more interesting and rewarding, as well as lightening your workload.

Make the most of the talents that other people have. It makes sense to allow them to operate fully within their competence, without undue duplication or interference. A major risk is that registrars, for example, are denied the opportunity to actually do anything, instead spending their time watching others, in the process neither acquiring skills nor delivering a service.

New ways of working are developing, which may permit more delegation of doctors' traditional tasks. Psychiatrists have for a long time assigned some assessment and follow-up duties to community psychiatric nurses. Clinical nurse specialists in medical subspecialties, usually working to well-defined protocols and guidelines, are now common. Continence promotion, community and interdepartmental liaison, tissue viability, pain management, diabetes mellitus and respiratory disease are areas where specialist nurses can help the elderly patient. Service development plans will often look more attractive if specialist nurses can be recruited rather than asking for extra consultants.

MEETINGS

Meetings are time consuming. You will be invited to go to a lot. Initially it feels good to be asked. Decide if you really need to be present. Insist on an agenda, a start and finishing time, and stick to them. You can agree or disagree with things at meetings, but rarely will you solve problems. It is difficult to keep everyone involved, and impossible to brainstorm solutions, where problems and potential answers have not been thought through. The worst meetings are those whose sole purpose is to demonstrate that 'consultation' has taken place.

Most of the work should be done before and after the meeting. A meeting without preparation is a waste of everyone's time. The chairperson has a special responsibility for preparation. Positions should be worked out in advance and you have to think about your response to challenges. Occasionally, you need to follow up points you have made with a letter to the chairperson, to make sure you have been heard.

You may be able to avoid meetings by offering written submissions to the chairperson, or by monitoring minutes for items of interest. But beware: unless you are careful, a meeting may decide something in your absence which could affect you.

MANAGING PAPERWORK

On becoming a consultant, piles of paperwork soon appear on your desk. A lot is rubbish, some of peripheral relevance, some potentially useful but not immediately so, some is important and needs sorting or filing. A tiny fraction of it is material of immense, urgent and crucial importance.

One approach is the 'single touch technique' – deal with it straight away or bin it. This means having dedicated time for clearing paperwork, but it is tempting to put some things off until you have thought more about them.

Another method is the 'bring forward file'. You need two filing cabinet drawers, one filled with dividers numbered for the days of the month, which represents the current month. The next is labelled with months of the year. As bits of paper come your way, asking you to go to things or do things, you put them in the appropriate slot for when you have to do it. At the end of the month, you redistribute next month's papers to the current month's drawer.

Your secretary can help. She needs to know what to do with your mail, including that marked personal, or private and confidential. Let her have charge of the filing. Be careful with paperwork that is sent for consultation, or which makes you formally aware of something, such as a colleague's absence. It may not be especially interesting, but may provide your only opportunity to respond.

Key points

1. Your time is limited and relatively expensive.
2. You cannot do everything, but have the responsibility of ensuring that your service runs smoothly.
3. You have to work around your job plan.
4. After that, decide what is important, what you want to do, and what cannot be avoided, and do it. Prioritize those tasks that are useful and interesting.

Continued

Key points   (Cont'd)

5. Try to delegate – but this may take some imagination and may not be easy.
6. If you can think of a better way of doing things, try to negotiate a change in your job plan with your clinical director.
7. If you are working at your limit, say no to things. But remember that every request is an opportunity, in which you may wish to invest some time.
8. Be brutal, but careful, with paperwork or it will overwhelm you.

USEFUL WEBSITES

http://www.bma.org.uk – see 'job planning standards of best practice'; under consultants/2003 contract/job planning

http://www.dh.gov.uk – see 'job planning standards of best practice'

http://www.modern.nhs.uk – NHS Modernisation Agency job planning guide

Chapter **52**

Dealing with complaints

Rowan H. Harwood

COMPLAINTS

NHS patients and their relatives have a right to complain, and complaints arise for many reasons. They may or may not be justified. They may reflect unrealistic expectations or they may be motivated by anger (perhaps as part of bereavement) or annoyance. But they may also tell you something you ought to know.

Complaints can be morale-sapping. They undermine your self-esteem. Most staff try their best in difficult circumstances, struggling with difficult diagnoses and management, sharing disappointing outcomes (death, disability, institutionalization), perhaps under-resourced and understaffed, and making judgments in good faith. Given all this, complaints can be hard to take and may provoke feelings of anger and injustice in the recipient.

The formal NHS complaints procedure is subject to 'statutory directions', which have the force of law, but verbal complaints directly to staff can be dealt with informally. The goals in dealing with complaints are:

- To reach a satisfactory conclusion as quickly as possible, using informal mechanisms if possible
- To discharge your legal responsibilities
- To minimize stress and discomfiture, for yourself, your teams, patients and relatives. Try to keep life as pleasant as possible for everyone

PREVENTION

Prevention is mostly common sense, good doctoring and an appreciation of human nature. The three areas giving rise to most complaints are:

- Clinical management
- Attitude of staff
- Communication and information

The importance of vigorous, proactive, and well-directed communication cannot be over-emphasized. This actually helps you manage complex problems more easily, and, in my view, improves clinical care. It also demonstrates a constructive and helpful attitude. I find that an initial 30–45 minute discussion can sort out even the most difficult cases:

- Pre-empt trouble. Spot the case that is going to need complicated discussions early and get on with it. This includes most patients with clinically significant cognitive impairment.
- Find out the background (previous cognitive and physical functioning, in particular).
- Clarify exactly what the problems are, new and long term, and how things have changed over time.
- What are the coping resources (physical environment, statutory and informal care)?
- Define objectives. What does everyone want? What does the patient think? Remember that

---

Box 52.1   Preventing complaints

- Good, up-to-date clinical practice
- Communication and courtesy, with patient, relatives and carers
- Listen to what they say, and respect the patient's autonomy
- Know your limits
- Manage expectations: do not promise the earth
- Ask colleagues if you are in doubt
- Make thorough, contemporaneous notes and letters

---

under the Mental Capacity Act 2005 patients lacking capacity to make a decision still have the right to be involved, and to have their stated opinions taken into account.

- Define what the health service can and cannot do to help.

Communicate primarily with the patient, but also identify and talk to other key carers, family members and stakeholders. Do not wait for face-to-face meetings. Use the telephone, if need be. Delegate to junior colleagues, nurses and therapists, but make sure you do your fair share (you will usually do it better). I also like to encourage relatives to be present during ward rounds, because of the opportunities that arise for discussion (Box 52.1).

WHOSE GOALS?

The consumerist philosophy welcomes complaints as important customer feedback and part of quality improvement. This may be true, at least in part, but your employer's objectives may not be the same as your own. Despite the vicarious legal liability of trusts for your actions, membership of a medical defence organization is still a necessity.

Employers want to:

- Meet their statutory duties (e.g. replying to complaints within a short time)
- Avoid expense (lawyers and court hearings are very expensive)
- Satisfy conditions of the Clinical Negligence Scheme for Trusts – The Clinical Negligence

Scheme for Trusts handles all clinical negligence claims against member NHS bodies. Although membership of the scheme is voluntary, all NHS trusts (including foundation trusts) and pimary care trusts (PCTs) in England currently belong to the scheme. The costs of the scheme are met by membership contributions

- Receive satisfactory inspection reports from the Healthcare Commission, a body which promotes improvement in the quality of the NHS and independent healthcare. It has a statutory duty to assess the performance of healthcare institutions, and to award annual performance ratings
- Maintain the image of the organization

Your own objectives may have more to do with:

- Personal, professional vindication
- Establishing and demonstrating the truth
- Avoiding being made the scapegoat for organizational or resourcing failures

MECHANICS OF COMPLAINTS

What you do depends on the route that the complaint arrives; a few ground rules follow:

- Complaints may be informal or formal. A letter to the chief executive or complaints manager will be treated as formal. A verbal complaint to the complaints manager will be transcribed and treated as written. However, each hospital trust also has a patient advocacy and liaison service (PALS), which is not part of the formal complaints procedures. They will try to direct complaints towards informal resolution if they can.
- You may be able to help explain something (helping a colleague elsewhere perhaps), but you can only properly respond to matters that are your own responsibility.
- The formal NHS complaints procedure can only deal with NHS services, but the trust may be responsible for coordinating a 'mixed sector' complaint it receives involving hospital care and other public services such as primary care or social services.

- Continuing care issues and the Mental Health Act have their own formal review procedure.
- If the complainant is not the patient, their written consent is required to pursue a formal complaint. If the patient lacks capacity, or has died, the trust complaints manager must decide if the complainant is a suitable person to initiate a complaint. A consultant should use common sense in judging this, if approached directly.
- Complaints must be made within 6 months, or within 12 months if delayed for a good reason (such as illness).
- The complaints procedure cannot be used if disciplinary or legal action has commenced.
- Foundation trusts can, in theory, introduce their own procedures.
- Scotland, Wales and Northern Ireland have different regulations, but their contents are almost identical to those in England.

Identify the key issues in a complaint. Sometimes, justified grievances come mixed up with ones that are not. You need to know what you are dealing with:

- What is being complained about, point by point (this may not be obvious from a letter)?
- At whom is the complaint directed?
- What does the complainant want?

RESPONDING TO COMPLAINTS

Aim to respond to (or otherwise defuse) the complaint at the earliest opportunity, informally if possible.

1. If the complaint is not justified, response is usually a matter of explanation. You may need to see (and accept) complaints as part of a grieving process. This can include a phase of anger and blame.

2. If the complaint is not against you, or those for whom you are directly responsible (such as ambulances, car parks, catering, nurses, a GP, or consultant colleague), either:
   - try not to get involved
   or
   - agree with the complainant if you think what is said is justified

You may, however, still need to support your team. 'Collective responsibility' has limits. Decisions are shared, but one individual has to remain accountable, usually the consultant. For example, a decision to attempt a trial of discharge is made by the 'team' and not the individual, but the consultant may be left to deal with the complaint when it goes wrong.

Moreover, it is unprofessional to undermine or blame colleagues (medical or otherwise), or appear to do so, with patients or relatives. Take a charitable view of others' actions. You cannot speak for what others have done in circumstances about which you have not been fully informed. For example, never say 'if only your GP had sent you in sooner'. However, if you identify a pattern of poor performance you may need to take this up (informally and quietly at first) with a nurse or therapy manager, or your clinical or medical director (possibly as part of your appraisal).

3. If the complaint is justified, there may be mitigating circumstances (e.g. staff were away, workload was too high) in which case:
   - Apologize
   - Inform the appropriate manager to try and find a solution
   - If you can, use complaints to help you fight other battles (such as over numbers of nurses or therapists)

4. If the complaint is against a member of staff for whom you have responsibility, primarily junior medical colleagues, you must decide if it is a training or a disciplinary matter.

   Training issues are far easier to manage. You must hear the trainee's version of events, tease out the core of the problem, and propose remedial action. This may be:
   - Awareness and reassurance about future performance
   - Increased levels of supervision
   - Additional training

   If you think disciplinary issues are involved, involve your clinical director and personnel department, director of postgraduate education, or postgraduate dean early. The process becomes quasi-judicial, and unless proper procedures are followed, the case may fail, and you risk being accused of one or other form of discrimination.

5. How do you deal with a justified complaint against yourself? Given the uncertainties that beset medicine, and the fine judgments that are often involved, it may not be easy to know if a complaint is justified or not. You must:
   - Provide an explanation
   - Apologize for the unfortunate outcome
   - Say you have learned from it, if you have made a mistake
   - Say what you propose doing to prevent a recurrence

It is important to know what redress the complainant wants. It is usually 'explanation and apology', but they may be moving towards litigation or a complaint to the GMC. If it seems to be getting serious:

- Involve a colleague to talk it through and for support
- Ask the advice of your medical defence organization

MEETINGS

Complainants are usually urged first to seek a meeting with the consultant involved:

- These can be arranged by patient advocacy and liaison services (PALS), who will also usually provide a note-taker.
- If ward or nursing issues are involved, it is useful to have a senior nurse from the ward present.
- If any other disciplines or individuals seem likely to be important, then invite them. Otherwise your failure to be able to comment on issues outside your jurisdiction and expertise could be interpreted as evasion or buckpassing.
- Make the meeting less intimidating by limiting the number of professional participants.
- Encourage the complainant to bring a friend or supporter. It may help to defuse tense situations, and enhance later recall of what was said. The supporter may be calmer, or otherwise an ally in judging the reasonableness of judgments.

THE FORMAL PROCEDURE FOR RESOLVING COMPLAINTS AGAINST THE NHS

Once a complaint is put in writing, a formal process commences:

- Trusts must have a complaints procedure, which must be publicized.
- They must have a designated complaints manager (who may go under various other names, such as 'consumer relations manager').
- The chief executive must respond in writing to any written, signed, complaint.
- Full investigation and resolution should occur within 20 working days, so requests for responses to complaints must be dealt with rapidly.

The process must demonstrate that:

- The complainants have been listened to
- Their concerns have been investigated
- Their concerns have been responded to, including an apology and measures to prevent recurrence, if appropriate

The procedure is designed to try to provide satisfaction in resolving grievances, and to reduce the amount of medical negligence litigation. It was introduced in 1996, and was revised in 2004. There are two parts:

- Local resolution
- Independent review

The process aims to be conciliatory, and most cases should be dealt with successfully through local resolution. Only if still not satisfied can the complainant call for an independent review.

Complainants may approach an independent complaints advisory service, which is contracted on a regional basis from a voluntary sector organization. They help complainants decide if they really want to complain (by working out what they are complaining about and considering what a good resolution might be) and then providing practical support (e.g. letter writing or attendance at meetings).

As part of the process, meetings may be arranged, but you will usually also have to prepare a written report (covering explanation, apology if appropriate and proposed remedial action), which will form the basis of a response letter written on behalf of the chief executive. You must therefore use plain language, and explain any technical terms. Some aspects of your report may get reworded or misinterpreted during this process. Ask to see the final response before it is sent, or ask that your response be forwarded verbatim with a cover letter from the chief executive.

At the end of the local resolution process (a final response letter from the chief executive), the complainant is informed that he or she has the right to ask for an independent review. Since 2004 these have been convened by the quasi-independent Healthcare Commission. Complainants must apply for review within 2 months of the final letter, using a form downloaded from the website (http://www.healthcarecommission.org.uk) or in leaflets:

- The Healthcare Commission will also review any complaint unresolved after 6 months.
- An initial review by a case manager will determine if there is a case to answer. The views of the complainant and the individual or organization complained against will be sought and correspondence and documents relating to the case considered. The case may be deemed inappropriate for action, dismissed, or referred back to the NHS trust for further efforts at resolution at this stage.
- Independent expert advisors will be appointed if needed (e.g. where clinical matters are concerned).
- The Healthcare Commission may then undertake a further investigation and produce a report with recommendations.
- If the complainant still is not happy, a review panel may be convened. This comprises three trained lay (non-NHS) people. They hear both sides of the case and will make a recommendation on resolution or improving services.
- In Scotland, this function is undertaken by the Scottish Public Services Ombudsman, in Wales by the Independent Review Secretariat, and in Northern Ireland by health boards.

If you have already given a full explanation of what occurred, apologized if something went wrong and stated what steps are being taken to prevent recurrence, there will be no independent review. Make sure you do these things first time around.

The independent review panel aims to resolve the grievance in a conciliatory way. The complainant and those complained against have a right to be heard by the panel, and accompanied by someone else for support, but may not be legally represented. Expert clinical evidence may be taken about the case and its management. The panel writes a report, which is confidential, detailing its conclusions, the evidence for them, and its recommendations.

If the complainant is still not satisfied, he or she can appeal to the Health Services Commissioner ('Ombudsman'), who may investigate further. Many complaints taken to the Ombudsman are about the fairness of the process of dealing with complaints. A sympathetic attitude can help avoid the impression of unfairness. As with a request for an independent review, the Ombudsman can opt not to consider a case if everything has already been done that should have been done.

You may feel that your time is better spent doing other things, especially if the complaint is wholly unjustified. Complaints form part of the system of 'accountability' for what we do, and cannot be ignored. They do not necessarily mean you are a bad doctor. Just accept that they will occur from time to time, and dealing with them is simply part of the job.

LEGAL PROCEEDINGS

The complainant may commence litigation at any stage, seeking damages for personal injury, on the basis that:

- The care received was negligent
- Loss has been incurred
- The loss was a result of the negligent actions

Other forms of legal proceedings may include charges of assault or manslaughter. If you are involved, contact your defence organization and trust solicitor for advice and guidance as soon as possible.

DISCIPLINARY ACTION

Disciplinary action is best avoided. In the case of trainee medical staff, if a problem can be seen as a training or counselling matter, and addressed

accordingly, life will be much easier than if disciplinary action is invoked.

Alleged misconduct may be:

- Professional (matters relating to medical practice, such as competence, confidentiality and
ethics – most notoriously, sexual ethics)
- Personal (matters of honesty, fraud, personal
and professional relationships)

Some issues, such as drug and alcohol abuse,
cut across both types. Sanctions include:

- Verbal or written warnings
- Suspension (said to be a neutral act, not imply-
ing guilt)
- Termination of your contract

You may become involved with allegations about
the conduct of one of your colleagues, junior staff
or one of the other professionals with whom you
work. Personal misconduct is generally dealt with
via policies and procedures set by the employer
or trust, and is quicker and easier to manage.
Professional misconduct is dealt with under
government-prescribed guidelines, and involves
the establishment of an independent committee
of inquiry. There are due processes to be gone
through, and, initially at least, it will be in the
trust's interest to resolve things amicably.

If you are making the accusations, or receive
accusations, involve your personnel department
and the postgraduate dean immediately. If you
are the subject of accusations, contact the British
Medical Association or your defence organization.

COMPLAINING AGAINST PATIENTS OR RELATIVES

Sometimes relationships break down. Abuse and
verbal or physical threats do occur. If a patient is
involved, we need to be sure that the unacceptable
behaviour is not part of the (psycho) pathology
we are dealing with, before we go any further. If
relationships break down to the extent that judgments are affected and further management is
impossible:

- Remember that professional responsibility and
legal duty of care override feelings of personal
hurt
- Talk to the GP. He or she may be able to add
valuable and unexpected background
- Try to arrange for a colleague to take over the
case

Relatives may be abusive, use threats or interfere
with other patients or the ward routine. This may
make their presence on the ward untenable:

- Unacceptable behaviour must be pointed out to
the offender
- Try to negotiate ground rules about conduct
- If problems persist, involve senior trust medical,
nursing and legal management (with a view to
avoiding or defending future complaints)
- If possible, give a written warning threatening
visiting time restrictions or exclusion from the
ward (relatives have no absolute right of access
to the hospital)
- If all else fails, carry out your threats (the
hospital security guards or police may have to
be involved)

Remember the possibility of physical assault on
yourself from an aggrieved complainant:

- Do not tolerate verbal or physical threats or
abuse
- If a meeting is getting bad tempered, suggest
that it be reconvened later on condition that the
complainant is willing to discuss things in a
civilized manner
- Otherwise, terminate the process, and refer it to
your trust complaints manager

FINALLY

Do not lie, do not cover up, and never try to alter
records. There are few ways of getting into real
trouble as a consultant, but these are among
them.

Key points

1. Prevent complaints by being competent, communicative and courteous.
2. Your employer's goals in dealing with complaints may not concur with yours. Membership of a medical defence organization protects your interests.
3. Unjustified complaints may be part of a grieving process.
4. Identify the core of a complaint, the key issues and who is responsible for them.
5. A complainant is entitled to an explanation, an apology if something went wrong, and a description of measure to prevent recurrence if appropriate, and within a short time.
6. Complaints may be dealt with verbally, but a formal 'local resolution procedure' is established for written complaints.
7. Try to make sure you deal with a complaint adequately first time. The system gets increasingly complicated and time consuming if you do not.
8. Training issues are easier to deal with than disciplinary issues.

USEFUL WEBSITES

http://www.healthcarecommission.org – see 'making a complaint about the NHS' and 'how the Healthcare Commission will handle complaints'

http://www.dh.gov.uk – see 'complaints policy' under policy and guidance

Chapter 53

Maintaining morale

Rowan H. Harwood

Happy workers tend to be good workers. However, maintaining morale can be a problem in the NHS. For an organization of its size and importance, the NHS is often poorly equipped, under-staffed, and at times, chaotically run. Salaries and working conditions for some staff are poor and we doctors get little thanks or appreciation from our political masters.

It helps if those around you are motivated and contented. There are two aspects to maintaining morale:

- Your own
- Other people's

Good working relationships are unlikely if you are rude, arrogant, lazy, or persistently late. Control these habits if you are prone to them. What you do when you see them in others requires first-rate people-management skills, tact, honesty and courage.

People need to feel valued and supported. They should:

- Have the right tools for the job (skills, manpower, equipment)
- Have someone who cares and fights for them if they do not (leaders)
- Know what is expected of them
- Know their job is worth doing (especially if it is not glamourous)
- Be proud of doing things that others cannot do (like nursing a delirious patient with pneumonia)
- Be told, congratulated and thanked when they get it right

Junior doctors in particular are not used to being thanked or congratulated. Often the only feedback they get is when there are problems. Feedback is both necessary and welcome. Fortunately with more formalized and regular appraisal this is increasingly available.

TEAMWORK

Many important ideas for maintaining morale come from the philosophy of team building and leadership. We belong to a web of different teams:

- Ward-based interdisciplinary teams, who have responsibility for planning and delivering treatment for patients, and ensuring safe discharge from hospital
- Teams with our medical colleagues, from the same discipline or others (old-age psychiatry, general medicine, orthopaedics)
- Subspecialty teams (stroke, continence)
- Management teams
- Educational teams
- Research teams

Teams that function well produce results that individuals working alone cannot. They are worth cultivating. Doctors, by virtue of their education, experience and responsibilities often assume the role of leader. Sometimes it may be more convenient for a social worker or nurse to lead. For example, our continence advisory service is 'nurse led', and 'medically supported'.

Some ground rules for successful leadership are:

- Leaders do not just give orders, they enable people to do their jobs better
- Team members enable their leaders to lead
- They do so because it is in their interest, making it easier for them to do their own jobs, and helping to achieve a worthwhile common goal

There are some specific leadership functions:

- Integrating information
- Maintaining momentum
- Helping to set goals
- Making or confirming decisions

Team members also need a set of working principles which are:

- Clear and agreed roles and duties
- Equal commitment
- Shared responsibility
- Identification and use of individuals' strengths
- Clear communication and sharing of information
- Honest, constructive feedback, including thanks and praise
- Mutual support (e.g. when things go wrong)

The leader has both to contribute something positive, and be seen to contribute. Doctors can get a little confused over this, especially team-working doctors like geriatricians. We exist neither to sort out social problems (families and social workers are better at it), nor to act as identikit generic rehabilitation workers. What we do (that others, by and large, do not do) is to:

- Make diagnoses, and explain them to others (patients, families, nurses, therapists)
- Prescribe specific preventative, curative or palliative medical treatments
- Make prognoses (although generally no one is very good at this)
- Refer on to other colleagues or specialties, when appropriate

Our main contribution to the team is to get the general medicine right. The team needs an explanation of what is going on, and what the future may hold, in biomedical terms. Only after that can we consider the disabilities (activity limitations), handicaps (participation restrictions), family, environmental and social issues. Diagnosis-free management is sometimes necessary, but is always beset with uncertainty and is unsatisfactory. Unless we understand our specific skills, we cannot contribute to the team, let alone lead it.

It is easy for some individuals to dominate a meeting, so it is important to be aware of who is contributing and who is not, so that the basic grade physiotherapist or junior student nurse can have their say. New or visiting members need a proper introduction and to be put at their ease. When it comes to decisions, these should be largely by consensus. If someone demurs, their position must be listened to (they may be right) and at the very least acknowledged and appreciated (even if not agreed with or acted upon), otherwise there will be resentment.

Healthcare teams are different from many other teams:

- Teams in industry are characterized by a line management structure. The leader has direct managerial responsibility over the team members.
- Doctors work with nurses, therapists and social workers, rather than managing them. The doctor is not in a position to tell a therapist what to do. He or she has to get them to agree.

This encourages a positive working style and removes some of the risk of being overbearing. For most of the things we ask our colleagues to do, there is usually no problem. However, demarcation issues sometimes arise, for example, over whether a nurse's duties involve counselling relatives, giving intravenous drugs, doing mini-mental state examinations, or wound debridement.

The teams we work with are inherently unstable. Staff turnover is high because of problems in recruitment and retention, and internal rotations of therapists. This has the virtue of the continual injection of fresh personalities and ideas, but means everyone must remain flexible. For example, the person who takes the lead over liaising with families about discharge arrangements may vary between doctor, occupational therapist and nurses.

PERSONAL MORALE AND STRESS

Being a member of positive, supportive, successful teams helps. Sometimes overwhelming external forces (personal, health, social, domestic) can dominate.

Personal goals vary. Elderly people, their situation and problems, may be the driving force into which you wish to channel all your personal abilities and energy. For others it is a job, to be done well, but to be kept firmly in its place. Some thinkers on this problem have defined three spheres:

- Work
- Domestic
- Personal

The attention each receives will vary from person to person, job to job, or with time. To ignore one completely, or to take up responsibilities in one area only to neglect those in another, is to invite problems. An obvious example is work squeezing out family; another is the combination of work and family excluding time for leisure. As a minimum, it is wise to be aware, at least, of your own responsibilities, commitments and goals in each domain.

Failure to address underlying tensions and conflicts results in stress. This is of concern to management and employers as well as the individual. Stress reduces work performance, results in increased complaints and sick leave, and stress has been the subject of personal injury litigation. Employers have a duty of care to minimize foreseeable work-related stress. Consultants live in something of a no-man's-land in this respect. They are both part of the establishment, the management structure, and yet are 'employees'. They are in a position to see both sides. We are not helped by the fact that throughout our lives we have been achieving, can-do, successful, coping types, and expect the same of our colleagues. We probably have greater resources than most to cope with life's difficulties, but it means that the environment is not always sympathetic when we run into trouble. Mild degrees of pressure can be a motivator and a defence against boredom. Where stress becomes troublesome will vary between individuals, so your colleague's ability to cope is not necessarily a sign that you should be able to cope (or vice versa).

> **Box 53.1 Dealing with stress**
>
> - Make it an acceptable issue for discussion
> - If you are stressed, admit it
> - Identify the sources of stress
> - Say 'no' if you are working to your limit
> - Make time for exercise and leisure activities
> - Beware caffeine, smoking, alcohol and overeating
> - Get enough sleep
> - Be positive and optimistic
> - Be sensitive to stress in others
> - Avoid the battleground mentality
> - Plan ahead and manage your time
> - Take sick leave if you need it

Stress is defined as:

- The emotional and physical distress which results from the inability of our coping mechanisms to deal adequately with the pressures of life.

There are plenty of pressures in medicine: workload, patients' expectations, competing demands (clinical, managerial, educational, research), inadequate resources, lack of appreciation. Like many such problems, stress is better addressed overtly and proactively rather than left to smoulder (Box 53.1).

HELPING

As a consultant, you will often be approached for help about non-clinical matters by junior medical staff, colleagues and other staff. They may need advice, to share ideas, to discuss a work problem, start a research project, or it may be something much more personal. Asking for help can be threatening, and may be perceived as weakness or inadequacy. Treat requests:

- Carefully – you may misjudge what is being asked
- Discretely – assume confidentiality is expected and respect it
- Sensitively – put people at their ease and see their point of view

In the counselling literature there are six different types of helping. Each can be useful at times and each will be the most appropriate response to some requests for help.

1. *Giving information* entails passing on facts or knowledge. Lack of information can make decision making impossible. Providing information is an easy solution.

2. *Advice* involves some degree of analysis and judgment of a problem, and the forming of an opinion as to the best response. This can be useful, but is limited by the amount of information on which the advice is based, and the possibility that the advisor has different values and priorities from the person seeking help.

3. *Direct action* means doing something – talking to someone, writing a letter or mediating in a dispute. This provides for an immediate need, but direct action is inevitably short term, and you cannot do everything for everyone yourself.

4. *Changing systems* may have a more far-reaching effect. Systems often limit how effectively we can work. One of the precepts of 'total quality management' is that you should not blame the workers for problems – they are probably doing their best in the circumstances. You need to look at the system to find out where improvements can be made.

5. *Teaching* involves helping someone to gain knowledge or skills that they need to do a job or accomplish some other objective.

6. *Counselling* is an empowering process of skilled listening, in which the listener enables the speaker to gain insight and understanding from what they are saying. The person is helped to explore problems and different ways of dealing with them, so they can decide what to do.

COUNSELLING

A good counsellor requires personal skill, and at least some training and direction. Doctors already have many of the necessary skills. We can adopt counselling methods as part of our everyday clinical and managerial repertoire. The intention is to help people understand themselves and cope better, function more effectively and gain in self-confidence.

Counselling aims:

■ To help someone explore and understand a problem for themselves
■ To help them to discover the most appropriate action or change

It does not aim to offer advice.

Some basic attitudes are important:

■ *Acceptance* – the person seeking help must trust you and feel that you accept them in their situation without prejudice or judgment. Negating or devaluing a perception or experience is unlikely to help
■ *Respect* – courtesy and attention, active listening and non-judgmentalism
■ *Empathy* – the ability to put yourself in their shoes
■ *Genuineness* – personal warmth (open posture, eye contact, smiling), appropriate self-disclosure (sharing similar situations from your own experience), and consistency between your verbal and non-verbal behaviour

There are also some specific skills to master. Some of these are similar to clinical history taking, but are more open-ended and less directive, since some of the benefits stem from the self-discovery process, as well as the solution identified:

1. Exploring and clarifying skills – to define the problems:
   ■ asking open questions
   ■ probing for details by repeating or reflecting key ideas
   ■ asking for specific, concrete examples, rather than vague generalizations
   ■ pointing out inconsistencies and discrepancies
   ■ summarizing the focus of the problems
2. Action skills – to help the person make plans and implement them

Gaining these skills can form a part of continuing professional development, and attending counselling courses would be a valuable use of study leave time in your early years as a consultant.

APPRAISAL

If you have people doing things for you, you cannot escape telling them how they are getting on. Appraisal is related to counselling, but focuses specifically on:

■ Work expectations
■ Work performance
■ Development needs

The same skills of respect, empathy and genuineness are required, and a process of active listening, clarifying, summarizing, objective setting and problem solving will be gone through. In contrast to personal counselling, the agenda is more set, and the interview is more appraiser-led.

The starting point for appraisal is an agreed set of goals or objectives. This means having a common understanding of what level of performance is expected, and what success might look like. Actual performance can then be compared with the standard. An appraisal is developmental rather than judgmental, and will only be effective if 'owned' by both appraiser and appraisee. A good appraisal should be supportive and enjoyable.

We should all have an annual appraisal and job plan review with our medical or clinical director. Participation should be active. Much of the time, however, we will be doing the appraising. You may undertake an appraisal with a trainee as a one-off, but ideally the process should be longer-term and iterative. The output of one appraisal feeds into the next. You may be mentor to a SHO going through a general medical rotation, providing continuity through an otherwise fragmented patchwork of training. Alternatively, you may have a staff grade, associate specialist or clinical assistant, with whom a longer-term relationship can be developed. Try to undertake appraisals 6-monthly or yearly.

In an appraisal:

■ The purpose should be clearly explained to reduce the sense of threat.
■ Pre-prepared questionnaires can provide focus and jog memories.
■ If you are lucky (or skillful), the appraisee will do most of the talking – and analysis of their own performance.
■ All feedback must concentrate on specific and observable behaviours – so behaviour is reinforced or can be changed.
■ Always start with something positive.
■ Strengths, weaknesses, successes and failures, objectives reached and needs-become-apparent are all discussed.
■ Solutions to problems can be negotiated.
■ You may tactfully have to confront aspects of unsatisfactory performance of which the trainee is unaware.
■ Negative feedback must be made helpful and never aggressive and destructive.
■ Concentrate on one or two important points if most of your appraisal is negative – do not let loose a deluge of criticism.
■ Criticisms should be justified with facts and concrete examples, not feelings and generalizations.

Good appraisal can help openness and trust to develop. It can help fulfil the basic requirements of good morale – knowing what is expected and how well this is being achieved.

SICK LEAVE

According to a recent statement by the NHS Director of Human Resources, doctors suffer from 'persistent presenteeism'. Whereas nurses spend about 5% of their time off sick, for doctors the figure is about 1%. When you take into account the few doctors with long-term problems with mental illness or bad backs, that means most of us are never off sick.

Remember, however, that being a consultant is playing a long game – 30 years or so. What you do has to be sustainable. Also, remember that if you are incapacitated or under the weather, your judgment and clinical performance might not be at its best. Take your sick leave if you need it.

Key points

1. Good morale is important for a service to work well. Morale should be actively managed, not left with a life of its own.
2. Being a team member with explicit, worthwhile, achievable goals helps morale.
3. Team members should clearly understand what they contribute to the team, and the leader should help members to do their jobs better and achieve more.
4. Stress is the emotional and physical distress which results from the inability of our coping mechanisms to deal adequately with the pressures of life.
5. Stress is avoided by resolving tensions and conflicts as they arise, in particular balancing the work, domestic and personal spheres. Where stress is a problem, its underlying causes must be identified and tackled.
6. Requests for help may be fulfilled by giving information, advice, taking direct action, changing systems, teaching or counselling.
7. Counselling aims to help people to understand their problems and explore solutions by creating a supportive, non-judgmental relationship, by probing and clarifying issues and identifying potential solutions. It will often be more effective or useful than other forms of helping.
8. Appraisal ensures that expectations are understood, that feedback on performance is given, and that training and development needs are identified. Junior doctors almost universally want more feedback on their performance, and do not know how to ask their consultants for it.

Chapter **54**

Keeping up to date

Rowan H. Harwood

One eminent British geriatrician has described our role as being a 'jack of all trades and master of one'. The breadth of interest and medical expertise we use in geriatric medicine is what attracted many of us into the specialty. The problem is knowing our limitations. Expert medicine is characterized by what goes on at the boundaries. The core should be reasonably well known, or fairly easy to find out about. The edges of knowledge are when familiarity and more narrowly defined expertise come in.

WHAT TO STUDY

How do we know what to concentrate on? Our current regimen of continuing medical education (CME) requires that we:

- Self-assess our abilities
- Compare with the needs of our clinical practice
- Arrange our educational activities accordingly

Unfortunately, most people attending most CME events do not need to be there. There are several reasons for this:

- We enjoy things we know we are interested in
- We never know when we are about to hear something new
- There is a social element to many meetings – we need informal interchange with like-minded people doing similar things to us in different places with different problems

If you are involved in providing a subspecialist service, or research, you will need to maintain greater depth than you will on other topics. From the service point of view, however, you will probably manage your specialist workload more impressively than something you might meet on a general medical take once a year. Patients (and, increasingly, the institutions of the NHS) demand the same quality of service for each.

Try to keep your medical education broad. Sometimes, you will learn things from paediatric or psychiatric meetings. If you keep going to the same general meetings year-in, year-out your return will be progressively less. Vary the special interests: stroke, osteoporosis, falls, Parkinson's disease, continence, blood pressure, rheumatology, psychiatry.

HOW TO LEARN

For life-long learners, there are two themes:

- Finding the information
- Assimilating it (or putting it somewhere where we can find it in a hurry)

There has been a revolution in adult learning methods in the past decade or two. Those of us involved with undergraduate teaching will have come across many of the themes:

- Student-centred, self-directed learning
- Superficial and depth learning
- Small group work on problem solving
- Mentors to keep you on the right track

The lecture is a pretty hopeless way of conveying useful information for retention. Variants, like case presentations, may score more highly on relevance to clinical practice, but being largely passive for the listener, they are not a good way of learning. Conferences have their place, especially if you are taking part, and for the breadth of coverage that a large meeting can give. But do not expect to retain much of what you hear. Going to conferences and listening to lectures is, however, how most of us get most of our CME.

Superficial learning is what we do before exams, and most of the knowledge temporarily gained goes the way of the anatomy and biochemistry we once knew. In-depth learning is what we are after. We acquire this by:

- Defining a problem
- Seeking information
- Using it – by writing it into a paper, research proposal or book chapter, applying it to a clinical case, or presenting it to our colleagues

One of the justifications for clinicians being involved with research is that it keeps them expert in their field. You will educate yourself best by giving CME rather than by receiving it. The 'educational prescription' is a variant on this – when seeing patients, write down a question to which you do not know the answer, on diagnosis, treatment or prognosis, and later answer it using the best available evidence (Sackett et al 1997).

It is not good practice to delegate every time it is your turn to do a departmental presentation, and if you do (as you should, since similar skills must be passed on to junior staff) then supervision should be active, not passive. When you have to present, choose a topic that is going to teach you something. Make it interesting – every talk is a performance. Taking part in SHO-directed teaching sessions is also a good demonstration of commitment. MRCP teaching is another good way of maintaining, and sometimes expanding, your knowledge.

FINDING INFORMATION

David Sackett, guru of the evidence-based medicine movement, suggests there are three ways of acquiring information, only one of which is a good way (Sackett et al 1991):

- Induction – remembering what worked before
- Deduction – looking for the best available evidence
- Seduction – asking someone, e.g. a colleague, an expert, or a drug company representative

Information varies in its intrinsic quality and changes with time as new ideas emerge and new research is done. Part of keeping up to date must involve scanning one or more general journals, and corresponding specialist journals. You will miss things. You may not see something, you will see it and not get round to reading it, or it will appear somewhere you have not looked. This means that at other times you will have to search for things. Be ready to appraise things for their relevance and quality. Sackett's books on evidence-based medicine (Sackett et al 1997) or clinical epidemiology (Sackett et al 1991) are particularly good if you need help on these.

Searchable databases are the future of information, and access to these is improving, e.g. libraries, websites such as those for the BMA (http://www.bma.org.uk) or Doctors (http://www.doctors.net.uk), and the National Library for Health (http://www.library.nhs.uk). You must learn how to use them if you cannot do so already. Depending on your computer skills, you will either hack around them until you get the idea, go on a course or ask your librarian.

For journal articles, you must learn how to search Medline, using a programme such as Ovid (available via the BMA website). The BMA website and locally provided electronic library resources also give you access to archives of electronic journals, allowing you to download and print single copies of articles rather than having to go to a library to find them. You can also do this via journal (or publishers') websites, but usually only for a subscription (or very expensive single use fee).

The Internet has revolutionized access to medical information. With computers on every ward, the quickest way to find out about something you do not know about is to enter its name on Google and press go. Unfortunately, you have no guarantee of the quality of what you find, but many university departments (especially American) and voluntary organizations have excellent (and free) information which should be reliable, and you can always visit a second site for a second opinion! In addition there are some specialist 'text book' sites, with regularly updated and peer-reviewed articles. Find out what your friends and colleagues use. I like http://www.emedicine. com. For drugs used in palliative care, have a look at http://www.palliativedrugs.com. The National Library for Health has 'Prodigy', but its coverage so far is very patchy (http://www.prodigy.nhs. uk). The Internet is also the best way of finding government documents (UK and elsewhere).

As a consultant, you are in many ways more isolated professionally than you have ever been before. You are less pluripotent and your field of expertise can expect to narrow progressively as your career progresses. Paper textbooks represent comprehensiveness and solidity, and still have a place. They go out of date quickly, but they are compact (especially the CD-ROM versions). It is still worth having one or two.

Key points

1. Geriatrics is unique in being broader than its parent discipline, general medicine.

---

2. This brings special challenges in both knowing your limits, and keeping up to date.
3. Effective education aims for 'depth' learning (assimilation and understanding) rather than 'superficial' learning (fact based).
4. Lectures are a very poor way of acquiring useful knowledge. Actively seeking and using information is far more effective (giving presentations, preparing clinical or research protocols).
5. You must be familiar with Internet resources, and searchable electronic databases, such as Medline and the Cochrane Database of Systematic Reviews.
6. You should be familiar with methods for appraising the quality of information.

REFERENCES

Sackett D L, Haynes R B, Guyatt G H et al 1991 Clinical epidemiology, a basic science for clinical medicine, 2nd edn. Little Brown, Boston
Sackett D L, Richardson W S, Rosenberg W et al 1997 Evidence based medicine: how to practice and teach EBM. Churchill Livingstone, Edinburgh

Chapter **55**

Making the most of information technology (IT)

Rob Morris and Rowan H. Harwood

INTRODUCTION

The *Oxford English Dictionary* defines information technology (IT) as:

- 'The use of processes (especially computers, microelectronics and communications) for storing, retrieving and sending information of all kinds (words, numbers, pictures etc.).'

Modern IT should allow us to do:

- Things we would not otherwise be able to do
- Routine things more easily

For doctors there are three tasks, which are to:

- Understand the technology and not be afraid of it. Most medical graduates now have grown up with computers, mobile phones, MP3 players, e-mail, digital cameras, and the Internet. But we still meet colleagues who say they are not 'computer types'
- Keep up to date. Technologies change very rapidly
- See the possibilities for using IT in healthcare and engaging in its introduction and use in everyday practice

This chapter is written from the perspective of computer-literate working clinicians, not IT specialists. Always remember:

- Computers do not speak our language and only do things if they receive the correct instructions

- We are the clever ones; we tell the machines what to do
- Computers do not have malicious streaks. They do exactly what they are told (unless they have broken down). If there is a problem, the most likely thing is that a human being (possibly you) overlooked something or made a mistake
- Ask 'How can I make the computer do what I want it to do?', not 'What can the computer do?'

THE PERSONAL COMPUTER (PC)

The PC is the way most people work with IT. If you have not got one, then you are not able to take advantage of the possibilities. There are plenty of PC magazines in the newsagents that include a glossary or 'jargon buster' section for the uninitiated. Otherwise most of us will know someone who will be pleased to explain the meaning of 'RAM' and 'ROM' and tell you how many gigabytes you need on your hard drive. Available computer power is far in excess of what you need most of the time.

Portable computers (laptops and notebooks) can do virtually everything that bigger desktop machines can (although the screen is smaller and some people find the keyboard less easy to use). They allow you to carry your work with you should you be bored on a train travelling to a conference.

PCs usually arrive with 'office' software pre-installed. These 'suites' provide a word processor,

Table 55.1	Useful software	
Type	**Examples**	**What it does**
Word processor	Word, WordPerfect, Word Pro	A sophisticated typewriter. Allows you to type and format text, and also integrate pictures, graphs, etc.
Desktop publisher	FrontPage, Pageplus	Produces publication quality documents, incorporating graphics. Modern word processors do much the same thing
Spreadsheet	Excel, 1-2-3	A way of storing and manipulating data in rows and columns
Graphics/Presentation	PowerPoint, Harvard Graphics, Freelance	Draws graphs, diagrams, makes slides and displays presentations
Database	Access, dBase, Approach	Stores data so they can be sorted and searched. Can produce formatted reports
Statistics	SPSS, Stata, SAS, Epi-info, Egret	Performs virtually every statistical calculation you will ever need and many more besides
Reference manager	Refman	Imports references and abstracts from Medline, stores them, is searchable, and can export them into a manuscript and reference list

spreadsheet, database, Internet and e-mail, desktop publishing and presentation functions. With a little effort in learning their language, you will be able to produce letters, posters, teaching materials and so on. The NHS currently has a deal with Microsoft to supply Microsoft Office (including Word, Excel and PowerPoint), and even if you are used to using something else, you should learn these as well. Your human resources, IT or training department will provide or advise on training courses. There are usually also very cut-price deals to allow you to use the same software at home – ask your IT department for details.

There is, of course, plenty of other software available. You can add applications according to personal need (Table 55.1).

■ Statistical software is essential if you do research, but also useful for clinicians, especially in the light of the need to audit and record performance. The catch is that you need to know your statistics before you can use the software properly. We recommend *Essentials of Medical Statistics* by Kirkwood (1988) (see Recommended reading. In fact, the programmes are so easy to use, that you run the risk of seriously abusing the statistics if you do not know what you are doing.

■ Reference manager software is also useful. You can download references from Medline, including an abstract, index, sort and retain those you want to keep, and then customize the citation and reference for output in a manuscript.

■ Databases are more for the enthusiast, but can be used for case registers. These can aid clinical management, including generating discharge summaries. You will probably need help with this sort of thing (buying in a commercial system, such as 'Dendrite', training your secretary, employing a data entry clerk). Audit, and patients suitable for drug trials, are two areas where clinical databases can be used.

The addition of a few extra devices (peripherals) allows you to use the 'multimedia' capabilities of your PC. Multimedia refers to different ways of presenting information, such as text, still pictures, moving pictures, sounds, animations, etc.

■ A scanner allows you to incorporate pictures and photographs into your work. You can scan a conventional photograph, or graphs and diagrams from a journal or book (it may be easier to photocopy them first).

■ Digital camera output can be fed straight into your PC. You can (just about) photograph

Table 55.2 Useful peripherals

Name	What it does
Printer	Prints computer text or images onto paper
Monitor	Allows you to see what the computer is doing, and respond to it
Scanner	Converts pictures or text into a form which the computer can store and manipulate
Modem (usually built in)	Allows your computer to communicate with others via telephone lines, and thereby gives access to the Internet
CD–ROM (usually built in)	Allows your computer to read data from CDs – and play them if they are the music sort
Floppy disk drive (built in)	Stores data to disks (1.44 MB)
USB disk storage ('flash drive')	Convenient portable memory connects via the universal serial bus port. Stores up to 1 Gigabyte, very useful for presentations
CD writer	Allows you to record very large quantities of data (650 MB) so that another computer can read it

X-rays and scans off a cold-light X-ray box, although the superior optics available to medical illustration departments will give a better result (and they will remove the name label for anonymization).

■ A digital video camera lets you incorporate action sequences (e.g. an abnormal gait) for teaching purposes away from the bedside. Medical illustration or postgraduate education centre staff will also be able to convert video tape into a digital format for display on a computer.

■ Optical character recognition software (often included with a scanner) allows you to scan text documents and import the result into a word processor for editing and storage (Table 55.2).

THE PERSONAL DESKTOP ASSISTANT (PDA, PERSONAL ORGANIZER)

These are mini hand-held computers. They include an office suite – word processing, spreadsheet and database. You can also download guidelines and some books (the British National Formulary [BNF], Kumar & Clark's *Clinical Medicine* textbook, the *Oxford Handbook of Clinical Medicine*).

They are designed to integrate with your desktop machine, allowing you to carry your electronic diary with you, and synchronize information added on the move with your diary on the office PC. Similarly, appointments, notes and so on can be added on the office PC by your secretary, and uploaded to the PDA. A paper diary cannot remind you of appointments or other commitments (by bleeping at you). Neither can a paper diary cope with appointments that fall next year. A personal organizer can. It must be admitted that a paper diary is slightly quicker to use, however.

PDAs may become the way we enter clinical information into electronic patient records, using infrared linkages via receivers on the ward or in the out-patient clinic to the main hospital computers.

NETWORKS

The key to many IT developments is networks – electronic systems made up of computers joined together. Understanding networks and the way data are moved around will inform issues like security and confidentiality.

A solitary PC is a PC, but two PCs joined by a connecting cable through which they can move information is a network. If more than two PCs are joined together in this way it is a bigger network. In this basic network, a group of people may decide to share access to information stored

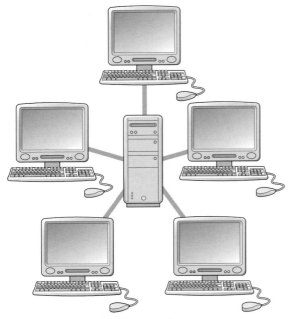

Figure 55.1   Client/server networking.

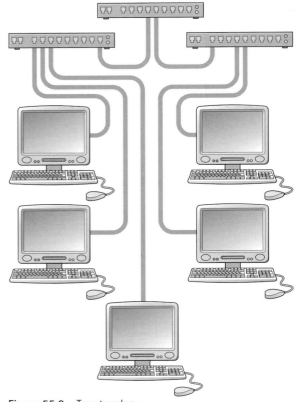

Figure 55.2   Tree topology.

on any of the participating PCs. Security is set by choosing which bits (files, programmes) of your own machine you want to share with others.

This arrangement works for small groups wishing to share resources but it gets difficult to manage if you join more than five PCs in this way. Security is poor and the machines must be in the same general geographical area.

Next is client/server networking (Figs 55.1 and 55.2). A server is the PC's big brother – it goes faster, has more memory, and built-in ways of storing information securely. Servers can back up their information constantly, so that, in the event of a disaster, no data are lost. Their greater power allows hundreds of users (clients) to connect their PC to the network and share information. Users can be widely dispersed around the hospital.

The server can carry messages between members of the network (electronic mail or e-mail) and gives everybody an identity (e-mail address). Networks of this size require someone to look after them (a network administrator). The network administrator can control the amount and type of information that users are allowed to see using

passwords, and how much storage space each is allowed to use. Copies of application programmes can be held on the server, which are then accessed and run on a client machine (Fig. 55.1).

Client PCs wishing to connect to the server require a cable. With the amount of information flowing around a network, you need 'clever' cables. These are actually a system of connection boxes (hubs) and switches (routers) joined up by telephone wires (Fig. 55.2).

This explains the telephone points in your new office, and the grey cabinets dotted around the hospital with glass fronts, lots of wires and flashing green lights. The components of the network are all in roughly the same place so this arrangement gets called a 'local area network' (LAN) or 'Intranet'.

There are two more types of network – wide area networks (WANs) and the Internet. Many general practitioners network PCs within the sugery as a small Intranet and have digital telephone lines (called 'ISDN') connections to other members of the local 'health community' (trusts, health authorities, each other) over a 'wide area', hence being part of a wide area network.

THE INTERNET

In the 1960s, American academics began sharing information this way. They developed servers, which would accept incoming telephone connections from other institutions giving access to resources. As more and more universities and other organizations got involved, they developed specific ways of communicating and identifying each other. This has grown over the years into what we call the Internet (worldwide web, www).

Using software called a web browser (e.g. Explorer) you can visit and view websites on computers maintained by other organizations – including the universities, BMA, BGS, Department of Health, journals, voluntary and commercial organizations. If you do this from home you subscribe to an Internet service provider (e.g. BT, AOL, NTL), who connects you up to their computer using your telephone line, gives you space to create your own website, and allows you to receive e-mail. 'Broadband' connections allow transmission of large quantities of data quickly. University and hospital computers allow you to connect to the Internet directly without going via a service provider.

E-mail allows you to send messages and computer files ('attachments') to other people very rapidly and cheaply. This is very useful if you have a group of collaborators who need to agree on a protocol, edit a manuscript, swap data files and so on. Unfortunately, usual e-mail is not sufficiently secure to send confidential patient data. If you have an urgent need to do this, either ask the patient's permission, or use information not readily identifiable (such as a hospital number).

Via the BMA and other sites you can search Medline, Embase and other databases. Many journals carry on-line versions, which allows you immediate access to their articles. Material from websites (e.g. a journal article) can be copied (downloaded) onto your own computer (see Ch. 54).

SEARCH ENGINES

To find specific information on the Internet you need to know where to look:

- If you know the Internet address (or uniform resource locator [URL]) you can type this in to your browser and go there. The site may then allow you to search further for what you are looking for.
- You can use a search engine. These scour web pages for the words you are looking for, and produce a list of possibilities. Recently Google (http://www.google.co.uk) has been dominant, but there are others. You type your topic of interest into the box and press 'go'. There are also software tools which combine the search results from a number of selected engines (e.g. http://www.copernic.com), so increasing the power of your enquiry.

Unfortunately, searching is not very precise. A search on 'dementia' identifies about 12 million pages. Some variations limit the search to pictures (images) or academic articles. Use 'advanced search options' to limit results by language or date, ensure hits contain your complete phrase (not just the individual words), exclude certain words, or search electronic books or academic papers. And remember that Google is paid to give preference to some commercial sites over others, so the apparent objectivity of the system is not complete (which is why you get told about off-site parking when you look for an airport website).

If you need a web page (or any other text) translated into English, try http://www.babel fish.com.

THE NATIONAL LIBRARY FOR HEALTH (NLH; HTTP://WWW. LIBRARY.NHS.UK)

This is a website that aims to provide easy access to best current knowledge in order to improve health and healthcare, patient choice and clinical practice. The content is quality controlled. Some access requires a username and password (contact your postgraduate library for details). It includes:

- A good selection of full text electronic journals (mostly downloadable as portable document format (pdf) files developed by Adobe Systems)
- Clinical research databases (Medline, Embase)
- The Cochrane Database of Systematic Reviews
- Links to NICE guidelines and National Service Frameworks
- Evidence-based reviews (Drugs and Therapeutics Bulletin, Bandolier)
- Electronic versions of textbooks and the British National Formulary
- NHS Direct Online (information for patients)

COMPUTER NASTIES

- *Viruses, Trojan horses, worms.* These are malicious programmes designed to damage or annoy. They self-replicate and spread via software or e-mails. Because of the risk, your hospital computer will probably not allow you to download or install software without a system administrator clearing it. Viruses can delete your data or slow down your machine. At home you need regularly updated commercial antivirus software (which spots and blocks the malicious programmes). Your hospital system will do the same.

- *Spam.* This is unsolicited advertising. Like all junk mail, if you send out a lot of something cheaply, you do not have to have many people respond to make it commercially worthwhile. However, it blocks up the system, wastes your time and is illegal in the EU. Commercial software (e.g. Norton) can attempt to filter it out, but may catch things you want as well, so you have to take a look at what it has found from time to time.

- *419 fraud (named after a section of the Nigerian penal code).* Ignore (delete or forward to your fraud prevention officer) e-mails offering to give you a cut of millions of dollars transferred from the bank accounts of deceased African businessmen, international lotteries and the like, in return for details of your bank account.

PRESENTATION SKILLS

A common example of how IT can help what you do is when giving lectures or making presentations. These can be scientific, educational, promotional or managerial. Some hospitals will ask you to make a presentation as part of your consultant interview.

Presentations create an impression. They are not a particularly good way of imparting information, and how you do it is what most people remember. Use IT, but do not let it dominate:

- Stand up, even in a small room.
- Talk slowly, with pauses, louder than you would normally, but just short of a shout.
- Talk to the audience, looking at individuals around the room as you do so.
- Do not read a script, or read your visual aids. You want the audience to look at you, not your slides.
- Prepare properly – unless you are very familiar with your material, talking off the cuff will not work
- Do not try to say too much. If appropriate to the situation, try to keep the audience involved. Ask questions, or opinions. Finish in good time.
- Never give apologies for what you are going to say – it puts people in the wrong frame of mind – if you do not have anything worth saying you should not be there.

Visual aids can enhance what you say. This, almost always now, will mean using a PowerPoint presentation:

- You can use a decorative background, but make sure it is effective and not distracting. Black on white or yellow on blue are safe bets.
- Funny noises between slides, or fancy transition effects, may be amusing the first time you try them, but soon become tiresome. If you use them, make sure you have a good reason.
- Keep slides brief – typically no more than five bullet points, but vary this if necessary. A crowded or busy slide will rarely be worth the amount it detracts from the overall impression. A single catch phrase or quotation may be all you need to 'talk to'.
- Use pictures. They add interest and variety, and are often better at explaining a point than text.

You can download these from the Internet (scans or diagrams), use digital photographs, or scan in a diagram from a book or journal.

- If discussing a paper, you can scan in the title to make an effective introduction. You can often download graphs or diagrams from electronic versions on the journal website (if you have access to an electronic subscription).
- CT and MRI scanners can download images that can be displayed in a presentation. This may be in a specialist radiology format (e.g. DICOM) or as a JPEG file (a compression algorithm invented by a standardization committee known as the Joint Photographic Experts Group).
- Video clips work well if done well, but be sure they will work well. A failed video clip is a dampener.
- If presenting elsewhere, you can e-mail your presentation ahead to check that it loads and projects correctly. If you have included a lot of pictures or video, your file will get very large. Take it on a flash drive or CD-ROM, or on your laptop hard drive.

VIDEOCONFERENCING AND TELEMEDICINE

A videoconference is a person-to-person or group discussion, in which participants are in different places, but can see and hear each other as though they were together in one place. Some videoconferences can take place over the Internet (but these can be slow). Otherwise they involve the use of a room at each geographic location with a special video camera, and document presentation facilities. In general, videoconferencing requires special telephone connections with a high capacity ('wide bandwidth', usually ISDN).

A simpler alternative to a videoconference is an audioconference, which is a similar meeting but with only voice connections. As with a videoconference, some special management is required to set up, control and ensure security for an audioconference.

One could imagine this sort of technology being used to convene a virtual case conference, enabling community nurses, social workers, reha-

bilitation staff or a GP to take part without having to travel to the hospital.

Telemedicine, according to two definitions is:

- The use of electronic information and communications technologies to provide and support healthcare when distance separates the participants
- The use of medical information exchanged from one site to another via electronic communications for the health and education of the patient or healthcare provider, and for the purpose of improving patient care

It includes a wide and expanding array of technologies and approaches for communicating patient data, voice or images, in order to assist, augment or replace in-person clinical consultations.

Telemedicine is employed for a variety of purposes:

- It provides or improve access to health services, especially for rural areas, oil rigs, Antarctic research stations and so on.
- Highly specialized services, such as neuro-radiology reporting, or neurosurgical opinions, can take place miles from the scanner by transmitting the images to a specialist centre.
- On a smaller scale, a GP can send a picture of a rash or a mole to a dermatologist for an opinion, or a histopathologist can send a slide to a colleague for a second opinion.

Telemedicine applications aim to improve the quality of care by improving communication and access to information. As yet, applications in geriatric medicine are few, but watch this space.

ASSISTIVE TECHNOLOGY (TELECARE)

Pendant alarm or call systems allow older or disabled people to call for help in a crisis, supporting independent living where fear of falls or sudden illness is a worry.

There is also an emerging related group of assistive technologies (termed 'telecare'). Tagging systems can monitor the movements of vulnerable elders living with dementia who are prone to wander. Devices can monitor the use of lights, or the opening of refrigerators, alerting carers if they are not used for a given time (suggesting a problem). Motion sensors can detect or prevent falls. Vital signs monitoring is also possible.

Government funds (£80 million, over 2 years from April 2006) are available to support telecare implementation through the Preventative Technology Grant. These aim to promote technology approaches in the delivery of health, social care and housing services and prevention strategies to enhance and maintain the well-being and independence of individuals.

COMPUTING IN THE NHS

Healthcare requires the storing of lots of data (administrative, clinical, operational, e.g. pharmacy stock control, and financial). Also, systems need to support the rapid transmission of information (pathology requests, handovers, referrals, communication with GPs). Computers should be ideally suited to do this but so far the potential is only slowly being realized.

The need for information sharing in the NHS has to be balanced against confidentiality and security. Would you want a teenaged hacker to have access to details of your medical history? To provide security, the NHS has a separate network (not part of the worldwide web, called NHSnet). This is currently being upgraded to one called N3. This is protected from the rest of the electronic world by filtering devices called firewalls. These prevent inward access from the Internet, but have secure outward connections. Ultimately, all organizations involved in the provision of healthcare services (GPs, social services, local authorities, hospitals, government agencies, etc.) will be connected.

Historically, the NHS has had many different computer systems. Originally these were based on 'mainframes' (big central computers) with 'dumb terminals' on wards and secretaries' offices. Some hospitals still have these. Newer systems are client/server networks based on PCs. Over the years, many different types of software have been used for different functions (such as patient administration or radiology and results reporting). The ability of these different programmes to work with each other is limited.

Until recently, the best IT in the NHS has been in primary care, where a number of successful systems have allowed some practices to become 'paperless', with clinical notes, test results, prescribing and referrals all catered for. Unfortunately, these systems are not yet able to interface with hospital systems.

THE NHS NATIONAL PROGRAMME FOR IT

The NHS has had a plan to modernize its IT since 1998, providing a system usable by all parts of the service, and with standard applications in different places so you do not have to learn a new one when you move hospital. Progress has been slow, but over the past 5 years almost all doctors now have access to a PC and the Internet, with an e-mail address, and hospital policies and information are available on an Intranet site. Electronic reporting of test results is widespread. A few hospitals have electronic records.

A government agency, called Connecting for Health, runs the National Programme for IT (NPfIT). It has commissioned private sector providers for infrastructure and national services (like the electronic record), and five large companies to provide local NHS computer systems.

These will include:

- The NHS electronic care record – a secure electronic patient record (eventually also accessible by the patient), planned to be fully functional by 2010
- An electronic booking service, Choose and Book, permitting on-line booking of out-patient referrals from a number of NHS and private providers of services
- Electronic prescribing
- A secure NHS e-mail service (called 'Contact')
- Picture archiving and communications system (PACS) for digital radiology (making images available as part of the care record)
- GP IT infrastructure (replacing current stand-alone systems)
- A secure private NHS national IT network ('N3')

A credit-card-style smart card will be used to gain access to the system and determine what type and level of information can be accessed.

Perhaps the most exciting development is the electronic care record. There will be three elements:

- The Detailed Care Record: containing the full electronic records for each NHS organization (hospital, GP practice, community service)
- The Summary Care Record comprising:
  - essential elements of a patient's record, extracted from general practice notes
  - essential elements relating to that person from other NHS departments (such as hospital discharge summaries)
- HealthSpace: where patients can add information, wishes or comments; also there will be a personal health organizer and protected link to their Summary Care Record

The Summary Care Record is intended to provide information in emergencies, unplanned contacts, or less complex care. It will contain details of a person's medical history, such as major diagnoses, procedures, current and regular prescriptions, adverse drug reactions and recent investigation results.

Access to the electronic record will be controlled, based on:

- Roles or jobs – some people (presumably including consultants) will have access to everything (or almost everything)
- Groups – some information will be available to groups (perhaps all members of a multidisciplinary team on a ward having access to each other's information)
- 'Legitimate relationships'. If you look at someone's record, you have to be able to demonstrate that you have a 'legitimate relationship', i.e. that the person is your patient and you have a need to know what is in it. All access to information will be logged, and the log made available to managers or the patient (if they wish to see it)

Ordinarily, if someone is referred to an NHS organization, staff will have access to that organization's Detailed Care Record, and consent for access to the Summary Care Record will be assumed. For more complex care, staff may want to access the Detailed Care Records from other organizations, but this will require explicit consent from the patient.

Current plans are that patients will be able to restrict access to their records. They will be:

- Able to limit who can see the Detailed Care Record, perhaps restricting it to one clinician or clinical team
- Allowed to opt out of having their Summary Care Record made widely available (e.g. parts not being made available, such as mental health diagnoses or genitourinary medicine, or parts only available with their specific consent, the 'sealed envelope')
- Able to opt out of having a Summary Care Record at all
- Able to have one that is only available in emergencies

Of course, it is unreasonable for a patient to expect to receive professional medical care without suitable records being kept at all. Whether a paper back up will be allowed for people refusing to have any electronic record is yet to be decided.

There will be limits to a person's ability to reduce their participation. They will not be able to restrict entries when to do so would put others or public health in danger (e.g. a history of violence towards health workers would be included regardless of the person's wishes). Doctors will be able to add information not accessible by the patient (another 'sealed envelope').

The new systems will bring some advantages:

- Better (and legible) access to information across organizational boundaries (primary–secondary care, between different GP practices or hospitals)
- Quicker (electronic) communication
- More secure prescribing (including drug history, adverse reactions and interactions identified)
- On-line decision support tools (pathways, protocols)
- Reduced duplication of information collected and tests ordered
- Fewer lost records

- Diagnostic imaging (scans and X-rays) will be available as part of the record and opinions from clinicians or radiologists remote from the patient will be easier
- Better access to management and cost data
- Fewer missed out-patient appointments (by letting patients choose their appointment time)

Disadvantages include:

- 800 000 staff will use the system, and will need training
- So far, planning has been more technical than clinical. The care record will only work if designed with the help of clinicians
- Choose and Book is overtly political ('choice'). Organizing clinics to fit its requirements will be challenging (referrals to the wrong sub-specialist, accommodating doctors' planned and unplanned leave, reduced flexibility to 'fit people in')
- Information overload. Just how much of a complex electronic record will you be able to read before your next out-patient walks through the door?
- Less targeted background information without traditional referral letters
- Insufficient account being taken of the needs of vulnerable groups. Elderly, depressed or demented people are of particular concern; because of clinical complexity, they stand to gain most from good records. Yet mental health diagnoses may be excluded from automatic inclusion in care records, perpetuating old stigmas and denying staff the benefit of a full clinical picture and knowledge of who else is involved in care
- The quality of other people's data will be uncertain

The National Programme for IT is not an end in itself, and will only prove its worth if it makes clinical care easier and better.

DATABASES

Plain text (such as a clinic letter or discharge summary) is an inefficient way of storing data. It is better to define 'fields' that contain a limited choice of responses.

There are already examples, such as diabetes registers, where a case register forms the main clinical record, including diagnostic history, complications, co-morbidities, treatments and annual review data.

Some information recording systems have been developed that may prove useful in developing electronic records (such as InterRAI's Minimum Data Sets for care homes, community care, including the Single Assessment Process in England, and acute hospital care). Much data will carry over from one setting to the next, avoiding the need to start from scratch.

Classification systems will need to be used more, including:

- International Classifications of Diseases (currently 10th edn, ICD-10)
- OPCS-4 (which records surgical procedures)
- The International Classification of Functioning, Disability and Health (http://www3.who.int/icf/icftemplate.cfm). One aim of this is to complement diagnosis and procedures information, by classifying disability and other consequences of ill health, and relevant contextual factors. This will be especially useful in chronic disease and rehabilitation-based specialties.

HOSPITAL INFORMATION

A lot of information is already collected by hospital computer systems. Most of it remains unanalysed and unused. Many doctors doubt its validity, which may or may not be true. This may be both the reason behind, and an effect of, the fact that no one is using it.

We suspect that data are not perfect, but are often good enough for most purposes. If you want some management information, such as how many patients you saw last year, trends in lengths of stay or differences between wards, it is worth seeing what your information department can come up with, before doing your own survey. What you find may enable you to change the way data are collected sufficiently to make the data more useful in future.

Clinical coding (what diagnoses, complications and co-morbidities your patients have) is routinely undertaken for all hospital in-patient episodes. It will form the basis of Healthcare Resource Groups that the government plans will determine hospital income (the 'tariff', under 'payment by results'). Making sure these are correct will become increasingly important.

A further aim of new IT systems is to provide better management and governance information (i.e. activity and quality). Clinical governance (see Ch. 49) makes it the responsibility of the chief executive to ensure that quality of clinical services is adequate. He or she is not going to do this alone, but will have to ensure there are systems in place to monitor quality.

We can expect 'benchmarked' comparisons of length of stay, mortality and complication rates, among other things. Interpretation will be difficult – these will be uncontrolled or inadequately controlled comparisons, and there will be numerous alternative explanations for differences between individual clinicians. The policy imperative to provide data is unstoppable. It is important that clinicians take an interest in the process early on in its development to make sure that what is produced is clinically sensible. Some epidemiological and statistical skills will also be at a premium.

THE DATA PROTECTION ACT (1998)

If you handle or store personal or medical data, you need to know about data protection legislation.

The legislation uses a few key terms:

- 'Data processing' is obtaining, recording or holding the information or data or carrying out any operation on the information.
- 'Personal data' is an all-encompassing term referring to any item of information held about a person, from complex disease-specific databases to a simple patient identification label.
- 'Data subjects' are people on whom data are kept.

There are eight principles:

1. 'Personal data shall be processed fairly and lawfully and, in particular, shall not be processed unless [certain specific conditions are met]' (e.g. that you have been given express permission to use it).

We must respect and protect the confidentiality of information obtained from patients. The common law of confidentiality must be complied with, so consent should be obtained for any use. Fortunately, Department of Health guidance is that confidentiality should not be construed in such ways as to disadvantage patients, and for many purposes consent is implied. There are circumstances you may have encountered where the information is of such importance that this issue becomes subject to 'the overriding public interest' (e.g. someone with epilepsy who will not stop driving).

2. 'Personal data shall be obtained only for one or more specified and lawful purposes, and shall not be further processed in any manner incompatible with that purpose or those purposes.'

Data recorded for one purpose cannot be used for anything else without the consent of the person involved, unless, exceptionally, there is an overriding public interest. This provision had the potential to forbid much research, published case series, epidemiological monitoring, cancer registries, contracting and audit, not to mention more commercial applications like the use of prescription data for marketing by pharmaceutical companies. Fortunately, there is already case law (the 'Source Informatics' case) establishing that anonymized, aggregated data (such as clinical case series for publication, or prescribing data) may be lawfully used for these additional purposes.

3. 'Personal data shall be adequate, relevant and not excessive in relation to the purpose or purposes for which they are processed.'

4. 'Personal data shall be accurate and, where necessary, kept up to date' and 'data are inaccurate if they are incorrect or misleading as to any matter of fact'.

5. 'Personal data … shall not be kept for longer than is necessary'.

6. 'Personal data shall be processed in accordance with the rights of data subjects under this Act.'

We must guard against any use of information which may cause unnecessary distress to the people to whom it refers. Examples would be refusing to give subjects access to the information, going against subjects' expressed wishes not to have their personal data used for specific purposes and using personal data for the purposes of direct marketing.

7. 'Appropriate technical and organisational measures shall be taken against unauthorised or unlawful processing of personal data and against accidental loss or destruction of, or damage to, personal data.'

   At first sight this is aimed at the managers and technical people, but what about notes left in your unlocked office or car boot?

8. 'Personal data shall not be transferred to a country or territory outside the European Economic Area, unless that country or territory ensures an adequate level of protection for the rights of data subjects in relation to the processing of personal data.'

   This effectively places limits on sharing personal data with colleagues in countries outside the EEA without the consent of the person involved. This is a minor point, but one of the reasons why there are standard protocols for international trial design and data collection.

In addition to these eight 'principles', the Data Protection Act gives seven rights to individuals in respect of their own personal data held by others. They are rights:

1. Of access to data
2. To prevent processing likely to cause damage or distress
3. To prevent processing for the purposes of direct marketing
4. In relation to automated decision taking (anything generated without it passing through human hands, and of relevance to life insurance enquires, credit rating and the like)
5. To take action for compensation if the individual suffers damage
6. To take action to rectify, block, erase or destroy inaccurate data
7. To make a request to the Data Protection Commissioner for an assessment to be made as to whether any provision of the Act has been contravened

---

Key points

1. Doctors must be computer literate.
2. Computers can make life easier for us – as a minimum, you should be familiar with word-processing and presentation software, searchable electronic databases and the Internet.
3. The NHS is investing in modernization of its IT and communications systems, so expect a period of rapid change over the next few years.
4. Respect the confidential personal data you access and make sure that you comply with the principles of the Data Protection Act.

RECOMMENDED READING

Books

Kirkwood B 1988 Essentials of medical statistics. Blackwell, Oxford

Wyatt J C, Sullivan F 1998 ABC of health informatics. BMJ Books, London. (Or http://bmj.bmjjournals.com)

Telecare

Building Telecare in England: http://www.dh.gov.uk

The Foundation for Assistive Technologies: http://www.fastuk.org

Integrated Community Equipment Services: http://www.icesdoh.org

Data Protection Act

http://www.opsi.gov.uk

http://www.dh.gov.uk

http://www.informationcommissioner.gov.uk

National Programme for Information Technology

http://www.connectingforhealth.nhs.uk – much of this reads like marketing rather than realistic planning, but gets more sensible when clinicians are involved

http://www.bma.org.uk – see under Information Technology

http://www.e-health-insider.com – independent NHS IT news stories

http://www.dh.gov.uk – UK Department of Health

Chapter 56

Professional issues

Nick Coni

HOW TO COPE WITH STRESS

Medicine can be a stressful, if rewarding, occupation. The condition we call stress is not sufficiently well defined to permit accurate epidemiological data, but there is fair agreement about its causes, its features, and about some of the strategies that can help people to cope with it.

Stress of one kind or another persists throughout a medical career, but some kinds stay the same and others change. The main sources of stress for trainees and consultants are as follows.

Trainees

- Working excessive hours
- Curtailment of social life, loss of friends
- Deaths, grieving relatives
- Being summoned to an emergency (or a triviality) while in the middle of another task
- Irritability of other staff
- Increasing responsibility, even if diminishing self-doubt
- Combining career with family/social life
- Career pressures – higher examinations, the next job, grand rounds, the need to publish
- Need to impress consultants

Consultants

- Combining medicine with family/social life
- Establishing/maintaining reputation – publishing, committees, etc.

- Accepting too many roles so that you fulfil them all less well than you would wish
- Complaints
- Conflicts with colleagues, managers and others
- Need to keep up to date
- Need/wish to impress patients, relatives, GPs, juniors, nurses, colleagues
- Grand rounds, giving papers and lectures
- Clinical governance

COPING STRATEGIES

There are different causes and different solutions, but a few general principles can be suggested:

1. Seek help – you are surrounded by people happy to give it, including nurses and other trainees.
2. At all stages of your career – make a conscious effort, when you walk out of the hospital entrance, to forget the place until you walk (or are called!) back in again: it will still be there.
3. If your bleeper keeps summoning you to different wards and departments, you have to set priorities. You cannot be in several places at once.
4. Consultants – try not to agree to take on so many tasks that you finish up doing none of them very well.
5. Try not to become ratty.
6. It is a big mistake to have recourse to alcohol or drugs. When off duty, music or some arduous exercise or a hobby is better for you.

7. Nobody thanks you for neglecting to take all the annual leave to which you are entitled.
8. A final thought: surely some degree of stress is not only unavoidable, but positively beneficial. Some people thrive on it, and most of us perform better when lecturing or teaching if not totally 'laid back'.

As can be appreciated, stress is a lifelong companion throughout a medical career. We all learn to live with it, and a few even enjoy it, or feel that it is necessary in order to achieve peak performance. In this respect, medicine is no different from a number of other demanding professions. We like to think that the stakes are higher, but they are pretty high for airline pilots and generals too.

HOW TO BE A GOOD TEACHER

This is not the place for a treatise on the theory of education, nor even its practice. Virtually all doctors will be called upon from time to time to teach, yet few receive any training in how to do it. The formality of the setting will vary from the house officer demonstrating a skill such as venepuncture to a few students, to a GP giving a talk to a first aid class, to a professor giving a Royal College lecture. In theory at least, the formal lecture to students is dead, and all teaching should be 'interactive'. The other dinosaur which stubbornly refuses to become extinct is the mixed business plus teaching ward round – there is general agreement that the two activities cannot be satisfactorily combined.

Teaching is one of the many human activities in which there are no good criteria by which a person's ability can be measured. Medical students are often in agreement as to which of their teachers are 'good' or 'bad', but often confuse this judgment with whose sessions they find fun or boring. However, perhaps stimulation does equate with good teaching.

RULE 1

'The function of the teacher is not to give out information but to inspire the student to do the work'

Despite the clamour by students for handouts for every seminar, the current emphasis is on medicine as a university education and not as a body of factual knowledge to be absorbed prior to its practical application as a house officer. Future students will therefore enjoy much greater latitude in which subjects they concentrate on, and in how much depth they research them. Perhaps the pendulum has swung too far in this direction, but any 50-plus-year-old doctor will testify that everything s/he learned as a student has since been superceded or rubbished.

RULE 2

This follows from rule 1. Teaching should be interactive – draw the student out, so they supply the answer from their own knowledge or intelligence. This is only possible in small group situations.

RULE 3

Never ridicule anyone in a teaching group, except in a kindly way. As a consultant, I was never able to fathom out why students expressed (anonymously, to the dean) a strong preference for being taught by a consultant, over being delegated to a registrar. One eventually explained to me: 'It's the art of gentle bullying – you make us realize we actually know more than we thought, but Dr X [the registrar] makes us realize we know less than we thought'.

RULE 4

Allow your enthusiasm for your subject to show through. If the teacher is not enthused, the students certainly will not be.

RULE 5

Rule 5 is for the set-piece lecture, or, for that matter, for presenting a paper. Do not start off in the manner typical of medical speakers. 'Chairman, ladies and gentlemen', they begin, and then swing round with their back to the audience and facing the screen, 'may I have the first slide, please' (usually followed by signs of total surprise, as though the slide is completely unfamiliar to them).

Eye contact is essential, so use prompting notes; do not read from a script, or you will sound like somebody reading from a script.

RULE 6

Finally, a popular teacher may not be necessarily the same as a good teacher – but it probably feels better!

HOW TO BE AN EFFECTIVE LEADER

There is increasing emphasis in medicine on inter-disciplinary teamwork, and a team generally requires a leader. It is normal for the leader of the clinical team to be a consultant, because s/he has undergone the longest and most rigorous training, is probably the most experienced member of the team, is likely to be the most permanent member of the team, and carries the ultimate legal responsibility for the patient. S/he also has the wider perspective of the bed situation and the pressures of demand – an onerous perspective shared by the registrar but not by the ward nursing and para-medical staff.

Consultants may have to show leadership qualities in other contexts too. They may become whole-time managers, as medical directors or chief executives, or as part-time clinical directors. They may be called upon to chair meetings or organize conferences. They may find themselves directing services. Whether leadership can be taught is a question best left to officer-cadet schools, but there are a few general rules which may help.

RULE 1

The leader generally expects that if there are different viewpoints, his or hers will prevail. In a hospital, this will only happen if you listen to the other views with respect and show that you value them. Unlike the military world, it is not sufficient simply to give orders.

RULE 2

A leader expects loyalty from the rest of the team. This is very much a two-way process, and s/he must in turn show loyalty to the others, and

spring to their defence if necessary. A consultant is fortunate in having, as junior colleagues, a group of highly intelligent, highly motivated young people. S/he is also fortunate in the close relationship, often over many years, s/he may enjoy with nursing staff, who are also extremely hard working and committed to their patients.

RULE 3

The consultant who shows genuine concern for the welfare of the patients will command respect.

RULE 4

Consultants who try to bluff their way out of situations beyond their competence will lose respect. A public admission of failure is far more impressive than repeatedly trumpeting one's successes.

RULE 5

Consultants who set a bad example will forfeit respect. This may take the form of poor timekeeping, or excessive devotion to private practice or golf, or discourtesy to patients, relatives, or staff.

RULE 6

Sir John Harvey-Jones, in his book *Making it Happen* (Harvey-Jones 2003), defines the qualities necessary for leadership as imagination, courage and sensitivity. He is describing the features of good management, and agrees that perhaps a good manager has to be decisive – but it helps if their decisions are the right ones.

The points listed above may stimulate some thought: it has to be admitted, however, that the subject of leadership is far from being evidence based, a characteristic which it shares with most human attributes.

HOW TO GET THE MOST OUT OF MEETINGS

Meetings that doctors attend fall into two categories – committee meetings, to try to make decisions about organizational matters, and academic meetings which vary from small departmental journal clubs to major international conferences.

Business meetings are what managers do all day, and have been described as 'meetings, bloody meetings'. If they are large, and you are not (in management speak) a 'key player', it is only too easy to get nothing out of them – unless you learn how to knit and emerge with a new pair of socks. It is important, however, for the trainee to attend a number of them, partly so that s/he can develop a feel for how organizational decisions are arrived at, partly so that s/he will be able to answer questions about that sort of thing at job interviews. Ideally, at some stage, the registrar should hold office in a committee in order to achieve a degree of management credibility on the CV.

When attending committee meetings as an observer, it is possible to avoid the apparently inevitable death by boredom, by using one's critical faculties. Does the committee fulfil any useful function, other than providing diversional therapy for ageing consultants? If you were elected chairman, would your first action be to dissolve it? Would you try to make it more effectual, and if so, how? Sometimes, the status quo has to be grudgingly accepted, even if the committee seems to be just a talking shop with no real executive function. For example, the former regional specialty advisory committee in geriatric medicine is discussing, in its usual paranoid way, the recurring theme of ageism in medicine. Dr Y, from Little Bumstead General, complains that his patients are being denied life-saving cancer treatment. After much nodding of greying heads, it is concluded that Dr Y is absolutely right, and the chairman is instructed to write to the clinical director of the regional cancer centre. The recently appointed Dr Z supports this suggestion, and points out that the Daily Loco has been running a campaign along these lines, and is keen to receive further ammunition. Might the chairman mention this in the letter, in such a way as to imply that Dr Y's information might be grist to the Loco mill? Unedifying, venal, informative, possibly effective – a lesson to be stored for future recall.

As far as small departmental academic meetings are concerned, if you are not getting much out of them, do not just stop going. Use your initiative to change them, thereby ensuring both that you do get something out of them, and that you get noticed by the consultants (always an item on your personal agenda). You will probably be volunteered to take over the organization of them, which is not actually a bad outcome, although a chore at the time.

What about conferences? It will become increasingly important, during the career of a registrar, that s/he attends certain conferences in the chosen specialty. Having done so, it is perfectly possible to return to base only to be asked 'What's new? What did you learn, then?' and to feel like replying 'Nothing, it was a complete waste of time'. Here then, are some suggestions for making sure you get *something* out of a conference, even if you do not learn anything specifically new:

1. Give a paper or show a poster. It *may* be published, you *may* get noticed, and anyway it is a rite of passage and good practice. You will meet fellow speakers and get to know them. Your consultant should help you with the preparation of your paper or poster.

2. Get a feel for what the 'movers and shakers' are thinking and talking about.

3. You *may* even hear a paper that impresses you, or stimulates an idea for a research project.

4. 'It's not what you know but who you know', so get to meet your contemporaries, and the heavies. Professor X may not give you such a hard time in the interview if you and he and a number of others got paralytic in the red light district of Barcelona a few weeks beforehand. He may, of course, give you a much harder time, particularly if you were ill-advised enough to disagree with his views on molybdenum metabolism and, even more unforgiveably, if you were right.

5. Listen to the tittle-tattle – what jobs are coming up, which are the good departments, and what is the general state of health of your chosen specialty.

6. At the very least, enjoy your time in Barcelona.

REFERENCE

Harvey-Jones J 2003 Making it happen: reflections on leadership. Profile Books, London

Chapter **57**

Research and audit

Nick Balcombe and Alan J. Sinclair

INTRODUCTION

Without research, many medical advances would not have been possible and current medical practice might still be limited to the use of leeches!

Geriatricians may feel that their primary role is clinical care and that research is unnecessary, if not distracting. This view is misplaced and, with the growing health needs of our ageing population, the impetus for research into age-related disorders and disabilities should be encouraged, especially by those delivering clinical care to older people.

Successful research requires hard work and determination. Everyone has the potential to be a competent researcher with the right help and support. The aim of this chapter is to provide a simple guide to the research process, from the initial planning through to the satisfaction of seeing your name in print.

Experience in clinical audit is also a mandatory part of training and an important part of life as a clinician. The ability to conduct and supervise audit projects is an essential requirement for consultants as part of clinical governance (see Ch. 49). This chapter will provide you with the basic principles of clinical audit.

One of the major aims of the recently created Postgraduate Medical Education and Training Board (PMETB: http://www.pmetb.org.uk) is to develop and promote postgraduate medical education and training. In order to achieve this they are counting on a collaborative approach; this is also as relevant to research as to specific training programmes, and as such we expect to see more evidence of research quality and assessment taking place in those institutions where research is conducted.

WHEN TO DO RESEARCH

Research can be done at any stage in your medical career. However, as a doctor progressing through the foundation programme or in the period shortly afterwards, it is likely that your attentions will have been directed towards preparing for the MRCP. Equally, you will find that, once a consultant, your attention will be directed to other pressing matters, such as provision of clinical care, educational supervision, teaching and clinical management. Therefore unless you have already demonstrated great motivation and/or ability in academic pursuits, the ideal time to undertake research is as a specialist registrar. There are different ways of doing research at this stage. You could try and do research as part of your clinical post or you could take time out to focus on your research as a research fellow or clinical lecturer (if a suitable university position is available). Which option you pursue will largely be driven by the presence of available opportunities, your social circumstances and financial considerations.

REGISTERING FOR A DEGREE

You may decide to do some research as a stand-alone project or as part of a higher degree. If the latter, you have two choices: a Masters degree or a Doctorate. An MSc comprises both learning elements and course work, as well as a dissertation (which usually includes presenting a single research project that you have undertaken). An MD comprises a series of related research studies that you have undertaken to address a particular area of research. While an MSc can be completed as a specialist registrar, an MD or PhD is only obtainable if you are in a more academically-focussed post, such as a research fellow or clinical lecturer.

HOW TO SET UP A RESEARCH PROJECT

CHOOSE YOUR TOPIC

Be realistic. Very few people win the Nobel prize and, while you might be one of them in the future, if you are reading this chapter now for advice, you are not yet in a position to win such an accolade. If you are having difficulties, reflect on clinical problems you encounter, go to conferences, listen to experts and keep up to date with medical journals. Ideas may emerge spontaneously after discussion with colleagues.

REVIEW THE LITERATURE

Explore the subject in depth to identify the gaps in knowledge and ensure that your ideas have not been followed by others already. Too many projects are 'me too' studies which waste time and effort and contribute little to the advancement of medical knowledge. Use the following search engines to help you:

- *Pubmed:* http://www.ncbi.nlm.nih.gov/entrez/query.fcgi
- *Cochrane:* http://www.cochrane.org
- *Embase:* http://www.embase.com
- *Ovid:* http://www.ovid.com/site/index.jsp

Employ the skills of medical librarians to help you with literature searches.

IDENTIFY YOUR RESEARCH QUESTION (HYPOTHESIS)

From your literature review, identify what gap in knowledge your research will attempt to fill. Identify the question you will attempt to answer. Be specific, clear and concise. A vague hypothesis is indicative of a muddled mind and this will lead to a hazy conclusion that is unlikely to advance knowledge and even less likely to result in successful publication. Do not attempt to answer too many questions in one research study.

PREPARE A PROTOCOL

This should be prepared according to set standards as follows:

Title of project

First impressions are always important so this is a vital part of the protocol. It should be short and clear and introduce the area of research, the research question and, in some cases, the study design. Try to be precise and avoid general terms (e.g. 'a case control study' or 'a randomized controlled trial of' is more informative than 'a study of').

Summary

This provides a map of the whole application and should explain why the research is needed and the main aim of the project. Provide brief details of the methodology (study design, nature and number of subjects and a broad description of the data to be collected) and describe the outcome measures and what implications the results may have.

Background (why you are doing this study)

Give the scientific background to the research and include a review of the current state of knowledge and highlight the gaps in knowledge. Clearly explain why your study is required.

Hypotheses

State them clearly. Include a *primary hypothesis* (your main question) and *secondary hypotheses* (other questions that may be answered). Aim for no more than one primary hypothesis and two secondary hypotheses.

Study design and methodology (what you are going to do)

This should detail how you are going to answer the hypothesis. Describe the study design:

Randomized
There are two groups, one treatment group and one control group. The treatment group receives the treatment under investigation, and the control group receives either no treatment or some standard default treatment. Patients are randomly assigned to all groups.

Cohort
A cohort study is a study in which patients who presently have a certain condition and/or receive a particular treatment are followed over time and compared with another group who are not affected by the condition under investigation.

Case controlled
Case controlled studies are studies in which patients who already have a certain condition are compared with people who do not. These studies produce less powerful evidence than randomized trials or cohort studies.

   Also include:

- The setting for the study *(hospital, ward, etc.)*
- Details of the study subjects *(inclusion criteria)*
- Details of subjects you are going to exclude *(exclusion criteria)*
- Recruitment details *(how you will recruit subjects)*
- Details of interventions to be performed *(what, are they valid?)*
- Details of the data to be collected *(what, how and when)*
- Details of outcome measures *(what and when)*

Duration of study

Describe how long the study is expected to last both for individual patients and the study as a whole. Provide a time plan for the project, including the following:

- Time to recruit subjects (depends on rate of recruitment and total sample size)
- Time to collect data (depends on time to recruit subjects and length of follow up)
- Time to analyse data (allow enough time for discussions with statistician)
- Time to disseminate results (time of next relevant conference, time to write up study)

Statistical support

Describe what statistical support will be available to help you. *We strongly recommend that you obtain input from a statistician when you are planning the methodology of your study.* This will ensure that you do not waste time pursuing a study that is not likely to yield relevant results because of inadequate sample size. Describe also details of statistical methods that will be used to analyse data.

Power calculation

For pilot studies and for qualitative research, a formal power calculation is not essential and may not be possible. This will help determine the number of patients you need to recruit to answer your hypotheses. Ensure that your power calculation is based on answering your primary hypotheses. Seek help from a statistician in order to obtain an accurate power calculation.

Qualitative research

This involves data collection methods which include in-depth interviews, focus group discussions, participant observation, etc. Data are thus rich in description. Although there is an element of subjectivity, qualitative studies allow you to develop concepts and may lead to one or more specific research questions being identified.

Funding

Explain where you have applied for funding for the study and list the major costings since this helps reviewers to assess the applicability and relevance of the funding proposal.

Feasibility of the project

Are the necessary equipment and expertise to conduct and successfully complete the study available? Can the appropriate numbers of patients be recruited? Ensure that you have identified at least one research supervisor.

OBTAIN ETHICAL APPROVAL

This will certainly be required if you are planning a study that involves direct patient contact. However, even studies which involve questionnaires only and do not involve blood sampling or drug administration will require the submission of an application form. You should also submit your protocol, patient information sheets, consent forms, data proforma and any questionnaires that you will be using to the local research ethics committee (LREC). Contact your LREC for the application packs and remember that the process of gaining ethical approval can take some time.

In addition, as a result of the recently introduced national research governance framework, it is also mandatory that all studies involving the NHS will require a *sponsor* who takes full medico-legal responsibility for the study. For pharmaceutical-sponsored studies, the pharmaceutical company will probably agree to undertake this role along with their financial responsibility for the study. For other studies, however, the researchers must usually convince their host institution (NHS trust or university) to take on this role. This will involve gaining approval from the local research and development office which can be a lengthy process (6–9 months in some cases). Occasionally, fees are demanded by the research and development office to provide the monitoring aspect of the study!

APPLYING FOR A GRANT

The competition for research money is intense and the aim of this section is to provide a basic introduction to preparing grant applications, the types of grant available and where to apply. All funding bodies have their own guidelines for the preparation of grant applications but all will require similar information to that already detailed in the research protocol. In addition, you will probably need to include the following information in support of your application:

BENEFICIARIES

Who will benefit from your proposed research? This may be patients with particular conditions or the NHS as a whole. Explain how your results will improve not only our knowledge but also directly make an impact on the way patients are cared for. It is also important to explain how generalizable your results will be.

BUDGET DETAILS AND JUSTIFICATION OF BUDGET

This section needs to explain fully what costs are going to be incurred and why. If the research requires additional staff, it is important to justify their salary by describing their exact role in the project. Consideration needs also to be given to pay rises, national insurance and superannuation contributions. Always ask the research finance department for help in providing this information for you. Other aspects to be considered include secretarial help, equipment, travel costs, the need to employ a statistician or health economist, and how much will be required for consumables such as stationery, photocopying, postage, computer equipment and software. Be precise in your estimates of cost, as this shows that you have carefully considered your research.

DISSEMINATION

Give brief details of how you intend to inform people of your findings, i.e. journal publication, poster presentation, platform presentation (locally or nationally).

CURRICULUM VITAE

This should be presented in a fashion that demonstrates you and your co-workers have the required experience and expertise to carry out the proposed project.

ETHICAL APPROVAL

A copy of the formal letter of approval from the ethics committee should be included in the grant application.

TYPES OF GRANT

Project grants

This is the most common type of grant. Project grants usually fund a specific single research project.

Programme grants

These are substantial awards given to support a series of related research questions, answered through a series of research studies. Few of these grants are awarded and they are only given to researchers and institutions with established reputation.

Fellowships

These are personal awards made to cover salary and associated research costs. They are given for 1–4 years. The main requirement of these fellowships is that the fellow must be part of an appropriate training programme. Training fellowships are usually based in university departments. More recently the Department of Health has introduced a scheme for establishing integrated training fellowships for specialist registrars as part of a new impetus to promote academic medicine training. These are particularly geared to those specialties where research has been waning and so geriatric medicine is a good candidate for this type of fellowship. Useful links for finding out more about these schemes are the UK Clinical Research Collaboration, The Wellcome Trust, Medical Research Council and Department of Health.

Where to seek grant funding

From whom you attempt to obtain funding will depend primarily on what sort of grant you require. For project grants, there are many potential sources of funding. If you work in a teaching hospital, the research and development (R&D) department may offer small grants to support local projects. Another good source of potential funding is the British Geriatrics Society, which offers start-up grants of up to £2000.

STATISTICAL ANALYSIS

'The difficulties many intelligent people have with "sums" are infinite'

(Greenwood 1948)

Medical statistics is, for most people, a difficult area to comprehend. Yet, it is a vital part of the research process. Most research projects can be competently analysed using a small number of basic tests. To determine which tests to use and how to present the results, talk to colleagues who have done research and look at the journals and, in particular, at papers that relate to yours. This section aims to give a basic overview of the types of tests that are commonly used.

VARIABILITY OF DATA

This can be simply described using frequency charts or histograms and will convey whether data are normally distributed. Quantification of variability can be achieved using descriptive statistics (mean, median, standard deviation, centiles, interquartile range, variance, confidence intervals). Whenever you quote a mean value, always quote the standard deviation and whenever you quote a median, always quote the interquartile range.

COMPARING GROUPS OF DATA

We may want to compare sets of data between different groups or within individuals over time. For data that are normally distributed (Fig. 57.1), parametric tests should be used (e.g. paired t tests, ANOVA), but for data that are not normally distributed, non-parametric tests should be used (e.g. Mann Whitney test, Chi squared).

In a normal distribution, the mean, median and mode are equal:

1 standard deviation from the mean includes 68% of the observations

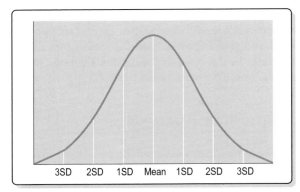

Figure 57.1   The normal distribution.

- 2 standard deviations from the mean include 95% of the observations
- 3 standard deviations from the mean include 99.7% of the observations

RELATIONSHIP BETWEEN SETS OF DATA

This can be described using correlation and regression. Correlation provides a numerical value of the relationship and ranges from +1 (perfect positive correlation) to −1 (perfect negative correlation). Regression provides a more detailed description of the relationship and enables a prediction to be made of the amount of change to be expected in one variable (dependent variable) as a result of changes in the other variable (independent variable).

DISSEMINATION OF RESULTS

WRITING FOR A MEDICAL JOURNAL

Different journals have different styles and requirements to which you will need to adhere. Read the 'information for contributors' details and do not be shy in discussing your paper with the editor. In this section, the aim is to provide basic hints on preparing papers for submission that may improve your chances of success. Submit your paper to a journal that has a good reputation and readers who will be most interested in your study.

CASE REPORTS

These fall into three sections: the reason for publication, the actual case report, and an explanation of the importance of the report. Around 600 words is the usual guideline on length and the case report itself should be the main focus of the article. It should be sufficiently detailed to allow the reader to feel confident that the correct diagnoses were reached or the right treatments given. Concentrate on positive findings and important negative findings. Do not try to build up the case as being indicative of a major medical breakthrough as case reports are considered to be lowly sources of evidence.

CLINICAL TRIAL REPORTS

The preparation of these should follow the IMRAD (introduction, methods, results and discussion) design:

Introduction and method (why you did the study and what you did)

These sections should be prepared as per the protocol.

Results (what you found)

Focus on the main aim of the project and present the data that are germaine to this. Do not give any interpretation of the results at this stage.

Discussion (what it means and where from here)

This section should be formally structured:

- Begin with a clear statement of the principal findings.
- State the strengths and weaknesses of your study. While criticizing your own study may not be particularly enjoyable, it is essential to maintain the trust of the reader.
- Relate your findings to previous work and explain any similarities or differences in results.

- Then give the implications of your findings. Do not attempt to claim too much. Let the reader decide how important the results are.
- Finally, discuss the remaining unanswered questions and say what further work is needed.

Abstract

Your final task is to prepare the first section of your paper. A good abstract should present a clear synopsis of the main features of your paper, including the reason for the study, the aim of the study, the study design, the major findings and the importance of the results.

POSTER PRESENTATIONS

Conferences are important for disseminating research findings. Most conferences will have specific guidance on the size and content of posters and it is important to follow such guidelines. For any poster you produce, the following advice should also be followed:

- Make sure the poster is clear, easy to follow and easy on the eye
- Make sure the title is clear
- Avoid overuse of text
- Where possible use short sentences and bullet points instead of long sentences
- Use large fonts to ensure easy readability
- Use lower case fonts where possible (these are easier to read than capitals)
- Define abbreviations, if used
- Ensure graphics are easy to understand
- Make sure the conclusions are readable and easy to understand

CLINICAL AUDIT (see Ch. 49)

'The purpose of audit should be educational and relevant to patient care'
(Royal College of Physicians 1989)

Research leads to the advancement of medical knowledge which has the potential to enhance standards of care. Clinical audit monitors the implementation of such advances. Many defini-

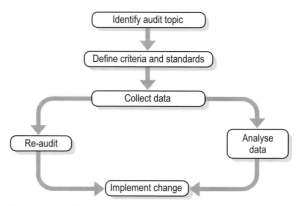

Figure 57.2 The audit cycle.

tions of clinical audit exist, but one of the more recent definitions is: 'systematic critical analysis of the quality of clinical care, including procedures used for diagnoses and treatment, the use of resources and the resulting outcome and quality of life for the patient'.

To perform a successful audit cycle, a systematic approach must be pursued, comprising the steps in Figure 57.2.

Factors contributing to audit failure include confusing audit with research, not setting standards, lack of interest from senior colleagues and failure to identify important and relevant topics. Audit projects require background reading, preparation and planning, cooperation of colleagues in the team and often assistance from audit staff.

Other difficulties include failing to have an adequate set of case notes from which to collect data, confusing an audit with a survey (which in essence is a collection of data without peer-review standards being applied), and not involving other team members such as nurses or therapists. Multidisciplinary audit should be the goal for most projects.

Most NHS trusts have departments of clinical audit (sometimes they are referred to as departments of quality and/or clinical effectiveness) and most directorates have identified clinical audit leads who can provide useful direction. Clinical audit departments are usually willing to provide some direction and guide you through the process of establishing your planned audit project. Remember, however, that resources are often tight and your request for assistance with an audit may be refused unless the topic has relevance to the priorities within the trust or directorate. It is always wise to get support from consultant colleagues when you wish to undertake an audit project.

RECOMMENDED READING

Altman D G 1997 Practical statistics for medical research. Chapman & Hall, Toronto

Armitage P, Berry G, Matthews J N S 2002 Statistical methods in medical research. Blackwell, Edinburgh and London

Blaxter L, Hughes C, Tight M 2000 How to research, 2nd edn. Open University Press, Buckingham

Crombie I K, du V Florey C 1998 The pocket guide to grant applications. BMJ Publishing Group, London

Dickinson E, Sinclair A J 1998 Clinical audit of health care. In: Pathy M S J (ed.) Principles and practice of geriatric medicine. John Wiley & Sons, Chichester

Shamoo A E, Resnik D B 2002 Responsible conduct of research. Oxford University Press, New York

USEFUL CONTACT ADDRESSES

Association of Medical Research Charities, 61 Grays Inn Road, London WC1X 8TL. Tel: 0207 269 8820, Fax: 0207 269 8821, Internet: http://www.amrc.org.uk

British Geriatrics Society, Marjory Warren House, 31 St John's Square, London EC1M 4DN. Tel: 0207 608 1369, Fax: 0207 608 1041, Internet: http://www.bgs.org.uk

Medical Research Council, 20 Park Crescent, London W1B 1AL. Tel: 0207 636 5422, Fax: 0207 436 6179, Internet: http://www.mrc.ac.uk

Research into Ageing, Help the Aged, 207–221 Pentonville Road, London, N1 9UZ. Tel: 0207 843 1571, Internet: http://www.ageing.org

Stroke Association, Stroke House, 240 City Road, London EC1V 2PR. Tel: 0845 3033 100, Internet: http://www.stroke.org.uk

Wellcome Trust, Gibbs Building, 215 Euston Road, London NW1 2BE. Tel: 0207 611 8888, Fax: 0207 611 8545, Internet: http://www.wellcome.ac.uk

SELF-ASSESSMENT QUESTIONS

Are the following statements true or false?

1. The following are essential in preparing any research protocol for ethical submission:
   a. Electronic database search
   b. Approval from your NHS trust R&D office
   c. Patient information sheets
   d. Power calculation

2. Clinical audit:
   a. Is intended to effect change in medical practice
   b. Can be performed where no guidelines exist
   c. Can be used to examine treatments but not investigations
   d. Requires ethics committee approval

3. In statistics:
   a. The variance is the square root of the standard deviation
   b. The Chi squared test is a non-parametric test
   c. A correlation coefficient of 0.1 indicates a good relationship
   d. The interquartile range is the difference between the 25th and 75th centiles

Answers to self-assessment questions

CHAPTER 1

1. a. F
   b. T
   c. F
   d. F
2. a. F
   b. F
   c. F
   d. T

CHAPTER 2

1. a. **F.** Elderly people are no more religious than their younger counterparts.
   b. **T.** A survey by Microsoft suggested that the over-60s spend more time on computers than younger age groups.
   c. **F.** About 15% of over-70s help with voluntary work.
   d. **F.**
2. a. **F.** High maternal mortality rates have previously adversely affected average life expectancy for women.
   b. **T.** Men generally die younger than their wives, leaving their widows to live alone.
   c. **F.** Women make up about two-thirds of the over-75s, and three-quarters of the over-85s.
   d. **F**

CHAPTER 3

1. a. F
   b. T
   c. F
   d. F
2. a. F
   b. F
   c. F
   d. T

CHAPTER 4

1. a. While CT head scan is mandatory to confirm the diagnosis, it is not essential to perform within 24 hours because he is already dependent and therefore has little potential for improvement.
   b. Taking into account the dependency and the likely poor prognosis associated with a complete middle cerebral artery territory infarction, it would not be appropriate to subject him to invasive investigations but to treat his anaemia empirically. This decision, however, should be made only after full discussion with other professionals and his family.
2. a. T
   b. F
   c. F
   d. T
   e. F

CHAPTER 5

1. a. F
   b. T
   c. F
   d. T
   e. T
2. a. F
   b. F. 40%
   c. T
   d. F. Older people's needs are complex; geriatricians need to adapt to a changing environment.
   e. T. It is hoped that they will be reduced in the long term.
3. a. T
   b. T
   c. T
   d. T
   e. T
4. a. T
   b. F
   c. T
   d. T
   e. F

CHAPTER 6

1. a. F. Geriatricians working in the community should have good access to hospital beds.
   b. T. It may be appropriate to support general practitioners with nursing home care generally or continuing healthcare residents in particular services.
   c. T. It is important that medical causes of need for intermediate care can be effectively assessed.
   d. T. A good working relationship between consultant and general practitioners is vital to maximize the benefit of community work.

2. a. F. The evidence base is patchy; more and robust evidence is required.
   b. T. Intermediate care can in part be considered to be a whole tier of services bridging home and hospital admission avoidance and early discharge schemes.
   c. T. Service development for intermediate care services should be jointly between social services, primary care trusts and geriatricians (among others).

   d. F. Intermediate care is a new word attempting to draw together what has often been many local ad hoc services under a new, organized tier of service provision.

CHAPTER 7

1. a. F
   b. F
   c. F
   d. F
   e. T
2. a. F
   b. F
   c. T
   d. F

CHAPTER 8

1. *Explanation:* Her life expectancy is about 11 years, so she is definitely not too old! Unless she has other risk factors or symptoms, it is not necessary to check for diabetes or lipid disorders. Hypertension and hearing impairment should definitely be sought. Evidence is inconclusive for screening for cognitive disorders. The best answer is **d**.

2. *Explanation:* At present there is insufficient evidence to make a firm recommendation. Rectal examination by a skilled examiner is reasonably specific for carcinoma, but insensitive (about 30%). PSA is recommended by some authorities, but false positives occur in benign prostatic hyperplasia and chronic prostatitis. Prostatic biopsy is uncomfortable and can be complicated by infection and haemorrhage. There is no evidence that early treatment prolongs life, and radical surgery or radiotherapy often result in incontinence and erectile dysfunction. Several large RCTs are underway to evaluate screening. The best answer is **c**.

CHAPTER 10

1. a. F
   b. T
   c. T

d. T
e. T
Stroke in an older person does not preclude further safe driving providing they have the necessary physical strength and dexterity, sensory input and cognitive skills to safely operate the vehicle, or are using an adapted vehicle to compensate for any disabilities. However, the patient is usually advised not to restart driving until at least 1 month after the stroke.

2. a. **F.** Their crash rates are the lowest of any age group.
   b. **F.** Driving cessation is associated with higher rates of isolation, loneliness and depression, and may expose the older person to further hazards as a pedestrian.
   c. **F.** No automatic assessment is necessary; driving assessment should be led by difficulty with the driving task.
   d. **F.** Automatic assessment can discourage older drivers from continuing to drive.
   e. **F.** Drivers with dementia should be assessed on the basis of their abilities and road usage as with any other condition. They often self-censor their driving habits to local areas at off peak times and may improve their safety by being accompanied.

CHAPTER 11

1. a. **F.** Since 2002, carers over 65 years are entitled to the carers' benefit.
   b. T
   c. **F.** It is worth more than £34 billion to the economy.
   d. **F.** The Carers' Recognition and Services Act 1995.
   e. F

CHAPTER 12

1. a. T
   b. F
   c. F
   d. F
2. a. F
   b. F
   c. T
   d. F

CHAPTER 13

1. a. F
   b. F
   c. T
   d. F
2. a. F
   b. T
   c. F
   d. T
3. a. F
   b. F
   c. T
   d. F
4. a. F
   b. F
   c. F
   d. F
   e. T

CHAPTER 14

1. a. T
   b. T
   c. F
   d. T
   e. F
2. a. F
   b. F
   c. F
   d. T
   e. T

CHAPTER 15

1. a. T
   b. F
   c. F
   d. T
2. a. F
   b. T
   c. F
   d. F

CHAPTER 16

2. a. F. It can be used cautiously on a prn basis.
   b. F. Lactulose is an osmotic laxative, and a combined softener and stimulant is required, such as codanthramer.
   c. T
   d. F. It is about half.
   e. F

CHAPTER 17

1. a. T
   b. F
   c. F
   d. F
   e. T
2. a. F
   b. F
   c. F
   d. T
   e. T

CHAPTER 18

1. a. T
   b. F
   c. F
   d. F

CHAPTER 20

1. a. F
   b. F
   c. T
   d. T
   e. F
2. a. F
   b. F
   c. T
   d. F
   e. F
3. a. F
   b. F

   c. F
   d. F
   e. T

CHAPTER 21

1. a. F. Bioavailability reflects both the amount of drug absorbed as well as pre-systemic (first-pass) metabolism.
   b. F. Renal clearance is best estimated by using the Cockroft and Gault equation, which uses serum creatinine.
   c. F. Changes in protein binding only become sufficient to affect volume of distribution for very highly protein-bound drugs.
   d. T. Reductions in total body water and muscle mass increase peak concentrations, requiring a reduction in the loading dose in elderly patients. The maintenance dose also needs reducing in view of the reduced renal clearance.

2. a. F. Increased sensitivity is due to the greater effect of warfarin on reducing functionally active vitamin K-dependent clotting factors in the elderly patient. There is no significant change in the volume of distribution or in plasma protein binding of the drug.
   b. T. The increased sensitivity manifests itself as impairment of balance hence increased likelihood of falling. There are also increased CNS effects. These effects are independent of the pharmacokinetic changes associated with ageing.
   c. F. Amiodarone is lipid soluble and has a high volume of distribution. The increase in the volume of distribution coupled with reduced clearance increase the elimination half-life, which may reach 3 months. Thus in some patients it may take as long as 15 months to clear (five times the elimination half-life).
   d. T. This is manifest as an increase in tremor.

CHAPTER 22

1. a. F
   b. F
   c. T
   d. T
   e. T
   f. F

CHAPTER 23

1. a. F
   b. T
   c. F
   d. F

CHAPTER 24

1. a. T
   b. F
   c. T
   d. F
   e. F

CHAPTER 25

1. a. F
   b. F
   c. F
   d. T
   e. T

A coronary heart disease risk of 1.5%/year is equivalent to a cardiovascular (CVD) risk of 2.0%/year. CVD risk (non-fatal myocardial infarction (MI) and stroke, coronary and stroke death and new angina pectoris) is accepted as a better way of deciding on whether to initiate treatment. This is because it takes a more global view of risk by including stroke disease rather than simply looking at the risk of coronary heart disease. Those who have a 10-year CVD risk of > 20% should be considered for treatment. In most Western countries there is an increase in systolic BP up to the age of 80 years for both men and women, but with men having lower values over the age of 55 years due to a steeper rise in post-menopausal women. In men, diastolic BP reaches a plateau at the age of 60 years and then tends to decline. The effect of sodium restriction on blood pressure increases with age.

2. a. F
   b. T
   c. T
   d. F
   e. F

In the major intervention trials (i.e. C+W, EWPHE, STOP-H, MRC, SHEP, Syst-Eur) total mortality has only been significantly reduced in STOP-H, where the reduction was 43%. In the others, the reductions ranged from 3–14% and were not significant. Cardiac mortality was reduced from 20–38%. It was only significantly reduced in EWPHE (38% reduction). In the C+W trial, there was a non-significant 1% increase. In all studies (apart from the MRC trial), stroke events were reduced by more than 35%. In the MRC trial, the reduction was 25% (still significant). The average reduction in SBP on treatment in these trials ranged from 12 mmHg in the SHEP trial to 23 mmHg in Syst-Eur. For the DBP it ranged from 4 mmHg in the SHEP trial to 11 mmHg in the C+W trial.

3. a. T
   b. T
   c. F
   d. T
   e. F

Casual hypertension is common in elderly people and its prevalence increases with age. Casual systolic hypertension (SBP > 159 mmHg on a single reading) is around 19% in men over 60 years but around 40% in men over 80 years. The corresponding values for women are 27% and 50% respectively. Several observational studies in very elderly subjects suggest an inverse relationship between blood pressure and survival, i.e. worse survival in subjects with low blood pressure levels. However, low blood pressure is also a consequence of disease and probably reflects a poor general health prior to death rather than an increased risk per se. A meta-analysis (Gueyffier et al 1999) of patients over 80 years in randomized controlled trials of antihypertensive treatment showed a 6% relative excess of death from all causes.

By 2020 the over-80s will account for around 4% of the total population in several European countries.

CHAPTER 26

1. a. T
   b. T
   c. T
   d. T
   e. T

2. a. T
   b. F
   c. T
   d. T
   e. T

3. a. T
   b. F
   c. F
   d. F
   e. T

CHAPTER 27

1. a. T
   b. F. 50%
   c. T
   d. F. 17-fold
   e. T
2. a. T
   b. F. 30%
   c. F. Rhythm control
   d. T
   e. F. 1B – not suitable
3. a. T
   b. F
   c. F. 1.8%
   d. F. 25%
   e. F
4. a. T
   b. T
   c. T
   d. F. Secondary prevention
   e. T

CHAPTER 28

1. a. F
   b. F
   c. T
   d. F
   e. T

CHAPTER 29

1. a. F
   b. T
   c. F
   d. F
   e. F
   f. F

CHAPTER 30

1. F
2. a. F
   b. T
   c. F
3. F. It is over 40%.
4. F. The oxygen requirements to propel a wheelchair are higher than those to walk over the same ground.
5. a. F
   b. F
   c. T
6. F. Although exercise testing is an invaluable aid in the assessment of such patients, the best method of assessing disability is to use a validated respiratory ADL scale such as the Manchester Respiratory ADL questionnaire or the London Chest ADL questionnaire.

CHAPTER 31

1. a. T
   b. T
   c. F
   d. F
   e. T
2. a. T
   b. T
   c. T
   d. F
   e. T

CHAPTER 32

1. F
2. T
3. F
4. F

CHAPTER 33

1. a. T
   b. T
   c. F
   d. F
   e. T

2. a. T
   b. T
   c. T
   d. F
   e. F
3. a. T
   b. F
   c. F
   d. T
4. a. F
   b. T
   c. T
   d. F. Not proven.
5. a. F
   b. F
   c. F
   d. T
   e. F
6. a. F
   b. F
   c. F
   d. T. Most urologists would treat this man.
   e. T

CHAPTER 34

1. a. T
   b. F
   c. F
   d. F
   e. T
2. a. T
   b. F
   c. F
   d. T
   e. F
3. a. F
   b. T
   c. F
   d. F
   e. T
4. a. F
   b. F
   c. T
   d. F
   e. F

CHAPTER 35

1. a. F
   b. F
   c. F
   d. T
   e. T
2. a. F
   b. F
   c. F
   d. T
   e. F

CHAPTER 36

1. a. F
   b. T
   c. F
   d. F

CHAPTER 37

1. The acute change in the patient's condition suggests delirium, and there could be a combination of contributing factors. It is important to exclude a septic arthritis or (unwitnessed) traumatic injury of the shoulder. The first step should be aspiration. The fluid should be sent for Gram stain and culture as well as polarized microscopy. An X-ray should also be requested. Pain from crystal arthropathy or soft tissue injury may also contribute to her agitation.

2. At this stage it is likely that the low tone of the shoulder girdle is creating unusual positioning of the glenohumeral joint, and consequently mechanical pain. Simple joint palpation will reveal if there is subluxation (X-ray to prove this is not helpful) or specific subacromial tenderness. Such patients have difficulty turning over in bed due to upper limb weakness, and may require extra attention overnight to achieve a comfortable position. During the day, the arm will have to be supported to reduce rotator cuff injury, and if this is not improved there may be benefit from strapping, electrical stimulation or steroid injection if there is marked tenderness on palpation. Oral analgesia may be helpful.

3. At this stage after stroke it is important to consider late mechanical complications (e.g. rotator cuff injury or subacromial bursitis from glenohumeral misalignment), the effect of increasing spasticity, and the onset of central post-stroke pain. Therefore assessment will have to include examination of the glenohumeral joint, assessment of upper limb tone, and mapping of sensory deficits. Rarely, reflex sympathetic dystrophy syndrome can present this early and although classically the affected limb has colour and temperature changes, it is often obvious by unexpected bony tenderness spreading distally to proximally (metacarpophalangeal joint palpation is particularly uncomfortable).

CHAPTER 38

1. a F
   b. F
   c. T
   d. F
2. a. F
   b. T
   c. F
   d. F

CHAPTER 39

1. a. F
   b. T
   c. T
   d. T
   e. F

CHAPTER 40

1. a. F
   b. F
   c. T
   d. F
   e. F
2. a. F
   b. F
   c. T

d. F
e. F
3. a. F
   b. F
   c. T
   d. F
   e. F

CHAPTER 41

1. a. F. Conjunctivitis is generally painless.
   b. F. For visual impairment registration the sight in the better eye is considered. About 5% of people have poor vision in one eye, usually due to amblyopia.
   c. T. Modern cataract surgery does not remove the posterior lens capsule. It may opacify months or years later.
   d. T. Surgery is simple and can sometimes be performed in an out-patient clinic.
   e. T. In acute glaucoma the cornea becomes hypoxic and cloudy so the view of the fundus is obscured.

2. a. F. Anticholinergic drugs very rarely precipitate acute glaucoma. Patients with a diagnosis of acute glaucoma will almost certainly have had bilateral iridotomies and therefore are not at risk of recurrent acute glaucoma. Anticholinergic drugs do not threaten vision or worsen chronic simple glaucoma.
   b. T. Topical beta-antagonist therapy can be equivalent to full dose systemic therapy. In the presence of bronchospasm, unstable left ventricular failure or bradycardia substitute alternatives to topical beta antagonists immediately. Refer to an ophthalmologist later.
   c. F. Cataract surgery is generally performed under local anaesthetic. So long as the patient can keep still and can lie fairly flat for half an hour surgery can be performed.
   d. F. PDT can be used to coagulate the membrane of 'wet' macular degeneration but only in a minority of cases. It has no role in 'dry' macular degeneration.
   e. T. Even small improvements in navigational vision and visual acuity may make a large difference to quality of life.

CHAPTER 42

1. **a. F.** Presbycusis is the commonest cause of sensorineural deafness.
   b. T
   c. F. It is 42%.
   d. F
   e. T
2. The question is based on the case study in the 10-minute consultation in Aung & Mulley (2002).
   a. F. This is now contraindicated.
   b. T. This is known as Arnold's reflex.
   c. T
   d. F
   e. T
3. **a. F**
   b. F. It is only a marker of hearing loss.
   c. F. It only causes tinnitus at high doses.
   d. T
   e. T

CHAPTER 43

1. **a. F**
   b. T
   c. F
   d. F
   e. F

CHAPTER 44

1. T
2. F
3. F
4. T
5. F

CHAPTER 45

1. **a. T**
   b. F
   c. T

2. **a. F**
   b. T
3. **a. F**
   b. T
   c. F

CHAPTER 46

1. **a F**
   b. F
   c. F
   d. T
   e. F
2. **a. T**
   b. F
   c. F
   d. F
   e. T

CHAPTER 47

1. **a. F**
   b. T
   c. F
   d. F
2. **a. F**
   b. F
   c. T
   d. T

CHAPTER 48

1. **a. F**
   b. T
   c. F
   d. F
   e. T
2. **a. T**
   b. T

c. T
d. F
e. F

CHAPTER 49

1. a. T
   b. T
   c. F
   d. F
   e. T
2. a T
   b. F
   c. F
   d. F
   e. T

CHAPTER 50

1. (a) and (c) are reasonable responses.

CHAPTER 57

1. a. T
   b. F
   c. T
   d. F
2. a. T
   b. T
   c. F
   d. F
3. a. F
   b. T
   c. F
   d. T

REFERENCES

Aung T, Mulley G P 2002 10 minute consultation; removal of earwax. British Medical Journal 325:27
Gueyffier F, Bulpitt C, Boissel J P 1999 Antihypertensive drugs in very old people: a subgroup meta-analysis of randomised controlled trials. INDANA Group. Lancet 353:793–796 **

Index

Research, 479–485
Residential care *see* Care homes;
    Nursing homes
Respiratory system
    asthma, 260–263
    COPD, 40–41, 260–263, 270, 271,
        272
    oral hygiene and, 282
    rehabilitation, 263, 269–272
    tuberculosis, 57, 265–267
Rest pain, ischaemic, 250
Restraint of patients, 49, 117
Resuscitation *see* Cardiopulmonary
    resuscitation
Retinal artery occlusion, 365
Retinal vein occlusion, 365
Retinopathy, diabetic, 364–365
Retirement, 11
Rheumatoid arthritis, 326
Rights legislation, 51, 474
Ripple mattresses, 205
Risedronate (Actonel), *316*, 317
Risperidone, 161
Rivermead Mobility Index, 238
Rivermead Visual Gait Assessment
    (RVGA), 238
Role-playing, 427–428
Romberg's test, 236
Royal College of Physicians, 436, 439
Royal Commission for Long-term
    Care ('With respect to old age'),
        39
Royal National Institute for the Blind,
    366
rt-PA, 192
Rubner's rule, 6
Rural carers, *84*

S

Saccades, 230–231
Saccharomyces boulardii, 389
Saccular aneurysm, *190*
Saliva, 276–277, 280, 281, 284
Scanners (PC peripheral), 464
Screening, 60, 61–62, 63–65
    breast cancer, 64, 338–339
    cervical cancer, 344
    colorectal cancer, 64, 344–345
    contractures, 333, *334*
    ethnic elders, 93
    fallers, 113–114
    lung cancer, 349–350
    MRSA, 394
    nutrition, 405
    ovarian cancer, 341–342
    prostate cancer, 65, 350–351
Scrotal itching, 377
Search engines, 467

Secondary prevention, 61, 63–64
    fragility fractures, 132, 319
Secretaries, 443, 445
Selective serotonin reuptake inhibitors
    (SSRIs), 155
Selegiline, 222
Self-harm, 155–156
Semi-permeable film dressings, 207
Senescence
    cell, 7–8
    pruritus of, 377
Senior house officers (SHOs), 421
Senna, 291
Sensory system
    falls, 110, 111, 114, 115
    screening tests, 64
    see also Hearing; Vision
Serious untoward incidents (SUIs), 433
Servers, PC networks, 466
Service development and planning,
    23–31, 431–432
    fallers, 118–119
    trauma patients, 132–133
    see also Community geriatric care
Service provision legislation, 50
Service user involvement, 26, 28–29,
    30
Sexuality, 309–312
Shoulder pain, 321–323
Sick leave, 458
Side-lying test, 231, *233*
Sigmoidoscopy, 344
Sikhism, *90*
Sildenafil (Viagra), 311
Situational syncope, 226
Skin care
    at end of life, 146
    foot, *326*, 328–329
    see also Pressure sores
Skin-fold thickness measurements,
    403, 404
Skin problems
    foot, 325, *326*, 328–329
    oral mucosal disease and, 277
    pruritus, 375–378
Skin tests, tuberculosis, 266
Sleep apnoea, *78*
Slough, leg ulcers, 383–384
Smoking
    asthma, 260
    cessation, 65–66, 270
    COPD, 260, 263, 270
    oral cancer, 277
    stroke patients, 196
    urinary incontinence, 100
Social aspects
    of ageing, 10–14
    oral health, 281
    of palliative care, 147–148
Social attitudes

ethnic elders, 89, *90–92*
    to ageing, 10–11
Social gerontology, 10–14
Social Indicators checklist, 175
Social services
    for dementia patients, 160
    ethnic elders, 94
    government policy, 38
    intermediate care, 29–30, 41
    projected long-term care needs, 37
    responsibilities, 34–35
    visual impairment, 366
    see also Local authorities
Social Work (Scotland) Act 1968, 50
Social workers
    Mental Health Act 1983 provisions,
        47, 48, 49
    service provision legislation, 50
    stroke patients, 194
Sodium picosulphate, 291
Software, 464, 468
Solifenacin, *103*
Sotalol, 255
Spam, 468
Spasticity, shoulder, *323*
Specialist registrars, 419, 421, 425–426,
    436, 479
Speech therapists, 194, 410
Spinal cord compression, 140
Spirometry, 261, 262, 271
Splinting, contractures, *335*
SSRIs, 155
Standardized assessment instruments,
    174–177
Staphylococcus aureus
    methicillin-resistant, 129, 386–387,
        391–395
    methicillin-susceptible, 387, 391
State benefits *see* Benefits system
Static mattresses, 204, *205*
Statins
    peripheral vascular disease, 250
    stroke patients, 196
Statistical software, 464
Statistics, research projects, 481,
    483–484
Stress, 456, 475–476
Stress urinary incontinence (SUI), 99,
    100, 104, 105
Stridor, 140
Stroke, 184–197
    acute medical treatment, *191*,
        192–194
    atrial fibrillation, 189, 196, *198*,
        253–254, 257
    blood pressure, 192–193, 195–196,
        241–242, 243, 244
    causes, 189, *190*
    cerebral haemorrhage, 185–186,
        188–189, 192, 193, *198*